Advances in Veterinary Dermatology
Volume 4

Advances in Veterinary Dermatology

Volume 4

Proceedings of the Fourth World Congress of Veterinary Dermatology, San Francisco, California, USA from 30 August to 2 September 2000

Edited by

Keith L. Thoday

The University of Edinburgh, The Royal (Dick) School of Veterinary Studies, Roslin, Midlothian, UK

Carol S. Foil

Louisiana State University, Baton Rouge, Louisiana, USA

and

Ross Bond

The Royal Veterinary College, University of London, North Mymms, Hatfield, Hertfordshire, UK

Blackwell
Science

Editorial Offices:
9600 Garsington Rd, Oxford OX4 2DQ, UK
Tel: +44 (0)1865 776868
Blackwell Science, Inc., 350 Main Street, Malden,
MA 02148-5020, USA
Tel: +1 781 388 8250
Iowa State Press, a Blackwell Publishing Company,
2121 State Avenue, Ames, Iowa 50014-8300, USA
Tel: +1 515 292 0140
Blackwell Publishing Asia Pty Ltd, 550 Swanston Street, Carlton
South, Melbourne, Victoria 3053, Australia
Tel: +61 (0)3 9347 0300
Blackwell Wissenschafts Verlag, Kurfürstendamm 57,
10707 Berlin, Germany
Tel: +49 (0)30 32 79 060

First published by Blackwell Science, 2002
Reprinted 2003

Library of Congress Cataloging-in-Publication Data is available

ISBN 0-632-05601-0

A catalogue record for this title is available from the British Library

Produced and typeset by Gray Publishing, Tunbridge Wells, Kent
Printed and bound in India by Thomson Press (I) Ltd, India

For further information on
Blackwell Publishing, visit our website: www.blackwellpublishing.com

Cover image: section of skin from a case of feline *Microsporum canis* infection kindly provided by Professor David Lloyd and Dr Joy Archer of the Royal Veterinary College, London and featured in the *Workshop on Dermatotechnology* (5.21, pages 341–344). The image was created using Montage Explorer (Synchroscopy) and illustrates how this technique is able to image a large area of tissue at high resolution and in a single plane of focus.

Contents

The Sponsors of the Fourth World Congress of Veterinary Dermatology

Principal Sponsors

Virbac Animal Health
DVM Pharmaceuticals, Inc.
Pfizer Animal Health
Merial Ltd
Novartis Animal Health
Purina
The Iams Company
Hill's Pet Nutrition, Inc.

Major Sponsors

Bayer
Waltham
Heska Corporation
Innovative Veterinary Diets
Pharmacia Animal Health

Supporting Sponsors

Janssen Pharmaceutica
Alpharma AS
Schering-Plough

Sponsors

Greer Laboratories
Veterinary Allergy Reference Laboratories
EVSCO
DermaPet

Officers and Organising Committees of the Fourth World Congress of Veterinary Dermatology

Officers

President	Dr Peter J. Ihrke (USA)
Secretary	Dr Stephen D. White (USA)
Treasurer	Dr Rod A. W. Rosychuk (USA)

Executive Organising Committee

The Officers and:

Dr Donna W. Angarano
Dr Bradley Baker
Dr Douglas J. DeBoer
Dr Craig E. Griffin
Professor Richard E. W. Halliwell
Dr Hans-Joachim Koch
Dr Wayne S. Rosenkrantz
Dr Candace A. Sousa
Dr Keith L. Thoday

Committees

Commercial Exhibition

Dr Craig E. Griffin (USA)	Chairperson

Finance and Fundraising

Dr Wayne S. Rosenkrantz (USA)	Chairperson
Professor David H. Lloyd (UK)	Co-chairperson
Dr Richard K. Anderson (USA)	
Dr Bradley Baker (Canada)	
Dr Hans-Joachim Koch (Germany)	
Professor Munetsugu Ogata (Japan)	
Dr Lloyd M. Reedy* (USA)	

*Deceased.

Local Organising Committee

Dr Candace A. Sousa (USA)	Chairperson
Dr Craig E. Griffin (USA)	
Dr Thelma Lee Gross (USA)	
Dr Helen T. Power (USA)	
Dr Susan I. Reinke (USA)	

Programme Committee

Dr Douglas J. DeBoer (USA)	Chairperson
Dr Leena Saijonmaa-Koulumies (Finland)	Co-chairperson
Dr Peter B. Hill (UK)	
Dr Thierry Olivry (USA)	
Dr Manon Paradis (Canada)	

Publications Committee

Dr Keith L. Thoday (UK)	Chairperson
Dr Ross Bond (UK)	
Dr Carol S. Foil (USA)	

Publicity Committee

Dr Donna W. Angarano (USA)	Chairperson
Dr Didier-Noël Carlotti (France)	Co-chairperson
Dr James O. Noxon (USA)	

Preface

The Fourth World Congress of Veterinary Dermatology was held in San Francisco, California, USA from 30 August to 2 September 2000. The Congress was organised by the American Academy of Veterinary Dermatology, the American College of Veterinary Dermatology, the Canadian Academy of Veterinary Dermatology, the European College of Veterinary Dermatology and the European Society of Veterinary Dermatology.

The First World Congress of Veterinary Dermatology was held in 1989 in Dijon, France, with the Second in Montreal, Canada (1992) and the Third in Edinburgh, Scotland (1996). The Fourth World Congress of Veterinary Dermatology represented a coming of age for the World Congress, presenting a greater range of dermatological topics than ever before. The interest in veterinary dermatology continues to grow exponentially, with this Congress attracting over 1000 registrants, the largest number yet, from 42 countries. The spacious San Francisco Hilton was an excellent venue for the first World Congress to be held in the USA. There were four plenary sessions with 21 state-of-the-art, supporting review and supporting original studies, 22 workshops, 81 free communications, 64 posters and a two-track clinical programme.

Advances in Veterinary Dermatology Volume 4 is the refereed proceedings of this Congress. It differs from some of its predecessors in that it does not include the abstracts of the free communications and the posters as, for the first time, these were published as a supplement to *Veterinary Dermatology* (Volume 11, Supplement 1, September 2000) which was provided both as a Congress document and, of course, to the journal's subscribers.

Planning for the Fourth World Congress of Veterinary Dermatology began almost immediately after the Edinburgh Congress, such is the amount of effort involved in the organisation of an event of this magnitude. It could not have happened without the enthusiasm, dedication, commitment and continued hard work of the officers and committee members. The Congress also would not have been possible without the very generous assistance of our colleagues in the pharmaceutical, pet food, diagnostic and parasite control industries. We are greatly indebted to our sponsors, listed on page viii, as friends and true supporters of veterinary dermatology throughout the world.

Keith L. Thoday
Roslin, UK

Carol S. Foil
Baton Rouge, USA

Ross Bond
North Mymms, UK

Part 1

Cutaneous biology

1.1
The dermal–epidermal basement membrane

M. Janoff MD[1] and M.P. Marinkovich MD[2]

[1] School of Medicine, University of California at Los Angeles, Los Angeles, California, USA
[2] VA Palo Alto Health Care System, and Department of Dermatology, Stanford University School of Medicine, Palo Alto, California, USA

Summary

Successful attachment of epithelia to their underlying substrate is the result of the careful coordination of complex interactions between numerous proteins in hemidesmosomes and the basement membrane zone. Intermediate filaments insert upon hemidesmosomes via plectin and BP230. Plectin and BP230, in turn, bind to the β_4-integrin and BP180 endodomains, respectively. The hemidesmosomal complex is further stabilized by co-association of the β_4-integrin and BP180 endodomains. Extracellular anchoring filaments, including laminins, facilitate epithelial attachment through connection with the hemidesmosomes at the exodomains of transmembrane proteins $\alpha_6\beta_4$-integrin and BP180. Further assembly of anchoring filaments takes place by association of $\alpha_6\beta_4$-integrin and possibly BP180 with laminin-5 or laminin-5/laminin-6 complex. The C-terminal regions of laminins-5 and -6 face the basal cell, while the N-terminal domains are oriented towards the lamina densa. The entire anchoring complex is linked with the lamina densa by the association of laminin-6 with nidogen which, in turn, is capable of binding collagen IV and perlecan. Through additional nidogen linkages, laminin-10 also assembles with collagen IV and perlecan. Anchoring filaments are linked to anchoring fibrils by a direct association between laminin-5 and the NC1 domain of collagen VII. In addition, the NC1 domain of collagen VII binds to collagen IV in the lamina densa. Finally, due to the flexible nature of collagen VII, anchoring fibrils wind around and entrap interstitial collagen and other molecules that serve to fasten the lamina densa onto the papillary dermis.

Introduction

Basement membranes are important interfaces for epithelia and deeper tissues throughout the body. Specific protein–protein interactions are required for the assembly and continued integrity of all basement membranes. In the highly specialized dermal–epidermal basement membrane zone (BMZ) an intricate and precise organization of many protein constituents is required to maintain dermal–epidermal cohesion. Disruption of this organized array of components, by either inherited (epidermolysis bullosa) (Marinkovich, 1999; Marinkovich *et al.*, 1999) or acquired (autoimmune bullous) diseases (Lin *et al.*, 1997), can result in extensive skin and mucosal blistering, both in humans and in animals (Olivry *et al.*, 1999a,c, 2000a–d). An authoritative reference on the BMZ can be a valuable resource for veterinarians who seek to understand the molecular pathophysiology of the many subepidermal bullous diseases that affect animals.

Ultrastructural organization of the dermal–epidermal BMZ

BMZ ultrastructure has traditionally been visualized by standard transmission electron microscopy. Through this technique, it can be appreciated that at the superior edge of the dermal–epidermal BMZ, intermediate filaments within the cell insert upon electron-dense condensations of the keratinocyte plasma membrane, called hemidesmosomes. The extracellular surfaces of hemidesmosomes are connected to the extracellular matrix by anchoring filaments. These thin, thread-like structures extend from the extracellular surface of hemidesmosomes, span the electron-lucent space in the BMZ termed the lamina lucida, and appear to connect hemidesmosomes to the lamina densa, the electron-dense portion of the extracellular BMZ (Ellison & Garrod, 1984).

Anchoring fibrils are banded structures that extend perpendicularly from the lamina densa into the adjacent superficial papillary dermis. Anchoring fibrils either extend back to reinsert onto the lamina densa or connect with anchoring plaques, electron-dense structures of the papillary dermis. In connecting to these structures, anchoring fibrils entrap interstitial collagen and other dermal molecules and help to attach the lamina densa firmly to the papillary dermis (Keene *et al.*, 1987).

Newer techniques in the analysis of tissues by electron microscopy combine high pressure, cryopreservation and freeze substitution to yield improved preservation of tissue architecture (Hippe-Sanwald, 1993). During the initial cryopreservation step, water in tissues is converted to non-crystalline ice through the combined application of very low temperature and very high pressure. Subsequently, absolute acetone or methanol with aldehyde or osmium is substituted for the ice, and cross-linking occurs at very low temperatures. This technique greatly reduces the loss of soluble substances such as proteoglycans and the increased integrity of preservation has furthered our understanding of the intricate architecture of the BMZ.

Recent studies with high-pressure freeze-substitution electron microscopy have demonstrated that the dermal–epidermal BMZ ultrastructure seen with conventional fixation may be artifactual (Keene & McDonald, 1993; Keene *et al.*, 1997). While hemidesmosomes and intermediate filaments are clearly visible with these techniques, anchoring fibrils and the lamina lucida appear to be absent. Instead, a continuous, felt-like matrix extends from the basal keratinocyte plasma membrane into the papillary dermis.

These studies suggest that the lamina lucida seen after conventional fixation may arise as a dehydration artifact caused by a shrinking away of the basal cell plasma membrane from the underlying dermis after the removal of water. The lamina densa, anchoring filaments and anchoring fibrils, may also appear owing to artifactual precipitation resulting from removal of proteoglycans and other soluble substances during conventional fixation methods. Therefore, conventional electron microscopy can be thought to pull artifactually the plasma membrane away from the basement membrane to expose interactions in a space that has been termed the lamina lucida, which normally would occur in the lamina densa, and to reveal the presence of anchoring filaments that normally exist hidden in the lamina densa. As long as one understands that it is an artifact, it is useful to speak of proteins that localize to the lamina lucida, as it enables one to understand how hemidesmosomes and anchoring filaments are connected. Therefore, the term lamina lucida is used here for further discussion.

Intermediate filament–hemidesmosome interactions

Basal keratinocyte intermediate filaments contain the acidic keratin-14 and the basic keratin-5. Initially these keratins combine together as polar coiled-coil dimers. The dimers go on to form staggered anti-parallel tetramers and then undergo additional lateral and end-to-end associations to form 2–3 nm diameter protofilaments and 4–5 nm diameter protofibrils. Finally, two to four protofilaments associate into a coiled-coil lattice to form 10 nm diameter intermediate filaments (Fuchs & Cleveland, 1998).

Recent studies have suggested that the non-helical keratin-5 head domain may be important in the anchoring of intermediate filaments to other structures (Smith & Fuchs, 1998). The desmosomal components desmoplakin, plakophilin-1 and plakoglobin all appear to interact with this domain. Intermediate filaments may also associate with hemidesmosomal components through the keratin-5 head domain, although this remains to be proven. The keratin-5 head domain is also suspected to be involved in the binding of intermediate filaments to melanosomes (Uttam *et al.*, 1996), as mutations that affect this domain are associated with epidermolysis bullosa simplex with mottled pigmentation.

Intracellular proteins

BP230

Hemidesmosomes contain plaque proteins, including BP230 (BPAG1) and plectin (HD1), both members of the plakin protein family. BP230 is a 230 kDa protein which consists of a central rod flanked by C-terminal and N-terminal globular domains (Sawamura *et al.*, 1991; Tanaka *et al.*, 1991; Tamai *et al.*, 1995; Tang *et al.*, 1996). BP230 has significant homology both to desmoplakin and to plectin in its two C-terminal repeating globular domains. This homologous region contains the keratin-binding domain.

Microscopic studies BP230 localizes to the inner plate on the cytoplasmic surface of the hemidesmosome and functions in the connection between hemidesmosomes and intermediate filaments. BP230-negative transgenic mice lack a hemidesmosomal inner plate and the connection between hemidesmosomes and intermediate filaments is severed. The creation of a cytoplasmic zone of mechanical fragility just above the hemidesmosomes results in intra-epidermal blistering (Guo *et al.*, 1995). In these mice neither hemidesmosome stability nor cell substratum adhesion appears to be weakened. Thus, BP230 does not appear vital for hemidesmosome or BMZ assembly.

Other related molecules BP230 also exists as an alternatively spliced neural isoform termed BPAG1n (dystonin). As a result of the ablation of the domains common for both BP230 and BPAG1n, BP230 knockout mice also develop severe dystonia and sensory nerve degeneration typical of dystonia musculorum (dt/dt) mice (Dowling *et al.*, 1997).

Disease BP230 is a major autoantigen targeted by sera of most patients with the autoimmune blistering disease bullous pemphigoid (Stanley, 1991), and it has been reported to be an autoantigen in patients with paraneoplastic pemphigus, an autoimmune blistering skin disease found in patients with cancer. BP230 has also been reported to be a target of autoantibodies in the serum of a patient with bullous systemic lupus erythematosus (Chan *et al.*, 1999). There have been recent reports that BP230 and plectin expression may be decreased in patients with dermatitis herpetiformis vulnerable to blistering (Leivo *et al.*, 1996), but further investigation is necessary to characterize the nature of the deficit.

Plectin

Plectin is a 500 kDa cytoskeletal linker protein (Liu *et al.*, 1996). Plectin associates with a variety of types of cytoskeletal structures including keratin, actin, vimentin, neurofilaments, microfilaments and microtubules. It shows a very widespread expression in the majority of tissues and cell types studied. In stratified epithelial cells plectin promotes intercellular adhesion by linking keratin-containing intermediate filaments with desmosomes. An additional role of plectin in promoting dermal–epidermal cohesion stems from its ability to link keratin to the hemidesmosomal plaque.

Microscopic studies Rotary shadowing electron-microscopic studies have shown that plectin, like many BMZ proteins, assumes a dumbbell shape and contains a central parallel 200 nm α-helical coiled-coil rod, which is flanked at either end by large globular domains (Wiche, 1998). Gel-permeation studies, which predict the molecular weight of plectin to be 1100 kDa, suggest that plectin exists as a dimer in solution. Immunogold electron-microscopic studies have demonstrated colocalization of plectin with intermediate filaments (Foisner *et al.*, 1995).

The C-terminal globular domain of plectin contains six repeating domains, each with approximately 300 amino acids. Each domain contains multiple copies of a 19 amino-acid tandem repeat. A 50 amino-acid segment bridges domains 5 and 6, and contains a cluster of basic amino-acid residues. This basic cluster is located in a bipartite nuclear localization sequence that functions as the intermediate filament binding site (Nikolic *et al.*, 1996). Near this site on domain 6 is a phosphorylation site for p34cdc2 protein kinase that may be involved with the dissociation of plectin from intermediate filaments during mitosis (Malecz *et al.*, 1996).

Study of the interaction of plectin with hemidesmosomes by immunogold electron microscopy with domain-specific antibodies (Foisner *et al.*, 1994) reveals a lack of specific orientation in plectin's association with intermediate filaments and hemidesmosomal plaques. In this study, the same domains were seen to insert both into keratin filaments and into hemidesmosomal plaques. These studies suggest that two binding sites exist on plectin that are each capable of interacting with other hemidesmosomal elements. These findings are consistent with direct ligand binding studies (Rezniczek *et al.*, 1998) that demonstrate that both the N- and C-terminal globular domains of plectin are capable of binding to the transmembrane protein β_4-integrin. Furthermore, plectin is capable of associating with two different regions of the β_4-integrin cytoplasmic domain. The N-terminal domain has been found to be structurally diverse, and this is the same area that contains the actin binding site for plectin (Geerts *et al.*, 1999). The significance of these multiple interactions remains to be elucidated.

Although studies have shown that the presence of plectin is not essential for hemidesmosome formation in the presence of laminin-5, the extracellular β_4-ligand, plectin does appear to be required for the assembly of hemidesmosomal clusters in its absence.

In plectin-negative cell lines, β_4-integrin is expressed diffusely and does not localize to the basal surface unless laminin-5 is present in the extracellular environment (Nievers *et al.*, 1999). Thus, proper localization of β_4-integrin to the basal surface and the formation of hemidesmosomes require the presence of either laminin-5 or plectin.

Other related molecules Plectin has been shown recently to exist in multiple isoforms generated by alternative splicing of the N-terminus (Elliott *et al.*, 1997). At least eight isoforms have been detected thus far. Isoform expression levels demonstrate an array of isoform expression in individual tissues, as shown by RNAse protection assays. The splicing diversity affects both coding and non-coding regions and may affect plectin function and/or expression. Other molecules, including HD1 (Heida *et al.*, 1992) and IFAP-300 (Skalli *et al.*, 1994), which show similarities with and differences from plectin in terms of tissue distribution and other parameters, may represent some of these alternatively spliced plectin isoforms, although this remains to be determined.

Disease Plectin-deficient patients show a blistering phenotype with intraepidermal separation of the skin occurring above the level of the hemidesmosome (Chavanas *et al.*, 1996; Gache *et al.*, 1996; McLean *et al.*, 1996; Smith *et al.*, 1996). Hemidesmosomes remain intact in these patients. Plectin-deficient patients have frequently been shown to have an associated muscular dystrophy, which accounts for the name given to the major disease caused by plectin deficiency: epidermolysis bullosa simplex with muscular dystrophy. Premature stop codon mutations of the plectin gene were found to be associated with the majority of these patients, although deletions have also been reported. In one case, a three amino-acid deletion was found in the N-terminal globular region. This region, as stated previously, is involved with the interaction of plectin with β_4-integrin and is likely to be important in plectin's function. An understanding of the pathogenesis of muscular dystrophy secondary to the absence of plectin in muscle is not yet complete.

A case of epidermolysis bullosa simplex with severe mucous membrane involvement due to nonsense mutations in exon 32 of plectin has also been reported (Kunz *et al.*, 2000). Muscle weakness need not appear concurrently with the blistering phenotype, and no signs of muscular weakness were observed during a 4 year follow-up. Plectin has also been reported to be among the autoantigens involved in paraneoplastic pemphigus (Proby *et al.*, 2000). Plectin knockout mice (Andrä *et al.*, 1997) demonstrated a blistering phenotype similar to the epidermolysis bullosa patients described above, but these mice show more extensive muscle pathology than their human counterparts.

Transmembrane proteins

$\alpha_6\beta_4$-Integrin

Hemidesmosomes also contain the transmembrane proteins BP180 and $\alpha_6\beta_4$-integrin (Figures 1.1.1, 1.1.2). The cytoplasmic portions of these molecules make up part of hemidesmosome dense plaques, whereas the extracellular portions of these molecules make up portions of anchoring filaments and may contribute to the structure known as the subbasal dense plate which underlies hemidesmosomes in the lamina lucida region. $\alpha_6\beta_4$-integrin serves as a crucial link between the intracellular and extracellular environments, and it has been shown that this molecule can communicate changes in the extracellular environment to the cytoskeleton (Giancotti, 1996; Giancotti & Ruoslahti, 1999).

$\alpha_6\beta_4$-Integrin is an essential and central component of the hemidesmosome (Sonnenberg *et al.*, 1991). Like all of the members of the family of molecules known as integrins (Hynes, 1992), it consists of two transmembrane subunits assembled in a non-covalent fashion (Sonnenberg *et al.*, 1990; Tamura *et al.*, 1990). The extracellular domains of these subunits combine to form a ligand-binding site, whereas the intracellular domain of β_4-integrin interacts with other hemidesmosomal components. β_4-Integrin is only known to combine with the α_6-subunit, whereas the α_6-subunit can combine with either β_4- or β_1-subunits. The $\alpha_6\beta_1$- and $\alpha_6\beta_4$-integrin combinations have been shown to act as receptors for laminin, and $\alpha_6\beta_4$-integrin acts as a receptor for laminin-5 (Niessen *et al.*, 1995).

Microscopic studies β_4-Integrin contains an especially large, approximately 1000 amino-acid, cytoplasmic domain that consists of two pairs of fibronectin repeats separated by a connecting segment. Replacement of β_4-integrin deletion constructs in β_4-integrin-negative keratinocytes revealed that a 27 amino-acid region of the connecting segment is required for hemidesmosome assembly (Niessen *et al.*, 1997). This region of β_4-integrin is critical in localizing plectin to hemidesmosomes, and a direct interaction between this

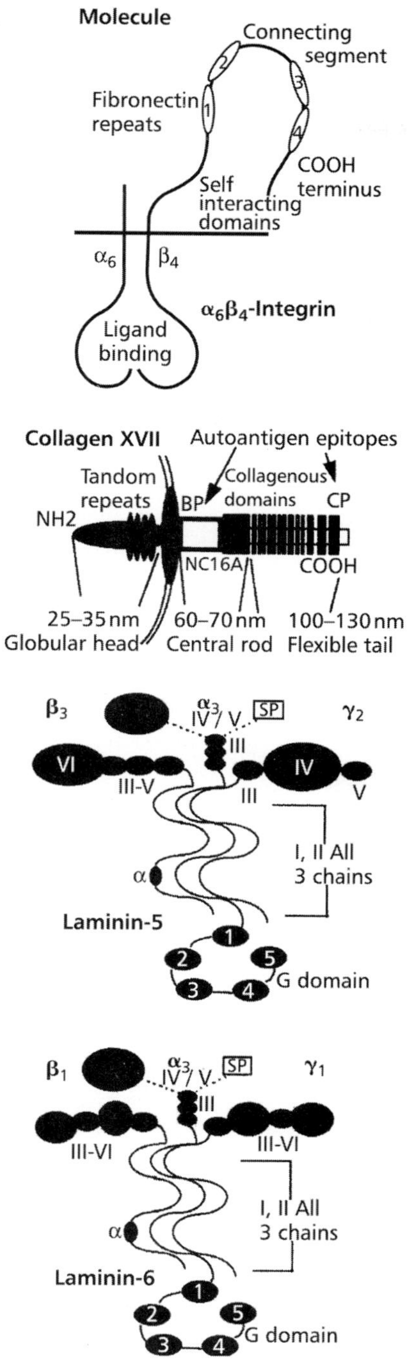

Domain	Function
β_4-integrin	
COOH terminus	Plectin binding
COOH terminus	Proximal endodomain binding
Connecting segment	Hemidesmosome assembly
Connecting segment	Plectin binding
Connecting segment	Tyrosine activation motif
Connecting segment and 3rd FN repeat	Collagen XVII binding
NH2 half, endodomain	COOH terminus binding
Exodomain	Extracellular ligand binding
α_6-Integrin	
Proximal exodomain	Collagen XVII binding
Exodomain	Extracellular ligand binding
NH2 terminus	Basal polarization
Endodomain	Interaction with β_4-integrin
Endodomain	Interaction with BPAG1
Transmembrane	Cell surface localization
NC16A	BP autoepitopes
NC16A	Interaction with α_6-integrin
NC16A	Processing site
Central rod	Coiled-coil assembly
Collagen domains	Triple helical assembly
Collagen domains	Collagenase cleavage sites
COOH terminus	CP autoepitopes
COOH terminus	Extracellular interactions
α_3 G1-3	Cell binding
α_3 G/I/II/III	CP autoepitope
α_3 G4-5	Heparin binding
α_3 G3-4	Proteolytic processing site
β_3 I/II	Coiled-coil assembly
β_3 VI	Association with laminin-6
γ_2 III, EGF 3	Proteolytic processing site
γ_2 I/II	Coiled-coil assembly
γ_2 III or β_3 III-IV or α_3 III	Collagen VII and Collagen XVII binding
α_3 G1-3	Cell binding
α_3 G/I/II/III	CP autoepitope
α_3 G4-5	Heparin binding
α_3 G3-4	Processing site
α_3 III, EGF 1	Disulfide bond laminin-5
α_3 I/II	Coiled-coil assembly
β_1 I/II	Coiled-coil assembly
γ_1 III, EGF 4	Nidogen binding
γ_1 I/II	Coiled-coil assembly

Figure 1.1.1. Structure and proposed functions of four key components of the dermal–epidermal basement membrane.

region of the β_4-integrin cytoplasmic domain and plectin has been demonstrated (Rezniczek *et al.*, 1998).

β_4-Integrin contains a tyrosine activation motif (TAM) in its connecting segment. Mutations involving the tyrosines in this motif have been shown to have variable effects. In one study, TAM mutations appeared to have only a minor effect on the localization of β_4 to hemidesmosomes (Borradori *et al.*, 1997).

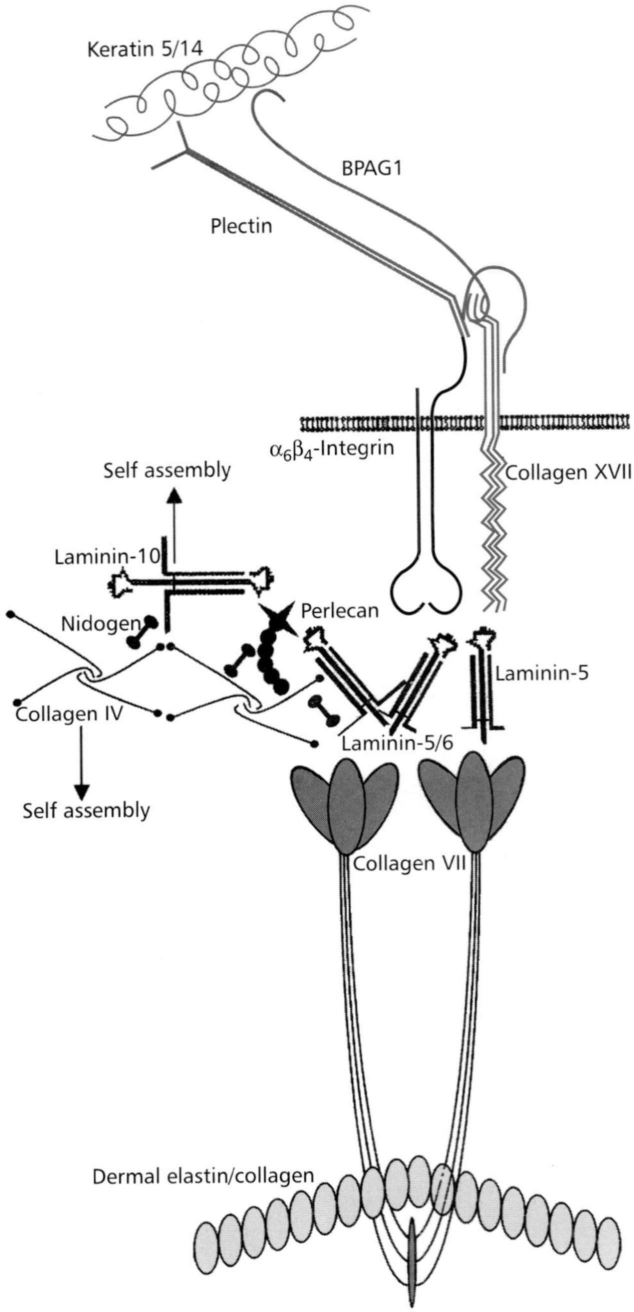

Figure 1.1.2. Schematic illustration showing the molecular organization of the dermal–epidermal basement membrane.

Other related molecules β_4-Integrin interacts directly with the cytoplasmic domains of BP180 (Borradori *et al.*, 1997; Schaapveld *et al.*, 1998) and influences its localization to hemidesmosomes. The sequences on β_4-integrin that appear to mediate this interaction lie on the C-terminal section of the connecting segment and in the third fibronectin repeat. In addition to binding BP180 and plectin, under some circumstances the β_4-integrin cytoplasmic domain may fold over and bind to itself. Ligand binding studies show that the C-terminal 85 amino acids of β_4-integrin can interact with and bind to the connecting segment and regions further towards the N-terminus. This folding appears to influence the affinity of β_4-integrin for plectin and may be involved in hemidesmosome assembly and disassembly.

New research indicates that a newly identified constituent of hemidesmosomes, CD151, may be an integral part of prehemidesmosomes. It is known to be a member of the tetraspan superfamily of proteins, which have not been found previously to localize to hemidesmosomes, but it recently has been shown to colocalize with $\alpha_3\beta_1$- and $\alpha_6\beta_4$-integrins on the basal surface of keratinocytes in conjunction with laminin-5. It appears to interact with the α-subunits of the integrins. The significance of this newly identified constituent of hemidesmosomes remains to be elucidated (Sterk *et al.*, 2000).

Disease As mentioned above, $\alpha_6\beta_4$-integrin is presumed to play a central role in hemidesmosome formation, since transgenic mice lacking the β_4-integrin show skin devoid of hemidesmosomes as well as blistering and severe deficits in cell adhesion (Dowling *et al.*, 1996). Patients with epidermolysis bullosa with pyloric atresia (EB-PA), in whom β_4-integrin (Vidal *et al.*, 1995) or α_6-integrin (Ruzzi *et al.*, 1997) is absent owing to underlying gene mutations, demonstrate only rudimentary hemidesmosome formation at best, and can develop widespread blistering and pyloric atresia.

BP180

BP180 (collagen XVII/BPAG2) is another transmembrane component of hemidesmosomes that helps to anchor the cell to its extracellular matrix. It is a collagenous triple-helical protein with a type II transmembrane orientation (Giudice *et al.*, 1992).

Microscopic studies Based on electron-microscopic and cross-linking studies, BP180 appears to assemble into a homotrimer (Schumann & Bruckner-Tuderman, 1996) and contains three main regions: an intracellular N-terminal globular head, a central rod and an extracellular flexible tail (Hirako *et al.*, 1996). The C-terminal portion of the molecule appears to be involved with polarization of the BP180 molecule to the basal surface of keratinocytes.

BP180 interacts with a number of hemidesmosomal proteins. As mentioned above, the cytoplasmic domain of BP180 colocalizes with and binds to the β_4-integrin in the hemidesmosome (Borradori *et al.*, 1998; Aho & Uitto, 1999). Some epidermolysis bullosa patients who lack BP180 expression also show a lack of localization of BP230 into hemidesmosomes (Borradori *et al.*, 1998). The N-terminus of BP180 has been shown to interact with the N-terminus of BP230 (Hopkinson & Jones, 2000), an interaction that is likely to be responsible for the proper localization of BP230. When expression of the endodomain of BP180 is restored, BP230 again localizes correctly in hemidesmosomes.

When BP180-deficient cells are transfected with wild-type human BP180, proper expression of BP180 can be restored (Seitz *et al.*, 1999). Analysis of deleted BP180 complementary DNA (cDNA) constructs suggests that the C-terminal half of the BP180 cytoplasmic domain is required for BP230 localization into hemidesmosomes. Thus, the BP180 endodomain has two important functions: interaction with BP230, which links intermediate filaments to the hemidesmosome, and interaction with the β_4-integrin endodomain, which in turn serves to localize BP180 correctly to the hemidesmosome.

The NC16A domain of BP180, a large, non-collagenous region near the transmembrane region, contains the epitopes recognized by bullous pemphigoid autoantibodies (Liu *et al.*, 1995). The central rod and flexible tail region of BP180 contains a number of interrupted collagenous domains that assemble into a triple helix. The most distal extracellular portion of this molecule contains epitopes recognized by autoantibodies from some patients with cicatricial pemphigoid (Balding *et al.*, 1996). Based on rotary shadowed electron-microscopic measurements, the extracellular portions of BP180 may extend up to 193 nm. It is therefore likely that BP180 extends the full length of the lamina lucida and inserts into the lamina densa. This is consistent with the observation that cicatricial pemphigoid autoantibodies recognize autoepitopes in the lamina densa region of the BMZ (Bédane *et al.*, 1997).

Other related molecules The anchoring filament component LAD-1 is a 120 kDa protein expressed by keratinocytes (Marinkovich *et al.*, 1996) which represents the non-degraded form of the previously identified 97 kDa linear immunoglobulin A (IgA) bullous dermatosis autoantigen (Zone *et al.*, 1990). The monoclonal antibody (mAb) 123, which recognizes

LAD-1, induces de-epithelialization of human skin *in situ*, suggesting that LAD-1 plays an important cohesive role in the dermal–epidermal BMZ (Marinkovich *et al.*, 1996). A previously described 125 kDa component of anchoring filaments which appears to be the bovine analog of LAD-1 was found to be the first protein to be expressed during the earliest phases of wound healing in an organ culture model (Klatte *et al.*, 1989).

There is now evidence that implicates LAD-1 as a proteolytic fragment of the BP180 exodomain. Originally, it was observed that linear IgA bullous dermatosis autoantibodies and a separate group of monoclonal antibodies reacted with LAD-1 extracted from skin and keratinocyte medium. These same antibodies did not show significant reaction with full-length BP180. It was hypothesized at that time that LAD-1 was a novel protein (Klatte *et al.*, 1989; Marinkovich *et al.*, 1996; Pas *et al.*, 1997; Zone *et al.*, 1998). Recent peptide sequencing studies, however, have shown that LAD-1 contains sequences homologous with BP180 (Zone *et al.*, 1998). Northern blot analysis has failed to confirm any alternatively spliced variants of BP180 (Schäcke *et al.*, 1998). Further, the absence of both LAD-1 and BP180 in patients with generalized atrophic benign epidermolysis bullosa (Marinkovich *et al.*, 1997) suggests that LAD-1 probably is not a separate gene product. Therefore, the most likely hypothesis is that LAD-1 is a proteolytic fragment of BP180, with proteolysis inducing a group of neoepitopes (Egan & Zone, 1999). Because these neoepitopes include those recognized by both linear IgA bullous dermatosis autoantibodies and mAb 123, which induces skin de-epidermalization *in situ*, the proteolysis of BP180 appears to be an important event in the development of disease.

N-terminal sequencing of processed BP180 isolated from skin suggests that the proteolytic cleavage occurs in the NC16A domain (Zone *et al.*, 1998). Processed BP180 appears to exist as a triple helix (Balding *et al.*, 1997) and contains domains that are collagenase sensitive but pepsin resistant (Schäcke *et al.*, 1998). In one study, proteolytic cleavage of a bacterial fusion protein containing the NC16A and its proximal collagenous domain was demonstrated using purified gelatinase B (Ståhle-Bäckdahl *et al.*, 1994). However, cleavage of native BP180 has not been demonstrated with this enzyme. In another study, inhibition of furin served to inhibit BP180 processing (Schäcke *et al.*, 1998). A furin consensus site is present in the NC16A region of BP180 and it is possible that this enzyme may be involved in BP180 processing in a membrane-associated form. Alternatively, it is known that furin proteolytically activates membrane-type metalloproteinase-1 and that this enzyme activates gelatinase A. Thus, it is also possible that either of these two enzymes may be responsible for BP180 processing.

A recent study noted the presence of two distinct COL17A1 gene transcripts that are hypothesized to be the result of differential splicing. It appears that the two transcripts are expressed at different rates in different cells, specifically in normal keratinocytes compared with squamous cell carcinoma cells (Molnar *et al.*, 2000). The significance of the differential splicing and the two transcripts is not yet known.

Disease Bullous pemphigoid is known to affect dogs as well as humans, and the NC16A domain has recently been described as the target of autoantibodies in a feline, a porcine and an equine model of bullous pemphigoid (Olivry *et al.*, 1999a, 2000a, c). Recent molecular work on canine BP180 shows approximately 85% homology between the human and canine proteins, and the canine antibodies have been shown to recognize the human proteins (Xu *et al.*, 1998). It is hoped that this discovery will foster greater collaborative research efforts in studies of humans and animal models.

In addition to its role in bullous pemphigoid and cicatricial pemphigoid, abnormalities in BP180 can lead to a number of other disease states, and many interesting cases have been described. BP180 assists in promoting epidermal adhesion, as evidenced by the widespread blistering that occurs in patients with generalized atrophic benign epidermolysis bullosa (GABEB) who lack this molecule. Retrovirally mediated BP180 gene replacement in primary GABEB keratinocytes corrected both adhesion defects *in vitro* and corrected blistering defects *in vivo* after grafting of these cells onto immunodeficient mice (Seitz *et al.*, 1999). In addition, revertant mosaicism for GABEB has been described caused by a mitotic gene conversion (Jonkman *et al.*, 1997).

A patient has also been described who was found to have mutations in both BP180 and laminin-5 that were responsible for his severe junctional epidermolysis bullosa (Floeth *et al.*, 1998). In addition, BP180 has been reported as a target of autoantibodies in the serum of one patient with lichen planus pemphigoides, in another with localized vulval pemphigoid of childhood and even in a case of pemphigoid gestationis without blisters (Hsu *et al.*, 2000; Schumann *et al.*, 2000; Skaria *et al.*, 2000).

Laminins of the dermal–epidermal BMZ

In addition to $\alpha_6\beta_4$-integrin and BP180, anchoring filaments contain the molecules laminin-5 (Carter *et al.*, 1991) and laminin-6 (Marinkovich *et al.*, 1992a) (Figure 1.1.1). Laminins are a family of heterotrimeric BMZ proteins that contain α-, β- and γ-chains (Burgeson *et al.*, 1994). Laminin-5 is made up of α_3-, β_3-, and γ_2-chains. All previously described laminins were shown to have three short arms and one long arm, forming a cross shape as shown by rotary shadowing analysis. In contrast, laminin-5 appears as a dumbbell shape as a result of severe truncations of the short arms. Each of these short arm reductions occurs primarily as a result of truncations of the genes coding for these subunits. Some of this reduction occurs post-translationally, however, as extracellular processing events on the α_3 and γ_2 short arms (Marinkovich *et al.*, 1992b). Because of these short-arm truncations, laminin-5 cannot polymerize or bind to nidogen. Instead, laminin-5 forms a disulfide-bonded complex with laminin-6 (Champliaud *et al.*, 1996).

Laminin-5: structure and function

Laminin-5 is initially synthesized and secreted by keratinocytes in an unprocessed form with an α_3-chain of 200 kDa, a β_3-chain of 140 kDa and a γ_2-chain of 155 kDa (Marinkovich *et al.*, 1992b). The domains I and II in all three chains are believed to adopt a helical coil conformation accounting for the rod-like central portion of the laminin molecule, and are essential for laminin assembly. βγ dimers accumulate intracellularly and assembly of these dimers with the α-chain appears to be the rate-limiting step in laminin assembly (Matsui *et al.*, 1995). Shortly after secretion, the α_3-chain becomes processed from 200 to 165 kDa. In addition, the γ_2-chain is processed from 155 to 105 kDa by the enzyme BMP-1 (Lee *et al.*, 1997). These processing steps occur both *in vitro* in cultured keratinocytes and *in vivo* in human tissues. An additional processing step predominantly occurs *in vivo* which results in the conversion of the α_3-chain from 165 to 145 kDa (Marinkovich *et al.*, 1992b). Analysis of laminin-5 extracted from human tissue shows that the former two steps occur to completion while the latter processing step occurs in approximately half of the laminin-5 molecules. In addition, further processing via MMP-2 of the γ_2-chain from 105 to 80 kDa occurs at the boundary of domains III and II in certain proliferative states, such as squamous cell carcinoma and the developing mammary gland (Giannelli *et al.*, 1997). This processing has only been demonstrated in rat tissues and appears to facilitate a promigratory epithelial phenotype. It remains to be shown whether this particular processing step occurs in human tissues.

The laminin α_3-chain contains an especially large C-terminal globular domain that consists of five repeating EGF-like segments. The G domain of laminin-5 α_3-chain contains the major cell binding activity, which enables laminin-5 to serve as the major attachment ligand for a number of epithelial cell types, including keratinocytes and squamous carcinoma cells. Processing of the α_3-chain from 200 to 165 kDa appears to occur near the junction of the G_3 and G_4 domains, and laminin-5 containing processed 165 kDa α_3-chain supports cell attachment (Rousselle & Aumailley, 1994; Rousselle *et al.*, 1995). Proteolytic processing of the α_3 globular domain is the key step in converting laminin-5 from a pro-motility protein to a catalyst for hemidesmosome formation (Goldfinger *et al.*, 1998).

These observations make it clear that the cell binding activity and the binding sites for integrins $\alpha_3\beta_1$ and $\alpha_6\beta_4$ are located somewhere in the G_1 to G_3 domains. Laminin-5 binding to $\alpha_3\beta_1$ is an important step in promoting migration, and binding to $\alpha_6\beta_4$ is important for regulating hemidesmosome formation. In the absence of laminin-5, however, $\alpha_3\beta_1$-integrin has been noted to associate with an alternative ligand (Ryan *et al.*, 1999). Furthermore, the monoclonal antibody BM165, which recognizes an epitope on the G_1 domain, has been shown to inhibit the attachment of keratinocytes to underlying culture substrate and to interfere with the attachment of epidermis to dermis (Rousselle *et al.*, 1991). It has also been shown in neonatal mice that anti-laminin-5 Fab fragments can induce subepidermal blistering (Lazarova *et al.*, 2000) and that human antibodies to laminin-5 induce subepidermal blistering in skin grafts onto SCID mice (Lazarova *et al.*, 1996). Research in this area has been complicated by the fact that human anti-laminin-5 antibodies do not bind to murine skin, but it is hoped that these newer models will allow for further investigation.

Laminin-5 additionally has heparin binding properties contained within the G_4 and G_5 domains (Sung *et al.*, 1997). The significance of the heparin binding is not yet clear. It is possible that before processing and insertion into the BMZ, laminin-5 may bind to perlecan, a BMZ heparan sulfate proteoglycan. Alternatively, the cell-surface heparan sulfate proteoglycan, syndecan may bind to laminin-5 and laminin-6 to influence BMZ formation and cell migration. The G_5 domain has been shown to have a promigratory activity (Sung *et al.*, 1997) and removal of this domain through processing appears to decrease the ability of laminin-5 to support cell migration and increase the ability of laminin-5 to support hemidesmosome formation (Goldfinger *et al.*, 1998).

Laminin-6: structure and function

Laminin-6, the other known anchoring filament laminin, contains α_3-, β_1- and γ_1-chains (Marinkovich *et al.*, 1992a), and based on sequence analysis it has been hypothesized that one of the unpaired cysteine residues in the laminin-6 α_3-chain domain 3 EGF1 region binds to an unpaired cysteine residue in the laminin-5 β_3 domain 6 region (Champliaud *et al.*, 1996). The α_3- and γ_2-chains of laminin-5 are processed completely and consistently when laminin-5 is complexed with laminin-6, and these processing steps are probably necessary in the covalent association of laminin-5 and laminin-6. Laminin-5 has also been shown to complex with another component, laminin-7, which contains the β_2 laminin chain; however laminin-7 does not appear to be present in skin to any significant extent. In addition, the N-terminal portion of the α_3-chain exists in two spliced variant forms (Ryan *et al.*, 1994). The functional significance of this alternative splicing is not yet clear. As laminin-6 also contains the α_3 G domain, it can theoretically combine with basal cell-surface receptors. This suggests that the laminin-5–laminin-6 heterodimer contains two cell binding regions per dimeric complex.

Laminins-5 and -6 together

The current data suggest that laminin-5 is orientated in the BMZ with its C-terminal G domain located adjacent to the basal cell surface and the N-terminal short arms facing the lamina densa complexing with laminin-6. Laminin-6, located in the lower lamina lucida and lamina densa, interacts with other BMZ components through linkage of its γ_1-chain with nidogen (Mayer *et al.*, 1993). Through this interaction, the divalent nidogen can link laminin-6 and the anchoring complex with its other known BMZ ligands, collagen IV and perlecan (Dziadek *et al.*, 1985). In addition to its interaction with laminin-6, laminin-5 is capable of binding with the NC1 domain of collagen VII (Chen *et al.*, 1997; Rousselle *et al.*, 1997), as determined by solid-phase binding assays and rotary shadowing analysis.

It is not entirely clear whether laminin-5 can associate simultaneously with both collagen VII and laminin-6. Even if laminin-5 were incapable of such a dual association, only approximately half of the laminin-5 purified from tissue is complexed with laminin-6. This would leave a significant portion of laminin-5 available to bind to collagen VII. The above model predicts that the N-terminal globular short-arm domains are probably the regions of laminin-5 that come in contact with collagen VII and thus these regions probably contain the binding sites. Preliminary studies have also demonstrated that the BP180 exodomain binds to laminin-5, indicating another possibly important interaction of laminin-5 with the extracellular BMZ. Because of its multiple interactions, laminin-5 is a molecule of central importance in the assembly of extracellular components of the dermal–epidermal BMZ.

The dermal–epidermal BMZ contains at least one other large laminin in addition to laminin-6, which contains β_1- and γ_1-chains as well as a chain recognized by mAb 4C7 (Engvall *et al.*, 1986). While it was originally believed that mAb 4C7 recognized laminin α_1-chain, recent evidence has shown that this mAb instead recognizes laminin α_5-chain (Tiger *et al.*, 1997). Therefore, it is likely that the dermal–epidermal BMZ contains the laminin combination, $\alpha_5\beta_1\gamma_1$, which has been termed laminin-10. Laminin-1 ($\alpha_1\beta_1\gamma_1$), in contrast, does not appear to be a significant constituent of the dermal–epidermal BMZ (Miner *et al.*, 1997).

Disease

The importance of laminin-5 in mediating epithelial adhesion is best illustrated by the widespread blistering, mucosal erosions and extracutaneous epithelial adhesion defects that occur in patients with Herlitz junctional epidermolysis bullosa, where laminin-5 expression is absent (Meneguzzi *et al.*, 1992; Marinkovich *et al.*, 1993) owing to underlying gene mutations (Uitto *et al.*, 1997). In addition, laminins-5 and -6 function as autoantigens in a subset of patients with the blistering disease cicatricial pemphigoid (Domloge-Hultsch *et al.*, 1992). The autoantibodies frequently recognize the processed laminin-5 α_3-chain (Kirtschig *et al.*, 1995) and thus the autoantibody must reside somewhere between the N-terminus and G domain 3 of this chain. Autoantibodies have also been reported against the β_3- and γ_2-chains of laminin-5 (Fujimoto *et al.*, 1999). As the autoantibodies disrupt skin cohesion, it is possible that the autoepitope site (or sites) is located in G domains 1–3 of the α_3-chain near the cell binding region. The inciting event for development of the autoantibodies is usually unknown, but a report of a gastric cancer that secreted laminin-5, with development of anti-laminin-5 antibodies in the patient, provides a possible model for inception of the autoimmune disease (Taniuchi *et al.*, 1999).

Anchoring complex–BMZ associations

General BMZs

All BMZs contain some type of laminin, collagen IV, nidogen and perlecan, a large heparan sulfate proteoglycan (Martin & Timpl, 1987). Several studies have demonstrated that these purified components are capable of assembling into structures resembling the lamina densa of the basement membrane (Yurchenco & O'Rear, 1994). This occurs through a number of interactions. Collagen IV, through a quaternary association via its 7-A regions and a binary association through its NC1 domain, can self-polymerize into an extended network that probably represents the central feature of the lamina densa (Yurchenco & O'Rear, 1994). Laminins also are capable of self-polymerizing and also contribute to the self-assembly capabilities of the BMZ. Linkages of collagen IV, laminins and perlecan with the 150 kDa linker protein nidogen (Dziadek *et al.*, 1985) are additional mechanisms that underlie the self-assembly of the lamina densa/lamina lucida in all BMZs.

Dermal–epidermal BMZ

In specialized BMZs such as the one at the dermal–epidermal junction, the assembly of the ubiquitous BMZ structures into a lamina densa–lamina lucida and the assembly of anchoring complex structures may occur independently. Impairment of anchoring complex but not lamina densa/lamina lucida formation is seen in knockout murine or EB-PA patient skin lacking $\alpha_6\beta_4$-integrin (Smith, 1993; Dowling *et al.*, 1996). In contrast, impairment of lamina densa–lamina lucida formation, but not anchoring complex formation, is seen in the skin of α_3-integrin knockout mice that lack the $\alpha_3\beta_1$-integrin. (Hodivala-Dilke *et al.*, 1998). These studies suggest that both $\alpha_6\beta_4$- and $\alpha_3\beta_1$-integrins perform important complementary functions in the development of the dermal–epidermal BMZ and that development of the ubiquitous and specialized portions of the dermal–epidermal BMZ may occur by separate mechanisms.

A primary mode of linkage of the specialized components of the anchoring complex with the rest of the ubiquitous BMZ structures probably occurs through association between nidogen and the fourth EGF repeat on domain III of the γ_1-chain of laminin-6 (Mayer *et al.*, 1993). Through this linkage with nidogen, laminin-6 and the anchoring complex may be adjoined directly to both collagen IV and perlecan, and indirectly to laminin-10 through repeated nidogen–ligand linkages. Another mode of association between the anchoring complex and the rest of the BMZ may occur through interaction of the heparin binding domains of the laminin α_3-chain G_4 and G_5 domains with perlecan, the high molecular weight heparan sulfate basement membrane proteoglycan. Interaction of perlecan with laminin-5 would theoretically occur only transiently, since the α_3-chain G_4 and G_5 domains are proteolytically removed during assembly into the basement membrane *in vivo* (Marinkovich *et al.*, 1992b).

One of the properties of laminins is the ability to polymerize with the responsible elements residing on the N-terminal portions of the molecule (Yurchenco & Cheng, 1993). While it is clear that the truncations that are present on all three short arms of the laminin-5 molecule prevent it from polymerizing, the ability of laminin-6 to polymerize had remained in question until a study examining the polymerization of laminin-6 with laminins-1 and -2 showed that truncations of the short arm of laminin-6 prevent it from self-polymerizing or polymerizing with laminins-1 and -2 (Cheng *et al.*, 1997). This study suggested that domains present on laminin α_1- and α_2-chains required for self-polymerization are lacking on the laminin-6 α_3-chain. Therefore, laminin polymerization does not appear to be a mechanism of association of the anchoring complex with the rest of the BMZ.

Collagen VII

Collagen VII is the major constituent of anchoring fibrils (Sakai *et al.*, 1986). The importance of collagen VII in dermal–epidermal cohesion is well demonstrated by dystrophic epidermolysis bullosa (DEB), a group of diseases resulting from the absence of collagen VII or functional defects in the protein due to underlying gene defects (Uitto *et al.*, 1994). In these diseases, sublamina densa separation of the skin and mucosa occurs as a result of a lack of intact anchoring fibrils.

Structure and function

Like all collagens, collagen VII assembles into a triple helix and requires sufficient ascorbic acid for proper conversion of proline to hydroxyproline, which is necessary for molecular stability. Analysis of the deduced amino-acid sequence of collagen VII (Parente *et al.*, 1991) reveals the presence of a long, central collagenous region characterized by repeating Gly-X-Y sequences. These sequences contain a number of non-collagenous interruptions, including a 39 amino-acid non-collagenous segment in the center of the helix corresponding to the 'hinge region' predicted by biochemical studies (Bachinger *et al.*, 1990). These interruptions account for the flexibility of the collagen VII molecule, and explain its ability to loop around and entrap dermal matrix molecules (Keene *et al.*, 1987), while anchoring the BMZ to the underlying papillary dermis. The 145 kDa N-terminal end of collagen VII contains the largest non-collagenous domain (Lunstrum *et al.*, 1986). This domain inserts onto the lamina densa and anchoring plaques. The C-terminal non-collagenous globular NC2 domain of the collagen VII molecule is processed prior to antiparallel dimer formation (Lunstrum *et al.*, 1987). Collagen VII triple helices are joined together at their processed NC2 globular domains to form antiparallel dimers (Morris *et al.*, 1986). When this step is prevented through mutations of this region of the collagen VII gene (Bruckner-Tuderman *et al.*, 1995), sublamina densa blistering and DEB result. Anchoring fibrils probably derive from lateral associations of the antiparallel dimers.

Other related molecules

Collagen IV in the lamina densa and anchoring plaques specifically binds to the collagen VII NC1 domain (Burgeson *et al.*, 1990). Anchoring fibrils were shown to extend as perpendicular projections in areas directly underlying anchoring filaments, and based on these findings it was suspected that a direct interaction between anchoring filaments and anchoring fibrils also existed. Recent studies have confirmed a specific interaction between the anchoring filament component laminin-5 and collagen VII NC1 domain. Colocalization of laminin-5 and the collagen VII NC1 domain has been demonstrated both in the lamina densa and in anchoring plaques of the dermal–epidermal BMZ (Rousselle *et al.*, 1997). The NC1 domain has been shown specifically to bind to both the β_3- and the γ_2-chain of laminin-5 (Chen *et al.*, 1997). These studies provide the first evidence of direct linkage between anchoring filaments and anchoring fibrils. A second component of anchoring fibrils has been identified recently (Gayraud *et al.*, 1997). This component is recognized by the mAb GDA-J/F3 and appears to be a 50 kDa protein that localizes to the junction of anchoring fibrils with the lamina densa.

Disease

As stated above, collagen VII defects have clearly been shown to cause dominant and recessive DEB, and over 100 mutations have been identified and reported. Research into collagen VII deficiencies is growing rapidly. The first case of DEB in sheep was described in the early 1990s (Bruckner-Tuderman *et al.*, 1991) and a case of decreased collagen VII immunoreactivity in a feline with DEB was reported recently (Olivry *et al.*, 1999b). Several mutations in collagen VII have been found to lead to a mild clinical disease or none at all (Bruckner-Tuderman *et al.*, 1999). Therefore, care must be exercised before prenatal diagnosis is undertaken. Collagen VII may also be the target of autoantibodies, and a case of canine bullous systemic lupus erythematosus that was linked to anti-collagen VII IgG was reported recently (Olivry *et al.*, 2000d).

Recent studies with mice that targeted the collagen VII gene for knockout revealed a more severe phenotype than that observed in humans, with the mice demonstrating severe subepidermal blistering (Heinonen *et al.*, 1999). The knockout mice all died during the first 2 weeks of life. Hopefully this model can be used to explore new therapies for DEB.

Conclusion

The dermal–epidermal BMZ is a region of intricate and precise interaction of highly specialized proteins working together in concert to facilitate successful dermal–epidermal cohesion. The disruption of these intricate interactions can lead to disease states with varying manifestations, both cutaneous and systemic, as detailed above. It is hoped that this paper may serve as an authoritative reference on the proteins of the BMZ and their interactions for veterinarians who seek to understand the molecular pathophysiology of the many subepidermal bullous diseases that affect animals.

Acknowledgement

The authors would like to thank the VA Palo Alto Health Care System for their assistance.

References

Aho, S. & Uitto, J. (1999) 180-kD bullous pemphigoid antigen/type XVII collagen: tissue-specific expression and molecular interactions with keratin 18. *Journal of Cellular Biochemistry*, **72**, 356–367.

Andrä, K., Lassmann, H., Bittner, R., Shorny, S., Fässler, R., Propst, F. & Wiche, G. (1997) Targeted inactivation of plectin reveals essential function in maintaining the integrity of skin, muscle, and heart cytoarchitecture. *Genes and Development*, **11**, 3143–3156.

Bachinger, H. P., Morris, N. P. & Lundstrum, G. P. (1990) The relationship of the biophysical and biochemical characteristics of type VII collagen to the function of anchoring fibrils. *Journal of Biological Chemistry*, **265**, 10095–10101.

Balding, S. D., Prost, C., Diaz, L. A., Bernard, P., Bedane, C., Aberdam, D. & Giudice, G. J. (1996) Cicatricial pemphigoid autoantibodies react with multiple sites on the BP180 extracellular domain. *Journal of Investigative Dermatology*, **106**, 141–146.

Balding, S. D., Diaz, L. A. & Giudice, G. J. (1997) A recombinant form of the human BP180 ectodomain forms a collagen-like homotrimeric complex. *Biochemistry*, **36**, 8821–8830.

Bédane, C., McMillan, J. R., Balding, S. D., Bernard, P., Prost, C., Bonnetblanc, J. M. *et al.* (1997) Bullous pemphigoid and cicatricial pemphigoid autoantibodies react with ultrastructurally separable epitopes on the BP180 ectodomain: evidence that BP180 spans the lamina lucida. *Journal of Investigative Dermatology*, **108**, 901–907.

Borradori, L., Koch, P. J., Niessen, C. M., Erkeland, S., Leusden, M. R. van & Sonnenberg, A. (1997) The localization of bullous pemphigoid antigen 180 (BP180) in hemidesmosomes is mediated by its cytoplasmic domain and seems to be regulated by the beta4 integrin subunit. *Journal of Cell Biology*, **136**, 1333–1347.

Borradori, L., Chavanas, S., Schaapveld, R. Q., Gagnoux-Palacios, L., Calafat, J., Meneguzzi, G. & Sonnenberg, A. (1998) Role of the bullous pemphigoid antigen 180 (BP180) in the assembly of hemidesmosomes and cell adhesion – reexpression of BP180 in generalized atrophic benign epidermolysis bullosa keratinocytes. *Experimental Cell Research*, **239**, 463–476.

Bruckner-Tuderman, L., Guscetti, F. & Ehrensperger, F. (1991) Animal model for dermolytic mechanobullous disease: sheep with recessive dystrophic epidermolysis bullosa lack collagen VII. *Journal of Investigative Dermatology* **96**, 452–458.

Bruckner-Tuderman, L., Nilssen, O., Zimmermann, D. R., Dours-Zimmermann, M. T. *et al.* (1995) Immunohistochemical and mutation analyses demonstrate that procollagen VII is processed to collagen VII through removal of the NC-2 domain. *Journal of Cell Biology*, **131**, 551–559.

Bruckner-Tuderman, L., Höpfner, B & Hammami-Hauasli, N. (1999) Biology of anchoring fibrils: lessons from dystrophic epidermolysis bullosa. *Matrix Biology*, **18**, 43–54.

Burgeson, R. E., Lundstrum, G. P. & Rokosova, B. (1990) The structure and function of type VII collagen. *Annals of the New York Academy of Sciences*, **580**, 32–43.

Burgeson, R. E., Chiquet, M., Deutzmann, R., Ekblom, P., Engel, J., Kleinman, H. *et al.* (1994) A new nomenclature for the laminins. *Matrix Biology*, **14**, 209–211.

Carter, W. G., Ryan, M. C. & Gahr, P. J. (1991) Epiligrin, a new cell adhesion ligand for integrin-3-1 in epithelial basement membranes. *Cell*, **65**, 559–610.

Champliaud, M. F., Lunstrum, G. P., Rousselle, P., Nishiyama, T., Keene, D. R. & Burgeson, R. E. (1996) Human amnion contains a novel laminin variant, laminin 7, which like laminin 6, covalently associates with laminin 5 to promote stable epithelial–stromal attachment. *Journal of Cellular Biology*, **132**, 1189–1198.

Chan, L. S., Lapiere, J. C., Chen, M., Traczyk, T., Mancini, A. J., Paller, A. S. *et al.* (1999) Bullous systemic lupus erythematosus with autoantibodies recognizing multiple skin basement membrane components, bullous pemphigoid antigen 1, laminin-5, laminin-6, and type VII collagen. *Archives of Dermatology*, **135**, 569–573.

Chavanas, S., Pulkkinen, L., Gache, Y., Smith, F. J., McLean, W. H., Uitto, J. *et al.* (1996) A homozygous nonsense mutation in the PLEC1 gene in patients with epidermolysis bullosa simplex with muscular dystrophy. *Journal of Clinical Investigation*, **98**, 2196–2200.

Chen, M., Marinkovich, M. P., Veis, A., Xiaoyan, C., Rao, C. N., O'Toole, E. A. & Woodley, D. T. (1997) Interactions of the amino-terminal noncollagenous (NC1) domain of type VII collagen with extracellular matrix components. *Journal of Biological Chemistry*, **272**, 14516–14522.

Cheng, Y. S., Champliaud, M. F., Burgeson, R. E., Marinkovich, M. P. & Yurchenco, P. D. (1997) Self-assembly of laminin isoforms. *Journal of Biological Chemistry*, **272**, 31525–31532.

Domloge-Hultsch, N., Gammon, W. R., Briggaman, R. A., Gil, S. G., Carter, W. G. & Yancey, K. B. (1992) Epiligrin, the major human keratinocyte integrin ligand, is a target in both an acquired autoimmune and an inherited subepidermal blistering skin disease. *Journal of Clinical Investigation*, **90**, 1628–1633.

Dowling, J., Yu, Q. C. & Fuchs, E. (1996) Beta4 integrin is required for hemidesmosome formation, cell adhesion and cell survival. *Journal of Cell Biology*, **134**, 559–572.

Dowling, J., Yang, Y., Wollmann, R., Reichardt, L. F. & Fuchs, E. (1997) Developmental expression of BPAG1-n: insights into the spastic ataxia and gross neurologic degeneration in dystonia musculorum mice. *Developmental Biology*, **187**, 131–142.

Dziadek, M., Paulsson, M. & Timpl, R. (1985) Identification and interaction repertoire of large forms of the basement membrane protein nidogen. *EMBO Journal*, **4**, 2513–2518.

Egan, C. A. & Zone, J. J. (1999) Linear IgA bullous dermatosis. *International Journal of Dermatology*, **38**, 818–827.

Elliott, C. E., Becker, B., Oehler, S., Castañón, M. J., Hauptmann, R. & Wiche, G. (1997) Plectin transcript diversity: identification and tissue distribution of variants with distinct first coding exons and rodless isoforms. *Genomics*, **42**, 115–125.

Ellison, J. & Garrod, D. R. (1984) Anchoring filaments of the amphibian epidermal–dermal junction traverse the basal lamina entirely from the plasma membrane of hemidesmosomes to the dermis. *Journal of Cell Science*, 163–172.

Engvall, E., Davis, G. E., Dickerson, K., Ruoslahti, E., Varon, S. & Manthorpe, M. (1986) Mapping of domains in human laminin using monoclonal antibodies: localization of the neurite promoting site. *Journal of Cell Biology*, **103**, 2457–2465.

Floeth, M., Fiedorowicz, J., Schäcke, H., Hammami-Hausli, N., Owaribe, K., Trüeb, R. M. & Bruckner-Tuderman, L. (1998) Novel homozygous and compound heterozygous COL17A1 mutations associated with junctional epidermolysis bullosa. *Journal of Investigative Dermatology*, **111**, 528–533.

Foisner, R., Feldman, B., Sander, L., Seifert, G., Artlieb, U. & Wiche, G. (1994) A panel of monoclonal antibodies to rat plectin: distinction by epitope mapping and immunoreactivity with different tissues and cell lines. *Acta Histochemica*, **96**, 421–438.

Foisner, R., Bohn, W., Mannweiler, K. & Wiche, G. (1995) Distribution and ultrastructure of plectin arrays in subclones of rat glioma C6 cells differing in intermediate filament protein (vimentin) expression. *Journal of Structural Biology*, **115**, 304–317.

Fuchs, E. & Cleveland, D. W. (1998) A structural scaffolding of intermediate filaments in health and disease. *Science*, **279**, 514–519.

Fujimoto, W., Toi, Y., Okazaki, F., Lazarova, Z., Yancey, K. B. & Arata, J. (1999) Anti-epiligrin cicatricial pemphigoid with IgG autoantibodies to the beta and gamma subunits of laminin 5. *Journal of the American Academy of Dermatology*, **40**, 637–639.

Gache, Y., Ohavana, S. S., Lacour, J. P., Witche, G., Owaribe, K., Meneguzzi, G. & Ortonne, J. P. (1996) Defective expression of plectin/HD1 in epidermolysis bullosa simplex with muscular dystrophy. *Journal of Clinical Investigation*, **97**, 2289–2298.

Gayraud, B., Hopfner, B., Jassim, A., Aumailley, M. & Bruckner-Tuderman, L. (1997) Characterization of a 50-kDa component of epithelial basement membranes using GDA-J/F3 monoclonal antibody. *Journal of Biological Chemistry*, **272**, 9531–9538.

Geerts, D., Fontao, L., Nievers, M. G., Schaapveld, R. Q., Purkis, P. E., Wheeler, G. N. *et al.* (1999) Binding of integrin alpha6beta4 to plectin prevents plectin association with F-actin but does not interfere with intermediate filament binding. *Journal of Cell Biology*, **147**, 417–434.

Giancotti, F. G. (1996) Signal transduction by the alpha 6 beta 4 integrin: charting the path between laminin binding and nuclear events. *Journal of Cell Science*, **109**, 1165–1172.

Giancotti, F. G. & Ruoslahti, E. (1999) Integrin signaling. *Science*, **285**, 1028–1032.

Giannelli, G., Falk-Marzillier, J., Schiraldi, O., Stetler-Stevenson, W. G. & Quaranta, V. (1997) Induction of cell migration by matrix metalloprotease-2 cleavage of laminin-5. *Science*, **277**, 225–228.

Giudice, G. J., Emery, D. J. & Diaz, L. A. (1992) Cloning and primary structural analysis of the bullous pemphigoid autoantigen BP180. *Journal of Investigative Dermatology*, **99**, 243–250.

Goldfinger, L. E., Stack, M. S. & Jones, J. C. (1998) Processing of laminin-5 and its functional consequences: role of plasmin and tissue-type plasminogen activator. *Journal of Cell Biology*, **141**, 255–265.

Guo, L. L., Degenstein, L., Dowling, J., Yu, Q. C., Wollmann, R., Perman, B. & Fuchs, E. (1995) Gene targeting of BPAG1: abnormalities in mechanical strength and cell migration in stratified squamous epithelia and severe neurological degeneration. *Cell*, **81**, 233–243.

Heida, Y., Nishizawa, Y., Uematsu, J. & Owaribe, K. (1992) Identification of a new major hemidesmosomal protein, HD1: a major high molecular mass component of isolated hemidesmosomes. *Journal of Cell Biology*, **116**, 1497–1506.

Heinonen, S., Männikkö, M., Klement, J. F., Whitaker-Menezes, D., Murphy, G. F. & Uitto, J. (1999) Targeted inactivation of the type VII collagen gene (Col7a1) in mice results in severe blistering phenotype: a model for recessive dystrophic epidermolysis bullosa. *Journal of Cell Science*, **112**, 3641–3648.

Hippe-Sanwald, S. (1993) Impact of freeze substitution on biological electron microscopy. *Microscopy Research and Technique*, **24**, 400–422.

Hirako, Y., Usukura, J., Nishizawa, Y. & Owaribe, K. (1996) Demonstration of the molecular shape of BP180, a 180-kDa bullous pemphigoid antigen and its potential for trimer formation. *Journal of Biological Chemistry*, **271**, 13739–13745.

Hodivala-Dilke, K. M., DiPersio, C. M., Kreidberg, J. A. & Hynes, R. O. (1998) Novel roles for alpha3beta1 integrin as a regulator of cytoskeletal assembly and as a trans-dominant inhibitor of integrin receptor function in mouse keratinocytes. *Journal of Cell Biology*, **142**, 1357–1369.

Hopkinson, S. B. & Jones, J. C. (2000) The N terminus of the transmembrane protein BP180 interacts with the N-terminal domain of BP230, thereby mediating keratin cytoskeleton anchorage to the cell surface at the site of the hemidesmosome. *Molecular Biology of the Cell*, **11**, 277–286.

Hsu, S., Ghohestani, R. F. & Uitto, J. (2000) Lichen planus pemphigoides with IgG autoantibodies to the 180 kd bullous pemphigoid antigen (type XVII collagen). *Journal of the American Academy of Dermatology*, **42**, 136–141.

Hynes, R. O. (1992) Integrins: versatility, modulation, and signaling in cell adhesion. *Cell*, **69**, 11–25.

Jonkman, M. F., Scheffer, H., Stulp, R., Pas, H. H., Nijenhuis, M., Heeres, K. *et al.* (1997) Revertant mosaicism in epidermolysis bullosa caused by mitotic gene conversion. *Cell*, **88**, 543–551.

Keene, D. R. & McDonald, K. (1993) The ultrastructure of the connective tissue matrix of skin and cartilage after high-pressure freezing and freeze-substitution. *Journal of Histochemistry and Cytochemistry*, **41**, 1141–1153.

Keene, D. R., Sakai, L. Y., Lunstrum, G. P., Morris, N. P. & Burgeson, R. E. (1987) Type VII collagen forms an extended network of anchoring fibrils. *Journal of Biological Chemistry*, **104**, 611–621.

Keene, D. R., Marinkovich, M. P. & Sakai, L. Y. (1997) Immunodissection of the connective tissue matrix in human skin. *Microscopy Research and Technique*, **38**, 394–406.

Kirtschig, G., Marinkovich, M. P., Burgeson, R. E. & Yancey, K. B. (1995) Anti-basement membrane autoantibodies in patients with anti-epiligrin cicatricial pemphigoid bind the α subunit of laminin 5. *Journal of Investigative Dermatology*, **105**, 543–548.

Klatte, D. H., Kurkapus, M. A., Grelling, K. A. & Jones, J. C. R. (1989) Immunochemical characterization of three components of the hemidesmosome and their expression in cultured epithelial cells. *Journal of Cell Biology*, **109**, 3377–3390.

Kunz, M., Rouan, F., Pulkkinen, L., Hamm, H., Jeschke, R., Bruckner-Tuderman, L. *et al.* (2000) Mutation reports: epidermolysis bullosa simplex associated with severe mucous membrane involvement and novel mutations in the plectin gene. *Journal of Investigative Dermatology*, **114**, 376–380.

Lazarova, Z., Yee, C., Darling, T., Briggaman, R. A. & Yancey, K. B. (1996) Passive transfer of anti-laminin 5 antibodies induces subepidermal blisters in neonatal mice. *Journal of Clinical Investigation*, **98**, 1509–1518.

Lazarova, Z., Hsu, R., Briggaman, R. A. & Yancey, K. B. (2000) Fab fragments directed against laminin 5 induce subepidermal blisters in neonatal mice. *Clinical Immunology*, **95**, 26–32.

Lee, S., Solow-Cordero, D. E., Kessler, E., Takahara, K. & Greenspan, D. S. (1997) Transforming growth factor-beta regulation of bone morphogenetic protein-1/procollagen C-proteinase and related proteins in fibrogenic cells and keratinocytes. *Journal of Biological Chemistry*, **272**, 19059–19066.

Leivo, I., Tani, T., Laitinen, L., Bruns, R., Kivilaakso, E., Lehto, V. P. *et al.* (1996) Anchoring complex components laminin-5 and type VII collagen in intestine: association with migrating and differentiating enterocytes. *Journal of Histochemistry and Cytochemistry*, **44**, 1267–1277.

Lin, M. S., Mascar, J. M., Jr, Liu, Z., España, A. & Diaz, L. A. (1997) The desmosome and hemidesmosome in cutaneous autoimmunity. *Clinical and Experimental Immunology*, **107** (Suppl. 1), 9–15.

Liu, C. G., Maercker, C., Cartanon, M. J., Hauptmann, R. & Wiche, G. (1996) Human plectin: organization of the gene, sequence analysis, and chromosome localization (8q24). *Proceedings of the National Academy of Sciences of the United States of America*, **93**, 4278–4283.

Liu, Z., Diaz, L. A., Swartz, S. J., Troy, J. L., Fairley, J. A. & Giudice, G. J. (1995) Molecular mapping of a pathogenically relevant BP180 epitope associated with experimentally induced murine bullous pemphigoid. *Journal of Immunology*, **155**, 5449–5454.

Lunstrum, G. P., Sakai, L. Y., Keene, D. R., Morris, N. P. & Burgeson, R. E. (1986) Large complex globular domains of type VII procollagen contribute to the structure of anchoring fibrils. *Journal of Biological Chemistry*, **261**, 9042–9048.

Lunstrum, G. P., Kuo, H. J., Rosenbaum, L. M., Keene, D. R., Glanville, R. W., Sakai, L. Y. & Burgeson, R. E. (1987) Anchoring fibrils contain the carboxyl-terminal globular domain of type VII procollagen, but lack the amino-terminal globular domain. *Journal of Biological Chemistry*, **262**, 13706–13712.

McLean, W. H., Pulkkinen, L., Smith, F. J., Rugg, E. L., Lane, E. B., Bullrich, F. *et al.* (1996) Loss of plectin causes epidermolysis bullosa with muscular dystrophy: cDNA cloning and genomic organization. *Genes and Development*, **10**, 1724–1735.

Malecz, N., Foisner, R., Stadler, C. & Wiche, G. (1996) Identification of plectin as a substrate of p34cdc2 kinase and mapping of a single phosphorylation site. *Journal of Biological Chemistry*, **271**, 8203–8208.

Marinkovich, M. P. (1999) Update on inherited bullous dermatoses. *Dermatologic Clinics*, **17**, 473–485, vii.

Marinkovich, M. P., Lunstrum, G. P., Keene, D. R. & Burgeson, R. E. (1992a) The dermal–epidermal junction of human skin contains a novel laminin variant. *Journal of Cell Biology*, **119**, 695–703.

Marinkovich, M. P., Lunstrum, G. P. & Burgeson, R. E. (1992b) The anchoring filament protein kalinin is synthesized and secreted as a high molecular weight precursor. *Journal of Biological Chemistry*, **267**, 17900–17906.

Marinkovich, M. P., Verrando, P., Keene, D. R., Meneguzzi, G., Lunstrum, G. P., Ortonne, J. P. & Burgeson, R. E. (1993) The basement membrane proteins kalinin and nicein are structurally and immunologically identical. *Laboratory Investigation*, **69**, 295–299.

Marinkovich, M. P., Taylor, T. B., Keene, D. R., Burgeson, R. E. & Zone, J. J. (1996) LAD-1, the linear IgA bullous dermatosis autoantigen, is a novel 120-kDa anchoring filament protein synthesized by epidermal cells [published erratum appears in *Journal of Investigative Dermatology* 1996; **106**: 1343]. *Journal of Investigative Dermatology*, **106**, 734–738.

Marinkovich, M. P., Tran, H. H., Rao, S. K., Giudice, G. J., Balding, S., Jonkman, M. F. *et al.* (1997) LAD-1 is absent in a subset of junctional epidermolysis bullosa patients. *Journal of Investigative Dermatology*, **109**, 356–359.

Marinkovich, M. P., Herron, G. S., Khavari, P. A. & Bauer, E. A. (1999) Hereditary epidermolysis bullosa. In: *Dermatology in General Medicine* (Eds I. M. Freedberg, A. Z. Eisen, K. Wolff, K. F. Austen, L. A. Goldsmith, S. I. Katz & T. B. Fitzpatrick), pp. 690–709. McGraw-Hill, New York.

Martin, G. R. & Timpl, R. (1987) Laminin and other basement membrane components. *Annual Reviews of Cell Biology*, **3**, 57–85.

Matsui, C., Wong, C. K., Nelson, C. F., Bauer, E. A. & Hoeffler, W. K. (1995) The assembly of laminin 5 subunits. *Journal of Biological Chemistry*, **270**, 23496–23503.

Mayer, U., Nischt, R., Poschl, E., Mann, K., Fukuda, K., Gerl, M. *et al.* (1993) A single EGF-like motif of laminin is responsible for high affinity nidogen binding. *EMBO Journal*, **12**, 1879–1885.

Meneguzzi, G., Marinkovich, M. P., Aberdam, D., Pisani, A., Burgeson, R. & Ortonne, J. P. (1992) Kalinin is abnormally expressed in epithelial basement membranes of Herlitz's junctional epidermolysis bullosa patients. *Experimental Dermatology*, **1**, 221–229.

Miner, J. H., Patton, B. L., Lentz, S. I., Gilbert, D. J., Snider, W. D., Jenkins, N. A. *et al.* (1997) The laminin alpha chains: expression, developmental transitions, and chromosomal locations of alpha1–5, identification of heterotrimeric laminins 8–11, and cloning of a novel alpha3 isoform. *Journal of Cell Biology*, **137**, 685–701.

Molnar, K., Van Der Steege, G., Jonkman, M. F., Nijenhuis, M., Husz, S., Van Der Meer, J. B. & Pas, H. H. (2000) Two type XVII collagen (BP180) mRNA transcripts in human keratinocytes: a long and a short form. *Clinical and Experimental Dermatology*, **25**, 71–76.

Morris, N. P., Keene, D. R., Glanville, R. W., Bentz, H. & Burgeson, R. E. (1986) The tissue form of type VII collagen is an antiparallel dimer. *Journal of Biological Chemistry*, **261**, 5638–5644.

Niessen, C. M., Hogervorst, F., Jaspars, L. H., Melker, A. A. de, Delwel, G. O., Hulsman, E. H. *et al.* (1995) The α6β4 integrin is a receptor for both laminin and kalinin. *Experimental Cell Research*, **211**, 360–367.

Niessen, C. M., Hulsman, E. H., Oomen, L. C., Kuikman, I. & Sonnenberg, A. (1997) A minimal region on the integrin beta4 subunit that is critical to its localization in hemidesmosomes regulates the distribution of HD1/plectin in COS-7 cells. *Journal of Cell Science*, **110**, 1705–1716.

Nievers, M. G., Schaapveld, R. Q. & Sonnenberg, A. (1999) Biology and function of hemidesmosomes. *Matrix Biology*, **18**, 5–17.

Nikolic, B., MacNulty, E., Mir, B. & Wiche, G. (1996) Basic amino acid residue cluster within nuclear targeting sequence motif is essential for cytoplasmic plectin–vimentin network junctions. *Journal of Cell Biology*, **134**, 1455–1467.

Olivry, T., Chan, L. S., Xu, L., Chace, P., Dunston, S. M., Fahey, M. & Marinkovich, M. P. (1999a) Novel feline autoimmune blistering disease resembling bullous pemphigoid in humans: IgG autoantibodies target the NC16A ectodomain of type XVII collagen (BP180/BPAG2). *Veterinary Pathology*, **36**, 328–335.

Olivry, T., Dunston, S. M. & Marinkovich, M. P. (1999b) Reduced anchoring fibril formation and collagen VII immunoreactivity in feline dystrophic epidermolysis bullosa. *Veterinary Pathology*, **36**, 616–618.

Olivry, T., Savary, K. C., Murphy, K. M., Dunston, S. M. & Chen, M. (1999c) Bullous systemic lupus erythematosus (type I) in a dog. *Veterinary Record*, **145**, 165–169.

Olivry, T., Borrillo, A. K. G., Xu, L., Dunston, S. M., Slovis, N. M., Affolter, V. K. *et al.* (2000a) Equine bullous pemphigoid IgG autoantibodies target linear epitopes in the NC16A ectodomain of collagen XVII (BP180, BPAG2) *Veterinary Immunology and Immunopathology*, **73**, 45–52.

Olivry, T., Dunston, S. M., Fahey, M., Nguyen, N. & Marinkovich, M. P. (2000b) Autoantibodies against the processed ectodomain of collagen XVII (BPAG2, BP180) define a canine homologue of linear IgA disease of humans. *Veterinary Pathology*, **37**, 302–309.

Olivry, T., Mirsky, M. L., Singleton, W., Dunston, S. M., Borrillo, A. K., Xu, L. *et al.* (2000c) A spontaneously arising porcine model of bullous pemphigoid. *Archives of Dermatology Research*, **292**, 37–45.

Olivry, T., Petersen, A., Dunston, S. M. & Chen, M. (2000d) Novel localised variant of canine epidermolysis bullosa acquisita. *Veterinary Record*, **146**, 193–194.

Parente, M. G., Chung, L. C. & Ryynanen, J. (1991) Human type VII collagen: cDNA cloning and chromosomal mapping of the gene (COL7A1) on chromosome 3 to dominant dystrophic epidermolysis bullosa. *American Journal of Human Genetics*, **24**, 119–135.

Pas, H. H., Kloosterhuis, G. J., Heeres, K., Meer, J. B. van der & Jonkman, M. F. (1997) Bullous pemphigoid and linear IgA dermatosis sera recognize a similar 120-kDa keratinocyte collagenous glycoprotein with antigenic cross-reactivity to BP180. *Journal of Investigative Dermatology*, **108**, 423–429.

Proby, C. M., Ota, T., Suzuki, H., Koyasu, S., Gamou, S., Shimizu, N. *et al.* (2000) Development of chimeric molecules for recognition and targeting of antigen-specific B cells in pemphigus vulgaris. *British Journal of Dermatology*, **142**, 321–330.

Rezniczek, G. A., Pereda, J. M. de, Reipert, S. & Wiche, G. (1998) Linking integrin alpha6beta4-based cell adhesion to the intermediate filament cytoskeleton: direct interaction between the beta4 subunit and plectin at multiple molecular sites. *Journal of Cell Biology*, **141**, 209–225.

Rousselle, P. & Aumailley, M. (1994) Kalinin is more efficient than laminin in promoting adhesion of primary keratinocytes and some other epithelial cells and has a different requirement for integrin receptors. *Journal of Cell Biology*, **125**, 205–214.

Rousselle, P., Lunstrum, G. P., Keene, D. R. & Burgeson, R. E. (1991) Kalinin: an epithelium-specific basement membrane adhesion molecule that is a component of anchoring filaments. *Journal of Cell Biology*, **114**, 567–576.

Rousselle, P., Golbik, R., Rest, M. van der & Aumailley, M. (1995) Structural requirement for cell adhesion to kalinin (laminin-5). *Journal of Biological Chemistry*, **270**, 13766–13770.

Rousselle, P., Keene, D. R., Ruggiero, F., Champliaud, M. F., Rest, M. & Burgeson, R. E. (1997) Laminin 5 binds the NC-1 domain of type VII collagen. *Journal of Cell Biology*, **138**, 719–728.

Ruzzi, L., Gagnoux-Palacios, L., Pinola, M., Belli, S., Meneguzzi, G., D'Alessio, M. & Zambruno, G. (1997) A homozygous mutation in the integrin alpha6 gene in junctional epidermolysis bullosa with pyloric atresia. *Journal of Clinical Investigation*, **99**, 2826–2831.

Ryan, M. C., Tizard, R., VanDevanter, D. R. & Carter, W. G. (1994) Cloning of the gene encoding the α3 chain of the adhesive ligand epiligrin. Expression in wound repair. *Journal of Biological Chemistry*, **269**, 22779–22787.

Ryan, M. C., Lee, K., Miyashita, Y. & Carter, W. G. (1999) Targeted disruption of the LAMA3 gene in mice reveals abnormalities in survival and late stage differentiation of epithelial cells. *Journal of Cell Biology*, **145**, 1309–1323.

Sakai, L. Y., Keene, D. R., Morris, N. P. & Burgeson, R. E. (1986) Type VII collagen is a major structural component of anchoring fibrils. *Journal of Cell Biology*, **103**, 1577–1586.

Sawamura, D. K., Li, K., Chu, M.-L. & Uitto, J. (1991) Human bullous pemphigoid antigen (BPAG1): amino acid sequence deduced from cloned cDNAs predicts biologically important peptide segments and protein domains. *Journal of Biological Chemistry*, **266**, 17784–17790.

Schaapveld, R. Q., Borradori, L., Geerts, D., Leusden, M. R. van, Kuikman, I., Nievers, M. G. *et al.* (1998) Hemidesmosome formation is initiated by the beta4 integrin subunit, requires complex formation of beta4 and HD1/plectin, and involves a direct interaction between beta4 and the bullous pemphigoid antigen 180. *Journal of Cell Biology*, **142**, 271–284.

Schäcke, H., Schumann, H., Hammami-Hauasli, N., Raghunath, M. & Bruckner-Tuderman, L. (1998) Two forms of collagen XVII in keratinocytes. A full-length transmembrane protein and a soluble ectodomain. *Journal of Biological Chemistry*, **273**, 25937–25943.

Schumann, H. & Bruckner-Tuderman, L. (1996) Isolation of collagen XVII/BP 180 from human keratinocytes as a native collagen (Abstract). *Journal of Investigative Dermatology*, **107**, 494.

Schumann, H., Baetge, J., Tasanen, K., Wojnarowska, F., Schacke, H., Zillikens, D. & Bruckner-Tuderman, L. (2000) The shed ectodomain of collagen XVII/BP180 is targeted by autoantibodies in different blistering skin diseases. *American Journal of Pathology*, **156**, 685–695.

Seitz, C. S., Giudice, G. J., Balding, S. D., Marinkovich, M. P. & Khavari, P. A. (1999) BP180 gene delivery in junctional epidermolysis bullosa. *Gene Therapy*, **6**, 42–47.

Skalli, O., Jones, J. C. R., Gagescu, R. & Goldman, R. D. (1994) IFAP 300 is common to desmosomes and hemidesmosomes and is a possible linker of intermediate filaments to these junctions. *Journal of Cell Biology*, **125**, 159–170.

Skaria, M., Jaunin, F., Hunziker, T., Riou, S., Schumann, H., Bruckner-Tuderman, L. *et al.* (2000) IgG autoantibodies from bullous pemphigoid patients recognize multiple antigenic reactive sites located predominantly within the B and C subdomains of the COOH-terminus of BP230. *Journal of Investigative Dermatology*, **114**, 998–1004.

Smith, E. A. & Fuchs, E. (1998) Defining the interactions between intermediate filaments and desmosomes. *Journal of Cell Biology*, **141**, 1229–1241.

Smith, F. J., Eady, R. A., Leigh, I. M., McMillan, J. R., Rugg, E. L., Kelsell, D. P. *et al.* (1996) Plectin deficiency results in muscular dystrophy with epidermolysis bullosa. *Nature Genetics*, **13**, 450–457.

Smith, L. T. (1993) Ultrastructural findings in epidermolysis bullosa. *Archives of Dermatology*, **129**, 1578–1584.

Sonnenberg, A., Linders, C. J. T., Daams, J. H. & Kennel, S. J. (1990) The α6β1 (VLA-6) and α6β4-protein complexes: tissue distribution and biochemical properties. *Journal of Cell Science*, **96**, 207–217.

Sonnenberg, A., Calafat, J., Janssen, H., Daams, H., Raaio-Helmer, L. M. H. van der, Falcioni, R. *et al.* (1991) Integrin α6β4 complex is located in hemidesomosomes, suggesting a major role in epidermal cell-basement membrane adhesion. *Journal of Cell Biology*, **113**, 907–917.

Ståhle-Bäckdahl, M., Inoue, M., Guidice, G. J. & Parks, W. C. (1994) 92-kD gelatinase is produced by eosinophils at the site of blister formation in bullous pemphigoid and cleaves the extracellular domain of recombinant 180-kD bullous pemphigoid autoantigen. *Journal of Clinical Investigation*, **93**, 2022–2030.

Stanley, J. R. (1991) Pemphigus and pemphigoid as paradigms of organ-specific, autoantibody-mediated diseases. *Journal of Clinical Investigation*, **83**, 1443–1448.

Sterk, L. M., Geuijen, C. A., Oomen, L. C., Calafat, J., Janssen, H. & Sonnenberg, A. (2000) The tetraspan molecule CD151, a novel constituent of hemidesmosomes, associates with the integrin alpha6beta4 and may regulate the spatial organization of hemidesmosomes. *Journal of Cell Biology*, **149**, 969–982.

Sung, U., O'Rear, J. J. & Yurchenco, P. D. (1997) Localization of heparin binding activity in recombinant laminin G domain. *European Journal of Biochemistry*, **250**, 138–143.

Tamai, K., Silos, S. A., Li, K., Korkeela, E., Ishikawa, H. & Uitto, J. (1995) Tissue-specific expression of the 230-kDa bullous pemphigoid antigen gene (BPAG1). Identification of a novel keratinocyte regulatory cis-element KRE3. *Journal of Biological Chemistry*, **270**, 7609–7614.

Tamura, R. N., Rozzo, C. & Starr, L. (1990) Epithelial integrin $\alpha 6\beta 4$: complete primary structure of $\alpha 6$ and variant forms of $\beta 4$. *Journal of Cell Biology*, **111**, 1593–1604.
Tanaka, T., Parry, D. A., Klaus-Kovtun, V., Steinert, P. M. & Stanley, J. R. (1991) Comparison of molecularly cloned bullous pemphigoid antigen to desmoplakin I confirms that they define a new family of cell adhesion junction plaque proteins. *Journal of Biological Chemistry*, **266**, 12555–12559.
Tang, H. Y., Chaffotte, A. F. & Thacher, S. M. (1996) Structural analysis of the predicted coiled-coil rod domain of the cytoplasmic bullous pemphigoid antigen (BPAG1). Empirical localization of the N-terminal globular domain-rod boundary. *Journal of Biological Chemistry*, **271**, 9716–9722.
Taniuchi, K., Takata, M., Matsui, C., Fushida, Y., Uchiyama, K., Mori, T. *et al.* (1999) Antiepiligrin (laminin-5) cicatricial pemphigoid associated with an underlying gastric carcinoma producing laminin 5. *British Journal of Dermatology*, **140**, 696–700.
Tiger, C. F., Champliaud, M. F., Pedrosa-Domellof, F., Thornell, L. E., Ekblom, P. & Gullberg, D. (1997) Presence of laminin alpha5 chain and lack of laminin alpha1 chain during human muscle development and in muscular dystrophies. *Journal of Biological Chemistry*, **272**, 28590–28595.
Uitto, J., Pulkkinen, L. & Christiano, A. M. (1994) Molecular basis of the dystrophic and junctional form of epidermolysis bullosa: mutations in the type VII collagen and kalinin (laminin-5) genes. *Journal of Investigative Dermatology*, **103**, 39S–45S.
Uitto, J., Pulkkinen, L. & McLean, W. H. (1997) Epidermolysis bullosa: a spectrum of clinical phenotypes explained by molecular heterogeneity. *Molecular Medicine Today*, **3**, 457–465.
Uttam, J., Hutton, E., Coulombe, P. A., Anton-Lamprecht, I., Yu, Q. C., Gedde-Dahl, T., Jr *et al.* (1996) The genetic basis of epidermolysis bullosa simplex with mottled hyperpigmentation. *Proceedings of the National Academy of Sciences of the United States of America*, **93**, 9079–9084.
Vidal, F., Aberdam, D., Miquel, C., Christiano, A. M., Pulkkinen, L., Uitto, J. *et al.* (1995) Integrin beta 4 mutations associated with junctional epidermolysis bullosa with pyloric atresia. *Nature Genetics*, **10**, 229–234.
Wiche, G. (1998) Domain structure and transcript diversity of plectin. *Biological Bulletin*, **194**, 381–383.
Xu, J., Zutter, M. M., Santoro, S. A. & Clark, R. A. (1998) A three-dimensional collagen lattice activates NF-kappaB in human fibroblasts: role in integrin alpha2 gene expression and tissue remodeling. *Journal of Cell Biology*, **140**, 709–719.
Yurchenco, P. D. & Cheng, Y. S. (1993) Self-assembly and calcium-binding sites in laminin. A three-arm interaction model. *Journal of Biological Chemistry*, **268**, 17286–17299.
Yurchenco, P. D. & O'Rear, J. J. (1994) Basement membrane assembly. In: *Methods of Enzymology* (Eds E. Ruoslahti & E. Engvall), pp. 489–518. Academic Press, New York.
Zone, J. J., Taylor, T. B., Kandunce, D. P. & Meyer, L. J. (1990) Identification of the cutaneous basement membrane antigen in linear IgA bullous dermatosis. *Journal of Clinical Investigation*, **85**, 812–820.
Zone, J. J., Taylor, T. B., Meyer, L. J. & Petersen, M. J. (1998) The 97 kDa linear IgA bullous disease antigen is identical to a portion of the extracellular domain of the 180 kDa bullous pemphigoid antigen, BPAg2. *Journal of Investigative Dermatology*, **110**, 207–210.

1.2

Collagen XVII (BP180, BPAG2) is the most common epidermal basement membrane autoantigen in humans and other animals

T. Olivry DrVet, PhD, DipACVD, DipECVD[1] and M.P. Marinkovich MD[2]

[1] Department of Clinical Sciences, College of Veterinary Medicine, North Carolina State University, Raleigh, North Carolina; and Department of Dermatology, School of Medicine, University of North Carolina, Chapel Hill, North Carolina, USA

[2] Program in Epithelial Biology and Department of Dermatology, Stanford University; and Palo Alto VA Health Care System, Palo Alto, California, USA

Summary

Collagen XVII (BP180, BPAG2) is now known to represent the most common skin basement membrane autoantigen in humans and other animals. It is one of the proteins targeted by autoantibodies from patients affected with bullous pemphigoid (BP), mucous membrane (cicatricial) pemphigoid (MMP) and linear immunoglobulin A (IgA) disease (LAD).

In humans and companion animals, BP lesions are characterized by blistering that occurs predominantly during adulthood. Microscopically, there is subepidermal vesiculation associated with neutrophilic and eosinophilic superficial dermal inflammation. Direct immunofluorescence reveals linear deposition of IgG and complement along the epidermal basement membrane. Indirect immunofluorescent methods confirm the presence of circulating IgG autoantibodies targeting cell-bound collagen XVII. The major antigenic epitope is situated in the NC16A domain, a non-collagenous segment situated just outside the keratinocyte's membrane.

Lesions of MMP affect predominantly mucous membranes and mucocutaneous junctions. In humans, dogs and cats, skin lesions consist of vesiculation, ulcerations and occasionally scarring in or around the oral cavity, eyes, genitalia or anus. Histological examination of skin biopsy specimens reveals ulceration and dermal scarring or subepidermal vesicles with few inflammatory cells. Immunological studies demonstrate that circulating IgG autoantibodies usually target various epitopes on cell-bound collagen XVII or on laminin-5.

In humans and dogs, lesions of LAD include vesiculation and ulceration distributed on the skin and mucous membranes. Microscopic skin lesions consist of subepidermal vesiculation with variable neutrophilic inflammation. Immunological studies demonstrate skin-fixed and circulating IgA (and sometimes IgG) autoantibodies that target LAD-1, the 120/97 kDa processed extracellular segment of collagen XVII.

Introduction

In humans and other animals, cutaneous vesiculation frequently occurs because of defective adhesion between basal keratinocytes and the epidermal basement membrane (Moll & Moll, 1998). In young patients, mutations of genes encoding basement membrane glycoproteins result in absent or abnormal protein production as seen in the various subsets of hereditary epidermolysis bullosa (Diaz & Giudice, 2000). The adhesive function of these basement membrane proteins also can be altered following binding of autoantibodies, thus producing dermoepidermal separation (Diaz & Giudice, 2000). In recent years, the classification of human and animal autoimmune subepidermal blistering dermatoses (AISBD) has been updated based on a combination of epidemiological,

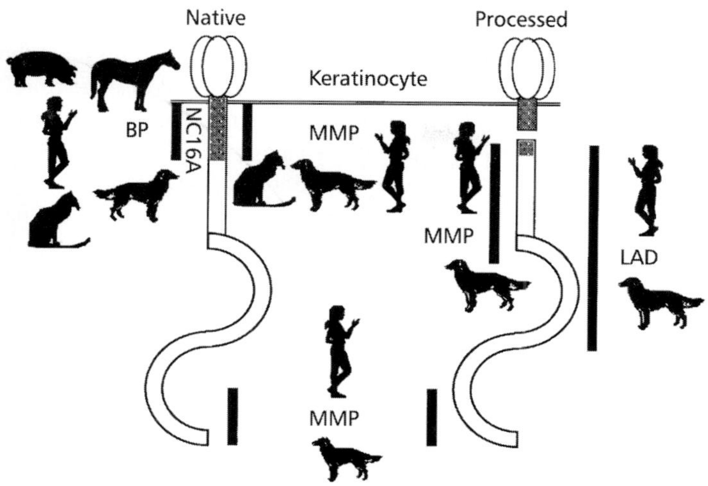

Figure 1.2.1. Epitope mapping of collagen XVII (BP180, BPAG2) in mammalian species. BP: bullous pemphigoid; LAD: linear IgA disease; MMP: mucous membrane pemphigoid; NC16A: 16th non-collagenous segment. Circulating autoantibodies from humans, dogs, cats, pigs and horses with BP recognize the NC16A domain. In patients affected with MMP, IgG antibodies recognize either the NC16A segment (humans, dogs and one cat), the collagenous mid-segment (humans, dogs) or the C-terminus of this glycoprotein (humans, one dog). LAD-affected patients exhibit IgA (±IgG) antibodies that bind to the processed extracellular segment of collagen XVII.

clinical and histopathological criteria together with the identification of targeted autoantigens (Zillikens, 1999; Diaz & Giudice, 2000).

Type XVII collagen, also known as BP180 or the second bullous pemphigoid antigen (BPAG2), has now emerged as the epidermal basement membrane protein that is most often targeted by autoantibodies in both humans and other mammalian species. Indeed, collagen XVII epitopes have been shown to be the target of autoantibodies in bullous pemphigoid (BP), mucous membrane (cicatricial) pemphigoid (MMP/CP) or linear immunoglobulin A (IgA) disease (LAD) (Figure 1.2.1). This review highlights the clinical and immunopathological findings of human and animal AISBD in which collagen XVII has been demonstrated to harbor autoantigenic epitopes. See Chapter 1.1 for a detailed review on the molecular biology of collagen XVII and its relationship to other proteins of the epidermal basement membrane.

Bullous pemphigoid

Bullous pemphigoid in humans

BP is the diagnosis made in 69% of people with AISBD (Bernard *et al.*, 1995). Its incidence has been estimated as approximately six new cases per million per year (Bernard *et al.*, 1995; Zillikens *et al.*, 1995; Jung *et al.*, 1999). BP usually affects elderly patients of both genders and its incidence increases dramatically with ageing (Jung *et al.*, 1999). Lesions of BP can persist, untreated, for many years and the patients may experience episodes of spontaneous remissions and exacerbations.

The typical lesions of BP are tense blisters that occur on either clinically normal or erythematous skin (Korman, 1998) (Plate 1). Vesiculation is seen primarily on the flexor surfaces of the limbs as well as the axillae, groin and abdomen (Korman, 1998). Oral lesions are seen rarely and, when present, are usually transient (Anhalt & Morrison, 1991; Korman, 1998; Nousari & Anhalt, 1999).

Microscopic examination of lesional skin biopsy specimens usually reveals a subepidermal vesicle that is rich in inflammatory cells including eosinophils and neutrophils (Korman, 1998; Courville *et al.*, 2000).

Immunofluorescence investigations reveal the presence of skin-fixed and circulating autoantibodies that recognize antigen(s) localized at the dermoepidermal junction (Zillikens, 1999). Complement is usually detected along the basement membrane zone (Zillikens, 1999).

Through the use of immunoblotting and immunoprecipitation, two BP autoantigens were identified (Anhalt & Morrison, 1991). BPAG1 (BP230), the autoantigen first identified in humans with BP (Stanley *et al.*, 1981), is a 230 kDa intracytoplasmic protein of the plakin family. It is believed to link keratin intermediate filaments to hemidesmosomal plaques in basal keratinocytes (Green & Jones, 1996; Hirako & Owaribe, 1998). Collagen XVII was subsequently recognized as the second BP autoantigen (Labib *et al.*, 1986). Epitope mapping studies have demonstrated that human collagen XVII-specific autoantibodies bind most commonly to linear peptide epitopes situated throughout the non-collagenous extracellular NC16A domain (Giudice *et al.*, 1993; Zillikens *et al.*, 1997; Perriard *et al.*, 1999).

This NC16A domain contains 77 amino acids and is situated immediately outside the basal keratinocyte membrane. Because rabbit antibodies directed against the mouse NC16A equivalent amino-acid sequence can induce dermoepidermal separation when passively transferred into neonatal mice, BPAG2 presently is suspected to be a true pathogenic BP autoantigen (Liu *et al.*, 1993). Passive transfer of NC16A antiserum into mouse neonates currently represents the experimental model most commonly used to study the immunopathogenesis of BP (Liu *et al.*, 1993, 1995, 1997a, b, 1998, 2000; Liu & Diaz, 1995).

Systemic corticosteroids remain a first-line therapy for pemphigoid subtypes and a primary therapy for herpes gestationis, the BP of gestation (see below) (Anhalt & Morrison, 1991; Lebrun-Vignes *et al.*, 1999). Most flares can be controlled with 1–2 mg/kg per day of prednisone divided into two doses. As blistering activity subsides, this daily dose can initially be tapered with meticulous assessment for blister recurrence. As the tapering proceeds, it is important to place patients on an alternate-day steroid regimen, as recurrences require an increase in the dose of prednisone to halt disease activity, sometimes back to initial levels, if the recurrence is severe. The goal is to reduce the steroid dose to the minimum or to eliminate it entirely, in order to reduce the widely recognized systemic effects. The ability to achieve this goal is variable, and often depends on fluctuations in disease activity in individual patients and the use of steroid-sparing agents listed below.

The use of a steroid-sparing agent reduces the side-effects encountered with systemic corticosteroids, but care needs to be taken to monitor for systemic toxicity of the steroid-sparing agents, including the increased risks of infection and malignancy. Probably the least toxic steroid-sparing regimen for bullous pemphigoid patients is the use of tetracycline 2 g/day and niacinamide 2 g/day. This regimen can be effective by itself for milder cases of BP or used in conjunction with steroids for more severe cases (Kolbach *et al.*, 1995).

Cyclophosphamide and azathioprine are potent steroid-sparing agents that can be used in the more recalcitrant cases of BP and MMP. Cyclophosphamide has significant potential systemic toxicity and patients must be carefully monitored during treatment, which usually consists of a single daily dose of 1–2 mg/kg. Side-effects include bone marrow suppression, urinary problems including bladder hemorrhage or fibrosis, pulmonary fibrosis, sterility and increased risk of hematological or bladder malignancies. It is especially important to encourage patients to increase their oral fluid intake. Azathioprine in general has less systemic toxicity than cyclophosphamide but it works more slowly. It is given at a dose of 1–3 mg/kg per day. Hepatotoxicity, sepsis and urinary complications are the most frequent serious complications and often occur within the first 1 or 2 weeks of therapy. Other steroid-sparing modalities that have shown efficacy for pemphigoid subtypes include cyclosporin (Curley & Holden, 1991), mycophenolic acid (Nousari *et al.*, 1998) and plasmapheresis (Roujeau, 1988; Guillaume *et al.*, 1993; Beckers *et al.*, 1995).

Herpes gestationis is an autoimmune bullous disorder affecting pregnant women which typically presents in the second and third trimester of pregnancy with a pruritic bullous eruption on the abdomen and limbs. The diagnosis is confirmed by the presence of complement-binding IgG antibasement membrane zone antibodies, which bind to the roof of salt-split skin. Immunopathologically, this disease is characterized by autoantibodies to collagen XVII-NC16 segment, making it a disease that is closely related to BP (Giudice *et al.*, 1993; Murakami *et al.*, 1996; Lin *et al.*, 1999; Zillikens & Giudice, 1999).

Bullous pemphigoid in animals

BP has been identified in dogs (Iwasaki *et al.*, 1995; Xu *et al.*, 2000), cats (Olivry *et al.*, 1999a), pigs (Olivry *et al.*, 2000c) and horses (Olivry *et al.*, 2000a). Even though BP is the most common AISBD diagnosed in people (69% of cases) (Bernard *et al.*, 1995), it represents 31, 50 and 100% of AISBD diagnosed in dogs, cats and horses, respectively (Table 1.2.1).

Whereas BP affects principally elderly people, this disease can afflict animals of any age, even before puberty. In a recently discovered porcine model of BP, initial blistering episodes develop in juvenile minipigs around 5 months of age (Olivry *et al.*, 2000c). Similarly, dogs and cats can exhibit skin lesions of BP around 1 year of age (Olivry *et al.*, 1999a). Conversely, horses identified with BP usually are geriatric patients (Olivry *et al.*, 2000a). Because young animals can be affected with BP, genetic factors are probably involved in the pathogenesis of the disease. This hypothesis is corroborated by the discovery of BP in genetically related male Yucatan minipigs (Olivry *et al.*, 2000c). In companion animals, however, too few cases of BP have been identified to provide meaningful information regarding any breed or sex predisposition for this dermatosis.

Clinical signs of BP appear similar in animals and are analogous to those seen in human patients. Lesions consist primarily of tense vesicles, erosions, ulcers and crusts (Iwasaki *et al.*, 1995; Olivry *et al.*, 1999a, 2000a, c) (Plate 2). The lesional distribution exhibits some variation across species, however. In dogs, the phenotype is usually mild as skin lesions can be seen, in grouped arrangement, on the concave ear pinnae, abdomen, axillae or mucocutaneous junctions (Iwasaki *et al.*, 1995). Oral vesicles and erosions, usually of mild severity, have been seen in five out of 12 cases of canine BP (T. Olivry, unpublished data). In cats, usually few lesions are present. Erosions predominate on the face and oral injuries are consistently observed (Olivry *et al.*, 1999a). In Yucatan minipigs, the vesicles are seen chiefly on the back and rump and there are no lesions in the oral cavity (Olivry *et al.*, 2000c). In horses, finally, there is a severe lesional phenotype because erosions and crusts exhibit a generalized pattern and the patients develop systemic illness (Olivry *et al.*, 2000a). In all horses so far diagnosed with BP, sloughing of the oral mucosa has been very severe.

The first step in the diagnosis of BP in animals involves histopathological examination of lesional skin biopsy specimens. In dogs and pigs with BP, subepidermal accumulation of neutrophil and eosinophil granulocytes is the earliest microscopic lesion seen (Iwasaki *et al.*, 1995; Olivry *et al.*, 2000c) (Figure 1.2.2).

Table 1.2.1. Relative frequency of autoimmune subepidermal blistering dermatoses

Disease	Humans (%)[a] (n = 100)	Dogs (%)[b] (n = 39)	Cats (%)[b] (n = 6)	Horses (%)[b] (n = 3)
BP	69	31	50	100
MMP/CP	12	44	25	0
PG	4	0	0	0
LAD	5	5	0	0
EBA	2	18	0	0
BSLE	2	3	0	0
Unclassified	6	0	25	0

[a] Bernard *et al.* (1995).
[b] Olivry: case studies of animals with antibasement membrane circulating autoantibodies (1995–2000).
BP: bullous pemphigoid; MMP: mucous membrane pemphigoid; CP: cicatricial pemphigoid; PG: pemphigoid of gestation; LAD: linear IgA disease; EBA: epidermolysis bullosa acquisita; BSLE: bullous systemic lupus erythematosus.

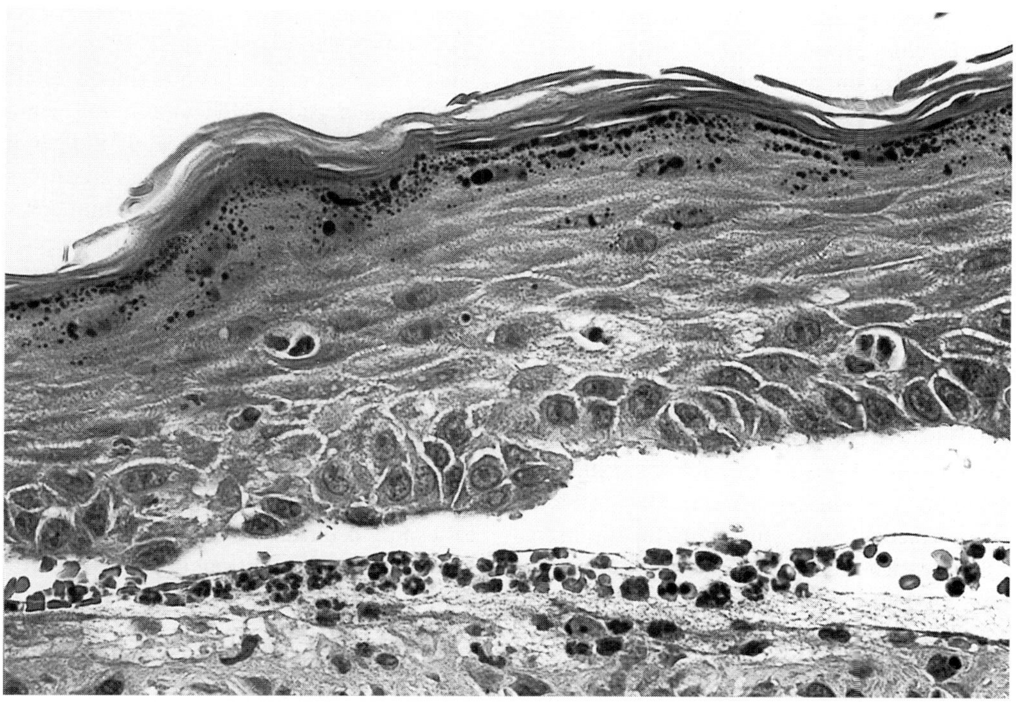

Figure 1.2.2. Bullous pemphigoid in a dog. Subepidermal clefting is associated with granulocytic inflammation. (Hematoxylin and eosin.)

Inflammatory subepidermal vesicles form secondarily. Many intact and degranulating eosinophils can be seen at the dermoepidermal junction of preblistered and blistered areas (Iwasaki *et al.*, 1995; Olivry *et al.*, 2000c). In cats and horses with BP, subepithelial vesicles exhibit fewer inflammatory cells than in dogs and pigs (Olivry *et al.*, 1999a). Special stains are usually needed to visualize degranulating eosinophils in feline BP (Olivry *et al.*, 1999a). In horses, conversely, special stains fail to identify superficial dermal eosinophils, a puzzling finding in light of the prominent skin eosinophilia seen usually in equine inflammatory dermatoses. In this species, the epidermis overlying vesicular lesions of BP usually contains many basal and suprabasal keratinocytes exhibiting microscopic characteristics of apoptosis. This discovery may indicate the occurrence of anoikis following the premature dissociation of epidermal integrin adhesion (Ruoslahti & Reed, 1994).

Direct immunofluorescent methods are used to visualize the deposition of autoantibodies in the perilesional skin of animal patients with BP. To date, direct immunofluorescent examination of skin biopsy specimens has revealed a fine linear and continuous deposit of IgG along the dermoepidermal junction in more than 90% of dogs, cats, horses and pigs with BP (Iwasaki *et al.*, 1995; Olivry *et al.*, 1999a, 2000a, c). In rare instances, faint IgG immunostaining can be found around basal keratinocytes (Olivry *et al.*, 1999a, 2000a). Basement-membrane binding of activated complement has been seen in some dogs.

In all animal patients with BP diagnosed to date, indirect immunofluorescent studies have revealed variable titers (1:20 to more than 1:5000) of circulating IgG autoantibodies that bind the basement membrane of intact animal or human gingival mucosae (Iwasaki *et al.*, 1995; Olivry *et al.*, 1999a, 2000a, c; Xu *et al.*, 2000). When salt-split epithelial substrates are used, however, the detection of basement membrane-specific circulating IgG appears to be enhanced. The latter method uses a normal skin specimen in which the epidermal basement membrane has been artificially cleaved within the lamina lucida after immersion in a 1 M solution of sodium chloride. This technique has been validated for the canine species (Iwasaki *et al.*, 1997). It has also proven useful in differentiating BP from other canine autoimmune subepidermal blistering dermatoses (Olivry *et al.*, 1998, 1999b, 2000d). When animal or human salt-split skin substrates are used, canine, feline, porcine and equine BP IgG autoantibodies label antigen(s) located on the epidermal side of artificial clefts, a pattern suggestive of BP in humans. In some cases, the IgG autoantibodies also bind, albeit with lower intensity, to the lateral and apical aspect of stratum basale keratinocytes. Such patterns of fluorescence are identical to those observed with antibodies specific for human or canine 180 kDa BP antigen (Hirako & Owaribe, 1998; Olivry *et al.*, 1999a; Xu *et al.*, 2000).

In animals, the diagnosis of BP should be confirmed by documenting that circulating IgG autoantibodies target one or both of the human BP antigens. Immunoblotting studies, performed with either canine, human or feline epidermal extracts, have established that canine and feline BP IgG solely identify a 180 kDa antigen of molecular size identical to BPAG2 (BP180), the transmembrane type XVII collagen (Iwasaki *et al.*, 1995; Olivry *et al.*, 1999a). In pigs and horses, circulating IgG autoantibodies bind to the recombinant full-length NC16A domain of human BPAG2 (Olivry *et al.*, 2000a, c). Moreover, when tested with enzyme-linked immunosorbent assay (ELISA) using synthetic oligopeptides spanning the human BPAG2-NC16A domain, IgG from dogs, cats, pigs and horses with BP recognize linear epitopes within this segment (Olivry *et al.*, 1999a, 2000a, c; Xu *et al.*, 2000). Similar findings were observed with an enzyme-linked immunosorbent assay (ELISA) using peptides based on the canine NC16A sequence (T. Olivry, unpublished data). These experiments undoubtedly establish type XVII collagen, and its NC16A non-collagenous extracellular section, as the principal BP antigen in animal species. Because this particular NC16A sequence exhibits some homology between humans and dogs (Xu *et al.*, 2000), it must demonstrate unique physicochemical properties that renders it immunogenic across species.

Too few cases of BP in animals have been diagnosed to provide meaningful information about the natural progression of the disease and its response to therapy. Nevertheless, long-term remission of BP has been seen in four dogs, one cat and in several pigs following short courses of corticosteroids (Olivry *et al.*, 1999a, 2000c). For example, blistering lesions in pigs usually resolve following the application of 2.5% hydrocortisone, twice daily for 2 weeks (Olivry *et al.*, 2000c). Some canine patients reportedly respond to a niacinamide–tetracycline combination regimen (500 mg *in toto*, orally, three times daily). These anecdotal findings suggest that, in these animal species, BP lesions usually respond to treatment and can exhibit self-limiting behavior. In contrast, BP in horses is extremely debilitating and can prompt the owner to request euthanasia of the patient.

Mucous membrane pemphigoid (cicatricial pemphigoid)

Mucous membrane pemphigoid in humans

Mucous membrane pemphigoid (MMP), previously known as cicatricial pemphigoid (CP), is an uncommon AISBD of humans characterized clinically by vesicles and erosions located preferentially on mucous membranes and mucocutaneous junctions. In spite of a characteristic phenotype, MMP in humans appears to be immunologically heterogeneous (Scully *et al.*, 1999).

MMP/CP is a chronic bullous disease with primarily mucosal involvement. Gingival and conjunctival mucosae are frequently affected, and scarring of mucosal surfaces is a common feature (Venning *et al.*, 1988; Anhalt & Morrison, 1991). Lesions of MMP/CP can also predominantly affect the eyes and extensive conjunctival scarring can lead to blindness (Hoang-Xuan *et al.*, 1999). Cutaneous lesions consisting of tense vesicles or bullae occur in about one-third of patients and are often found on the face, neck and scalp. Rupture of the vesicles results in erosions that often heal with or without atrophic scars.

Immunopathologically, this disease is heterogeneous. Autoantibodies to laminin-5 (previously termed epiligrin), laminin-6 (Kirtschig *et al.*, 1995; Chan *et al.*, 1997), collagen XVII (BP180) (Balding *et al.*, 1996; Bédane *et al.*, 1997) and several other poorly characterized autoantigens have been described to be associated with MMP/CP. Associated solid tumors have been described in many cases of anti-laminin CP (Taniuchi *et al.*, 1999).

Direct immunofluorescent microscopy of a perilesional biopsy of skin or mucosa is the most effective way to make the diagnosis of MMP/CP, in combination with clinical findings. The immunoreactants may localize to either the dermal or epidermal sides of salt-split skin.

Lesions of MMP/CP rarely go into spontaneous remission and this disease often follows a chronic and progressive course (Yancey, 1999). Treatment of human patients will depend on the severity of the mucosal lesions and their related morbidity. If lesions are restricted to one mucosa, morbidity may be minimal and treatment could be limited to corticosteroid mouthwash or eye-drops with or without oral tablets (Anhalt & Morrison, 1991; Vincent *et al.*, 1993; Scully *et al.*, 1999; Yancey, 1999). The efficacy of dapsone remains the subject of controversy (Scully *et al.*, 1999; Yancey, 1999). If lesions cannot be controlled with topical and systemic corticosteroids, then adjunctive immunosuppressive agents will be used, as proposed for patients with BP (Anhalt & Morrison, 1991; Yancey, 1999).

Mucous membrane pemphigoid in animals

The authors have now identified 17 dogs and two cats with clinical signs and autoantibodies identical to those seen during MMP/CP in humans (Olivry *et al.*, 2001). MMP appears to represent the most common subset of AISBD in dogs (Table 1.2.1).

Clinically, companion animals with MMP exhibit varying degrees of depigmentation, erythema, turgid clear or hemorrhagic vesicles and bullae, erosions, ulcers and crusts. These lesions predominate in the oral cavity and can also affect the mucocutaneous junctions of the gingival, genital, anal and ocular mucosae (Plate 3). Surprisingly, lesions commonly affect the nasal planum and perinasal skin. Rarely, vesicles and ulcers are also seen on the hairless concave aspect of the ear pinnae. The treatment and prognosis of canine MMP overall appear similar to those of BP in this species.

Microscopic examination of lesional mucosal biopsy specimens reveals subepidermal blistering that occurs with no vesicular inflammation or with few eosinophils, neutrophils or mononuclear cells in the blister cavity. Hemorrhagic clefts sometimes can be seen. In some patients, intact vesicles are not seen and ulcers delineated by the basement membrane are observed. Because biopsy specimens are obtained from mucosae, there is often a non-specific superficial dermal band-like infiltrate of plasma cells and lymphocytes. When mucosal ulcers are present, dermal inflammation can be intense and exhibits characteristics of granulation tissue.

Direct immunofluorescent examination of perilesional mucosa is indistinguishable from that seen in canine or feline BP skin samples. IgG and associated complement (C3 fraction) are visualized linearly and continuously along the dermoepidermal junction. Indirect immunofluorescence confirms the existence of circulating IgG autoantibodies that recognizes basement membrane antigen(s). When salt-split epithelial substrates are utilized, however, two opposite patterns can be seen. In most dogs, autoantibodies label the epidermis in a pattern identical to canine BP. Further investigations have confirmed that, in most cases, the 'epidermal' autoantibodies target the NC16A ectodomain of canine or human collagen XVII, a pattern analogous to that obtained with BP IgG. In rare patients, circulating autoantibodies bind to the dermal side of salt-split clefts. In one of these animals, IgG was shown to recognize antigenic epitopes located within a 30 kDa segment at the C-terminus of human BPAG2. In one cat with MMP, immunological investigations suggest that the autoantibodies target the α_3-chain of human laminin-5 (T. Olivry *et al.*, unpublished data).

Similarly to its human counterpart, canine MMP exhibits unique clinical and histological characteristics, albeit being immunologically heterogeneous. Further studies are awaited to provide explanations about the singular localization of vesicles to mucosae in light of an autoimmune response that can mirror that of BP.

Linear IgA disease

Linear IgA disease in humans

LAD is an acquired autoimmune subepidermal blistering dermatosis that affects human children and adults (Wojnarowska *et al.*, 1994; Egan & Zone, 1999; Zillikens & Giudice, 1999).

The childhood variant of LAD, known as chronic bullous disease of childhood (CBDC), has a mean age of onset of 4–5 years and rarely persists beyond puberty. Onset is often abrupt and vesicles or erosive lesions involve the face and perineum with subsequent generalization to the trunk and the extremities. In adults, LAD presents with a mean age of onset of 60–65 years. The trunk is almost always involved (Plate 4), but LAD lesions also frequently affect the limbs, face, scalp, hands and feet. The majority of children and adults present with mucosal involvement (60–80%). This may manifest as oral ulcers and erosions, which may scar and therefore be difficult to differentiate from MMP/CP. LAD has been associated with an increased risk of developing various malignancies, especially lymphoproliferative types such as Hodgkin's or B-cell lymphoma (Godfrey *et al.*, 1990). A subset of patients has been described with drug-induced linear IgA disease. Intravenous vancomycin has been the drug most consistently implicated (Whitworth *et al.*, 1996).

The histology of perilesional or lesional skin in LAD typically reveals a subepidermal bulla with a predominantly neutrophilic superficial inflammatory infiltrate. In this aspect, LAD may be difficult to distinguish from other subepidermal diseases based on histology alone. The gold standard for diagnosis of LAD is direct immunofluorescence of perilesional skin and must demonstrate linear IgA deposition along the epidermal basement membrane. This is in contrast to the granular superficial deposit of IgA seen in patients affected with dermatitis herpetiformis. In BP, linear IgG deposition is seen, usually in conjunction with complement; however, in a minority of cases the presence of both linear IgA and IgG antibody deposition complicates the diagnosis. Indirect immunofluorescent testing of LAD sera on salt-split skin has shown the majority of patients to have purely epidermal binding of autoantibodies, while the minority show a purely dermal pattern, and a few exhibit a mixed epidermal and dermal binding pattern. Western immunoblotting has been shown a more sensitive method than indirect immunofluorescence to detect autoantibodies in LAD.

Initial studies identified a 97 kDa protein extracted from both epidermis and dermis, which was thought to be different from the BP and epidermolysis bullosa acquisita (EBA) antigens on the basis of molecular weight and tissue distribution (Zone *et al.*, 1990). It was later shown that the 97 kDa antigen shared immunological identity with a 120 kDa protein, termed LAD-1, produced by cultured keratinocytes. This was accomplished through the use of monoclonal antibody 123 and the same LAD sera, which reacted to both the 97 and 120 kDa proteins. Moreover, monoclonal antibody 123 induced dermo-epidermal separation of human skin *in situ* and localized to the epidermal side of salt-split skin along with LAD-1 (Marinkovich *et al.*, 1996). Recent studies have suggested that LAD-1 is likely to be the processed BP180 extracellular segment, and that collagen XVII processing may produce or expose pathological neoepitopes recognized by LAD autoantibodies (Zone *et al.*, 1998).

Dapsone is considered the standard drug of choice to treat human patients with LAD. Therapy is begun at low dosages (<0.5 mg/kg) and is slowly increased to a dosage higher than 1 mg/kg with a target maintenance of 100–200 mg/day in an adult and 25–50 mg/day in children. Common early side-effects which should be routinely screened for include hemolytic anemia, which can be severe in patients at risk for glucose-6-phosphate dehydrogenase (G6PD) deficiency, and methemoglobinemia, which can cause symptoms from benign cyanosis to weakness, dyspnea, tachycardia and angina. An alternative treatment is sulfapyridine, usually given at a dose of 1.0–3.0 g/day. This dose may require frequent adjustment owing to its irregular absorption. Sulfamethoxypyridazine (adult dose 1.0–1.5 g/day) may also be used and is often better tolerated. In patients in which skin lesions cannot be adequately controlled by the maximally tolerated dose of a single drug, the addition of corticosteroids is recommended and can lead to disease remission.

Linear IgA disease in the dog

A spontaneous animal homologue of LAD in humans has been recently identified in 2 dogs (Olivry *et al.*, 2000b). Dogs with LAD exhibit ulcerative lesions in the oral cavity, face and on the extremities. In these patients, vesiculation was not seen macroscopically. Microscopic examination of hematoxylin and eosin-stained sections reveals subepidermal vesiculation with no inflammatory cells or with few neutrophils. There are no intact or degranulated eosinophils in the vesicles and superficial dermis of dogs with LAD, in marked contrast to the eosinophil-rich infiltrate of canine BP skin sections (Olivry *et al.*, 2000b).

Direct immunofluorescence reveals a strong linear and continuous deposit of IgA and/or IgG along the epidermal basement membrane zone of canine LAD skin. Indirect immunofluorescence, using normal canine or human lip substrates, demonstrates that circulating IgG and IgA autoantibodies bind to epithelial basement membranes in a fine linear and continuous pattern. When canine and human salt-split substrates are used, IgG or IgA autoantibodies label antigen(s) located on the basal aspect, and not lateral sides, of stratum basale epidermal keratinocytes (Olivry *et al.*, 2000b).

Immunoblotting studies have established that circulating IgA and IgG from dogs with LAD recognize a soluble 120 kDa antigen present in a keratinocyte culture conditioned medium but not in cell membrane-rich fractions. The canine LAD antigen was determined to be LAD-1, since autoantibodies from both dogs were shown recently to bind to a fusion protein corresponding to the processed extracellular domain of human BPAG2 (MP Marinkovich, unpublished results) (Olivry *et al.*, 2000b). Of interest is that canine patients with IgA deposition at the basement membrane zone were identified almost 20 years ago (Scott *et al.*, 1982). However, the described patients differed in their clinical signs and microscopic skin lesions and they were given the diagnosis of either BP, discoid lupus erythematosus or subcorneal pustular dermatitis (Scott *et al.*, 1982). More recently, a dog with epidermolysis bullosa acquista was shown to exhibit *in vivo* and circulating IgG and IgA antibodies that targeted type VII collagen (Olivry *et al.*, 1998). Hence, basement-membrane IgA autoantibodies can be seen in a variety of canine dermatological entities.

For comparative purposes, the authors therefore propose to restrict usage of the name LAD to the dermatosis that affects dogs with cutaneous macrovesicles or microvesicles and IgA, with or without IgG circulating autoantibodies that target LAD-1, the 120/97 kDa processed extracellular type XVII collagen.

Conclusion

The application of 'modern' immunological methods recently has permitted the recognition of new AISBD in animals. Moreover, determination of the antigen(s) targeted by autoantibodies led to a revision of the nosology of autoimmune vesicular dermatoses in various animal species. It is remarkable to observe that companion animals can be affected by blistering diseases that are exquisitely similar to those afflicting humans and that in all species, collagen XVII seems to be the most common basement membrane autoantigen. The availability of these current spontaneous natural animal models of AISBD could provide medical clinical and basic investigators with outstanding material for researching the pathogenesis and therapy of these severe diseases of humans.

Acknowledgements

The authors would like to acknowledge the funding of the Office of Research and Development, Palo Alto VA Health Care System (MPM), and NIH grant P01-AR4401 (MPM).

References

Anhalt, G. J. & Morrison, L. H. (1991) Bullous and cicatricial pemphigoid. *Journal of Autoimmunity* **4**, 17–35.

Balding, S. D., Prost, C., Diaz, L. A., Bernard, P., Bedane, C., Aberdam, D. & Giudice, G. J. (1996) Cicatricial pemphigoid autoantibodies react with multiple sites on the BP180 extracellular domain. *Journal of Investigative Dermatology*, **106**, 141–146.

Beckers, R. C., Brand, A., Vermeer, B J. & Boom, B. W. (1995) Adjuvant high-dose intravenous gammaglobulin in the treatment of pemphigus and bullous pemphigoid: experience in six patients. *British Journal of Dermatology*, **133**, 289–293.

Bédane, C., McMillan, J. R., Balding, S. D., Bernard, P., Prost, C., Bonnetblanc, J. M. *et al.* (1997) Bullous pemphigoid and cicatricial pemphigoid autoantibodies react with ultrastructurally separable epitopes on the BP180 ectodomain: evidence that BP180 spans the lamina lucida. *Journal of Investigative Dermatology*, **108**, 901–907.

Bernard, P., Vaillant, L., Labeile, B., Bédane, C., Arbeille, B., Denoeux, J.-P., Lorette, G. *et al.* (1995) Incidence and distribution of subepidermal autoimmune bullous skin diseases in three French regions. *Archives of Dermatology*, **131**, 48–52.

Chan, L. S., Majmudar, A. A., Tran, H. H., Meier, F., Schaumburg-Lever, G., Chen, M. *et al.* (1997) Laminin-6 and laminin-5 are recognized by autoantibodies in a subset of cicatricial pemphigoid. *Journal of Investigative Dermatology*, **108**, 848–853.

Courville, P., Kupfer, I., Gilbert, D., Thomine, E., Metayer, J. & Joly, P. (2000) Histological criteria of bullous pemphigoid. Correlation with immunoblot analysis. *Annales de Pathologie*, **20**, 564–569.

Curley, R. K. & Holden, C. A. (1991) Steroid-resistant bullous pemphigoid treated with cyclosporin A. *Clinical and Experimental Dermatology*, **16**, 68–69.

Diaz, L. A. & Giudice, G. J. (2000) End of the century overview of skin blisters. *Archives of Dermatology*, **136**, 106–112.

Egan, C. A. & Zone, J. J. (1999) Linear IgA bullous dermatosis. *International Journal of Dermatology*, **38**, 818–827.

Giudice, G. J., Emery, D. J., Zelickson, B. D., Anhalt, G. J., Liu, Z. & Diaz, L. A. (1993) Bullous pemphigoid and herpes gestationis autoantibodies recognize a common non-collagenous site on the BP180 ectodomain. *Journal of Immunology*, **154**, 5742–5750.

Godfrey, K., Wojnarowska, F. & Leonard, J. (1990) Linear IgA disease of adults: association with lymphoproliferative malignancy and possible role of other triggering factors. *British Journal of Dermatology*, **123**, 447–452.

Green, K. J. & Jones, J. C. R. (1996) Desmosomes and hemidesmosomes: structure and function of molecular components. *FASEB Journal*, **10**, 871–881.

Guillaume, J. C., Vaillant, L., Bernard, P., Picard, C., Prost, C., Labeille, B. *et al.* (1993) Controlled trial of azathioprine and plasma exchange in addition to prednisolone in the treatment of bullous pemphigoid. *Archives of Dermatology*, **129**, 49–53.

Hirako, Y. & Owaribe, K. (1998) Hemidesmosomes and their unique transmembrane protein BP180. *Microscopy Research and Technique*, **43**, 207–217.

Hoang-Xuan, T., Robin, H., Demers, P. E., Heller, M., Toutblanc, M., Dubertret, L. & Prost, C. (1999) Pure ocular cicatricial pemphigoid – a distinct immunopathologic subset of cicatricial pemphigoid. *Ophthalmology*, **106**, 355–361.

Iwasaki, T., Olivry, T., Lapière, J. C., Chan, L. S., Peavey, C., Liu, Y. Y. *et al.* (1995) Canine bullous pemphigoid (BP) – identification of the 180 kD canine BP antigen by circulating autoantibodies. *Veterinary Pathology*, **32**, 387–393.

Iwasaki, T., Isaji, M., Yanai, T., Kitagawa, H. & Sasaki, Y. (1997) Immunomapping of basement membrane zone macromolecules in canine salt-split skin. *Journal of Veterinary Medical Science*, **59**, 391–393.

Jung, M., Kippes, W., Messer, G., Zillikens, D. & Rzany, B. (1999) Increased risk of bullous pemphigoid in male and very old patients: a population-based study on incidence. *Journal of the American Academy of Dermatology*, **41**, 266–268.

Kirtschig, G., Marinkovich, M. P., Burgeson, R. E. & Yancey, K. B. (1995) Anti-basement membrane autoantibodies in patients with anti-epiligrin cicatricial pemphigoid bind the alpha subunit of laminin 5. *Journal of Investigative Dermatology*, **105**, 543–548.

Kolbach, D. N., Remme, J. J., Bos, W. H., Jonkman, M. F., Dejong, M. C. J. M., Pas, H. H. & Vandermeer, J. B. (1995) Bullous pemphigoid successfully controlled by tetracycline and nicotinamide. *British Journal of Dermatology*, **133**, 88–90.

Korman, N. J. (1998) Bullous pemphigoid – the latest in diagnosis, prognosis and therapy. *Archives of Dermatology*, **134**, 1137–1141.

Labib, R. S., Anhalt, G. J., Patel, H. P., Mutasim, D. F. & Diaz, L. A. (1986) Molecular heterogeneity of bullous pemphigoid antigens as detected by immunoblotting. *Journal of Immunology*, **136**, 1231–1235.

Lebrun-Vignes, B., Roujeau, J. C., Bernard, P., Delaporte, E., Joly, P., Prost, C. *et al.* (1999) Prednisone is more effective than prednisolone metasulfobenzoate in the treatment of bullous pemphigoid (Letter). *Archives of Dermatology*, **135**, 89–90.

Lin, M. S., Gharia, M., Fu, C. L., Olague-Marchan, N., Hacker, M., Harman, K. E. *et al.* (1999) Molecular mapping of the major epitopes of BP180 recognized by herpes gestationis autoantibodies. *Clinical Immunology*, **92**, 285–292.

Liu, Z. & Diaz, L. A. (1995) Molecular mapping of a pathogenically relevant BP180 epitope associated with experimentally induced murine bullous pemphigoid. *Journal of Immunology*, **155**, 5449–5454.

Liu, Z., Diaz, L. A., Troy, J. L., Taylor, A. F., Emery, D. J., Fairley, J. A. & Giudice, G. J. (1993) A passive transfer model of the organ-specific autoimmune disease, bullous pemphigoid, using antibodies generated against the hemidesmosomal antigen, BP 180. *Journal of Clinical Investigation*, **92**, 2480–2488.

Liu, Z., Giudice, G. J., Swartz, S. J., Fairley, J. A., Till, G. O., Troy, J. L. & Diaz, L. A. (1995) The role of complement in experimental bullous pemphigoid. *Journal of Clinical Investigation*, **95**, 1539–1544.

Liu, Z., Giudice, G. J., Zhou, X. Y., Swartz, S. J., Troy, J. L., Fairley, J. A. *et al.* (1997a) Major role for neutrophils in experimental bullous pemphigoid. *Journal of Clinical Investigation*, **100**, 1256–1263.

Liu, Z., Roopenian, D. C., Zhou, X. O., Christianson, G. J., Diaz, L. A., Sedmak, D. D. & Anderson, C. L. (1997b) Beta(2)-microglobulin-deficient mice are resistant to bullous pemphigoid. *Journal of Experimental Medicine*, **186**, 777–783.

Liu, Z., Shipley, J. M., Vu, T. H., Zhou, X. Y., Diaz, L. A., Werb, Z. & Senior, R. M. (1998) Gelatinase B-deficient mice are resistant to experimental bullous pemphigoid. *Journal of Experimental Medicine*, **188**, 475–482.

Liu, Z., Shapiro, S. D., Zhou, X. Y., Twining, S. S., Senior, R. M., Giudice, G. J. *et al.* (2000) A critical role for neutrophil elastase in experimental bullous pemphigoid. *Journal of Clinical Investigation*, **105**, 113–123.

Marinkovich, M. P., Taylor, T. B., Keene, D. R., Burgeson, R. E. & Zone, J. J. (1996) LAD-1, the linear IgA bullous dermatosis autoantigen, is a novel 120-kDa anchoring filament protein synthesized by epidermal cells. *Journal of Investigative Dermatology*, **106**, 734–738.

Moll, R. & Moll, I. (1998) Epidermal adhesion molecules and basement membrane components as target structures of autoimmunity. *Virchows Archiv*, **432**, 487–504.

Murakami, H., Amagai, M., Higashiyama, M., Hashimoto, K., Chorzelski, T. P., Bhogal, B. S. *et al.* (1996) Analysis of antigens recognized by autoantibodies in herpes gestationis. Usefulness of immunoblotting using a fusion protein representing an extracellular domain of the 180 kD bullous pemphigoid antigen. *Journal of Dermatological Science*, **13**, 112–117.

Nousari, H. C. & Anhalt, G. J. (1999) Pemphigus and bullous pemphigoid. *Lancet*, **354**, 667–672.

Nousari, H. C., Griffin, W. A. & Anhalt, G. J. (1998) Successful therapy for bullous pemphigoid with mycophenolate mofetil. *Journal of the American Academy of Dermatology*, **39**, 497–498.

Olivry, T., Fine, J.-D., Dunston, S. M., Chasse, D., Pascal Tenorio, A., Monteiro-Riviere, N. A. *et al.* (1998) Canine epidermolysis bullosa acquisita: circulating autoantibodies target the aminoterminal noncollagenous (NC1) domain of collagen VII in anchoring fibrils. *Veterinary Dermatology*, **9**, 19–31.

Olivry, T., Chan, L. S., Xu, L., Chace, P., Dunston, S. M., Fahey, M. & Marinkovich, M. P. (1999a) Novel feline autoimmune blistering disease resembling bullous pemphigoid in humans: IgG autoantibodies target the NC16A ectodomain of type XVII collagen (BP180/BPAG2). *Veterinary Pathology*, **136**, 328–335.

Olivry, T., Savary, K. C. M., Murphy, K. M., Dunston, S. M. & Chen, M. (1999b) Bullous systemic lupus erythematosus (type I) in a dog. *Veterinary Record*, **145**, 165–169.

Olivry, T., Borrillo, A. K. G., Xu, L., Dunston, S. M., Slovis, N. M., Affolter, V. K. *et al.* (2000a) Equine bullous pemphigoid IgG autoantibodies target linear epitopes in the NC16A ectodomain of collagen XVII (BP180, BPAG2). *Veterinary Immunology and Immunopathology*, **73**, 45–52.

Olivry, T., Dunston, S. M., Fahey, M., Nguyen, N. & Marinkovich, M. P. (2000b) Autoantibodies against the processed ectodomain of collagen XVII (BPAG2, BP180) define a canine homologue of linear IgA disease of humans. *Veterinary Pathology*, **37**, 302–309.

Olivry, T., Mirsky, M. L., Singleton, W., Dunston, S. M., Borrillo, A. K. G., Xu, L. *et al.* (2000c) A spontaneously arising porcine model of bullous pemphigoid. *Archives of Dermatological Research*, **292**, 37–45.

Olivry, T., Petersen, A., Dunston, S. M. & Chen, M. (2000d) Novel localized variant of canine epidermolysis bullosa acquisita. *Veterinary Record*, **146**, 193–194.

Olivry, T., Dunston, S. M., Schachter, M., Xu, L., Nguyen, N., Marinkovich, M. P. & Chan, L. S. (2001) A spontaneous canine model of mucous membrane (cicatricial) pemphigoid, an autoimmune blistering disease affecting mucosae and mucocutaneous junctions. *Journal of Autoimmunity*, **16**, 411–421.

Perriard, J., Jaunin, F., Favre, B., Budinger, L., Hertl, M., Saurat, J. H. & Borradori, L. (1999) IgG autoantibodies from bullous pemphigoid (BP) patients bind antigenic sites on both the extracellular and the intracellular domains of the BP antigen 180. *Journal of Investigative Dermatology*, **112**, 141–147.

Roujeau, J. C. (1988) Plasmapheresis therapy of pemphigus and bullous pemphigoid. *Seminars in Dermatology*, **7**, 195–200.

Ruoslahti, E. & Reed, J. C. (1994) Anchorage dependence, integrins and apoptosis. *Cell*, **7**, 477–478.

Scott, D., Manning, T. & Lewis, R. (1982) Linear IgA dermatoses in the dog: bullous pemphigoid, discoid lupus erythematosus and a subcorneal pustular dermatitis. *Cornell Vet*, **72**, 394–402.

Scully, C., Carrozzo, M., Gandolfo, S., Puiatti, P. & Monteil, R. (1999) Update on mucous membrane pemphigoid – a heterogeneous immune-mediated subepithelial blistering entity. *Oral Surgery, Oral Medicine, Oral Pathology, Oral Radiology and Endodontics*, **88**, 56–68.

Stanley, J. R., Hawley-Nelson, P., Yuspa, H., Shewach, E. M. & Katz, S. I. (1981) Characterization of bullous pemphigoid antigen: a unique basement membrane protein of stratified squamous epithelia. *Cell*, **24**, 897–903.

Taniuchi, K., Takata, M., Matsui, C., Fushida, Y., Uchiyama, K., Mori, T. *et al.* (1999) Antiepiligrin (laminin 5) cicatricial pemphigoid associated with an underlying gastric carcinoma producing laminin 5. *British Journal of Dermatology*, **140**, 696–700.

Venning, V. A., Frith, P. A., Bron, A. J., Millard, P. R. & Wojnarowska, F. (1988) Mucosal involvement in bullous and cicatricial pemphigoid. A clinical and immunopathological study. *British Journal of Dermatology*, **118**, 7–15.

Vincent, S. D., Lilly, G. E. & Baker, K. A. (1993) Clinical, historic, and therapeutic features of cicatricial pemphigoid – a literature review and open therapeutic trial with corticosteroids. *Oral Surgery, Oral Medicine and Oral Pathology*, **76**, 453–459.

Whitworth, J. M., Thomas, I., Peltz, S. A., Sullivan, B. C., Wolf, A. H. & Cytryn, A. S. (1996) Vancomycin-induced linear IgA bullous dermatosis (LABD). *Journal of the American Academy of Dermatology*, **34**, 890–891.

Wojnarowska, F., Allen, A. & Collier, P. (1994) Linear IgA disease: a heterogeneous disease. *Dermatology*, **189** (Suppl. 1), 52–56.

Xu, L., O'Toole, E. A., Olivry, T., Hernandez, C., Peng, J., Chen, M. & Chan, L. S. (2000) Molecular cloning of canine bullous pemphigoid antigen 2 cDNA and immunomapping of NC16A domain by canine bullous pemphigoid autoantibodies. *Biochimica et Biophysica Acta – Molecular Basis of Disease*, **1500**, 97–107.

Yancey, K. B. (1999) Cicatricial pemphigoid. In: *Dermatology in General Medicine CD-ROM.* (Eds I. M. Freedberg, A. Z. Eisen, K. Wolff, K. F. Austen, L. A. Goldsmith, S. I. Katz & T. B. Fitzpatrick). McGraw-Hill, New York.

Zillikens, D. (1999) Acquired skin diseases of hemidesmosomes. *Journal of Dermatological Science*, **20**, 134–154.

Zillikens, D. & Giudice, G. J. (1999) BP180 type XVII collagen: its role in acquired and inherited disorders or the dermal–epidermal junction. *Archives of Dermatological Research*, **291**, 187–194.

Zillikens, D., Wever, S., Roth, A., Weidenthaler-Barth, B., Hashimoto, T. & Bröcker, E. B. (1995) Incidence of autoimmune subepidermal blistering dermatoses in a region of central Germany. *Archives of Dermatology*, **131**, 957–958.

Zillikens, D., Rose, P. A., Balding, S. D., Liu, Z., Olague-Marchan, M., Diaz, L. A. & Giudice, G. J. (1997) Tight clustering of extracellular BP180 epitopes recognized by bullous pemphigoid autoantibodies. *Journal of Investigative Dermatology*, **109**, 573–579.

Zone, J. J., Taylor, T. B., Kadunce, D. P. & Meyer, L. J. (1990) Identification of the cutaneous basement membrane zone antigen and isolation of antibody in linear immunoglobulin A bullous dermatosis. *Journal of Clinical Investigation*, **85**, 812–820.

Zone, J. J., Taylor, T. B., Meyer, L. J. & Petersen, M. J. (1998) The 97 kDa linear IgA bullous disease antigen is identical to a portion of the extracellular domain of the 180 kDa bullous pemphigoid antigen, BPAg2. *Journal of Investigative Dermatology*, **110**, 207–210.

1.3

Distribution and expression of desmosomal proteins, desmoglein-1 and -3, in normal canine skin and mucous membrane

M. Aoki DVM,[1] K. Nishifuji DVM,[1] M. Amagai MD, PhD,[2] T. Nishikawa MD, PhD,[2] S. Park DVM[1] and T. Iwasaki DVM, PhD[1]

[1] Veterinary Medical Teaching Hospital, Gifu University, Gifu, Japan
[2] Department of Dermatology, Keio University, Tokyo, Japan

Summary

Pemphigus is an autoimmune skin disease of humans and other animals. Autoantibodies against desmoglein-1 (Dsg1) and Dsg3 are thought to play a pathogenic role to induce loss of epidermal cell adhesion. The differences between lesions in pemphigus foliaceus (PF) and pemphigus vulgaris (PV) relate to the distribution and expression of desmogleins in human pemphigus. In this study, the expression of Dsg1 and Dsg3 in normal canine epidermis and mucosal epithelia was investigated by immunofluorescence and immunoblotting to determine a possible relationship between clinical involvement and the expression of desmogleins.

In indirect immunofluorescent studies, Dsg1 was expressed in all stratified squamous epithelia, whereas Dsg3 was expressed in only the oral cavity, oesophagus and anus. In immunoblot studies, the 160 kDa bands were denser in the muzzle and oral mucous membrane than in the extracted proteins from abdomen and esophagus. Dense bands at 130 kDa appeared in the extracted proteins from the oral mucous membrane and esophagus, whereas those from the muzzle were faint.

It is conceivable that canine PF mainly affects the muzzle and pinna because the distribution of Dsg1 in these areas is dense compared with other regions of epidermis or mucosal epithelia. In contrast, there was intense expression of Dsg3 in the oral cavity and anus, suggesting that these areas may be mainly affected in canine PV.

Introduction

Keratinocytes are tightly bound to each other by adhesion units. The desmosome is a major adhesive structure in epithelia and heart muscles. It is composed of desmogleins and desmocollins as transmembrane components, with desmoplakins, plakoglobins and band 6 proteins as cytoplasmic components. Desmogleins are classified into three isoforms called desmoglein-1 (Dsg1), Dsg2 and Dsg3. It is reported that expression of Dsg1 and Dsg3 in humans is restricted to basically stratified squamous epithelia, whereas Dsg2 is detected in all desmosome-possessing tissues including simple epithelia and myocardium (Schäfer *et al.*, 1994). Desmogleins are Ca^{2+}-dependent transmembrane glycoproteins and belong to the cadherin supergene family. Their basic structure is similar to that of classic cadherins. These cadherins have four cadherin repeats consisting of about 110 amino acids in the extracellular domain (Koch *et al.*, 1990).

Pemphigus has two major subtypes, pemphigus foliaceus (PF) and pemphigus vulgaris (PV). Human PF is clinically characterized by small flaccid blisters, scaly and erythematous lesions in the scalp, chest, face and upper back. Histopathologically, the blisters occur in the subcorneal granular cell layer of the epidermis. Human PV shows flaccid blisters and widespread erosions of face, scalp and groin, oral and mucocutaneous junctions of lips, eyelids, prepuce, vulva and anus, and the blisters develop in the suprabasal layer of the epidermis. Recently, another type of pemphigus has been reported as a paraneoplastic pemphigus (de Bruin *et al.*, 1999).

Canine PV was first reported in 1975 (Hurvitz & Feldman, 1975) and PF in 1977 (Halliwell & Goldschmidt, 1977). PF is the most common of all autoimmune skin diseases in dogs (Scott & Lewis, 1981). Skin lesions are characterized by crusting and pustules in the muzzle, periocular region, ears and footpads. Histopathologically, pustules contain acantholytic cells with numerous neutrophils and/or eosinophils in the subcorneal region of the epidermis. Canine PV is characterized by erosions and firm vesicles of the mucous membrane and mucocutaneous junctions such as the oral cavity and anus. Acantholysis occurs in the lower epidermis, and the cleft localizes just above the basal cell layer (Werner *et al.*, 1983; Ihrke *et al.*, 1985; Day *et al.*, 1993).

When autoantibodies bind to desmoglein, it causes disruption of intercellular junctions. In human medicine, the pathogenesis of pemphigus has been studied since antiepidermal intercellular antibodies in human PV sera were detected by immunofluorescent studies using normal human skin as the substrate (Beutner & Jordon, 1964). The autoantigens in pemphigus have been extensively investigated and shown to be desmosomal glycoproteins. It has also been demonstrated that PF antigen is a 160 kDa protein, which has been shown to be Dsg1, whereas the PV antigen is a 130 kDa protein, which was later shown to be Dsg3 (Koulu *et al.*, 1984; Eyre & Stanley, 1987, 1988; Hashimoto *et al.*, 1990, 1995). In the past few years, recombinant Dsg1 and Dsg3 proteins were produced by baculovirus, and these proteins were found to absorb and eliminate pathogenic autoantibodies from PF and PV sera (Amagai *et al.*, 1994, 1995). Most human PV sera include both anti-Dsg3 and anti-Dsg1 autoantibodies, so it is possible to produce a specific antibody against Dsg3 or Dsg1 by immunoabsorption with recombinant human Dsg1 (Dsg1-Ig-His) and Dsg3 (Dsg3-Ig-His). The distribution and expression of Dsg1 and Dsg3 have been investigated in humans, and it has been reported that Dsg1 was expressed most intensively in the upper layer of the skin, whereas Dsg3 was expressed in only the suprabasal layer. In contrast, in mucous membranes, the Dsg3 expression was most intense throughout the epithelia, whereas the expression of Dsg1 was very low. These results showed that the distribution and expression of desmogleins may relate to the localization of lesions (Amagai *et al.*, 1996; Ishi *et al.*, 1997; Shirakata *et al.*, 1998).

Canine keratinocytes cultured in high-calcium conditions showed fluorescent deposits in intercellular spaces by indirect immunofluorescent testing using sera from canine and human pemphigus as a primary antibody. In an immunoblotting study, canine PF and PV sera were found to recognize the 160 kDa and 130 kDa proteins, respectively. Therefore, the target antigens directed by canine PF and PV autoantibodies have been considered as being Dsg1 and Dsg3 (Suter *et al.*, 1993; Iwasaki *et al.*, 1996, 1997).

Clinically, canine PF usually affects the skin and is characterized by acantholysis in the upper layer of the epidermis, whereas canine PV patients have mucosal involvement characterized by suprabasal acantholysis. These differences in the distribution pattern of lesions and the depth of acantholysis between canine PF and PV may relate to the distribution and expression of desmogleins, as in humans. In the present investigation, the distribution of Dsg1 and Dsg3 was studied in several epidermal sites and in oral and some other sites of mucous membrane using immunofluorescence and immunoblotting with Dsg-isotype-specific antibodies.

Materials and methods

Antibodies

Immunofluorescence studies used anti-Dsg1-specific and anti-Dsg3-specific sera produced by immunoabsorbed human PV sera with recombinant Dsg3 and Dsg1 baculoprotein. PV sera were obtained from Keio University Hospital. Immunoblot studies used anti-Dsg1 mouse monoclonal antibody (DG3.10; PROGEN, Heidelberg, Germany) (Koch *et al.*, 1990) and anti-Dsg3-specific sera produced by immunoabsorbed human PV sera with recombinant Dsg1 baculoprotein. The index against Dsg1 or Dsg3 of these human PV sera was 100–120 or 70–90 by enzyme-linked immunosorbent assay (ELISA), respectively, where Index = [(OD of patients' sera − OD of negative control)/(OD of positive control − OD of negative control)] × 100 (Amagai *et al.*, 1999).

Immunoabsorption of human PV sera with recombinant Dsg1 and Dsg3 baculoprotein

Human PV sera were used as a Dsg1-specific or Dsg3-specific antibody. Human PV sera contained antibodies against both Dsg1 and Dsg3. Dsg1-specific antibody was prepared by immunoabsorbed human PV sera with

Table 1.3.1. Protocol of immunoabsorption for indirect immunofluorescence

	1:20	1:80
Anti-Dsg1 antibody	5 μl human PV sera + 95 μl Dsg3-Ig-His	25 μl 1:20 diluted PV sera + 75 μl Dsg3-Ig-His
Anti-Dsg3 antibody	95 μl Dsg1-Ig-His	75 μl Dsg1-Ig-His
Positive control	95 μl High Five sup.	75 μl High Five sup.
Negative control	47.5 μl Dsg3-Ig-His + 47.5 μl Dsg1-Ig-His	37.5 μl Dsg3-Ig-His + 37.5 μl Dsg1-Ig-His

PV: pemphigus vulgaris; Dsg1: desmoglein-1; Dsg3: desmoglein-3; Dsg3-Ig-His: recombinant human Dsg3 (absorbs only anti-Dsg3 autoantibody in human PV sera); Dsg1-Ig-His: recombinant human Dsg1 (absorbs only anti-Dsg1 autoantibody in human PV sera); High Five sup.: uninfected culture supernatants. These diluted human sera were used after leaving at 4°C overnight.

recombinant Dsg3 baculoprotein (Dsg3-Ig-His) and Dsg3-specific antibody was prepared by immunoabsorbing human PV sera with recombinant Dsgl baculoprotein (Dsgl-Ig-His), as described previously (Amagai *et al.*, 1994, 1995, 1996; Shirakata *et al.*, 1998). In brief, human PV sera were serially diluted to 1:20 and 1:80 for immunofluorescence with culture supernatants containing Dsg3-Ig-His or Dsgl-Ig-His (Table 1.3.1), and 1:10 for immunoblotting with culture supernatants containing Dsgl-Ig-His. They were then incubated at 4°C overnight. Human PV sera were also incubated with uninfected culture supernatants (High Five sup.) as positive controls. Human PV sera absorbed with culture supernatants containing both Dsg3-Ig-His and Dsgl-Ig-His were used as a negative control.

Immunofluorescence

Indirect immunofluorescence was performed on skin of normal dogs obtained from the muzzle, ear, shoulder, lumbar region, abdomen and footpad, and normal canine mucous membrane obtained from the buccal mucosa, esophagus, anus, trachea, small intestine and urinary bladder. These specimens were collected from four dogs immediately after death. The specimens were embedded in OCT compound (Miles, Elkhart, IN, USA) and frozen to −80°C. Normal skin from human axillae and oral mucous membrane (kind gifts from Dr Kamiya, Department of Dermatology, Gifu University, Gifu, Japan) were used as positive controls.

Indirect immunofluorescent studies were performed as described previously (Iwasaki *et al.*, 1995, 1996). In brief, 5 μm cryosections were obtained from each sample and the sections were first incubated with absorbed human PV sera for 45 min at room temperature in a moist chamber. Then they were incubated with fluorescein isothiocyanate (FITC)-conjugated goat anti-human immunoglobulin G (IgG) (Cappel, West Chester, PA, USA) diluted 1:160 with 1% bovine serum albumin (BSA)/phosphate-buffered saline (PBS) for 25 min at room temperature. The slides were then washed with PBS and observed by fluorescence microscopy (Olympus, Tokyo, Japan).

Epidermal extraction

Epidermal extracts were collected as described previously (Hashimoto *et al.*, 1990; Shirakata *et al.*, 1998). In brief, samples from the muzzle, abdomen, oral cavity, esophagus, trachea and urinary bladder were obtained from two dogs and from human axillary skin (a kind gift from Dr Kamiya, Department of Dermatology, Gifu University, Gifu, Japan) were cut into 1–2 cm slices and incubated with 250 U of dispase (Goudou-Shusei, Tokyo, Japan) in Dulbecco's modified Eagle's medium (DMEM; Gibco BRL, Grand Island, NY, USA) at 4°C overnight. The epidermis was separated and homogenized on ice with 0.5 ml of 1.5% sodium dodecyl sulfate (SDS)-0, 0625 M Tris–HCl buffer, pH 6.8, supplemented with 10 mM calcium chloride, 5% 2-mercaptoethanol and complete protease inhibitor (Boehringer Mannheim, Germany). Samples were then boiled for 5 min and centrifuged at 8000 *g* for 30 min. The supernatant was harvested and stored at −80°C until use.

Immunoblotting

The total protein in the extracted proteins from canine and human epidermis was estimated by Bradford's method. The same amount of protein (25 μg) on each lane was separated by 7.5% sodium dodecyl sulfate–polyacrylamide gel electrophoresis (sodium dodecyl sulfate–PAGE) (Laemmli, 1970) and electrophoretically transferred to a nitrocellulose membrane (MSI, Westboro, MA, USA) according to the method described by Towbin *et al.* (1979). Strips of membrane were blocked with 3% skimmed milk in Tris–HCl-buffered saline (TBS) for 2 h at room temperature. Samples were then incubated with DG3.10 (1:200 with TBS), anti-Dsg3-specific human PV sera (1:10 with Dsg1-Ig-His) or human normal sera (1:10 with uninfected culture supernatant) at 4°C overnight, and subsequently incubated with alkaline phosphatase (AP)-conjugated goat anti-mouse IgG or goat anti-human IgG (Zymed, South San Francisco, CA, USA) for 1 h at room temperature. The reaction was visualized with nitroblue tetrazolium and 5-bromo-4-chloro-3-indolyl phosphate (Sigma, St Louis, MO, USA). A computer system was used for the quantitative analysis of Western blotting. Each lane was captured and dot numbers were calculated for each band.

Results

The results of the indirect immunofluorescent studies are summarized in Table 1.3.2. The expression of Dsg1 in the shoulder, loins and abdomen, which have stratified squamous epithelia, was weaker than in other regions of the epidermis. Anti-Dsg1 antibodies stained most intensely all layers of the epidermis from the muzzle, pinna and footpad by indirect immunofluorescence. In the upper layer of the epidermis, the intensity of the reaction against anti-Dsg1 was strong compared with that in the middle and lower epidermis (Figure 1.3.1a). Some samples from the muzzle,

Table 1.3.2. Expression of desmoglein-1 and -3 (Dsg1 and Dsg3) in canine epidermis and mucosal epithelia

Tissue	Dsg1	Dsg3
Shoulder	+	±
Loins	+	±
Abdomen	+	±
Muzzle	++	±
Ear	++	±
Footpad	++	+
Oral cavity	++	++
Esophagus	+	+
Anus	++	++
Trachea	–	–
Small intestine	–	–
Urinary bladder	–	–

Staining intensity was arbitrarily assessed on a four-level scale: –, ±, +, ++.

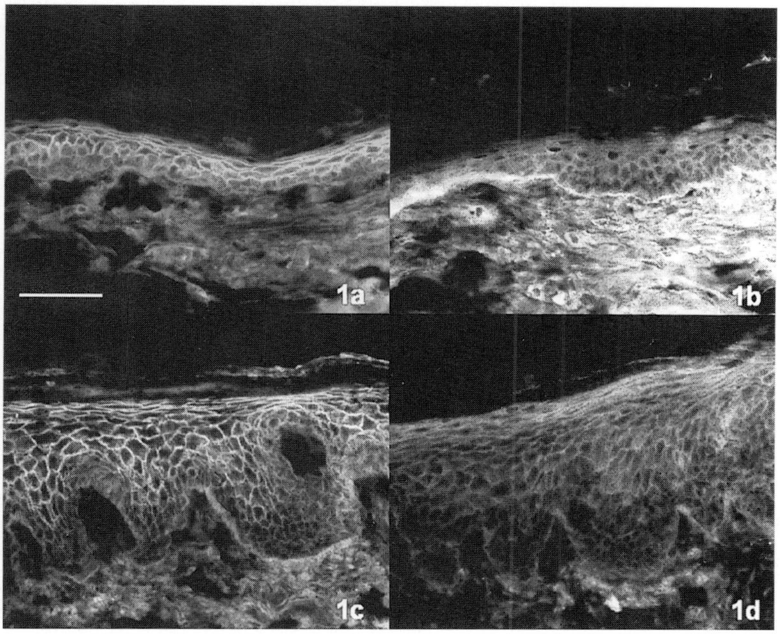

Figure 1.3.1. Comparison of expression between desmoglein-1 and -3 (Dsg1 and Dsg3) by immunofluorescence staining in the muzzle skin and oral mucous membrane. Anti-Dsg1 antibodies (a, c) and anti-Dsg3 antibodies (b, d) were used to stain muzzle skin (a, b) and oral mucous membrane (c, d). White scale bar = 50 μm.

pinna and footpad showed faint Dsg3 expression in the lower layer of the epidermis, but most of these samples did not reveal the reaction against anti-Dsg3 (Figure 1.3.1b). The epidermis of shoulder, loins or abdomen was very thin and anti-Dsg1 antibody stained only the upper layer of the epidermis. The distribution and expression of desmogleins were investigated in the mucous membrane of oral cavity, anus and esophagus, which have stratified squamous epithelia different from other mucous membranes. In oral mucous membrane and anus, anti-Dsg3 antibody stained intensely all layers of the mucosal epithelia (Figure 1.3.1d). However, in dogs, Dsg1 was also expressed in the middle layer of the oral mucous membrane, as opposed to the results in humans (Figure 1.3.1c). In the esophagus, the distribution of desmogleins was similar to that in the canine oral cavity and anus, but the reaction was weak. In the trachea, small intestine and urinary bladder, these tissues are not stratified squamous epithelia, so neither Dsg1 or Dsg3 was expressed.

To confirm the difference in expression level of Dsg1 and Dsg3 observed by immunofluorescence, proteins were extracted from the epidermis and mucous membrane and subjected to immunoblot analysis. The 160 kDa bands were detected strongly by anti-Dsg1 antibody in the extracted proteins from the muzzle, which is mainly affected in canine PF (Figure 1.3.2, lane 3). In the muzzle, 130 kDa bands were also detected by anti-Dsg3 antibody, but the bands were faint (Figure 1.3.3, lane 3). The 160 kDa bands were also detected in the extracted proteins from the abdomen, which is mainly not affected in canine PF, but the bands were less intense than those of the muzzle (Figure 1.3.2, lane 2). In the oral cavity, the region mainly affected in canine PV, dense 130 kDa bands were detected by anti-Dsg3 antibody (Figure 1.3.3, lane 4). However, 160 kDa bands were also detected strongly in the proteins extracted from the oral cavity (Figure 1.3.2, lane 4). In proteins extracted from the esophagus, both 160 kDa and 130 kDa bands were detected by anti-Dsg1 and anti-Dsg3 antibody, respectively (Figures 1.3.2, lane 5, 1.3.3, lane 5). Neither band was detected in the trachea or urinary bladder.

Discussion

Canine pemphigus is classified into two major forms, PF and PV. It is considered that there may be clinical, histological and immunological differences between the two PFs. The clinical signs shown in canine PF occur chiefly in skin of the muzzle, pinna and the periocular region, and are characterized by pustules, erosions and crust formation. The clinical signs of canine PV are distributed in the oral mucous membrane, mucocutaneous junctions, axillae and groin, with erosions and vesicles (Scott *et al.*, 1996). Histologically, the separation of epidermis and the formation of pustules in canine PF are usually located at the subcorneal to upper epidermis with acantholytic cells and polymorphonuclear leukocytes. The separation of epidermis in

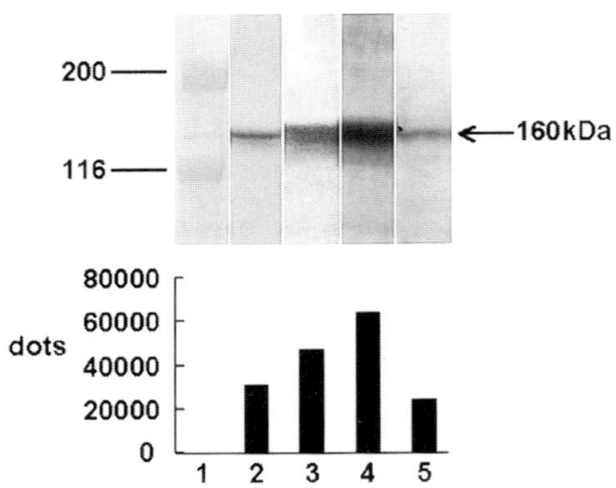

Figure 1.3.2. Anti-desmoglein-1 (Dsg1) antibody showed a faint 160 kDa band against proteins extracted from the skin of canine abdomen and esophagus (lanes 2, 5). Anti-Dsg1 also reacted strongly with 160 kDa protein extracted from the skin of canine muzzle and oral mucosa (lanes 3, 4). Lane 1: molecular weight standard.

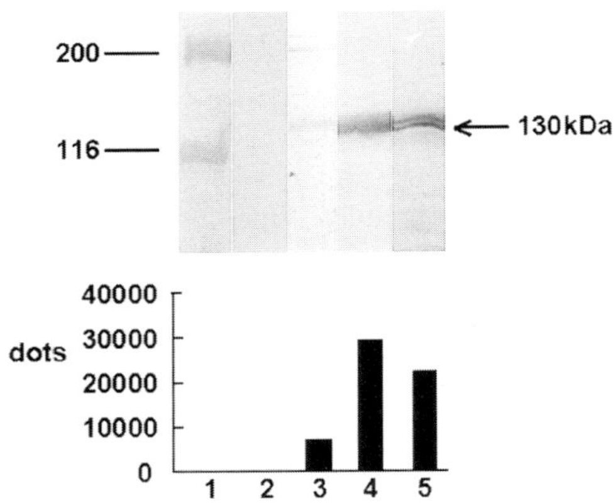

Figure 1.3.3. Anti-desmoglein-3 (Dsg3) strongly detected 130 kDa bands with proteins extracted from canine oral mucosa (lane 4) and esophagus (lane 5). Anti-Dsg3 antibody also showed a faint 160 kDa band against proteins extracted from the skin of canine muzzle (lane 3). Anti-Dsg3 did not show any proteins extracted from the skin of canine abdomen (lane 2). Lane 1: molecular weight standard.

canine PV occurs in the suprabasal cell layer. Immunologically, the proteins targeted by the autoantibody of canine PF are considered to be Dsg1, since patient sera from PF recognized 150–160 kDa bands of proteins extracted from canine cultured keratinocytes or epidermis by immunoblotting (Suter *et al.*, 1993; Iwasaki *et al.*, 1997). Similarly, the autoantigen of canine PV is thought to be the 130 kDa Dsg3 (Iwasaki *et al.*, 1997).

This study attempted to determine whether the distribution pattern of the predilection sites and the location of the separation within the epidermis could be attributed to a difference in expression of Dsg1 and Dsg3 in canine skin.

The expression of Dsg1 in canine skin was intense in the muzzle, pinna and footpads, and weak in the abdomen. The upper epidermis tended to show an intense reaction compared with the lower epidermis. Dsg1 expressions in canine mucous membrane were moderate to intense in the oral cavity and anus, but weak in the esophagus. These results may suggest that the clinical predilection site of canine PF corresponds to a Dsg1-rich region besides the oral cavity and anus. Therefore, it is conceivable that the occurrence of lesions in PF may depend on the amount of autoantigen, Dsg1. The intense expression of Dsg1 in upper layers of the epidermis may contribute to pustule formation in the upper epidermis in canine PF. However, clinical oral or anal involvement in canine PF is not common, despite the fact that these lesions are rich in Dsg1. Desmosomes are composed of several types of transmembranous adhesive protein. Distinct isoforms of desmocollin, another type of desmosome protein, are assembled in the same desmosome (North *et al.*, 1996) and similar mechanisms may be present for desmogleins. When anti-Dsg1 autoantibodies block the intercellular adhesive function of Dsg1 in oral mucous membrane, the function of Dsg3 within the same desmosomes may compensate the cell–cell adhesion (Mahoney *et al.*, 1999).

The expression of Dsg3 in canine skin was weak or faint in the muzzle, pinna, footpads and abdomen, whereas those in the mucous membranes, oral cavity and anus were intense. These results indicate that the distribution and the amount of Dsg3 may correlate with the involvement of blister formation in canine PV. However, Dsg1 was coexpressed with Dsg3 in the oral mucous membrane, where blister formation is common. The distribution of Dsg1 in the oral mucous membrane is dense in the middle layer and faint in the suprabasal portion, where the separation of epithelia occurs. In canine PV, it is suggested that Dsg1 expression in the lower mucous membrane may not suffice to compensate for the loss of numerous Dsg3 adhesions, and produces suprabasal separation.

Conclusion

The results of this study demonstrated that the distribution pattern of clinical signs and the location of intraepidermal clefts in canine PF and PV may depend on the expression of Dsg1 and Dsg3.

References

Amagai, M., Hashimoto, T., Shimizu, N. & Nishikawa, T. (1994) Absorption of pathogenic autoantibodies by extracellular domain of pemphigus vulgaris antigen (Dsg3) produced by baculovirus. *Journal of Clinical Investigation*, **94**, 59–67.

Amagai, M., Hashimoto, T., Green, K. J., Shimizu, N. & Nishikawa, T. (1995) Antigen-specific immunoabsorption of pathogenic autoantibodies in pemphigus foliaceus. *Journal of Investigative Dermatology*, **104**, 895–901.

Amagai, M., Koch, P. J., Nishikawa, T. & Stanley, J. R. (1996) Pemphigus vulgaris antigen (desmoglein 3) is localized in the lower epidermis, the site of blister formation in patients. *Journal of Investigative Dermatology*, **106**, 351–355.

Amagai, M., Komai, A., Hashimoto, T., Shirakata, Y., Hashimoto, K., Yamada, T. *et al.* (1999) Usefulness of enzyme-linked immunoabsorbent assay using recombinant desmoglein 1 and 3 for serodiagnosis of pemphigus. *British Journal of Dermatology*, **140**, 351–357.

Beutner, E. H. & Jordon, R. E. (1964) Demonstration of skin antibodies in sera of patients with pemphigus vulgaris by indirect immunofluorescent staining. *Proceedings of the Society for Experimental Biology and Medicine*, **117**, 505–510.

Bruin, A. de, Muller, E., Wyder, M., Anhalt, G. J., Lemmens, P. & Suter, M. M. (1999) Periplakin and envoplakin are target antigens in canine and human paraneoplastic pemphigus. *Journal of the American Academy of Dermatology*, **40**, 763–766.

Day, M. J., Hanlon, L. & Powell, L. M. (1993) Immune-mediated skin disease in the dog and cat. *Journal of Comparative Pathology*, **109**, 395–407.

Eyre, R. W. & Stanley, J. R. (1987) Human autoantibodies against a desmosomal protein complex with a calcium-sensitive epitope are characteristic of pemphigus foliaceus patients. *Journal of Experimental Medicine*, **165**, 1719–1724.

Eyre, R. W. & Stanley, J. R. (1988) Identification of pemphigus vulgaris antigen extracted from normal human epidermis and comparison with pemphigus foliaceus antigen. *Journal of Clinical Investigation*, **81**, 807–812.

Halliwell, R. E. W. & Goldschmidt, M. H. (1977) Pemphigus foliaceus in the canine: a case report and discussion. *Journal of the American Animal Hospital Association*, **13**, 431–436.

Hashimoto, T., Ogawa, M. M., Konohana, A. & Nishikawa, T. (1990) Detection of pemphigus vulgaris and pemphigus foliaceus antigens by immunoblot analysis using different antigen sources. *Journal of Investigative Dermatology*, **94**, 327–331.

Hashimoto, T., Amagai, M., Garrod, D. R. & Nishikawa, T. (1995) Immunofluorescence and immunoblot studies on reactivity of pemphigus vulgaris and pemphigus foliaceus sera with desmoglein 3 and desmoglein 1. *Epithelial Cell Biology*, **4**, 63–69.

Hurvitz, A. I. & Feldman, E. (1975) A disease in dogs resembling human pemphigus vulgaris: case reports. *Journal of the American Veterinary Medical Association*, **166**, 585–590.

Ihrke, P. J., Stannard, A. A., Ardans, A. A. & Griffin, C. E. (1985) Pemphigus foliaceus in dogs: a review of 37 cases. *Journal of the American Veterinary Medical Association*, **186**, 59–66.

Ishi, K., Amagai, M., Hall, R. P., Hashimoto, T., Takayanagi, A., Gamou, S. *et al.* (1997) Characterization of autoantibodies in pemphigus using antigen-specific enzyme-linked immunosorbent assays with baculovirus-expressed recombinant desmogleins. *Journal of Immunology*, **159**, 2010–2017.

Iwasaki, T., Olivry, T., Lapiere, J. C., Chan, L. S., Peavey, C., Liu, Y. Y. *et al.* (1995) Canine bullous pemphigoid (BP): identification of the 180 kDa canine BP antigen by circulating autoantibodies. *Veterinary Pathology*, **32**, 387–393.

Iwasaki, T., Shimizu, M., Obata, H., Ogata, M., Nagata, M., Yanai, T. *et al.* (1996) Effect of substrate on indirect immunofluorescence test for canine pemphigus foliaceus. *Veterinary Pathology*, **33**, 332–336.

Iwasaki, T., Shimizu, M., Obata, H., Isaji, M., Yanai, T., Kitagawa, H. & Sasaki, Y. (1997) Detection of canine pemphigus foliaceus autoantigen by immunoblotting. *Veterinary Immunology and Immunopathology*, **59**, 1–10.

Koch, P. J., Walsh, M. J., Schmelz, M., Goldschmidt, M. D., Zimbelmann, R. & Franke, W. W. (1990) Identification of desmoglein, a constitutive desmosomal glycoprotein, as a member of the cadherin family of cell adhesion molecules. *European Journal of Cell Biology*, **53**, 1–12.

Koulu, L., Kusumi, A., Steinberg, M. S., Klaus-Kovtun, V. & Stanley, J. R. (1984) Human autoantibodies against a desmosomal core protein in pemphigus foliaceus. *Journal of Experimental Medicine*, **160**, 1509–1518.

Laemmli, U. K. (1970) Cleavage of structural proteins string assembly of the head of bacteriophage T4. *Nature*, **277**, 680–685.

Mahoney, M. G., Wang, Z., Rothenberger, K., Koch, P. J., Amagai, M. & Stanley, J. R. (1999) Explanation for the clinical and microscopic localization of lesions in pemphigus foliaceus and vulgaris. *Journal of Clinical Investigation*, **103**, 461–468.

North, A. J., Chidgey, M. A., Clarke, J. P., Bardsley, W. G. & Garrod, D. R. (1996) Distinct desmocollin isoforms occur in the same desmosomes and show reciprocally graded distributions in bovine nasal epidermis. *Proceedings of the National Academy of Sciences of the United States of America*, **93**, 7701–7705.

Schäfer, S., Koch, P. J. & Franke, W. W. (1994) Identification of the ubiquitous human desmoglein, Dsg2, and the expression catalogue of the desmoglein subfamily of desmosomal cadherins. *Experimental Cell Research*, **211**, 391–399.

Scott, D. W. & Lewis, R. M. (1981) Pemphigus and pemphigoid in dog and man: comparative aspects. *Journal of the American Academy of Dermatology*, **5**, 148–167.

Scott, D. W., Miller, W. H. & Griffin, C. E. (1996) Pemphigus complex. In: *Small Animal Dermatology*, 5th edn, pp. 558–573. W. B. Saunders, Pennsylvania, PA.

Shirakata, Y., Amagai, M., Hanakawa, Y., Nishikawa, T. & Hashimoto, K. (1998) Lack of mucosal involvement in pemphigus foliaceus may be due to low expression of desmoglein 1. *Journal of Investigative Dermatology*, **110**, 76–78.

Suter, M. M., Ziegra, C. J., Cayatte, S. M., Smith, C. A. & Crameri, F. M. (1993) Identification of canine pemphigus antigens. In: *Advances in Veterinary Dermatology*, Vol. 2 (Eds P. J. Ihrke, I. S. Mason & S. D. White), pp. 367–380. Pergamon Press, Oxford.

Towbin, H., Staehelin, T. & Gordon, J. (1979) Electrophoretic transfer of proteins from polyacrylamide gels onto nitrocellulose sheets: procedure and some applications. *Proceedings of National Academy of Sciences of the United States of America*, **76**, 4350.

Werner, L. L., Brown, K. A. & Halliwell, R. E. W. (1983) Diagnosis of autoimmune skin disease in the dog: correlation between histopathologic, direct immunofluorescent and clinical findings. *Veterinary Immunology and Immunopathology*, **5**, 47–64.

1.4

Age- and breed-related differences in canine skin surface lipids and pH

R.W. Dunstan DVM, MS, DACVP,[1] T.H. Herdt DVM, MS,[2] B. Olivier DVM, PhD, DACVC,[3] B.S. Mei,[2] K.M. Credille DVM, PhD, DACVP,[1] R.A. Kennis DVM, DACVD,[4] R.L. Maier DVM,[1] B. Olivier DVM, PhD, DACVC,[3] S. Castle BS,[1] G.A. Reinhart PhD[5] and G.M. Davenport PhD[5]

[1] Department of Veterinary Pathobiology, Texas A&M University, College Station, Texas, USA
[2] Animal Health Diagnostic Laboratory and Department of Large Animal Clinical Sciences, College of Veterinary Medicine, Michigan State University, East Lansing, Michigan, USA
[3] Department of Small Animal Medicine and Surgery, College of Veterinary Medicine, Michigan State University, East Lansing, Michigan, USA
[4] Department of Small Animal Medicine and Surgery, Texas A&M University, College Station, Texas, USA
[5] The Iams Company, Lewisburg, Ohio, USA

Summary

Surface lipids and pH were measured at intervals between 10 and 81 weeks of age in male, age-matched Siberian huskies, Labrador retrievers and miniature poodles. The major surface lipids identified were cholesterol, cholesterol esters and wax esters. In general, cholesterol and triglycerides/free fatty acids decreased over the course of the study, whereas cholesteryl esters remained relatively constant and wax esters increased. The surface lipids of Labrador retrievers had the lowest percentage of cholesterol and triglycerides/free fatty acids, but the highest percentage of cholesteryl and wax esters. All breeds had a smaller amount of surface lipids than in matched sites from humans; however, the quantity of surface lipids was much lower in miniature poodles than in the other breeds examined. Labrador retrievers and Siberian huskies had alkaline skin surfaces, whereas the skin of miniature poodles tended to be neutral or slightly acidic. The results suggest that the skin surface environment of dogs is markedly different from that of humans and that in the future clinicians should consider breed differences in formulating topical therapies.

Introduction

Skin surface lipids provided by sebum and the intercellular lipids of the stratum corneum are important components of the barrier function provided by the skin. Not only are they important to selective permeability, but free fatty acids provided by these lipids play a major role in determining skin surface pH. Although there are reports of the quantity and composition of skin surface lipids in dogs as well as reports of skin surface pH, there is little known about whether they are affected by breed or age. The purpose of this study was to quantify the skin surface lipids and determine the surface pH in male, age-matched Siberian huskies, Labrador retrievers and miniature poodles from 10 to 81 weeks of age.

Materials and methods

All procedures dealing with animal care, handling and treatment in this study were reviewed, approved and subjected to continual monitoring by the Animal Use Committee, Texas A&M University.

This study was performed on a colony of 36 male, purebred dogs consisting of 12 Siberian huskies, 12 Labrador retrievers and 12 miniature poodles. These dogs were brought into the colony between the months of June and August when they were 7–8 weeks old. All dogs were housed indoors in air-conditioned and heated runs maintained at a constant temperature (20°C) with 12 h light/dark cycles. The dogs were given at least 2 weeks to adjust to the new environment before any procedures were performed. These dogs were part of a study to define the effects of diet on the skin. Thus, half of the dogs in each breed were fed a high-quality diet and the other half a lower quality diet. Because diet had no significant effect on the two groups (Dunstan *et al.*, in preparation) for the purposes of this report, data are included for all 12 dogs in each breed group.

The study was divided into two phases. In both phases, samples were collected at 3 week intervals. Phase 1 started when the dogs were 10 weeks old and concluded when they were 28 weeks old. Phase 2 started when the dogs were 63 weeks old and concluded when they were 81 weeks old. In an attempt to avoid diurnal variation, samples were collected between 09:00 and 12:00 h. During week 45 of the study, one of the Labrador retrievers was euthanized for a reason unrelated to the investigations being performed. Thus, phase 2 data for Labrador retrievers were based on 11 dogs.

The assays performed on the dogs were: (1) qualitative skin surface lipid analysis (phases 1 and 2); (2) quantitative skin surface lipid measurement (phase 2); and (3) skin surface pH measurement (weeks 3, 6, 12, 15 and 18 of phase 2).

Qualitative skin surface lipid analysis

For all dogs, samples were obtained from the interscapular skin. The sampling technique was a variation of the method described by Burton *et al.* (1992). Basically, the interscapular area from each dog was closely clipped with a beautician's clipper to insure that the hair was a short, consistent length. The shaved area was defatted by gently wiping with 70% isopropyl alcohol-soaked cotton pads. Once the skin had dried, three strips of Sebutape (CuDerm, Dallas, TX, USA) were applied to the clean skin. The strips were covered with gauze pads and taped firmly to the trunk using Elasticon Tape (Johnson and Johnson). To insure that the sites were not traumatized, the taped dogs were maintained in a portable, size-appropriate kennel and the Sebutape was allowed to contact the skin for 1 h. After this period, the Sebutape was removed from the skin and transferred to cryotubes. These tubes were placed on dry ice during transport and were subsequently stored at −70°C until used for thin layer chromatography (TLC).

For TLC, the central portion of each strip to be analyzed was placed in vials containing 10 ml of a 2:1 mixture of chloroform and methanol. Vials were sealed and agitated. The tapes were removed and rinsed with an additional 2.5 ml of the chloroform and methanol solvent to extract any residual lipids. The effluent was combined with the original 10 ml of solution. Potassium dihydrogen phosphate (2%, 5 ml) was added to each vial, mixed thoroughly and allowed to stand overnight. The next day, the upper phase was removed by pipetting and the volume of the lower phase reduced through evaporation. The solutions were then dried over sodium sulfate, filtered into 4 dram vials, evaporated to dryness and reconstituted with 3 μl of chloroform.

TLC was performed on prewashed, 20 × 20 cm TLC plates coated with a 0.25 ml layer of silica gel containing an inorganic binder (Anatech, Newark, DE, USA). Reconstituted canine sebum and working standards [squalene (a cholesterol precursor), cholesterol, cholesterol palmitate (a cholesterol ester), tristearin (a triglyceride) and stearic acid (a free fatty acid)] at concentrations ranging from 400 to 200 ng/μl were applied to the TLC plates using 5 μl/spot. The plates were developed vertically using three solvent systems: heptane (eluent 1), toluene–hexane (eluent 2) and hexane–diethyl ether-acidic acid (eluent 3). The plates were dried for 10 min after each development, sprayed with sulfuric acid (25%, 7 ml) and charred at 250°C for 15 min. The charred plates were analyzed with a scanning densitometer (CAMAG TLC Scanner II; CAMAG, Muttenz, Switzerland) and calibration plots were generated using Cats 3.18 (CAMAG Software, Muttenz, Switzerland). For each sampling period, the mean ± standard error of the mean (SEM) were determined for each breed of dog.

Quantitative skin surface lipid measurement

For this and all subsequent assays, the skin over the right scapula was sampled. A Sebumeter SM 810 (Courage & Khazaka, Koln, Germany) was used for this measurement. Samples were obtained from unwashed, closely clipped skin. Three measurements from different but proximate locations were performed on each dog. Data were expressed as μg surface lipids/cm^2. For each interval, the mean ± SEM were determined.

Skin surface pH evaluation

The pH was determined using a Skin-pH-Meter PH 900 (Courage & Khazaka, Koln, Germany) with a flat, glass electrode. The device was calibrated as recommended with standard buffers at pH 4.0 and 7.0. The electrode was washed in standard buffer after each use and briefly dried before application. Three measurements from different but proximate locations were performed on each dog. For each sampling interval, the mean ± SEM were determined based on breed.

Statistical analysis

Statistical comparisons for the effects of breed and age and their interactions were made using a grouped, repeated measures ANOVA with breed and age. Huynh–Feldt adjusted *p*-values were used for the applicable repeated measures factors to lessen the impact of any departures from compound symmetry. Statistically significant ANOVA breed effects were followed by linear contrasts for the three paired breed comparisons. An α-value of 0.05 was chosen as the nominal threshold for statistical significance.

Results

The results demonstrated that the major surface lipids in the dog were cholesterol, wax diesters and cholesteryl esters. Triglycerides (triacylglycerols) and free fatty acids were also present, but in lower amounts. Triglycerides and free fatty acids were added together because the values of these lipids were generally inversely related: high triglyceride values were correlated with low free fatty acid values and vice versa. This was partially expected because, on the skin surface, free fatty acids are largely derived from bacterially hydrolyzed triglycerides (Downing *et al.*, 1999). To permit comparisons of data, TLC data were expressed as a percentage of the total lipids in the sample. This allowed the determination of whether alterations in a lipid value changed in relation to the other lipids.

Examining time with breed as a percentage of total lipids indicated that there was a significant decrease in cholesterol and a significant increase in wax esters during phase 1 but not phase 2, and although there was a downward trend for triglycerides/fatty acids during phase 1, significant differences were not established. Cholesterol esters remained relatively constant for the duration of the study and no significant differences were noted over time (Figure 1.4.1a–d). Breed differences independent of time were not noted. During phase 2, the percentage of cholesterol was lower in Labrador retrievers than in Siberian huskies and miniature poodles. Labrador retrievers also had lower percentages of triglycerides/fatty acids in phase 2 than the other breeds examined. In contrast, they had a higher percentage of cholesteryl esters than miniature poodles and a higher percentage of wax esters than both miniature poodles and Siberian huskies through most of phase 2; however, significant differences between Labrador retrievers and the other breeds in this study could not be established.

The quantity of surface lipids measured using the Sebumeter during phase 2 demonstrated that values increased significantly over the course of the study for all breeds and that miniature poodles had significantly lower levels of surface lipids than the other two breeds examined (Figure 1.4.2). Although Siberian huskies had more surface lipids than Labrador retrievers during most of the periods of measurement, significantly higher differences were not established.

Marked differences in surface pH were identified. Both huskies and Labrador retrievers had alkaline skin (pH > 8.0). Although the trends suggested that the skin of Labradors was slightly more alkaline than that of Siberian huskies no significant differences were defined between these two breeds. In sharp contrast were the miniature poodles, whose pH varied from neutral to slightly acidic and was significantly lower than both Labrador retrievers and Siberian huskies (Figure 1.4.3). In all breeds there was a progressive and significant decline in pH.

Discussion

This study is part of an ongoing investigation to define a dynamic but largely ignored area of the skin, the surface of the stratum corneum. Although preliminary results are presented, the trends provide some insights into the surface of the canine skin.

The assays confirmed that the major surface epidermal lipids in the dog were cholesterol, wax diesters and cholesteryl esters, as reported previously by Nicolaides *et al.* (1968), Sharaf *et al.* (1977), Wheatley (1986) and Burton *et al.* (1992). The results also showed that the relative amount of skin surface cholesterol decreased, while that of wax esters increased between 10 and 81 weeks of age. In addition, cholesterol decreased

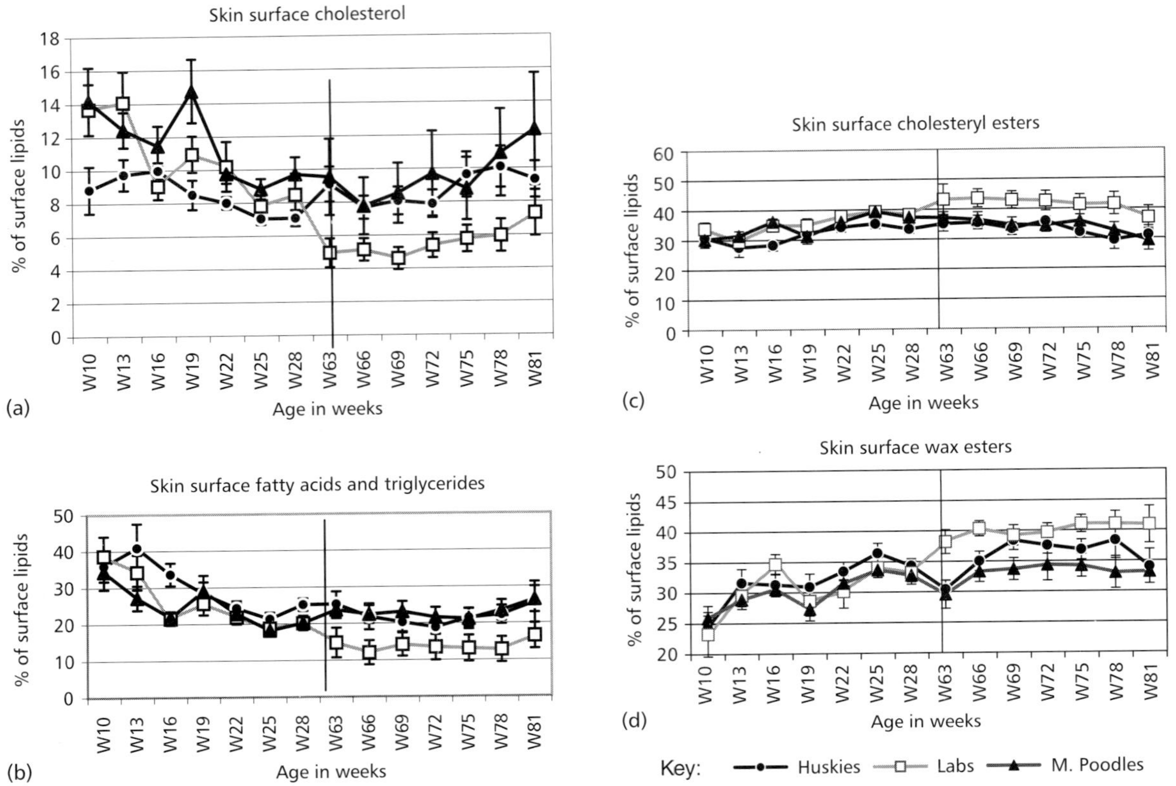

Figure 1.4.1. (a–d) Differences in the major epidermal surface lipids over time. Each datum point represents the mean ± SEM for 12 Siberian huskies, 12 Labrador retrievers and 12 miniature poodles for phase 1 of the study. Because one of the Labrador retrievers died during the period between phase 1 and phase 2, means for the Labrador retrievers were based on 11 dogs in phase 2 for this breed. The line through the center separates phase 1 from phase 2 of the study. During the course of the study, skin surface cholesterol decreased significantly during phase 1 ($p < 0.00001$) and wax esters increased significantly ($p < 0.00001$).

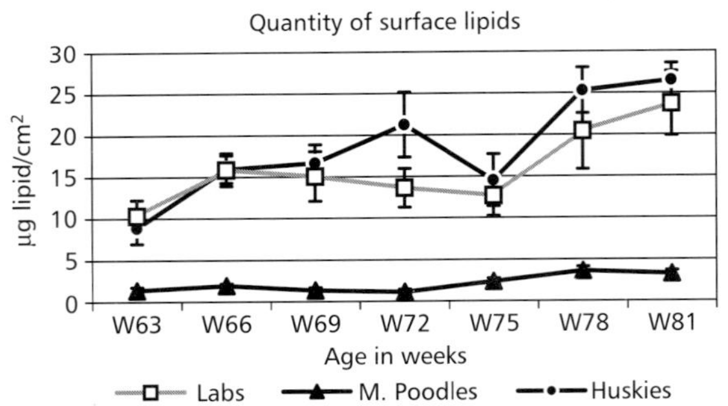

Figure 1.4.2. Differences in the quantity of skin surface lipids over time. Each datum point represents the mean ± SEM for 12 Siberian huskies, 11 Labrador retrievers and 12 miniature poodles. As a trend, skin surface lipids increased significantly for all dogs in the study over time ($p < 0.0009$) and miniature poodles had significantly lower skin surface lipids than either huskies ($p < 0.0009$) or Labrador retrievers ($p < 0.002$).

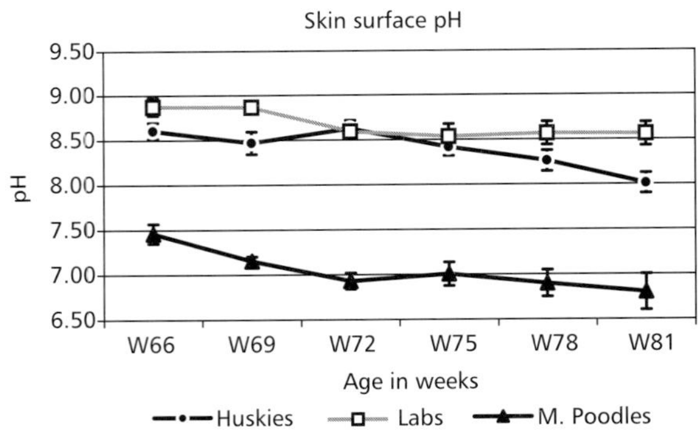

Figure 1.4.3. Differences in the skin surface pH over time. Each datum point represents the mean ± SEM for 12 Siberian huskies, 11 Labrador retrievers and 12 miniature poodles. Skin surface pH decreased significantly over the course of the study ($p < 0.000001$) and by breed ($p < 0.0083$). Poodles had significantly lower skin surface pH than either huskies ($p < 0.0101$) or Labrador retrievers ($p < 0.0024$).

significantly as a percentage of total surface lipids, while wax esters significantly increased. A similar finding has been reported in humans during puberty, where an increasing wax ester to cholesterol ratio is used as a sign of maturation and greater activity of sebaceous glands (Cunliffe & Simpson, 1998; Downing *et al.*, 1999). With the current sample size, no significant breed differences in sebum composition were demonstrated. However, the trends suggested that there are breed differences in the composition of sebum and that Siberian huskies and miniature poodles have more in common regarding the percentage of the different surface lipids than Labrador retrievers (the breed that consistently had the lowest cholesterol and trigylcerides/free fatty acids and the highest cholesteryl esters and wax esters).

Dogs have a much lower concentration of epidermal lipids on their truncal skin than do humans. Sebumeter values from the backs of humans normally range from 55 to 130 $\mu g/cm^2$ (data from manufacturers). None of the dogs in the present study had mean values as high as this. The low quantity of sebum on the canine trunk was further confirmed by the inability to use Sebutape as a means to quantitate sebum. In humans, sebum absorbed onto this tape forms visible spots from almost any site on the body, making Sebutape the most widely used semiquantitative method in humans for determining the amount of sebum on the epidermal surface. The amount of sebum is given a grade based on the size of these spots by comparing the results from graded examples provided by the manufacturer. In the authors' experience, the application of Sebutape on dogs five to 10 times longer than is recommend by the manufacturer for humans failed to absorb grossly detectable surface lipids (data not shown) (Pierard & Pierard-Franschimont, 1992; Clarys & Barel, 1995; Downing *et al.*, 1999).

Even though the three breeds examined in this study had a lower quantity of surface lipids than has been reported in humans, breed differences were still apparent. Siberian huskies and Labrador retrievers produced much more detectable epidermal lipid than the miniature poodle, whose mean superficial lipid values never exceeded 5 $\mu g/cm^2$. In humans, when the surface lipid quantity is lower than 10 $\mu g/cm^2$, no sebum is thought to be present; rather, this level of lipid represents that contributed solely by the epidermis (Cunliffe & Simpson, 1998). This does not appear to be true for dogs, where the sebum-specific wax esters were always a major component of the surface lipids examined (even in miniature poodles). In short, sebum was isolated and detected by the techniques described even in low ranges.

A reasonable question to ask is why dogs, which have greater follicular density than humans and sebaceous glands that approximate the size of sebaceous glands on non-facial human skin, have quantitatively lower skin surface lipids than humans. It may be hypothesized that this is because the Sebumeter, the instrument used to measure surface epidermal lipids in the dog, uses a grease spot photometer method. This method measures lipid quantity by determining the increased clarity of a lipid-absorbent membrane of known area. The clearer the membrane postexposure, the greater the quantity of surface lipids. This method may give the highest readings for species in which the major skin surface lipids are oily like humans, where the predominant epidermal lipids are free fatty acids and triacylglycerols. This may not be true for species such as dogs in which the major skin surface lipids are waxes and cholesterol esters, molecules that may be quite solid at room temperature (personal communication, R. Homan, Pfizer Co., September 2001). Further testing needs to be performed to confirm this hypothesis.

This study also defined breed variability in surface pH: Siberian huskies and Labrador retrievers had a highly alkaline skin surface (pH 8.0–9.0), with Labrador retrievers having the highest pH through most of the study period. In contrast, the pH for miniature poodles was significantly lower, varying from neutral to slightly acidic. The finding of such alkaline skin surface pH values for Labrador retrievers and Siberian huskies is at odds with some reports but in agreement with others. According to Scott *et al.* (1995) and Draize (1977), the pH of normal feline and canine skin is in the range of 5.5–7.5. Recently, Campbell & Bibus (1999) described the pH of beagle dogs as also being quite alkaline (range 8.5–7.5). Whether the high pH of the skin surface is real is subject to debate. Meyer & Neurand (1991) reported that the pH of the skin surface of dogs (beagles and Great Danes) could increase by more than 1.0 pH unit within 1 min after they became very anxious. Although the possibility exists that the present results in Labrador retrievers and Siberian huskies and those by Campbell & Bibus (1999) are spuriously elevated because the samples were taken from excited dogs, if this is true, then there is no way of sampling a 'normal' dog. As with all dogs, those used in this study responded differently to being handled. Although some were more excited than others, the degree of excitability could not be associated with increased pH values. In addition, miniature poodles, the breed with the lowest mean skin surface pH were not found to be less excitable than the other breeds studied. The progressive and significant decline in pH during the period when these values were obtained may be explained by a similar increase in skin surface lipids and assumedly free fatty acids, even though free fatty acids/triglycerides decreased as a percentage of the other lipids measured by TLC. However, other factors not measured in this investigation, such as increased lactic acid through sweat production, may have played a role in the decline in pH.

That the skin surface of some breeds of dogs may have such an alkaline pH raises questions about the basic physiology of the canine skin. If true, then the concept of the acid mantle that is purported to serve as a protective mechanism in the skin of mammals is not present in dogs (Marchionini & Hausknecht, 1938). In addition, if the enzymes of the stratum corneum of humans, some of which have been associated with desquamation, typically function in an acidic range, how do these enzymes function in dogs (Laube, 1956; Ohman & Vahlquist, 1993)? Finally, a pH in the range of what was concluded to be normal for Labrador retrievers and Siberian huskies is associated with increased permeability in humans (Berardesca *et al.*, 1998).

Conclusion

This study suggests that much more work needs to be done to understand the dynamic environment of the skin surface in dogs. Furthermore, the differences between dogs and humans regarding skin surface lipids and pH are so marked that topical treatments not specifically designed for and tested on dogs may not be optimally effective. Finally, breed differences suggest that truly optimized topical treatments may need to be done on an individual breed basis.

Acknowledgement

This study was funded by the Iams Company.

References

Berardesca, E., Pirot, T., Singh, M. & Maibach, H. (1998) Differences in stratum corneum pH gradient when comparing white caucasian and black African–American skin. *British Journal of Dermatology*, **138**, 855–857.

Burton, D. E., Bailey, D. L., Jeromin, A. M., Wyder, W. E., Hollenbach, E. J. & Johnson, G. R. (1992) Quantitative determination of canine sebaceous lipids by thin layer chromatography. *Journal of Planar Chromatography*, **5**, 179–183.

Campbell, K. L. & Bibus, D. (1999) Effects of α-linolenic acid on the skin and plasma phopholipids of beagle pups. In: *15th Proceedings of AAVD/ACVD Meeting*, pp.105–106.

Clarys, P. & Barel, A. (1995) Quantitative evaluation of skin surface lipids. *Clinics in Dermatology*, **13**, 320–321.

Cunliffe, W. J. & Simpson, N. B. (1998) Disorders of the sebaceous glands. In: *Rook/Wilkinson/Ebling Textbook of Dermatology*, 6th edn (Eds R. H. Champion, J. L. Burton, D. A. Burns & S. M. Breathnach), pp. 1927–1984. Blackwell Scientific, Oxford.

Downing, D. T., Stewart, M. E. & Strauss, J. S. (1999) Lipids of the epidermis and the sebaceous glands. In: *Dermatology in General Medicine*, 5th edn (Eds I. M. Freedburg, A. Z. Eisen, K. Wolff, K. F. Austen, L. A. Goldsmith, S. I. Katz & T. B. Fitzpatrick), pp. 144–155. McGraw-Hill, New York.

Draize, J. H. (1977) The determination of the pH of the skin of man and common domesticated animals. *Journal of Investigative Dermatology*, **5**, 77–85.

Laube, F. (1956) Die Veranderung des pH, der Alkaliresistenz, der Alkali- und Saure-Nettralisation der Haut nach verschiedenen Reinigungsbadern. *Dermatologica*, **112**, 454–467.

Marchionini, A. & Hausknecht, W. (1938) Sauremantel der Haut und Baketerienabwehr. *Klinik Wochenschrift*, **17**, 663–666.

Meyer, W. & Neurand, K. (1991) Comparison of skin pH in domesticated and laboratory animals. *Archives of Dermatological Research*, **283**, 16–18.

Nicolaides, N., Fu, H. C. & Rice, G. R. (1968) The skin surface lipids of man compared with those of eighteen species of animals. *Journal of Investigative Dermatology*, **51**, 83–89.

Ohman, V. & Vahlquist, A. (1993) *In vivo* studies concerning a pH gradient in human stratum corneum and upper epidermis. *Acta Dermatologica Venereologica (Stockholm)*, **74**, 375–379.

Pierard, G. & Pierard-Franchimont, C. (1992) The Sebutape technique for monitoring androgen dependent disorders. *European Journal of Medicine*, **1**, 109–112.

Scott, D. W., Miller, W. H. & Griffin, C. E. (1995) *Miller and Kirk's Small Animal Dermatology*, 5th edn, p. 4. W. B. Saunders, Philadelphia, PA.

Sharaf, D. M., Clark, S. J. & Downing, D. T. (1977) Skin surface lipids of the dog. *Lipids*, **12**, 786–793.

Wheatley, V. R. (1986) *The Physiology and Pathophysiology of the Skin, Vol. 9, The Sebaceous Glands* (Ed. A. Jarrett), pp. 2763–2796. Academic Press, London.

1.5

What happens when a dog loses its puppy coat? Functional, developmental and breed-related changes in the canine hair follicle

K.M. Credille DVM, PhD, DACVP,[1] C.J. Lupton PhD,[2] R.A. Kennis DVM, DACVD,[3] R.L. Maier DVM,[1] J. Dziezyc DVM, DACVO,[3] K.A. Tucker BS,[1] G.A. Reinhart PhD,[4] G.M. Davenport PhD[4] and R.W. Dunstan DVM, MS, DACVP[1]

[1] Department of Veterinary Pathobiology, Texas A&M University, College Station, Texas, USA
[2] Texas A&M Agricultural Research Extension Center, San Angelo, Texas, USA
[3] Department of Small Animal Medicine and Surgery, Texas A&M University, College Station, Texas, USA
[4] Research and Development, The Iams Company, Lewisburg, Ohio, USA

Summary

This study attempted to define anatomical and functional differences in the hair follicle associated with age and breed in a colony of 36 intact, male dogs (12 Siberian huskies, 12 miniature poodles and 12 Labrador retrievers). Between 10 and 28 weeks of age, the dogs were periodically sampled and follicular morphology was assessed using the following techniques: (1) DermScope examination of the eruptive morphology of the hair shafts; (2) histological and morphometric examination of site-matched, horizontally sectioned 6 mm skin biopsy samples and (3) Optical-based Fibre Diameter Analyser (OFDA) evaluation to determine the diameter and curvature of hair shafts. Morphometric evaluation of the number of hair follicles and the hair cycle showed that the mean number of hair follicles per follicular unit increased in all breeds. The percentage of follicles in telogen in the miniature poodles decreased throughout the study, whereas the number of telogen follicles increased in Siberian huskies. At the end of the study, both Siberian huskies and Labrador retrievers had approximately 50% of their follicles in telogen. In contrast, the miniature poodles had only 12% of their follicles in telogen. The OFDA data showed that Labrador retrievers had the largest mean hair shaft diameter. Siberian huskies had the greatest mean curvature. DermScope examination visually confirmed these observations. The results indicate that 'loss of the puppy coat' is best thought of as a gain in the adult coat and that this process is extremely breed specific.

Introduction

The importance placed on the hair coat by dog owners is evidenced by the diversity of coat types that have evolved over the centuries. With the arguable exception of the contours of a dog's body provided by the musculoskeletal system, the feature that most distinguishes the different canine breeds is the hair coat. Thus, it is no surprise that every breed has standards by which the coat is assessed in the show ring (American Kennel Club, 1997). The hair coat is also important in establishing the animal–human bond; animals are enjoyable to view, but also to 'pet'. Therefore, diseases associated with hair loss are of concern to most dog owners. Not only do their pets have a less attractive appearance, but the pets are also handled less frequently. These concerns ultimately are transferred to veterinarians who are asked to improve the coat of an alopecic dog.

With the importance that the hair coat plays in establishing the identity of a breed and the human– animal bond, it is surprising that there has been no substantive advancement in defining breed differences in the canine hair coat for over 40 years (Gair, 1928; Brunsch, 1956). This lack of knowledge of breed-associated differences in the hair coat is more than just a cosmetic issue. For dermatopathologists, the morphological assessment of the severity of hair loss is dependent on how the biopsy sample differs from normal. Because little information is available regarding breed-related differences, all biopsy samples are viewed as a generic representative of the species, not of the breed.

The authors are currently involved in an ongoing study to define breed-related differences in the skin of dogs and to apply this knowledge to understand better the role that factors such as nutrition play in maintaining a healthy hair coat. This report describes the pelage differences in three canine breeds (Siberian huskies, Labrador retrievers and miniature poodles) that occur between the ages of 10 and 28 weeks. During this time, the fine, soft 'puppy' coat of many breeds is transformed into the hair coat that characterizes the adult dog; however, little is known about how this process occurs.

Materials and methods

All procedures dealing with animal care, handling and treatment in this study were reviewed, approved and monitored by the Animal Use Committee, Texas A&M University.

This study was performed on a colony of 36 male, purebred dogs consisting of 12 Siberian huskies, 12 Labrador retrievers and 12 miniature poodles. These dogs were brought into the colony between June and August 1998 when they were 7–8 weeks old. All dogs were housed indoors in individual runs (Siberian huskies and Labrador retrievers) or runs shared by three dogs (miniature poodles) maintained at a constant temperature (20°C) with 12 h light/dark cycles. The dogs were given at least 2 weeks to adjust to the new environment before any procedures were performed. These dogs were part of a study to define the effects of diet on the skin. Thus, half of the dogs in each breed were fed a high-quality diet and the other half a lower quality diet. For the purposes of this report, data are included for all 12 dogs in each breed group and dietary effects were ignored.

Samples of clipped hair and punch biopsy samples were collected at 3 week intervals starting when the dogs were 10 weeks old and continuing for 18 weeks. Because of size limitations of the puppies, different sites were used for sample collection (see below).

The assays performed on the dogs were: (1) DermScope evaluation; (2) histological and morphometric assessment of skin biopsy samples; and (3) Optical-based Fibre Diameter Analyser (OFDA) analysis.

The DermScope is a portable, external microscope that produces a high-quality digital image. In this study, it was used as an external scanning microscope, allowing qualitative examination of the clipped hair coat at magnifications of up to 600×. For each dog, DermScope evaluation was performed on the dorsal lumbar area. To prepare the site for the DermScope evaluation, the area was closely clipped and wiped gently with an alcohol-soaked cotton pad.

Skin biopsy samples were obtained from the middle to caudal dorsolateral thoracic area. Two 6 mm skin biopsy samples were used for morphological and morphometric assessment of the hair follicles. Biopsy samples were obtained under local anesthetic using standard surgical techniques. To avoid inflammation and scarring related to previous biopsy sites, samples were taken a minimum of 4 cm apart from other sites. Samples were fixed in 10% neutral buffered formalin and, after fixation, one biopsy sample was trimmed vertically. The other biopsy sample was sectioned horizontally as described by Headington (1984). Samples were routinely processed, embedded cut side down, sectioned at 5 μm and stained with hematoxylin and eosin. Routine descriptive morphological evaluation was performed on the vertically sectioned samples. The horizontally sectioned samples were step-sectioned until the isthmus region of all the hairs in five follicular units could be assessed. A follicular unit was defined as the anatomical aggregation of compound hair follicles that occurs in dogs. Most follicular units consist of three compound follicles adjacent to each other with the middle compound follicle containing the largest (primary) hair shaft. The horizontally sectioned samples were evaluated routinely and morphometrically. The morphometric analysis took two forms: (1) the stage of the hair cycle was defined for each follicle in the five follicular units evaluated; and (2) the number of hairs/follicular unit was counted. A hair follicle was considered in anagen when an inner sheath surrounded the hair shaft at the level of the follicular isthmus. A hair follicle was considered in 'haired' telogen when trichilemmal cornification surrounded the hair shaft at the isthmic region. A follicle was considered in 'hairless' telogen when the hair follicle at the level of the isthmus was devoid of a hair shaft and either had luminal trichilemmal cornification but no hair shaft or was simply an epithelial tube with no luminal cornification (Nixon, 1993). Because catagen hairs are impossible to recognize consistently on horizontal sections and are uncommon, no attempt was made to identify them in this study.

The OFDA is a computerized microscope with attached video camera that captures digitized images of a moving sample of cleaned hair shafts that have been cut into 2 mm lengths. The hair snippets are randomly spread onto a hinged glass slide using an automatic spreader. No mounting liquid is used, and after measurement the fibers are vacuumed off. The width (diameter) and degree of curvature of each captured fiber image is measured. The advantages of using the OFDA to evaluate hair shafts are in its accuracy (the instrument is capable of a resolution of 1 μm and can determine diameters in the range of 4–300 μm) and speed (>10 000 fibers can be measured per minute) (Lupton, 1995). For OFDA analysis, the hair in an area approximately 4 × 4 cm over the left scapula was clipped and stored until the hair was ready to be cleaned (Baxter *et al.*, 1992). Because the samples evaluated were from clippings of hair obtained every 3 weeks, what was actually measured by OFDA analysis was the diameter and curvature of the hair shafts that had erupted during the 3 week interval between sampling periods.

Results

The DermScope examination visually defined differences in the number and pattern of hair shafts erupting through the follicular opening. The 200× lens provided sufficient detail to allow for assessment of the cuticular pattern of erupting hair. Differences were noted both between breeds and over time. Siberian huskies had the largest number of hair shafts with the greatest visible differences between the size of primary and secondary hairs. Miniature poodles and Labrador retrievers had approximately the same number of hair shafts per follicular opening, but there was considerable interbreed variability in diameter. The hair shafts of the miniature poodles were much finer with smaller diameters and the hair shafts from Labrador retrievers were coarser with larger diameters.

At the end of the study, when the dogs were 28 weeks old, the pelage of the Siberian huskies had a marked increase in the number of secondary hairs and a slight and subjective increase in the diameter of primary hairs. The differences in the number of hair shafts were more difficult to discern in miniature poodles and Labrador retrievers. Miniature poodles appeared to have a slight increase in the number of hair shafts, but no discernible difference in hair shaft diameter compared with 10 weeks of age. Labrador retrievers had no discernible increase in the number of hairs, but had a striking increase in the diameter of hair shafts.

The DermScope was also used to evaluate the epidermis qualitatively. In all dogs, the epidermis was non-pigmented and opaque, allowing visualization of the dermis and, to some extent, the base of pigmented hairs. Occasionally, tylotrich pads, localized neuroreceptor organs associated with follicles, were identified, especially in Siberian huskies. Tylotrich pads appeared as slightly raised, white thickenings of the epidermis.

Histological and morphometric assessment of vertically sectioned skin biopsy samples revealed that the dermis became somewhat thicker in each breed from the beginning of the study to the end. Sebaceous glands also became larger. The overall follicular morphology was difficult to discern by this method of trimming. However, even here, breed differences were at least suggested in that the Siberian huskies had many more hair shafts in the infundibula and the Labrador retrievers had fewer and coarser hairs. The miniature poodles (the only breed in the group with curly primary hairs) had primary hairs that were vaguely curved. Miniature poodle primary and secondary hair shafts appeared smaller than the other two breeds and were less numerous than in the Siberian huskies.

A diagram of the microscopic appearance of a horizontally sectioned skin biopsy sample is presented in Figure 1.5.1. The compound follicles had a distinct anatomical orientation with a single, large anterior follicle and multiple smaller posterior follicles. Because of this orientation, the largest anterior follicle in a compound follicle was called an anatomical primary follicle. All other follicles were considered anatomical secondary follicles. Most follicular units were composed of three compound follicles, but occasionally, follicular units composed of one to five compound follicles were

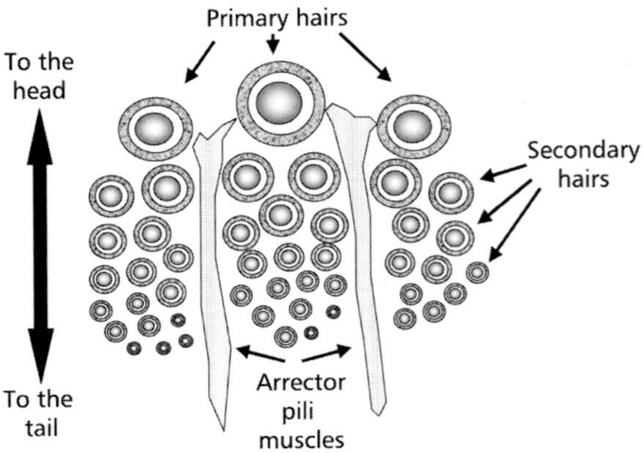

Figure 1.5.1. Canine follicular unit examined by horizontal sectioning. Follicular units usually consist of groupings of three compound hair follicles, each with its own follicular opening. In each compound follicle there is a large, anterior primary hair flanked by secondary hairs that become smaller caudally.

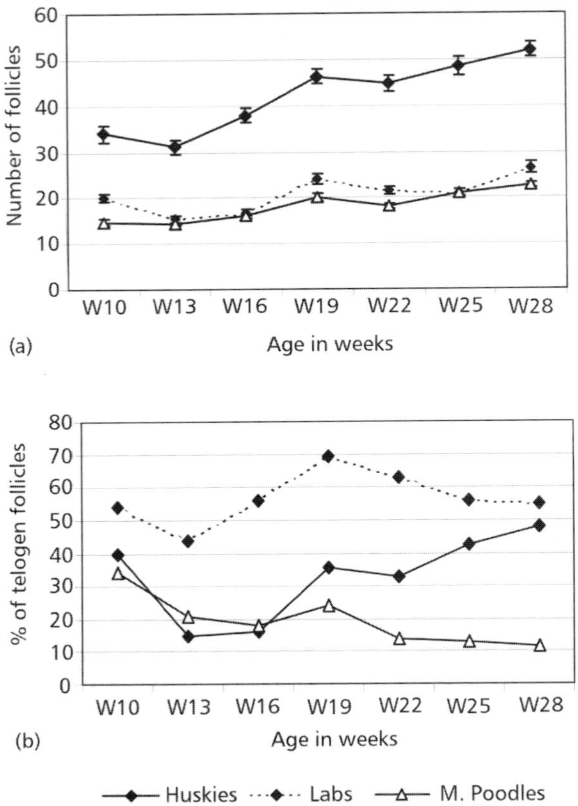

Figure 1.5.2. (a) Mean number of hair follicles per follicular unit for Siberian huskies, Labrador retrievers and miniature poodles. Each data point represents the mean ± SEM of 12 dogs. (b) Percentage of telogen follicles for Siberian huskies, Labrador retrievers and miniature poodles.

noted. In general, the more compound follicles in a follicular unit, the larger the central anatomical primary follicle and the hair shaft it produces.

The morphometric evaluation of the number of hair follicles and the hair cycle is presented in Figure 1.5.2a and b, respectively. For each breed, the mean number of hair follicles per follicular unit increased over the course of the study. The increase was most dramatic for Siberian huskies and miniature poodles (approximately 50%) and less for Labrador retrievers (approximately 30%). The percentage of follicles in telogen in the miniature poodles decreased throughout the study, whereas the number of telogen follicles increased in Siberian huskies. For Labrador retrievers, the mean number of telogen follicles decreased from week 10 to week 16 and then the number increased. At the end of the study, both Siberian huskies and Labrador retrievers had approximately 50% of their follicles in telogen. In contrast, the miniature poodles examined had only 12% of their follicles in telogen.

The data obtained from OFDA analysis defined marked breed differences in both diameter (Figure 1.5.3a) and curvature of hair shafts (Figure 1.5.3b). As was noted on the DermScope images and examination of horizontal histological sections, Labrador retrievers had the largest mean diameter, with Siberian huskies having a slightly larger mean diameter than miniature poodles. These differences were slightly less noticeable at week 10 than at week 28. For the Labrador retrievers, the mean diameters increased from week 10 to 16 and then approached the week 10 level at the end of the study. In contrast, the mean diameters of the Siberian huskies and miniature poodles decreased over the course of the study, with a greater rate of decline in the Siberian huskies.

Of the three breeds studied, hair samples from Siberian huskies had the greatest mean curvature. In addition, the curvature in this breed increased from week 13 to 19 and then decreased slightly. Miniature poodle hair had only a slightly greater mean curvature than Labrador retrievers. Hair samples from the miniature poodles did not change substantively during the course of the study. The hair samples from the Labradors decreased in curvature from week 13 to 19, increased by week 22 and then remained constant for the final two measurement periods.

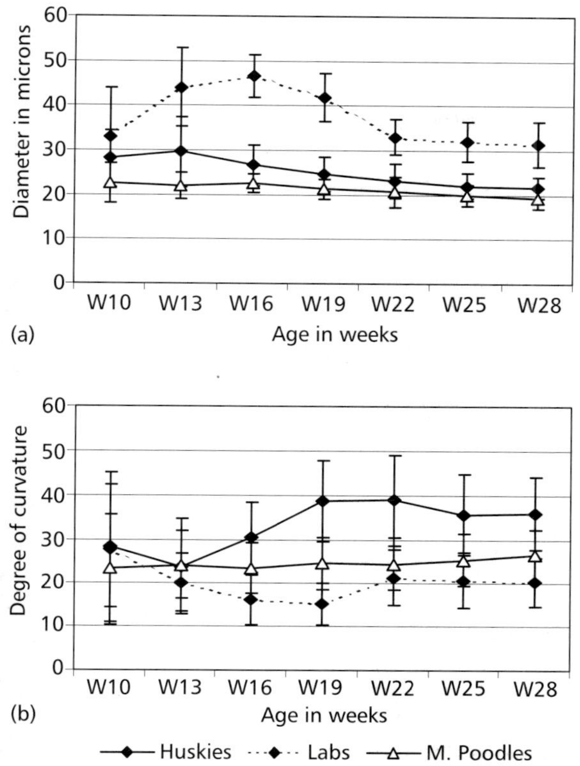

Figure 1.5.3. (a) Optical-based Fibre Diameter Analyser (OFDA) results of mean hair diameter for Siberian huskies, Labrador retrievers and miniature poodles. (b) OFDA results of mean degree of curvature for Siberian huskies, Labrador retrievers and miniature poodles. Each data point represents the mean ± SEM of 12 dogs.

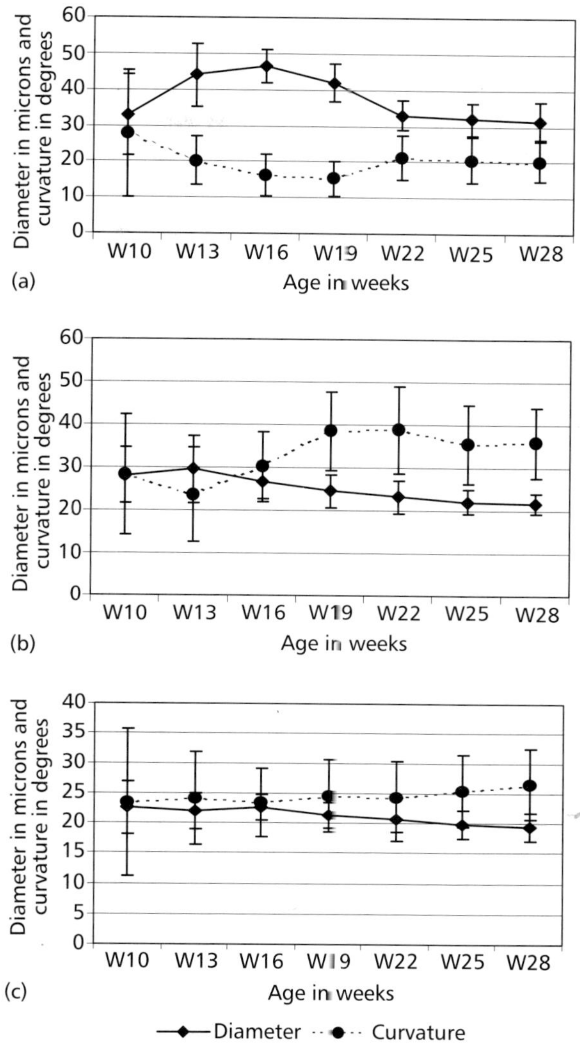

Figure 1.5.4. (a) Optical-based Fibre Diameter Analyser (OFDA) results of mean hair shaft diameter and degree of curvature for Labrador retrievers. (b) OFDA results of mean hair shaft diameter and degree of curvature for Siberian huskies. (c) OFDA results of mean hair shaft diameter and degree of curvature for miniature poodles. Each data point represents the mean ± SEM of 12 dogs.

The presence of a relationship between hair diameter and curvature is defined by graphing these data together for each breed (Figures 1.5.4a–c). For Labrador retrievers, the increase in diameter correlated with a decrease in curvature; for Siberian huskies, the hair diameter decreased as the curvature increased; for miniature poodles, the differences appeared negligible, with only a slight increase in curvature and a slight decrease in diameter.

Discussion

In this study, multiple techniques were used to assess the morphology of the canine hair follicle, the hairs it produced, the number of hairs shafts per follicular unit, the number of follicles in telogen, and the diameter and degree of curvature of these hairs. In combination, these techniques provide a better means of assessing the pelage of the dog than previously used methods. These techniques were applied in an attempt to understand what happens when a dog loses its puppy coat.

Based on this analysis, the maturational changes that occur in the hair follicles are breed specific and what has been described as the 'loss of a puppy coat' is better thought of as the 'gain of an adult coat'. In the three breeds examined, the period of 10–28 weeks of age is associated with an increase in the number of hair follicles and a change in the type of actively growing hairs that are produced, as described below.

In Siberian huskies, during the 18 week period examined, the growing follicles are predominantly those that produce smaller diameter hair shafts that are highly curved. These data indicate that for Siberian huskies, the gain of an adult coat is associated with an increase in the number of highly twisted hair shafts that make up the dense, air-filled undercoat of this breed.

A very different pattern of 'puppy coat loss' occurs in Labrador retrievers. At the start of the study, the coat of the Labrador retrievers had fewer hairs per follicular unit than Siberian huskies, but the diameter and degree of curvature were quite similar. Over the course of the investigation, there was a period in which relatively straight, large-diameter hair shafts were produced. This corresponds to the replacement of the fine, soft and moderately curly Labrador retriever puppy coat with the coarse pelage that defines the adult hair coat of the breed.

In miniature poodles, only minimal changes were identified in the diameter and curvature of hair shafts over the 18 weeks of investigation. Thus, in this breed, it seems that the gain of an adult coat is associated with an increase in the number of follicles, but the diameter of these follicles remains fairly constant.

That Siberian huskies had the largest number of follicles per follicular unit was expected; however, it was surprising that miniature poodles and Labrador retrievers had approximately the same number of follicles per follicular unit, as it was thought that miniature poodles would have a denser pelage. It is possible that the number of follicles per follicular unit may not be the only indicator of the density of the hair coat. In this study, no attempt was made to determine how close the follicular units were to each other. If the follicular units of the miniature poodle are closer together than those of the Labrador retriever, then the coat of miniature poodles would have been denser even though each follicular unit produced the same number of hair shafts. It was also surprising that the mean curvature of the hair from miniature poodles was closer to a Labrador than a Siberian husky. However, on closer inspection, the curvature of undercoat (anatomical secondary follicles) from adolescent Siberian huskies is curlier than the primary and secondary hair shafts from adolescent miniature poodles. However, this is a transient stage of follicular growth. Ongoing studies by the authors have shown that as miniature poodles age, their hair shafts eventually become curlier than those of even Siberian huskies (data not shown), as one would expect.

Another unexpected finding was that at the conclusion of the study, approximately 50% of the follicles in Labrador retrievers and Siberian huskies were in telogen. This observation has profound implications on the histological assessment by pathologists who may consider a dog with >50% of its follicles in telogen to be abnormal. In the authors' experience, most adult dogs that do not require hair cuts will have the majority of their follicles in telogen (Credille *et al.*, 2002). Similarly, because miniature poodles have <10% of their follicles in telogen, observations of >10% of telogen hairs in this breed may indicate an underlying pathological condition.

Finally, although all the techniques used in this study were of value in defining the morphology of the canine hair follicle, the single most important technique was horizontal sectioning of biopsy samples. Although seldom used by veterinary dermatopathologists, this method of histological evaluation of the hair follicle is critical for accurate morphological assessment.

References

American Kennel Club (1997) *The Complete Dog Book*, 19th edn. Howell Book House, New York.

Baxter, B. P., Brims, M. A. & Taylor, T. B. (1992) Description and performance of the optical fibre diameter analyser. *Journal of the Textile Institute*, **83**, 507–526.

Brunsch, A. (1956) Vergleichende Untersuchungen am Harrkleid von Wildcaniden und Haushunden. *Zeitschrift für Tiersucht und Zuchtungs Biologie*, **67**, 205–240.

Credille, K. M., Slater, M. R., Nachreiner, R. F., Tucker, K. A. & Dunstan, R. W. (2001) The effects of thyroid hormones on the skin of beagle dogs. *Journal of Veterinary Internal Medicine*, **15**, 539–546.

Gair, R. (1928) Die Wuchsformen des Haarkleides bei Haustieren nach Untersuchungen beim Hunde. *Zeitschrift für Tiersucht und Zuchtungs Biologie*, **11**, 57–58.

Headington, J. T. (1984) Transverse microscopic anatomy of the human scalp. A basis for a morphometric approach to disorders of the hair follicle. *Archives of Dermatology*, **120**, 449–456.

Lupton, C. J. (1995) Standard deviation of fiber diameter and other characteristics of United States wool. *Sheep and Goat Research Journal*, **3**, 11–121.

Nixon, A. J. (1993) A method for determining the activity state of hair follicles. *Biotechnic and Histochemistry*, **68**, 316–325.

1.6

Evaluation of radiography, otoscopy, pneumotoscopy, impedance audiometry and endoscopy for the diagnosis of otitis media in the dog

L.K. Cole DVM, MS, K.W. Kwochka DVM, M. Podell DVM, MS, A. Hillier BVSc and D.D. Smeak DVM

Department of Veterinary Clinical Sciences, College of Veterinary Medicine, The Ohio State University, Columbus, Ohio, USA

Summary

Forty-five dogs with chronic recurrent otitis externa were evaluated for otitis media using radiography, otoscopy, pneumotoscopy, tympanometry and the acoustic reflex. The results of these diagnostic tests were compared with the results of culture and cytology from the middle ear obtained by myringotomy. The diagnosis of otitis media was made if infection was detected by either method.

Of the 90 ears evaluated, 80 (88.9%) ears had concurrent otitis media and the tympanic membrane was intact in 58 of 80 (72.5%) ears. Seventeen different organisms were isolated from the horizontal ear canal and 16 organisms from the middle ear. The high false-negative rates of all the tests resulted in low sensitivities and negative predictive values; therefore, many ears with otitis media were not identified and myringotomy appears to be the optimum technique for the diagnosis of otitis media. However, in the ears with an abnormal test, over 90% had otitis media. Therefore, otitis media should be suspected when an abnormal test is obtained radiographically, otoscopically, pneumotoscopically or by impedance audiometry in a dog with chronic recurrent otitis externa.

Introduction

In one study it was found that in dogs with chronic otitis externa, 82.6% have undiagnosed concurrent otitis media (Cole *et al.*, 1998). Evaluation of chronic otitis in the dog may include a medical history, physical examination, otoscopic examination of the external ear canal and tympanic membrane, radiographs, computed tomography or magnetic resonance imaging of the tympanic bulla, cytology and culture and susceptibility of the horizontal ear canal and middle ear, impedance audiometry, biopsies of the middle ear and myringotomy (Neer & Howard, 1982; Harvey, 1985; Shell, 1988; Remedios *et al.*, 1991; Bruyette & Lorenz, 1993; Rosychuk, 1994).

Studies have been performed in dogs which assess radiography (Remedios *et al.*, 1991; Hoskinson, 1993), otoscopy (Little & Lane, 1989) and impedance audiometry (Penrod, 1980; Forsythe, 1985; Sims *et al.*, 1986; Sims, 1988; Little & Lane, 1989) as individual diagnostic techniques for evaluation of the canine ear. No one study has been conducted to evaluate all three techniques for the diagnosis of otitis media in dogs with chronic otitis externa. To the authors' knowledge, there have been no studies published evaluating the use of pneumotoscopy or endoscopy in the dog for the diagnosis of otitis media.

The purpose of this study was to assess and correlate radiography, otoscopy, pneumotoscopy, impedance audiometry and endoscopy with the presence of otitis media diagnosed by myringotomy in dogs with chronic recurrent otitis externa.

Materials and methods

Inclusion criteria

Ohio State University Veterinary Teaching Hospital Board approval was obtained for the study procedures and informed consent was obtained from the owners. Forty-five dogs with chronic bilateral otitis externa referred consecutively to The Ohio State University Veterinary Teaching Hospital were entered into the study. There were no age, breed or sex requirements. Chronic otitis externa was defined as recurrent or continuous external ear infections of at least 6 months' duration. A diagnosis of otitis media was made on the basis of exudate in the middle ear and cytological or culture evidence of bacterial or yeast infection. Previous or concurrent topical, oral or parenteral treatment did not exclude a dog from the study. All dogs had been given numerous medications; however, none of the dogs was given medication the day they entered the study.

Diagnostic tests

The dogs were hospitalized for 2 days for the diagnostic procedures. Swab specimens for cytological examination and bacterial culture and susceptibility testing (C/S) were taken from the horizontal canal of each ear. Blood was drawn for a complete blood count (CBC) and serum biochemical analysis as preanesthetic screening tests.

On the following day each dog was premedicated and placed under general anesthesia with isoflurane for the procedures, which were performed in the order listed below. The choice of anesthetic premedication was made on the basis of age, disposition and health status of each dog.

Bulla radiographs were performed to visualize the bone integrity of the tympanic bulla along with soft-tissue changes in the external auditory canal. The views included were the dorsoventral, open mouth rostral caudal, and right and left lateral obliques. The radiographs were interpreted by one of two board-certified radiologists or by one of two radiology residents under direct supervision of one of the radiologists. Radiographic signs deemed to represent or be suspicious of otitis media included thickening of the bulla, lysis of the bulla or petrous temporal bone, opacity in the bulla, or sclerosis and bony proliferation of the petrous temporal bone. The presence and severity, or absence, of external or middle ear disease was recorded.

Each ear was soaked for 10 min with a ceruminolytic ear cleaner (Pan-Otic, Pfizer Animal Health, Exton, PA, USA). The ears were subsequently flushed with warmed sterile isotonic saline (0.9% NaCl) solution, using a disposable bulb syringe. The horizontal ear canal was examined using a hand-held otoscope (Welch Allyn diagnostic closed head otoscope; Welch Allyn, Skaneateles Falls, NY, USA) with a gas-sterilized otoscopic cone (Welch Allyn specula, Welch Allyn). A final flush was performed with isotonic saline solution infused through the otoscopic cone using an 8 F polypropylene urinary catheter (Sovereign polypropylene catheter; Sherwood Medical, St Louis, MO, USA) cut to a length of 9 cm and attached to a 12 ml syringe. The ear canal was dried by passing an open-end Tom cat catheter attached to a 12 ml syringe through the otoscopic cone to aspirate as much fluid as possible from the canal.

Otoscopy was performed using a hand-held diagnostic head otoscope and otoscopic cone to visualize the tympanic membrane. The tympanic membrane was classified as present (intact, partial tear) or absent. In some cases, the horizontal ear canal was so stenotic that the tympanic membrane was recorded as not visualized.

Pneumotoscopy was performed using a hand-held diagnostic head otoscope and otoscopic cone fitted with a pneumatic bulb to assess directly the compliance of the tympanic membrane. The otoscope was placed into the external ear canal and air pressure in the external ear canal was increased and decreased with the pneumatic bulb while observing the motion (compliance) of the tympanic membrane (Gates, 1986). The compliance was subjectively assessed as present or absent in those ears in which the tympanic membrane was visualized.

Impedance audiometry procedures consisted of tympanometry and induction of the acoustic reflex. These tests were performed using a middle ear analyzer (GSI 33 Middle-Ear Analyzer; Grayson-Stadler Inc., Littleton, MA, USA) as described previously (Cole *et al.*, 2000). Tympanometry is the measurement of changes in the ear drum compliance as pressure in the external ear canal is changed (Sims, 1988).

The acoustic reflex is the involuntary action of the middle ear muscles in response to a sound stimulus, resulting in a decrease in tympanic membrane compliance (Sims, 1988). Ipsilateral acoustic reflexes were tested at the ear canal pressure at which a peak was present in the tympanogram corresponding to maximum compliance, or at 0 daPa if there was no peak pressure. At each stimulus, the change in compliance was recorded in milliliters. An acoustic reflex was classified as present with a negative deflection on the meter and a 0.02 ml or greater change in compliance.

The endoscope (Storz 2.7 mm pediatric endoscope; Karl Storz Veterinary Endoscope-America Inc., Kennett Square, PA, USA) was placed into the external ear canal and advanced as far into the horizontal ear canal as possible to evaluate the tympanic membrane. The tympanic membrane was classified as present (intact, partial tear) or absent. In some cases, the horizontal ear canal was so stenotic that the tympanic membrane was recorded as not visualized.

If the tympanic membrane was visualized and present (intact, partial tear), a myringotomy was performed by passing a sterile culture swab (Calgiswab Type 1; Spectrum Microgon, Laguna Hills, CA, USA) through a new gas-sterilized otoscopic cone into the caudoventral quadrant of the tympanic membrane. The first swab was used to perform the myringotomy and obtain a sample from the middle ear for bacterial C/S. A second swab was passed through the original incision to obtain a sample for cytological analysis. A diagnosis of a 'false middle ear' was made when the swab was unable to penetrate what appeared to be an intact tympanic membrane into the middle ear cavity. This was not a cholesteatoma, since a mass was not found in the ear canal. If the tympanic membrane was absent, the two sterile culture swabs were passed consecutively into the middle ear cavity for bacterial C/S and cytological analysis, respectively.

If the tympanic membrane was not visualized because of stenosis of the horizontal ear canal, two sterile swabs were blindly passed consecutively into the middle ear cavity for bacterial C/S and cytological analysis, respectively. The tympanic membrane was recorded as intact if the first swab was felt to pass through the tympanic membrane into the middle ear cavity. If no membrane was felt prior to reaching the middle ear cavity, then the tympanic membrane was recorded as absent. All swab specimens were examined to determine whether there was exudate in the middle ear and the color was recorded.

Morphological identification of the yeast, *Malassezia pachydermatis* (Ihrke, 1996), and bacterial organisms (Cole *et al.*, 1998) by light microscopy has been described previously. The sample was rolled onto a glass microscope slide and stained (Diff-Quik Fixative; Baxter Healthcare Corporation Dade Division, Miami, FL, USA) after heat-fixing. Yeast or bacterial organisms were counted from 10 consecutive, random, oil-immersion fields (1000×) and the mean number of organisms per field was calculated. If the mean number of yeast or bacterial organisms per oil-immersion field was ≥4, the yeast or bacterium was considered a significant pathogen (Ihrke, 1996; Cole *et al.*, 1998).

Swab samples taken for bacterial C/S were plated on blood agar and MacConkey's medium and incubated at 35°C for 18–24 h. Organisms were identified by routine biochemical testing.

After sample collection, the middle ear was flushed with warmed 0.9% NaCl. Exudate on the sterile culture swab along with cytological or microbial culture evidence of bacteria or yeast from the middle ear established the diagnosis of otitis media.

Statistical analysis

Chi-squared tests for independence using a 2 × 2 contingency table (GBStat; Dynamics System, Silver Spring, MD, USA) for the diagnosis of otitis media between radiography, otoscopy, pneumotoscopy, tympanometry, acoustic reflex and myringotomy were applied. A *p*-value of less than 0.05 was considered significant.

The sensitivity, specificity, positive predictive value, negative predictive value and accuracy of radiography, otoscopy, pneumotoscopy, tympanometry, and the acoustic reflex for the diagnosis of otitis media compared to results from myringotomy were calculated.

Results

Demographic data

In total, 27 (60.0%) female dogs (25 spayed) and 18 (40.0%) male dogs (nine castrated) were entered into the study. Breeds represented included Labrador retriever (*n* = 11), cocker spaniel (11), German shepherd dog (6), golden retriever (2), giant schnauzer (2), old English sheepdog (1), beagle (1), basset Hound (1), English bulldog (1), Dalmatian (1), West Highland white terrier (1), akita (1), English springer spaniel (1) and sealyham terrier (1). Four mixed-breed dogs were identified.

Dogs ranged in age from 1.5 to 12 years old (median 5 years). The duration of the chronic otitis externa ranged from 7 months to 10.5 years (median 2 years). Age at onset of the otitis ranged from 2 months to 10.5 years (median 2.5 years).

Clinical signs

The most common clinical signs of otitis reported by the owners were shaking the head and scratching the ears. In 11 of 45 (24.4%) dogs, the only dermatological abnormality was the otitis externa, while 34 of 45 (75.6%) dogs had clinical signs of concurrent skin problems reported by the owner, which included pruritus, licking or chewing the feet, pyoderma, seborrhea sicca or fleas.

Ears diagnosed with otitis media

Of the 45 dogs with chronic bilateral otitis externa, 39 had bilateral otitis media, one had unilateral otitis media, three did not have otitis media in either ear, one had a unilateral 'false middle ear' and unilateral otitis media, and one had bilateral 'false middle ears'. Therefore, of the 90 ears evaluated with chronic recurrent otitis externa, 80 (88.9%) ears had concurrent otitis media. When the sterile culture swab was passed into the middle ear for sample collection, the tympanic membrane was found to be intact in 58 of 80 (72.5%) ears with otitis media.

Test results

Seventeen different organisms were isolated from the horizontal ear canal and 16 organisms from the middle ear (Table 1.6.1).

Analysis for independence between myringotomy and each test employed (radiography, otoscopy, pneumotoscopy, tympanometry, acoustic reflex) demonstrated no relationship between these tests ($p > 0.05$). Therefore, each test was treated separately for sensitivity and specificity analysis.

Radiographic signs suggestive of external ear disease were found in 75 of 90 (83.3%) ears with clinical otitis externa and included narrowing of the external auditory canal in 41 of 75 (54.7%) ears, calcification of the external auditory canal in 28 of 75 (37.3%) ears, and obliteration of the external auditory canal by a soft-tissue opacity in 22 of 75 (29.3%) ears. The data for radiography from the ears with a diagnosis of a 'false middle ear' were not analyzed. Thirteen of 87 (14.9%) ears had radiographic signs of otitis media, including thickening of the bulla in 11 of 13 (84.6%) ears, lysis of the bulla in one of 13 (7.7%) ears, and opacity in the bulla in seven of 13 (53.8%) ears. The results from radiography were compared with the results from myringotomy for the diagnosis of otitis media (Tables 1.6.2, 1.6.3).

Table 1.6.1. Organisms isolated from swab specimens obtained from the horizontal ear canal and middle ears of 45 dogs with chronic otitis externa

Organism	% of all isolates		% of all ears	
	HEC	ME	HEC	ME
Staphylococcus intermedius	23	21.3	56.7	45
Yeast	21.4	12	58.9	28
Pseudomonas aeruginosa	14.5	19.1	27.8	31.3
Enterococcus spp.	8.9	9.3	20	21.3
Proteus spp.	8.5	12.6	20	25
β-Hemolytic streptococcus	7.7	8.2	17.8	18.8
Corynebacterium spp.	6.9	7.7	17.8	15
Escherichia coli	2.4	3.8	6.7	7.5
Group D non-enterococcus	1.2	NI	3.3	NI
Moraxella spp.	1.2	0.5	3.3	1.3
Pseudomonas spp.	0.8	0.5	1.1	1.3
Staphylococcus aureus	0.8	0.5	2.2	1.3
Pasteurella spp.	0.8	0.5	1.1	1.3
α-Hemolytic streptococcus	0.8	NI	2.2	NI
Coagulase-negative staphylococcus	0.4	0.5	1.1	1.3
Citrobacter spp.	0.4	0.5	1.1	1.3
Non-group D streptococcus	0.4	2.2	1.1	5
Lactobacillus spp.	NI	0.5	NI	1.3

HEC: horizontal ear canal; ME: middle ear; NI: not isolated.

Visualization to the level of the tympanic membrane was possible in 65 of 87 (74.7%) and 58 of 87 (66.7%) ears otoscopically and endoscopically, respectively, with an overall agreement between the two methods in 48 of 58 (82.8%) ears (Table 1.6.4). The results from otoscopy were compared with those from myringotomy for the diagnosis of otitis media (Tables 1.6.2, 1.6.3).

Pneumotoscopy was performed in the 61 ears in which the tympanic membrane was present. The data for pneumotoscopy from the ears with a diagnosis of a 'false middle ear' were not analyzed. The results from pneumotoscopy were compared with those from myringotomy for the diagnosis of otitis media (Tables 1.6.2, 1.6.3).

In the ears with otitis media, the exudate on the culture swab or in the flush from the middle ear was brown ceruminous in 37 of 80 (46.3%) ears, yellow ceruminous

Table 1.6.2. Results of radiography, otoscopy, pneumotoscopy, tympanometry and acoustic reflex compared with the results from myringotomy for the diagnosis of otitis media

Test results	Myringotomy diagnosis (no. of ears)	
	Otitis media	No otitis media
Radiography		
Otitis media	13	0
Normal	67	7
Otoscopy		
Non-intact tympanic membrane	11	0
Intact tympanic membrane	47	7
Pneumotoscopy		
No compliance	25	2
Compliance	29	5
Tympanometry		
Abnormal	27	2
Normal	25	5
Acoustic reflex		
Absent	30	2
Present	22	5

Table 1.6.3. Sensitivity, specificity, positive-predictive value, negative-predictive value and overall accuracy of radiography, otoscopy, pneumotoscopy, tympanometry and acoustic reflex compared with the results from myringotomy for the diagnosis of otitis media

Variable × 100% (formula)	Rad	Oto	Pneu	Tymp	AR
Sensitivity (TP/TP + FN)	16.3	19	46.3	51.9	57.7
Specificity (TN/TN + FP)	100	100	71.4	71.4	71.4
Positive-predictive value (TP/TP + FP)	100	100	92.6	93.1	93.8
Negative-predictive value (TN/TN + FN)	9.5	13	14.7	16.7	18.5
Overall accuracy (TP + TN/Total)	23	27.7	49.2	54.2	59.3

Rad: radiography; Oto: otoscopy; Pneu: pneumotoscopy; Tymp: tympanometry; AR: acoustic reflex; TP: true positive; FN: false negative; TN: true negative; FP: false positive.

in 36 of 80 (45%) ears, not recorded in three of 80 (3.8%) ears, mucoid in two of 80 (2.5%) ears, yellow purulent in one of 80 (1.2%) ears, and white in one of 80 (1.2%) ears.

Tympanometry and the acoustic reflex were performed on all ears. For tympanometry, if the pressure was less than −170 daPa in conjunction with a flat or sloped tympanogram, the pressure and compliance

Table 1.6.4. Comparison of endoscopic and otoscopic visualization of the tympanic membrane

Otoscopy (no. of ears)	Endoscopy (no. of ears)			
	Intact	Partial tear	Not intact	Not visualized
Intact	40	9	0	5
Partial tear	1	6	0	0
Not intact	0	0	2	2
Not visualized	0	0	0	22

peak values for that ear were changed to no compliance pressure reading and no compliance peak value, respectively. If the ear canal volume was greater than 5 ml in conjunction with an abnormal tracing, the data from that ear for tympanometry and the acoustic reflex were not analyzed, since those results were artifactual. The data for tympanometry and the acoustic reflex from the ears with a diagnosis of a 'false middle ear' or ears in which the tympanic membrane was not visualized were not analyzed. The results from tympanometry and the acoustic reflex were compared with those from myringotomy for the diagnosis of otitis media (Tables 1.6.2, 1.6.3).

Discussion

The results of this study indicate that infectious otitis media was present in 80 of 90 (88.9%) ears in dogs with chronic recurrent otitis externa and 58 of 80 (72.5%) ears had an intact tympanic membrane. This finding differs from a previous report of dogs with chronic otitis externa, in which 100 ears were examined at necropsy, and it was determined that 52 of those ears had tympanic membrane rupture and concurrent otitis media (Spreull, 1964). In that study, myringotomy was not performed in the remaining 48 ears to determine whether otitis media existed. In dogs with otitis externa, if otitis media exists and it is not diagnosed and treated, it is possible that the otitis will recur. Therefore, it is recommended that all dogs with chronic recurrent otitis externa be evaluated for concurrent otitis media.

Radiography, otoscopy, pneumotoscopy, tympanometry and acoustic reflex were evaluated for the diagnosis of infectious otitis media. Owing to the high false-negative rates of the procedures, resulting in low sensitivities and negative predictive values, many ears with otitis media were not identified and, therefore, none of these diagnostic tests would be recommended in place of performing a myringotomy in dogs with chronic otitis. However, when pneumotoscopy, tympanometry and acoustic reflex are used in children for the diagnosis of middle ear effusion, the sensitivity of the combined tests is 97% (Cantekin *et al.*, 1980). There are three reasons for the discrepancy in sensitivity of these three tests between dogs and humans. These tests evaluate compliance of the tympanic membrane either directly (pneumotoscopy) or indirectly (tympanometry, acoustic reflex), and fluid behind the tympanic membrane will result in non-compliance (Sims, 1988). In humans, otitis media is usually effusive, resulting in a non-compliant tympanic membrane; however, in this study, only three of 80 (3.8%) ears had an effusive otitis media. In the dogs' ears without effusion with a non-compliant tympanic membrane, it is possible that the non-compliance was due to a thickening or fibrosis of the tympanic membrane due to the chronic recurrent otitis externa. Furthermore, these tests are more difficult to perform in dogs than in humans, because of the shape of the external ear canal and the chronic changes that occur in dogs' ears with otitis.

However, in the ears in this study with an abnormal test, over 90% had infectious otitis media. Therefore, infectious otitis media should be suspected when an abnormal test is obtained radiographically, otoscopically, pneumotoscopically or by impedance audiometry in a dog with chronic otitis externa. In the clinical situation, otoscopy and pneumotoscopy would be the recommended diagnostic tests, since both are easy to perform and require minimal equipment.

Chronic recurrent otitis externa may lead to stenosis and hyperplasia of the horizontal ear canal, along with ulcerations from secondary infections. Owing to the stenosis of the horizontal ear canal, examination to the level of the tympanic membrane was possible otoscopically in only 65 of 87 (74.7%) ears. In some ears, the otoscopic examination caused the ears to become more stenotic and to bleed. Thus, when the endoscopic examination was performed after the otoscopic examination, visualization was possible in only 58 of the ears. However, in nine of the 58 (15.5%) ears, otoscopy misidentified the ear as having an intact tympanic membrane, while endoscopy revealed a partial tear. Therefore, endoscopy may be a better indicator of the patency of the tympanic membrane than otoscopy, but with both procedures, visualization may be impaired if stenosis or hemorrhage is present.

The diagnosis of infectious otitis media was made based on exudate in the middle ear and positive cytological or culture evidence of yeast or bacterial organisms. The assumption was made that in the ears in which the tympanic membrane was not visualized, the myringotomy swab was placed into the middle ear cavity. However, since the tympanic membrane was not visualized, it is possible that the exudate obtained on the myringotomy swab was obtained from the horizontal ear canal beyond the stenosis, before entry into the middle ear cavity. Furthermore, in the ears in which the tympanic membrane was not visualized, it was possible that there was a small tear in the tympanic membrane that was not evident when the myringotomy swab was passed into the middle ear cavity. Therefore, in the 22 ears in which the tympanic membrane was not visualized, there may be a question as to where the exudate was obtained and the patency of the tympanic membrane. However, this study was meant to replicate the types of clinical situation that practitioners face, in which the tympanic membrane may not be visualized owing to stenosis of the ear canal.

It has been suggested that in cases of chronic otitis externa with occlusion of the ear canal, a pocket of tympanic membrane may bulge into the middle ear cavity and adhere to the inflamed mucosa of the middle ear, resulting in a 'false middle ear' (Griffin, 1993; Logas, 1994). In this study, the diagnosis of a false middle ear was made based on the inability to pass the myringotomy swab through what appeared to be an intact tympanic membrane into the middle ear cavity. This diagnosis would need to be confirmed histopathologically. Because of the nature of the study, which used client-owned animals for the procedures, histopathology was not performed.

Conclusion

Infectious otitis media is common in dogs with chronic recurrent otitis externa. An abnormal test radiographically, pneumotoscopically or by impedance audiometry, or a non-intact tympanic membrane otoscopically is a good predictor of otitis media. However, owing to the poor sensitivity of these tests, none of them can be recommended to replace myringotomy.

Acknowledgements

This study was sponsored by Bayer Animal Health and The Ohio State University Canine Research Funds.

References

Bruyette, D. S. & Lorenz, M. D. (1993) Otitis externa and otitis media: diagnosis and medical aspects. *Seminars in Veterinary Medicine and Surgery (Small Animal)*, **8**, 3–9.

Cantekin, E. I., Bluestone, C. D., Fria, T. J., Stool, S. E., Beery, Q. C. & Sabo, D. L. (1980) Identification of otitis media with effusion in children. *Annals of Otology, Rhinology and Laryngology*, **89**, 190–195.

Cole, L. K., Kwochka, K. W., Kowalski, J. J. & Hillier, A. (1998) Microbial flora and antimicrobial susceptibility patterns of isolated pathogens from the horizontal ear canal and middle ear in dogs with otitis media. *Journal of the American Veterinary Medical Association*, **212**, 534–538.

Cole, L. K., Podell, M. & Kwochka, K. W. (2000) Impedance audiometric measurements in clinically normal dogs. *American Journal of Veterinary Research*, **61**, 442–445.

Forsythe, W. B. (1985) Tympanographic volume measurements of the canine ear. *American Journal of Veterinary Research*, **46**, 1351–1353.

Gates, G. A. (1986) Differential otomanometry. *American Journal of Otolaryngology*, **7**, 147–150.

Griffin, C. E. (1993) Otitis externa and media. In: *Current Veterinary Dermatology* (Eds C. E. Griffin, K. W. Kwochka & J. M. McDonald), pp. 244–262. Mosby Year Book, St Louis, MO.

Harvey, C. E. (1985) Diseases of the middle ear. In: *Textbook of Small Animal Surgery* (Ed. D. H. Slatter), pp. 1915–1923. W. B. Saunders, Philadelphia, PA.

Hoskinson, J. J. (1993) Imaging techniques in the diagnosis of middle ear disease. *Seminars in Veterinary Medicine and Surgery (Small Animal)*, **8**, 10–16.

Ihrke, P. J. (1996) Malassezia dermatitis and hypersensitivity. *Proceedings, North American Veterinary Conference*, Orlando, FL, January 15, 1996, pp. 45–48.

Little, C. J. L. & Lane, J. G. (1989) An evaluation of tympanometry, otoscopy, and palpation for assessment of the canine tympanic membrane. *Veterinary Record*, **124**, 5–8.

Logas, D. B. (1994) Diseases of the ear canal. *Veterinary Clinics of North America: Small Animal Practice*, **24**, 905–919.

Neer, T. M. & Howard, P. E. (1982) Otitis media. *Compendium on Continuing Education*, **4**, 410–417.

Penrod, J. P. (1980) The diagnostic uses of impedance audiometry in the dog. *Journal of the American Animal Hospital Association*, **16**, 941–948.

Remedios, A. M., Fowler, J. D. & Pharr, J. W. (1991) A comparison of radiographic versus surgical diagnosis of otitis media. *Journal of the American Animal Hospital Association*, **27**, 183–188.

Rosychuk, R. A. W. (1994) Management of otitis externa. *Veterinary Clinics of North America: Small Animal Practice*, **24**, 921–952.

Shell, L. G. (1988) Otitis media and otitis interna: etiology, diagnosis, and medical management. *Veterinary Clinics of North America: Small Animal Practice*, **18**, 885–899.

Sims, M. H. (1988) Electrodiagnostic evaluation of auditory function. *Veterinary Clinics of North America: Small Animal Practice*, **18**, 913–944.

Sims, M. H., Weigel, J. P. & Moore, R. E. (1986) Effects of tenotomy of the tensor tympani muscle on the acoustic reflex in dogs. *American Journal of Veterinary Research*, **47**, 1022–1031.

Spreull, J. S. A. (1964) Treatment of otitis media in the dog. *Journal of Small Animal Practice*, **5**, 107–152.

Part 2

Infectious and parasitic diseases

2.1

Changing trends in ectoparasite control

B.L. Blagburn PhD

College of Veterinary Medicine, Department of Pathobiology, Auburn University, Alabama, USA

Summary

The 1990s brought astounding advances in the knowledge, treatment and control of ectoparasitic diseases of companion animals. Successful flea control has been the primary target of pharmaceutical companies. This was achieved with topical or systemic adulticidal formulations of phenylpyrazole (fipronil), nitroguanidine (imidacloprid) and avermectin (selamectin) compounds. Formulations of ovicidal and/or larvicidal benzoylphenyl urea (lufenuron), pyridine (pyriproxyfen) and terpenoid (methoprene) compounds have also contributed to successful flea control. Use of these novel compounds has revolutionized our approaches to flea control and has rechannelled pet owners' interests towards the ethical veterinary product market. Certain trends are evident in the development of recent ectoparasiticides. Newer products clearly target a broader spectrum of parasites. Many of the newer products also possess claims against important nematode parasites such as heartworms and intestinal worms. This trend is likely to continue and will eventually yield products that target a variety of ectoparasites and many helminths including nematodes, flatworms such as tapeworms, and perhaps some flukes.

One challenge that confronts this industry is the need to develop strategies for deterrence of resistance to available agents. A recent industry/academic collaborative monitoring initiative is an excellent first step in dealing with this resistance challenge. Another challenge faced by parasite control experts is to quieten the increasingly loud voice of advocates for over-the-counter delivery of ectoparasiticides. The veterinary community can better monitor the efficacy, development of resistance, non-compliance and safety of these products if they remain under its supervision.

Introduction

The 1990s brought astounding advances in the understanding, treatment and control of several ectoparasitic diseases of companion animals. Although flea control remained the primary subject of developmental efforts by pharmaceutical companies, advances were also made in the treatment and control of other ectoparasite-induced diseases. This was achieved primarily by the development and introduction of newer, more effective anthelmintics, insecticides and acaricides. As we move into the first decade of the new millennium, several dominant trends are emerging that are likely to affect our approaches to ectoparasite control. Both opportunities and potential pitfalls are apparent in these trends. In this presentation, the intention is to discuss several of these trends and to review our progress in the control of selected companion animal ectoparasites. The review is not intended to be all-inclusive, nor should these comments be regarded as representing the views of all researchers in parasitology and dermatology.

Trends in companion animal ectoparasitology

Changes currently underway in the discipline of ectoparasitology can be viewed with optimism and opportunism or, in some instances, as potential threats or as negative impacts. Some of the general trends that may impact parasite control strategies in the near future are discussed briefly. Clearly, one trend that is seen in the development and marketing of companion animal parasiticides is an increase in the spectrum of activity exhibited by many of the newer agents. Many products now carry label claims for nematode, cestode, trematode and arthropod parasites (reviewed by Blagburn & Lindsay, 1995; Courtney & Roberson, 1995; Roberson & Courtney, 1995). This is achieved either by combining existing parasiticides or by introducing newer single-entity agents with broad-spectrum properties. Use of such agents allows veterinarians to target several potentially problematic parasites without the necessity of using multiple treatments. Many of these newer agents also are administered at convenient intervals (e.g. monthly) to promote compliance and to emphasize prevention and control strategies. In addition, products available for control of endoparasites and ectoparasites are more likely to be marketed in a greater variety of formulations. Oral, topical and injectable formulations are now available to provide the veterinarian with options to deal with individual pet and pet owner situations and circumstances. These trends of broad-spectrum emphasis and diversity of formulations are likely to continue, given the positive responses that such products have received.

There also is an increasing interest in potentially zoonotic parasites of companion animals and the need to prevent the transmission of the these parasites from pet animals to people (Blagburn, 1999). Because of this interest, it could be viewed as an opportunity to include ectoparasite control into this strategy. The combined use of agents or the use of broad-spectrum endectocides (except for cestodes), whether for the control of zoonotic internal parasites or for their ectoparasiticidal properties, could increase the use of these products and aid the control efforts.

Few would disagree that the domestic cat remains unexploited in terms of preventive veterinary medicine in many parts of the world. Certainly, veterinary care providers in North America see fewer cats than dogs on a regular basis. The reasons may be that pet owners think that cats do not acquire parasite-induced diseases as frequently as do dogs or that, because they generally are restricted to indoor habitats, cats are not exposed to potentially infectious agents, as dogs are. Nonetheless, many of the new agents, because of their spectrum of activity and convenience of use, can aid greatly in increasing the numbers of cats placed on parasite prevention or control regimens.

Another opportunity that enhances our development and use of parasiticides is the growth in communication afforded by the Internet and the World Wide Web. One can speak with colleagues, exchange case and treatment information, e-mail photographs and consult expert sources of information by simply logging onto a computer. The numbers and diversity of websites available to veterinary parasitologists and dermatologists is extensive and growing (Noxon, 1999). These sites, together with the growing numbers of specialty group lists created to facilitate intradisciplinary and interdisciplinary communication, has had a great effect on the approach to diagnosis and treatment of parasitic diseases. One can only imagine what future technologies will add to this already indispensable resource.

In addition to opportunities for advances in these disciplines, there exist some perceived threats or causes for concern. Among them are the ever-increasing numbers of excellent products available for parasite control. Although viewed as a resource or opportunity by many people, the many products may cause some confusion as to which products to use in different circumstances. It remains the responsibility of the veterinary community to remain knowledgeable of the efficacy and safety profiles of marketed parasiticides and to recommend actively the most effective products and regimens based on individual pet situations. Similarly, with the introduction of many new vaccines and flea and tick prevention products, pet owners are faced with an ever-increasing array of preventive products. Strategies need to be identified to deal with the possible attitude of 'overprevention'. It may be that practitioners must become more discretionary and develop priorities for prevention recommendations, and be prepared to justify them. They must also remain informed of the 'over-the-counter' pet parasiticide market. Although many of the products that are sold directly to consumers can be used effectively and safely, pet owners often lack the training and knowledge in parasite biology and behavior that is necessary to develop successful treatment and control strategies.

Current trends in flea control

Flea infestation and the allergic dermatitis that it may cause remain among the more difficult of canine and feline dermatological conditions to control (Carlotti & Jacobs, 2000). During the past decade, several safe, effective and convenient on-animal and environmental flea control agents have been introduced. These products have led to a level of flea control that was not possible with previous agents. Why have these newer products been so successful? The answers are quite simple. First, the biological behavior of the cat flea (*Ctenocephalides felis*) is now better understood. Veterinarians are more knowledgeable and pet owners are better informed as to how flea behavior can affect successful flea control. Secondly, the convenience of use and improved efficacy of the new products have resulted in much better pet owner compliance and persistence in the implementation of flea eradication and control initiatives.

The approach to the control of fleas and flea allergy dermatitis is not likely to change dramatically in the coming decade. What is likely to change is the spectrum of products and product formulations (i.e. topical, oral, injectable) available and either the combination of agents or the identification of novel new agents that will allow product label claims to be broadened. Regarding the latter, many future products will be active against common endoparasites and ectoparasites and will retain the safety and convenience of current products. Examples of this latest trend are seen in some of the products discussed below. One additional point that must be addressed in the near future is the potential impact of insecticide resistance on the efficacy of available products and successful flea control. The development of resistant populations of fleas could mean a return to the previous situation, with fleas and flea-induced disease once again being a difficult or unmanageable problem.

Lessons from flea biology

A considerable body of information is now available on the developmental cycle of fleas in general and the common cat flea in particular (Rust & Dryden, 1997). However, the information most relevant to successful flea control may be condensed into a few points. First, the vast majority of life stages (eggs, larvae and pupae) of the flea remain off the host and inaccessible in many cases to on-animal agents. This is particularly important for the resting adults in the pupa (cocoon). Latent, unstimulated adults can emerge over extended developmental periods, leaving the unknowing pet owner with the false presumption that control efforts are having little effect. This is particularly true when these stages are in locations where the pet spends time, unbeknownst to the pet owner. Secondly, the life cycle of the flea is driven by abiotic factors such as temperature and relative humidity, and these conditions impose differential effects on the length of the life cycle, depending on geographical location. Cooler, drier climates result in longer life cycles, while warmer, humid climates support shorter cycles. Thirdly, *C. felis* demonstrates a lack of host specificity. The presence of cat fleas on many mammalian species, including some urban-adapted wildlife, can create sources of fleas in the pet's environment that are not immediately apparent to the pet owner. Finally, the female flea has prolific egg-laying capabilities. A small residual population of surviving fleas can produce many eggs in a short period. Fleas survive even the most effective of agents as their residual activity diminishes, and these fleas can serve as a continuing environmental source of reinfestation. If veterinarians remember and communicate these points to pet owners, many of their inquiries about perceived lack of efficacy will be eliminated.

The agents

Most of the recent success in the control of fleas is the result of newer safe, convenient and effective products. The traditional carbamate, organophosphate and botanical insecticides and their derivatives (Table 2.1.1) have given way to new chemical classes of insect growth regulators (IGRs), insect development inhibitors (IDIs) and residual adulticides. These agents, together with some new chemistry currently in development in many laboratories, will form the foundation for future treatment strategies.

Insect growth regulators/insect development inhibitors

Lufenuron, methoprene, pyriproxyfen and other IGRs/IDIs exert their effects on flea eggs or larvae (Blagburn, 1996). They do so either by interfering with the development of chitin or chitinous structures or by disrupting the hormonal signals necessary for successful development and molting. These agents are administered either orally, by injection (lufenuron) or topically (pyriproxyfen, methoprene) and as such provide long-term (generally 30 days or more) ovicidal and larvicidal effects. Because these agents have no exploitable effect on adult fleas, many veterinarians and pet owners have abandoned them for the agents that kill adult fleas. However, these agents should not be abandoned too quickly, as there is continuing convincing evidence of their successful control of fleas in many situations. Lufenuron is available as a single entity product (Program; Novartis Animal Health, Greenboro, NC, USA) for dogs or cats and is combined with milbemycin oxime (Sentinel; Novartis Animal Health) to provide broad-spectrum internal parasite control as well as heartworm prevention and intestinal nematode control for dogs. It is also available in an injectable formulation for use in cats. Pyriproxyfen is available in spray,

Table 2.1.1. Insecticides used for on-animal and/or environmental control of canine or feline flea infestations

Chemical class	Mode(s) of action	Compounds	Properties/comments
Organochlorines	Inhibition of cytochrome oxidase; inhibition of GABA	Lindane, methoxychlor	Persistent in environment; toxic to cats; not universally available
Organophosphates	Irreversible inhibition of acetylcholinesterase	Chlorpyrifos, cythioate, dichlorvos, diazinon, fenthion and others	Some may be toxic; some have short residual activity; available in systemic and topical formulations
Carbamates	Reversible inhibition of acetylcholinesterase	Carbaryl, propoxur	Some have short residual activity; potentially toxic
Plant derivatives			
Citrus extract	Similar to pyrethrins (see below)	D-Limonene	Virtually non-toxic to warm-blooded animals
Derris extract	Inhibits respiratory enzymes (acts between NAD^+ and coenzyme Q)	Rotenone	Minimal efficacy against fleas; potentially toxic to cats
Pyrethrins	Modulate neurotransmission via sodium channels	Mixture of several natural extracts	Very quick kill; little residual activity
Synthetic pyrethroids	Modulate neurotransmission via sodium channels and by inhibition of GABA	Bioallethrin, cyfluthrin, cypermethrin, deltamethrin, permethrin and others	Very quick kill; residual activity better than prototype pyrethrins; some are toxic to cats
Phenylpyrazoles	Modulate neurotransmission via GABA-gated chloride channels	Fipronil	Quick kill of fleas; activity includes fleas and ticks; excellent residual activity
Neonicotinoids			
Nitroguanidines	Modulate neurotransmission via postsynaptic binding to nicotinic receptors	Imidacloprid	Very quick kill; good residual activity
Nitroenamines		Nitenpyram	Extremely quick kill; short residual activity
Avermectins	Modulate neurotransmission via glutamate-gated chloride channels	Selamectin	Broad spectrum, includes fleas, ticks and mites; good residual activity
Insect growth regulators	Inhibit embryogenesis and molting by competing with endogenous developmental hormones	Methoprene, fenoxycarb, pyriproxyfen, cyromazine and others	No exploitable effects on adult fleas; often used in environmental products; can be used with adulticides to shorten period required to control infestations; good residual activity; very safe
Insect development inhibitors	Inhibit chitin biosynthesis or deposition	Lufenuron, diflubenzuron and others	No exploitable effects on adult fleas; good residual activity; can be used with adulticides to shorten period required to control infestations; very safe
Activated orthoboric acid	Desiccation; toxicity to insect gut	Sodium polyborate	For use indoors or in sheltered outdoor areas; only effective against larval stages; good residual activity
Mineral insecticides	Desiccation; damage to insect cuticle	Silica gel, diatomaceous earth	For environmental use

Modified from Carlotti & Jacobs (2000).
GABA: γ-aminobutyric acid; NAD^+: oxidized form of nicotinamide-adenine dinucleotide.

spot-on and collar formulations for both dogs and cats. The collar formulation can be particularly appealing because it provides long-term ovicidal effects without the need for periodic treatment. A likely future trend is the combination of these agents with products that kill adult fleas. The strength of such combinations is two-fold. First, they are likely to decrease the time necessary to control flea infestations. This is particularly important in the case of heavy flea infestations or when pet owners are experiencing flea bites. Secondly, when used in combination with adulticidal compounds, the likelihood of development of resistance is diminished considerably, since the flea life cycle is being disrupted at different points and by entirely different mechanisms.

Adulticides

The traditional insecticides, including carbamates, organophosphates, organochlorines, pyrethrins and pyrethroids, have largely given way to the safer, more effective agents discussed below. Although they remain as active ingredients in a number of ethical and over-the-counter products, as well as in many environmental products, they are no longer used with the frequency that they once were. A brief summary of these agents is given in Table 2.1.1.

Imidacloprid (Advantage; Bayer Animal Health, Shawnee Mission, KS, USA) is a member of the nitroguanidine subclass of neonicotinoid insecticides (Table 2.1.1). It is currently marketed as a 9.1% w/w solution which, when applied topically at 10 mg/kg, is completely distributed over the animal's body within 24 h. It has potent activity against adult fleas, but lacks any apparent repellent activity. Imidacloprid is among the fastest acting flea adulticides. When applied topically to dogs at approximately 10 mg/kg, imidacloprid achieved an 86.6% level of flea control within 6 h of application. Efficacy improved to 97.6% within 12 h (Everett *et al.*, 2000). The efficacy of imidacloprid is retained at 97.8–100% for dogs and 90–96% for cats until day 28 (Hopkins *et al.*, 1997). Imidacloprid does not prevent fleas from feeding for the short time that they survive on the dog or cat host (Marsella, 1999). However, in fairness it would be difficult for any topical insecticide to possess such properties since it is known that fleas feed generally within 1 h after placement on the host. Frequent bathing, particularly with medicated shampoos, can reduce the residual activity of imidacloprid. Consequently, it is the opinion of some that reapplication of the product is necessary in animals that are frequently bathed or wetted (Marsella, 1999).

The safety of imidacloprid in companion animals is outstanding. This is due in part to the greater number of imidacloprid receptors in target fleas than in the dogs and cats that host them, and to the increased binding affinity of imidacloprid for the flea receptor compared with its mammalian counterpart. These features have allowed the administration of imidacloprid to puppies and kittens (minimum age 8 weeks), and to pregnant and lactating dogs and cats at exaggerated doses without evidence of toxicity. One additional advantage of imidacloprid is that it can be administered as frequently as once weekly. This is particularly helpful for animals with severe flea-associated dermatitis.

Nitenpyram (Capstar, CGA 246916; Novartis Animal Health) is the newest of the neonicotinoid (nitroenamine) flea adulticides. It is similar chemically to imidacloprid, but differs from it in that it is administered orally rather than topically at a minimum target dose of 1 mg/kg (Schenker & Barnett, 2000). Nitenpyram is marketed as a rapid, but short-acting flea-removal adulticide. Studies indicate that it removes over 95% of adult fleas from cats and dogs 4–6 h after oral administration. Nitenpyram is rapidly eliminated following oral administration. Peak blood levels are achieved in approximately 1 h. Nitenpyram is eliminated from dogs, mostly by urinary excretion, within 24 h. Complete elimination requires slightly more time in the cat. Because of its rapid elimination, nitenpyram is remarkably safe in both dogs and cats (Witte *et al.*, 2000). It is likely to be marketed in conjunction with lufenuron (Program, Sentinel; Novartis Animal Health) for rapid removal and long-term control of on-animal and environmental flea infestations.

Fipronil (Frontline; Merial, Duluth, GA, USA) is a phenylpyrazole insecticide/acaricide (Table 2.1.1) currently marketed as a 0.29% w/w alcohol-based spray, and as a 9.7% w/w solution for spot-on administration to dogs and cats. The target dosage for the spray formulation is approximately 7.5 mg/kg (3 ml/lb). The spot-on is admini-stered at a minimum target dosage of approximately 10 mg/kg. Both the spray and spot-on formulations provide excellent residual activity. Both are capable of effecting a 95% or greater removal of fleas for 37 days or longer (Tanner & Romano, 1997). Use of the spray product usually extends the period of residual activity beyond what is observed for the spot-on formulation. The spray formulation can result in significant drying of the skin and can irritate inflamed or excoriated skin surfaces. These same formulations also control the four common genera of ticks found on dogs and do so for 1 month or more in most situations. As with imidacloprid, frequent bathing, particularly when using degreasing and antiseborrheic shampoos, can reduce the residual activity compared with non-bathed or less frequently bathed animals. However, the solubility of fipronil in water (2 mg/l) suggests that it is likely to have good residual activity on animals, a property confirmed by field use. The safety of fipronil is exceptional (Consalvi *et al.*, 1996). Long-term field use has confirmed the previously documented safety of fipronil. The incidence of adverse reactions following use of the spray formulation was reported to be less than 1 in 200 000 and involved more than 3 million treatments (Consalvi *et al.*, 1996). Fipronil also has reported (and approved) activity against some parasitic mites, although this information is not included on the product label in all countries.

Selamectin (Revolution; Pfizer Animal Health, New York, USA) is a semisynthetic avermectin compound, derived from doramectin (Evans *et al.*, 1999). It is marketed as a isopropanol/dipropylene glycol monomethyl ether-based topical liquid (6% or 12% w/v active) for spot-on application to both dogs and cats. Selamectin is the first broad-spectrum, single-entity endectocide (effective against both endoparasites and ectoparasites) available in a topical formulation. Selamectin is positioned principally as a topical heartworm preventive (in heartworm endemic areas) and flea-control agent for use in both dogs and cats at a minimum target dose of 6 mg/kg. In field veterinary patient studies, its efficacy against fleas in both dogs and cats was greater than 90% after the first month of administration and exceeded 99% on day 90, following three monthly administrations (Boy *et al.*, 2000). Selamectin also carries a label claim against flea eggs in the US market. Based on research published to date, bathing or wetting appears to have little effect on the efficacy of selamectin as long as it is delayed for at least 2 h after treatment.

US claims in the dog, in addition to heartworm and fleas (including flea eggs), include *Sarcoptes scabiei*, *Otodectes cynotis* and *Dermacentor variabilis*. However, claims in other countries may vary and may omit parasites that are on the US label or include additional ones. Efficacy against *Otodectes* and *Sarcoptes* is pronounced. One or two applications usually result in complete elimination of mites and resolution of lesions. There appear to be varying reports on the capability of selamectin to control *D. variabilis* infestations on dogs. Efficacy against *Rhipicephalus sanguineus* has been demonstrated experimentally, although this species is not included on the product label (Chieffo *et al.*, 1999). The author has been told of both enthusiastically positive results against ticks (species often unknown) on some dogs and disappointingly poor results on others. Such variations in client experiences are probably due to several factors, including differences in species of the offending tick, somewhat slower rate of kill for selamectin than certain other products, severity of environmental tick challenge and the extent to which pet owners monitor pets for ticks.

Claims in the cat, again in addition to heartworm, fleas and flea eggs, include *Otodectes cynotis*, adult intestinal roundworms (*Toxocara cati*) and hookworms (*Ancylostoma tubaeforme*). One particular strength of selamectin is its capability to provide broad-spectrum external and internal parasite control for cats in a convenient and safe formulation.

The safety of selamectin has been documented in numerous studies in both dogs and cats. Field use of this product did not result in observable adverse events in studies conducted in both the USA and Europe (McTier *et al.*, 2000; Six *et al.*, 2000). Additional studies have confirmed the safety of selamectin in ivermectin-sensitive collies (Novotny *et al.*, 1999).

Integrated pest management

Integrated approaches to flea control incorporate both mechanical and chemical methods applied to the pet and the pet's indoor and outdoor environments (Marsella, 1999). Indoor methods include rigorous vacuuming of floor and furniture surfaces, together with washing of rugs, pet bedding, bed clothing and furniture coverings to remove the immature stages. This is usually combined with targeted treatments of the same areas with pump sprays or inverted aerosol formulations. Total release room foggers cannot be recommended because of their inability to reach sheltered areas. Outdoor areas should be cleared of leaf litter and vegetative debris and treated with directed insecticides as suggested for the indoor areas. It is important to focus on those areas that show evidence of frequent pet visits. These are the areas where the majority of flea stages reside. Traditional integrated pest management (IPM) methods should not be used except in extreme, almost desperate, levels of flea infestations. These would include flea allergy in one or more pets in the household, and symptoms or complaints of flea allergy or flea bites in pet owners. As mentioned previously, pharmaceutical, academic and private laboratories continue to collaborate to provide safe, effective and convenient on-animal flea control agents. It is imperative that these products are exploited to achieve and maintain successful and sustained flea control. Because many of these products contain adulticidal, as well as ovicidal or larvicidal claims, they allow some elements of IPM to be practiced without the difficulties and inconveniences imposed by a comprehensive IPM program. To recommend IPM approaches to flea control in all situations and circumstances would impose a level of inconvenience that could lead to the frustrations and non-compliance that were experienced before the new flea-control agents became available.

Flea resistance to insecticides and the recent interinstitutional resistance monitoring initiative

Insecticide resistance has had an impact on the commercial rearing of foodstuffs and livestock on several continents. Although resistance of fleas to older, commercially available insecticides has been documented (Brossard *et al.*, 1998; Dryden *et al.*, 2000), there has been no organized effort to establish monitoring or resistance control initiatives for fleas. This is due in part to the limited effects of documented resistance on the practice of companion animal ectoparasite control, and on the apparent lack of interest in flea resistance as a potential problem. Most instances of either real or perceived flea-control product failures represent one or more of the following: pet owner non-compliance, the presence of unknown or unsuspected sources of fleas, greater challenge from the environment than experienced previously, or change in pet owner perception or expectations. Factors that contribute to the development of flea resistance include short developmental cycle, year-round development in some regions of the world, the existence of closed genetic populations of fleas, the continuous application of the same or similar agents, and the failure to monitor flea populations for resistant phenotypes. Disinterest in flea resistance may be the result of one or more of the following: lack of belief in the importance and potential impact of resistance, the belief that the problem can be solved by simply changing insecticides, the belief that there exists an inexhaustible reserve of insecticides, and the belief that industry will solve the problem. Certainly, given the excellent products now available for flea control, there is a need to address the issue of flea insecticide resistance and to develop control strategies should it emerge. Towards that end, an international team of research scientists, in collaboration with scientists from Bayer Animal Health, has set about to establish a comprehensive resistance monitoring initiative (Jacobs *et al.*, 2000). The first of its kind for fleas, the initiative will first develop and validate *in vitro* assays using available laboratory strains of fleas and imidacloprid as the test compound. Having established and confirmed robust and reproducible assays, the team will seek field strains of fleas from throughout Europe, Australia and the USA. Should resistant strains of fleas emerge, they can be colonized in the laboratory and their resistance traits confirmed by *in vivo* tests. Further molecular characterizations would follow, with the objective of better understanding the molecular or biochemical mechanisms underlying their resistance traits. Ultimately, this information could be used to enhance the efficacies of existing insecticides, but perhaps also to identify new flea-control agents (Hansen *et al.*, 2000).

Current trends in the control of acariases of companion animals

The control of ticks and tick-borne diseases remains a substantial practice effort for veterinarians in many regions of the world. Some of the products (permethrin, fipronil) previously discussed as flea-control agents are, also active against many or most of the species of ticks that commonly parasitize companion animals (Table 2.1.1). With the exception of selamectin, little in the way of new chemistry has been introduced recently and, to the author's knowledge, none is currently under development. In addition to those already discussed, the formamidine compound amitraz (Preventic; Virbac), formulated as a long-acting topical in-collar formulation, has provided excellent control of ticks in many situations (Estrada-Pena & Ascher, 1999). Amitraz, permethrin and the topical and spray formulations of fipronil, remain the cornerstones of tick control in most regions of the world. The author is often asked whether the incidence of tick infestation on dogs is increasing in the south-eastern USA. In response, although we do seem to hear more about tick infestations of pets and premises, this probably has little to do with performance or efficacies of the available acaricides. People often prefer to live, if possible, in rural environments. Residing more closely to nature increases the likelihood of exposure to ticks. People often prefer not to alter natural habitats surrounding their homes, often because they want to encourage visits from wildlife. Such practices, as is known from the biological behavior of ticks, are likely to enhance human and pet exposure to ticks, particularly those that develop in woodland habitats and utilize many alternative hosts during their developmental cycles (Sonenshine, 1991).

With the exception of amitraz, fipronil (some world markets) and selamectin (Tables 2.1.1, 2.1.2), few new compounds have been developed and marketed as approved miticides. Most approved therapies have used traditional insecticides/acaricides such as pyrethrins, organophosphates and sulfurated lime (Blagburn & Lindsay, 1995). With the introduction of the avermectins for dogs in the 1980s, and milbemycin oxime and

Table 2.1.2. Selected treatments for mite-induced dermatoses of companion animals[a]

Parasite	Treatment	Comments	Reference
Otodectes cynotis	Selamectin (canine and feline): 6 mg/kg applied topically for one or two treatments	Treatments administered 1 month apart; label approved in some countries; infestations controlled with monthly administration	Six *et al.* (2000)
	Ivermectin (canine and feline): 200–400 μg/kg administered either orally or subcutaneously	Two subcutaneous treatments administered 14 days apart; three oral treatments, 7 days apart (off-label use)	Gram *et al.* (1994), Scott *et al.* (1995), Paradis (1998)
	Ivermectin (feline): 500 μg applied topically to each ear	Multiple treatments every 7–14 days necessary to eliminate mites; some recurrence observed (off-label use)	Jeneskog & Falk (1990)
	Moxidectin (canine): 200 μg/kg administered orally or subcutaneously	Two treatments, 10 days apart (off-label use)	Bourdeau *et al.* (1998)
	Moxidectin (canine): 400 μg/kg administered orally	Seven treatments, 3 days apart (off-label use)	Bourdeau *et al.* (1998)
	Fipronil 0.25% spray (canine)	Two treatments, 4 weeks apart (off-label)	Coleman & Atwell (1999)
Sarcoptes scabiei	Amitraz dip	Bi-weekly (approved in some countries)	Scott *et al.* (1995)
	Ivermectin: 200–400 μg/kg administered orally or subcutaneously	Oral treatments every 7 days for 4–6 weeks; subcutaneous treatments every 14 days for 4–6 weeks (off-label)	Paradis (1998)
	Milbemycin oxime: 2 mg/kg administered orally	Every 7 days for three to five treatments (off-label)	Miller *et al.* (1996)
	Milbemycin oxime: 1 mg/kg administered orally	Every 2 days for eight treatments (off-label)	Christensson (1999)
	Moxidectin: 250 μg/kg administered subcutaneously	Weekly for 3 weeks (off-label)	Wendelberger & Wagner (1998)
	Fipronil 0.25% spray	As used to control fleas and ticks	Saridomichrlakis *et al.* (1999)
	Selamectin: 6 mg/kg administered topically	Every 30 days (label approved)	Sture *et al.* (1999), McTier *et al.* (2000)
Cheyletiella spp.	Ivermectin: 300 μg/kg administered orally or subcutaneously (canine and feline)	Weekly oral treatments for 6–8 weeks; subcutaneous treatments administered every 14 days for 6–8 weeks	Paradis (1998)
	Fipronil 0.25% spray (canine)	Two applications administered 4 weeks apart	Chadwick (1997)
Demodex spp. (canine)	Amitraz: various treatments; see specific approved labels	Dosages and regimens vary; numerous off-label protocols have been used	Paradis (1999)
	Ivermectin: numerous protocols have been used; common regimen is 300–600 μg/kg administered orally	Administered daily until lesions resolve and mites are not recovered; responses vary, generally requires 10–40 weeks	Paradis (1999)
	Milbemycin oxime: several protocols proposed; 2.2 mg/kg administered orally appeared most effective	Administered daily for 9–26 weeks (off-label)	Miller *et al.* (1995)
	Moxidectin: 400 μg/kg administered orally	Administered daily for 3–7 months	Bensignor & Carlotti (1998)

[a] Many of these regimens are not label approved. Adverse events may occur following the use of certain agents in some animals (e.g. high doses of ivermectin in some types of dogs). Consult specific references for details of product use. These tabulated products and regimens are intended as examples of those published in the scientific literature or presented at scientific meetings. This is not intended to be an exhaustive list.

moxidectin in the 1990s, significant research demonstrated the potent and exploitable miticidal properties of these compounds (Table 2.1.2). Their demonstrated activities, particularly against *Demodex*, *Otodectes* and *Sarcoptes* spp., have led to numerous off-label regimens that have allowed certain cases to be successfully treated and controlled that were not controlled with approved miticides. Selamectin represents the first of the avermectins to carry regulatory label claims for important acarines of companion animals (Evans *et al.*, 1999; McTier *et al.*, 2000; Six *et al.*, 2000). Given the interest in the development and marketing of products with broadened label claims, it is likely that similar product trends will be seen in the coming decade.

Vaccines for the control of ectoparasites

Vaccination strategies for the control of fleas and ticks are based on the induction of antibodies (or other factors) that attack and destroy 'concealed' or 'hidden' gut antigens (Heath *et al.*, 1994; Willadsen & Jongejan, 1999). These strategies presume that moieties from the midgut of fleas and ticks are not revealed to the host during feeding and engorgement (thus 'hidden' antigens). They are isolated, purified and introduced into target animals, together with adjuvant substances to enhance contact with immune competent cells. Although some success has been achieved using these strategies for both ticks of production animals (Willadsen & Jongejan, 1999) and fleas of companion animals (Heath *et al.*, 1994), the levels of efficacy achieved so far would probably be unsatisfactory to veterinarians and pet owners. Continued improvements in molecular methods of identification, isolation and delivery of putative immunogens may eventually lead to the development and marketing of such vaccines in dogs and cats. This author's opinion is that they are more likely to be useful as agents to prevent accumulations of environmental stages of fleas or ticks, given that their principal effects are to reduce engorgement, and hence egg-laying, by the female arthropod. They also may be useful in reducing the transmission of arthropod-borne diseases if the period of feeding and engorgement can be reduced sufficiently.

References

Bensignor, E. & Carlotti, D. N. (1998) Essai de traitement de la démodécie généralisée du chien par la moxidectine: résultats préliminaires (18 cas). In: *Proceedings of GEDAC/GTVB*, Lille, France, 1998, pp. 554–555.

Blagburn, B. L. (1996) Advances in ectoparasite control: insect growth regulators and insect development inhibitors. *Veterinary Medicine* (Suppl., June), **91**, 9–14.

Blagburn, B. L. (1999) A case for continuous internal parasite control: compliance with CDC, NCID, and AAVP guidelines. *Compendium on Continuing Education for the Practicing Veterinarian*, **21** (Suppl.), 46–50.

Blagburn, B. L. & Lindsay, D. S. (1995) Ectoparasiticides. In: *Veterinary Pharmacology and Therapeutics*, 7th edn (Ed. H. R. Adams), pp. 984–1003. Iowa State University Press, Ames, IA.

Bourdeau, P., Baudry, J. & Lecanu, J. M. (1998) The probable role of environmental conditions in the efficacy of treatment of *Otodectes* infestation in dogs: an example with moxidectin (Cydectin) in 50 dogs. In: *Proceedings of the 15th Annual Congress of the ESVD/ECVD*, Maastricht, The Netherlands, September 1998, p. 149.

Boy, M. G., Six, R. H., Thomas, C. A., Rowan, T. J. & Jernigan, A. (2000) Field efficacy and safety of selamectin against fleas on dogs and cats in North America. In: *Proceedings of the 45th Annual Meeting of the American Association of Veterinary Parasitologists*, Salt Lake City, UT, July 2000, p. 65.

Brossard, R. L., Hinkle, N. C. & Rust, M. K. (1998) Review of insecticide resistance in cat fleas (Siphonaptera: Pulicidae). *Journal of Medical Entomology*, **35**, 415–422.

Carlotti, D. N. & Jacobs D. E. (2000) Therapy, control and prevention of flea allergy dermatitis in dogs and cats. *Veterinary Dermatology*, **11**, 83–98.

Chadwick, A. J. (1997) Use of a 0.25 per cent fipronil pump spray formulation to treat canine cheyletiellosis. *Journal of Small Animal Practice*, **38**, 261–262.

Chieffo, C., McTier, T., Hair, J., Krautmann, M. J., Wang, C. S., Rowan, T. G. *et al.* (1999) Efficacy of selamectin against adult *Rhipicephalus sanguineus* ticks on dogs. In: *Proceedings of the 44th Annual Meeting of the American Association of Veterinary Parasitologists*, New Orleans, LA, July 1999, p. 59.

Christensson, D. A. (1999) Milbemycin oxime for treatment of infection with *Sarcoptes scabiei* in the dog. In: *Proceedings of the 16th Annual Meeting of the ESVD/ECVD*, Helsinki, Finland, August 1999, p. 153.

Coleman, G. T. & Atwell, R. B. (1999) Use of fipronil to treat ear mites in cats. *Australian Veterinary Practitioner*, **29**, 166–168.

Consalvi, P. J., Arnaud, J. P., Jeanin, P. & Keister, M. (1996) Safety of a 0.29% w/w fipronil solution (Frontline Spray) in dogs and cats/results of a pharmacovigilance survey one year after launch. In: *Proceedings of the 41st Annual Meeting of the American Association of Veterinary Parasitologists*, Louisville, KY, July 1996, p. 53.

Courtney, C. H. & Roberson, E. L. (1995) Antinematodal drugs. In: *Veterinary Pharmacology and Therapeutics*, 7th edn (Ed. H. R. Adams), pp. 885–932. Iowa State University Press, Ames, IA.

Dryden, M. W., Blagburn, B. L., Bledsoe, D. L., Denholm, I., Dryden, M. W., Hansen, O. *et al.* (2000) Susceptibility of fleas to control agents: development of a monitoring system. In: *Proceedings of the 45th Annual Meeting of the American Association of Veterinary Parasitologists*, Salt Lake City, UT, July 2000, p. 36.

Estrada-Pena, A. & Ascher, F. (1999) Comparison of an amitraz-impregnated collar with topical administration of fipronil for prevention of experimental and natural infestations by the brown dog tick (*Rhipicephalus sanguineus*). *Journal of the American Veterinary Medical Association*, **214**, 1799–1803.

Evans, N. A., Bishop, B. F., Bruce, C. I., Goudie, A. C., Gration, K. A. F., Gibson, S. P. *et al.* (1999) Discovery and biological spectrum of selamectin. In: *Symposium on the Ectoparasitic Activity of Selamectin, 17th International Conference of the World Association for the Advancement of Veterinary Parasitology*, Copenhagen, Denmark, August 1999, p. 11.

Everett, R., Cunningham, J., Arther, R., Bledsoe, D. & Mencke, N. (2000) Comparative evaluation of the speed of kill of Advantage (Imidacloprid) and Revolution (Selamectin) on dogs. In: *International Flea Control Symposium. Compendium on Continuing Education for the Practicing Veterinarian*, **22** (Suppl.), pp. 9–14.

Gram, D., Payton, A. J., Gerig, T. M. & Bevier, D. E. (1994) Treating ear mite in cats: a comparison of subcutaneous and topical ivermectin. *Veterinary Medicine*, **89**, 1122–1125.

Hansen, O., Blagburn, B. L., Bledsoe, D. L., Denholm, I., Dryden, M. W., Hansen, O. *et al.* (2000) Outlook in the future:

new perspectives to safeguard insecticides. In: *Proceedings of the 45th Annual Meeting of the American Association of Veterinary Parasitologists*, Salt Lake City, UT, July 2000, p. 39.

Heath, A. W., Arfsten, A., Yamanaki, M., Dryden, M. W. & Dale, B. (1994) Vaccination against the cat flea (*Ctenocephalides felis felis*). *Parasite Immunology*, **16**, 187–191.

Hopkins, T. J., Kerwick Gyr, P. & Woodley, I. (1997) Efficacy of imidacloprid to remove and prevent *Ctenocephalides felis* infestations on dogs and cats. *Compendium on Continuing Education for the Practicing Veterinarian*, **19** (Suppl.), 11–16.

Jacobs, D. E., Blagburn, B. L., Bledsoe, D. L., Denholm, I., Dryden, M. W., Hansen, O. *et al.* (2000) Development of bioassays to determine susceptibility to an insecticide: standardization of laboratory methods. In: *Proceedings of the 45th Annual Meeting of the American Association of Veterinary Parasitologists*, Salt Lake City, UT, July 2000, p. 38.

Jeneskog, T. & Falk, K. (1990) The effect of local ivermectin treatment on ear mite infestation in a cat breeding colony. *Scandinavian Journal of Laboratory Animal Science*, **1**, 17–22.

McTier, T. L., Six, R. H., Clemence, R. G., Thomas, C. A., Behan, S., Boy, M. G. *et al.* (2000) Field efficacy and safety of selamectin against *Sarcoptes scabiei* on dogs in the United States and Europe. In: *Proceedings of the 45th Annual Meeting of the American Association of Veterinary Parasitologists*, Salt Lake City, UT, July 2000.

Marsella, R. (1999) Advances in flea control. *Veterinary Clinics of North America/Small Animal Practice*, **29**, 1407–1424.

Miller, W. H., Jr, Scott, D. W. & Cayatte, S. M. (1995) Clinical efficacy of increased dosages of milbemycin oxime for treatment of generalized demodicosis in adult dogs. *Journal of the American Veterinary Medical Association*, **207**, 1581–1584.

Miller, W. H., Jr, Jaham, C. de, Scott, D. W. & Cayatte, S. M. (1996) Treatment of canine scabies with milbemycin oxime. *Canadian Veterinary Journal*, **37**, 219–221.

Novotny, M. J., Krautmann, M. J., Ehrhart, J., Goden, C. S., Evans, E. L., McCall, J. W. *et al.* (1999) Clinical safety of selamectin in dogs. In: *Proceedings of the 44th Annual Meeting of the American Association of Veterinary Parasitologists*, New Orleans, July 1999, p. 61.

Noxon, J. O. (1999) Dermatology and the World Wide Web. *Veterinary Clinics of North America/Small Animal Practice*, **29**, 1461–1473.

Paradis, M. (1998) Ivermectin in small animal dermatology. Part II. Extralabel applications. *Compendium on Continuing Education for the Practicing Veterinarian*, **20**, 459–469.

Paradis, M. (1999) New approaches to the treatment of canine demodicosis. *Veterinary Clinics of North America/Small Animal Practice*, **20**, 1425–1436.

Roberson, E. L. & Courtney, C. H. (1995) Anticestodal drugs. In: *Veterinary Pharmacology and Therapeutics*, 7th edn (Ed. H. R. Adams), pp. 933–954. Iowa State University Press, Ames, IA.

Rust, M. K. & Dryden, M. W. (1997) The biology, ecology, and management of the cat flea. *Annual Review of Entomology*, **42**, 451–473.

Saridomichelakis, M., Soubasis N., Koutinas, A. F., Bornstein, S. & Laipi, M. (1999) Treatment of canine sarcoptic mange with fipronil monitored clinically and serologically. In: *Proceedings of the 16th Congress of the ESVD/ECVD*, Helsinki, Finland, August 1999, p. 161.

Schenker, R. & Barnett, S. (2000) Simulated home trials to compare nitenpyram flavored tablets in combination with Program (lufenuron) to Program alone for the control of *C. felis* on cats and dogs. In: *Proceedings of the 44th Annual Meeting of the American Association of Veterinary Parasitologists*, New Orleans, LA, July 1999, p. 92.

Scott, D. W., Miller, W. H., Jr & Griffin, C. E. (1995) Parasitic skin diseases. In: *Muller and Kirk's Small Animal Dermatology*, 5th edn, pp. 392–468. W. B. Saunders, Philadelphia, PA.

Six, R. H., Clemence, R. G., Thomas, C. A., Boy, M. G., Watson, P., Benchoui, H. *et al.* (2000) Field efficacy and safety of selamectin against *Otodectes cynotis* on dogs and cats in the United States and Europe. In: *Proceedings of the 45th Annual Meeting of the American Association of Veterinary Parasitologists*, Salt Lake City, UT, July 2000, p. 66.

Sonenshine, D. E. (1991) *Biology of Ticks.* Oxford University Press, New York.

Sture, G. H., Clements, P. J. M., Jones, R. L., Smith, D. G., Rowan, T. G. & Jernigan, A. D. (1999) Efficacy of selamectin against natural infestations of *Sarcoptes scabiei* on dogs in the UK. In: *Proceedings of the 16th Congress of the ESVD/ECVD*, Helsinki, Finland, August 1999, p. 152.

Tanner, P. A. & Romano, N. M. (1997) Comparative studies to investigate the flea control efficacy of Frontline Topspot and Advantage flea adulticide in the dog and cat. In: *Proceedings of the 42nd Annual Meeting of the American Association of Veterinary Parasitologists*, Reno, NE, July 1997.

Wendelberger, U. & Wagner, R. (1998) Moxidectin: an alternative to ivermectin? In: *Proceedings of the 15th Annual Congress of the EVSD/ECVD*, Maastricht, The Netherlands, September 1998, pp. 149–150.

Willadsen, P. & Jongejan, F. (1999) Immunology of the tick–host interaction and the control of ticks and tick-borne diseases. *Parasitology Today*, **15**, 258–262.

Witte, S. T., Luempert, L. G. III, Goldenthal, E. I., Schardein, J. L. & Johnson, B. E. (2000) Safety of nitenpyram in dogs. In: *Proceedings of the 44th Annual Meeting of the American Association of Veterinary Parasitologists*, New Orleans, LA, July 1999, p. 92.

2.2

Pathogenesis of *Malassezia* dermatitis

R. Bond BVMS, PhD, DVD, MRCVS, DipECVD

Dermatology Unit, Department of Small Animal Medicine and Surgery, Royal Veterinary College, University of London, Hatfield, UK

Summary

The yeast *Malassezia pachydermatis* is a normal inhabitant of canine skin and mucosa. It has long been recognised as a cause of canine otitis externa, but more recently it has been shown to be a common cause of canine dermatitis. The clinical signs associated with *M. pachydermatis* are variable, but pruritus, erythema and greasy exudation are commonly encountered. However, the factors that determine whether colonisation or infection occurs, and the mechanisms by which the yeast induces dermatitis, are poorly understood. The organism has been shown to produce an array of enzymatic substances when cultured *in vitro* and to adhere to canine stratum corneum cells in an *in vitro* model. Thus, proliferation of the organism within the stratum corneum may be associated with liberation of enzymes and metabolites which may induce cutaneous inflammation, particularly in cases where yeast population densities are high. Concurrent proliferation of staphylococci may also be important in some cases. Hypersensitivity responses, particularly immediate, reaginic-antibody-mediated processes, may occur, particularly in dogs with atopic disease. However, some dogs show delayed intradermal test reactivity without immediate reactions to *Malassezia* antigens, indicating that other mechanisms are important. Further studies on the physical and chemical properties of the canine stratum corneum in relation to *M. pachydermatis* colonisation are required. Investigations into the interactions between the yeast and the skin immune system may ultimately explain the susceptibility of individual dogs and the recurrent nature of the disease in such cases, and allow the development of novel therapeutic and prophylactic strategies.

Introduction

The lipophilic yeast *Malassezia pachydermatis* is part of the normal cutaneous microflora of most warm-blooded vertebrates. The fungus was first described as *Pityrosporum pachydermatis* in 1925, having been isolated from an Indian rhinoceros with exfoliative dermatitis (Weidman, 1925). The genus has recently been the subject of taxonomic revision and six other lipid-dependent species (*M. furfur*, *M. sympodialis*, *M. globosa*, *M. restricta*, *M. obtusa* and *M. slooffiae*) are now recognised (Guillot & Guého, 1995; Guého *et al.*, 1996).

It is now widely accepted that *M. pachydermatis* is an opportunistic pathogen of the dog, with an important role in both otitis externa (Gustafson, 1955) and dermatitis (Dufait, 1983). The presence of high population densities of the yeast in lesional skin in dogs with dermatitis refractory to antibacterial and anti-inflammatory therapy, and the clinical response following antifungal treatments and the associated reduction in yeast numbers provide good evidence for a pathogenic role (Dufait, 1983; Mason & Evans, 1991; Bond *et al.*, 1995a). However, the pathogenic mechanisms involved in canine *Malassezia* dermatitis remain poorly understood. The clinical spectrum of signs seen in terms of lesion type, distribution, severity and course, and the presence or absence of various concurrent diseases suggest that multiple mechanisms may be important. This paper reviews aspects of the limited information available with emphasis on studies relating to dogs.

Malassezia pachydermatis populations in canine skin in health and disease

Malassezia pachydermatis is a normal inhabitant of healthy canine skin and mucosae (Gustafson, 1955; Hajsig *et al.*, 1985; Bond *et al.*, 1995b; Kennis *et al.*, 1996). In one study of 40 healthy dogs (Bond *et al.*, 1995b), the yeast was most commonly isolated from the lip region (80% of dogs), interdigital skin (60%), anal mucosa (52.5%) and external ear canal (32.5%). In a preliminary temporal study of *M. pachydermatis* carriage in eight healthy beagles, 'resident' carriage, defined in this study as yeast isolation on at least five out of six occasions at intervals of 2 weeks, was identified in the external ear canal and anus of seven and three dogs, respectively (Bond, 1996).

Dogs with skin disease associated with *M. pachydermatis* may have 100–10 000-fold increases in skin population densities in comparison to healthy dogs (Bond & Lloyd, 1997). Skin populations in healthy basset hounds, a breed predisposed to '*Malassezia* dermatitis', were also found to exceed those of healthy dogs of other breeds, which may reflect the susceptibility of this breed to the disease (Bond & Lloyd, 1997). *Malassezia pachydermatis* populations at the nose, prepuce and vulva in affected dogs also exceeded those of healthy dogs, indicating that the factors that enable the development of abnormally high cutaneous populations also permit proliferation of the yeast at certain mucosal sites (Bond & Lloyd, 1997). Some atopic dogs have abnormally high *M. pachydermatis* populations in both affected (Bond *et al.*, 1994) and unaffected areas (White *et al.*, 1998). The factors that make the skin of some atopic dogs more favourable to yeast colonisation are not clear, although the potential roles of altered temperature, humidity and epidermal barrier function associated with allergic inflammation warrant further study.

Malassezia pachydermatis adherence *in vitro* to canine corneocytes from healthy and affected dogs

Adherence, the specific attachment of micro-organisms to cells and tissues, is thought to play an important role in the colonisation and infection of mammals by pathogenic fungi (Kennedy, 1988). The adherence of *M. pachydermatis* to canine corneocytes (stratum corneum cells) *in vitro* was found to be dependent upon dose, time and yeast cell growth phase (Bond & Lloyd, 1996). Pretreatment of the yeasts with 0.1% trypsin for 30 min reduced ($p < 0.01$) the adherence of four out of five strains, and trypsin pretreatment of the corneocytes reduced ($p < 0.01$) the adherence of two out of five strains, suggesting that trypsin-sensitive proteins or glycoproteins are involved in adherence in this system. Pretreatment of canine corneocytes with concanavalin A (10 μg/ml) inhibited ($p < 0.01$) the adherence of one out of six *M. pachydermatis* strains. This effect was abrogated by preincubating concanavalin A with its hapten inhibitor (6% methyl α-D-mannopyranoside), suggesting that mannosyl-bearing carbohydrate residues on the epithelial cells serve as ligands for adhesins expressed by this strain (Bond & Lloyd, 1998a).

An assay of *M. pachydermatis* adherence to canine corneocytes *in vitro* was used to examine whether the adhesive capacities of the epithelial cells could be related to population sizes of the yeast in the skin of seborrhoeic and healthy basset hounds, and in healthy Irish setter control dogs (Bond & Lloyd, 1998b). The *M. pachydermatis* population sizes in the healthy basset hounds ($n = 5$) were significantly greater ($p < 0.001$) than those in the Irish setters ($n = 6$) but were significantly lower ($p < 0.001$) than those in the seborrhoeic basset hounds ($n = 6$). The numbers of adherent yeast cells of the two *M. pachydermatis* strains tested were significantly greater ($p < 0.001$) on corneocytes taken from the healthy basset hounds, compared with corneocytes derived from healthy Irish setters and seborrhoeic basset hounds. The inverse relationship between population densities *in vivo* and corneocyte adherence *in vitro* suggests that increased corneocyte receptivity for the yeast is not important in the pathogenesis of seborrhoeic dermatitis associated with *M. pachydermatis* in basset hounds. These findings are similar to those reported in a previous investigation of *M. furfur* adherence in humans with seborrhoeic dermatitis; the yeast was better able to adhere to stratum corneum cells from healthy individuals than to cells from patients with seborrhoeic dermatitis (Bergbrant & Faergemann, 1994).

The ability of six *M. pachydermatis* strains obtained from healthy dogs and six from affected dogs to adhere to canine corneocytes *in vitro* was compared using a previously developed assay (Bond & Lloyd, in preparation). Although highly significant differences between strains have been identified, overall the adherence of strains from the two groups of dogs was comparable. It is possible that adherence to corneocytes represents a virulence factor in the sense of the ability to colonise the host. However, these findings do not support the hypothesis that strains apparently capable of inducing skin disease are more adherent than strains that induce no disease, although studies involving larger numbers of strains are warranted.

Evaluation of potential virulence determinants of *Malassezia pachydermatis in vitro*

Microbial products expressed in the cell wall or released into the local environment for homoeostatic purposes may have a detrimental effect on mammalian hosts. Laboratory investigations can be useful in establishing the biochemical products of microbes and enable comparisons to be made between strains. However, substances produced under laboratory conditions may not necessarily be expressed *in vivo*. Subtle changes in cultural conditions may also affect the metabolism of the organism. The results of laboratory studies must be interpreted with caution.

Genetic heterogeneity has been demonstrated among *M. pachydermatis*. Ribosomal large subunit sequencing identified seven 'sequevars', designated Ia–Ig (Guillot *et al.*, 1997). Some of these variants are host specific, suggesting that this species is in the course of differentiation and adaptation to specific animal hosts (Guillot *et al.*, 1997). Other molecular techniques such as restriction fragment length polymorphism (Anthony *et al.*, 1994), and random amplification of polymorphic DNA (RAPD) and chitin synthetase 2 gene sequences (Aizawa *et al.*, 1999) have been used to differentiate strains. However, a relationship between these genetic differences and strain 'virulence' has not been established.

Sodium dodecyl sulfate–polyacrylamide gel electrophoresis (SDS–PAGE) has been used to examine and compare concentrated broth culture supernatants from strains obtained from healthy dogs and from dogs with dermatitis (R. Bond & D. H. Lloyd, unpublished data). Complex patterns of up to 14 proteins ranging from 229 to 20 kDa have been identified. Proteins of approximately 172, 104, 90, 65, 60 and 55 kDa were present in the majority of samples. Although considerable variability between strains has been seen, no clear association between the origin of the strain (healthy or affected dog) and the expression of a particular protein or proteins has been identified.

In a similar study, Coutinho *et al.* (1997) compared the protein profiles of 15 isolates obtained from dogs with otitis externa with 15 isolates from dogs with dermatitis, using SDS–PAGE. Protein bands ranging from 15 to 146 kDa were resolved, but no statistically significant differences were observed in the patterns obtained from the two groups.

The semiquantitative enzyme detection system API ZYM (bioMérieux, Marcy l'Etoile, France) has been used to evaluate enzymatic activity in the culture supernatants described above, and in cell suspensions collected from the same cultures (R. Bond & D. H. Lloyd, unpublished data). Alkaline phosphatase, C4 esterase, esterase lipase, leucine arylamidase, acid phosphatase, napthol-AS-BI-phosphohydrolyase and β-glucosidase activities were commonly detected in both the supernatants and cell pellets. Alkaline phosphatase and esterase lipase activities were significantly greater ($p < 0.05$) in the culture supernatants than in the cell suspension, indicating that enzymes with these activities are readily liberated extracellularly, whereas the other enzymes detected had comparable activities in both samples. Cell suspensions of strains derived from healthy dogs expressed significantly greater ($p < 0.01$) C4 esterase activity than did suspensions of strains from affected dogs. Otherwise, no significant differences were found in enzyme activities in samples derived from the two groups of dogs. The enzyme profiles obtained from the isolates studied were broadly similar to those of previous reports, although the *M. pachydermatis* isolates tested by Reynaud & Chauve (1983) and Bastide *et al.* (1988) using the same commercial kit did not show leucine arylamidase and esterase lipase activity.

Malassezia furfur was shown to produce lipase and phospholipase but not keratinase and gelatinase when cultured on a variety of solid media at various temperatures and pH (Muhsin *et al.*, 1997). Protease, lipase, urease and phosphatase activity was demonstrated when *M. pachydermatis* isolates obtained from dogs' ears were cultured on various solid and liquid media (Mathieson, 1998). Coutinho & Paula (2000) reported production of proteinase and chondroitin sulfatase by 30 strains of *M. pachydermatis* isolated from dogs with otitis or dermatitis. Hyaluronicase and phospholipase were also produced by all strains except for one isolated from the ear. Quantities of these enzymes produced by strains from either site did not vary significantly.

In many cases of *Malassezia* dermatitis in dogs, populations of pathogenic staphylococci, principally *S. intermedius*, are also markedly elevated. Cytological techniques such as tape-stripping may demonstrate the presence of coccoid bacteria. Detergent scrub techniques have shown median population densities in affected basset hounds of approximately 10^6 colony-forming units per square centimetre of skin (Bond *et al.*, 1995a). Bacterial infection may also play an important role in the pathogenesis of some cases, and the use of topical or systemic antibacterial agents, in addition to antifungal drugs, may be beneficial (Mason & Stewart, 1993). The interaction between *M. pachydermatis* and staphylococci in such cases is not understood.

Thus, in common with other cutaneous microbes, *M. pachydermatis* can produce a range of enzymatic substances which are probably involved in its nutrition. Liberation of enzymes by the fungus may ensure that a local supply of appropriate nutrients can enter the cell in a form suitable for further metabolism. These substances may induce host immune and inflammatory responses; however, the relative importance of the various enzymatic products from *M. pachydermatis* in inducing cutaneous inflammation has not been established.

Immunological aspects of *Malassezia*-associated skin disease

In humans, *M. furfur* and related lipid-dependent yeasts are the cause of pityriasis versicolor and are implicated in the pathogenesis of seborrhoeic dermatitis and some cases of atopic dermatitis. Immediate and delayed hypersensitivity responses to *Malassezia* antigens have been reported in humans with the head–neck form of atopic dermatitis (Kieffer *et al.*, 1990). Immunoblotting studies using human sera have shown that 39 proteins may be stained by immunoglobulin E (IgE) (Lintu *et al.*, 1997). However, some patients who showed serological (IgE) responses to fungal proteins did not show skin-prick test reactivity to fungal extracts, indicating that caution is warranted when interpreting the clinical significance of serological responses (Nissen *et al.*, 1998). Tengvall Linder *et al.* (2000) patch-tested 15 atopic dermatitis patients, eight seborrhoeic dermatitis patients and eight healthy controls with an extract of *Pityrosporum orbiculare* on non-lesional, tape-stripped skin of the back. Thirteen atopic patients but none of the others had *Malassezia*-specific IgE in their serum. Eight of these 13 atopic patients showed positive patch-test reactions with a maximal reaction at 48 h; CD4-positive T-cells and eosinophils were observed histologically at the reactive test sites. The remaining patients did not react to patch testing. *Malassezia*-specific IgE titres were significantly higher in those atopic patients who showed patch-test reactivity than in those who did not. This study provides further evidence for a role of *Malassezia* spp. in triggering or exacerbating atopic dermatitis in humans.

The immunomodulatory properties of lipid-dependent *Malassezia* species have been investigated (Kesavan *et al.*, 1998, 2000). Under certain conditions, the incubation of yeast cells with human peripheral blood mononuclear cells reduced the expression of the proinflammatory cytokines interleukin-6 (IL-6), IL-1β and tumour necrosis factor-α compared with control cultures (Kesavan *et al.*, 1998). A depressive effect on proinflammatory cytokine production may confer a biological advantage to a saprophytic yeast; prevention of the induction of an inflammatory response may allow the yeast to persist in the stratum corneum. In a follow-up investigation, Kesavan *et al.* (2000) showed that chloroform/methanol extraction of the surface lipids of *M. sympodialis*, *M. globosa* and *M. restricta* reversed the capacity of the yeast cells to reduce proinflammatory cytokine production. The authors hypothesised that absence of or alterations in the lipid microfibrillar layers of the yeast cells may occur in skin diseases such as seborrhoeic dermatitis, leading to inflammatory changes within the skin.

Studies of cellular immunity in dogs

Peripheral blood mononuclear cell proliferative responses following exposure to *M. pachydermatis* antigen (500 μg/ml) *in vitro* in seven healthy basset hounds exceeded ($p < 0.05$) those in eight seborrhoeic basset hounds with high populations of *M. pachydermatis* and eight Irish setters with gluten-sensitive enteropathy (Bond *et al.*, 1998). Stimulation indices in the latter two groups and eight healthy beagles were comparable. Stimulation indices following *M. pachydermatis* exposure at 50 μg/ml and to the mitogen phytohaemagglutinin in the four groups of dogs did not vary significantly. These findings are analogous to the reduced lymphocyte transformation responses to *M. furfur* reported in humans with pityriasis versicolor (Bergbrant *et al.*, 1999). Further studies are required to determine whether the reduced peripheral blood mononuclear cell proliferative responses to *M. pachydermatis* in affected basset hounds, in comparison to healthy hounds, are a cause or an effect of this disease.

Studies of humoral immunity in dogs

Serum titres of *M. pachydermatis*-specific IgG and IgA measured by enzyme-linked immunosorbent assays (ELISAs) in 21 seborrhoeic bassets and 11 affected dogs of various breeds exceeded ($p < 0.01$ for IgG; $p < 0.05$ for IgA) those of 14 healthy basset hounds and eight healthy beagles (Bond *et al.*, 1998). These results indicate that high serum IgG and IgA titres do not prevent *M. pachydermatis*-associated seborrhoeic dermatitis in basset hounds and other breeds. Total serum IgA concentrations in healthy bassets, seborrhoeic bassets and affected dogs of mixed breeds were significantly greater ($p < 0.01$) than those in beagles. Concentrations in affected basset hounds exceeded ($p < 0.01$) those in the Irish setters. These data indicate that serum IgA deficiency is not a factor in the pathogenesis of the disease.

Western immunoblotting was used to investigate further and compare humoral immune responses in healthy dogs and dogs with *Malassezia* dermatitis by blotting of *M. pachydermatis* antigens separated by SDS–PAGE (R. Bond & D. H. Lloyd, unpublished). Nitrocellulose membranes were incubated with sera used in the previous ELISA studies and probed with peroxidase-conjugated anti-dog IgG antibody. In total, 14 bands of immunoreactivity were identified with approximate molecular weights of 219, 204, 132, 110, 76, 71, 66, 60, 50–54, 43–50, 42, 37–40, 35 and 32 kDa. The number of bands (mean ± SEM) of immunoreactivity observed in the seborrhoeic basset hounds (10.7 ± 0.4) was significantly greater ($p < 0.01$) than those in beagles (3.0 ± 1.0), Irish setters (5.5 ± 1.1) and healthy basset hounds (5.6 ± 0.7). Band numbers in the mixed-breed affected dogs (9.4 ± 0.9) were significantly greater than those in beagles ($p < 0.01$), healthy basset hounds ($p < 0.01$) and Irish setters ($p < 0.05$). There were no significant differences between beagles, Irish setters and healthy basset hounds. In general, staining intensity was greatest in specimens where multiple bands were evident.

There were clear differences in the individual protein bands recognised between groups. Most dogs displayed immunoreactivity towards the 132, 66 and 50–54 kDa proteins and few dogs recognised the 204 and 76 kDa proteins. The majority of affected dogs showed reactivity towards the 219, 110, 71 and 42 kDa proteins, whereas reactivity to these proteins was seldom detected in healthy dogs. Less well-defined differences between groups were seen with the 40–37, 35 and 32 kDa proteins. There was a highly significant positive correlation ($r_s = 0.76$, $p < 0.001$) between the number of bands identified and the titre of *M. pachydermatis*-specific IgG antibodies in each sample as determined previously using ELISA.

Intradermal testing with Malassezia pachydermatis *antigens in dogs*

Immediate intradermal test reactivity has been observed in atopic dogs following the injection of *M. pachydermatis* extracts at concentrations that cause no reaction in healthy dogs, suggesting that hypersensitivity responses to yeast allergens may be involved in the pathogenesis in some cases of atopic disease (Morris *et al.*, 1998). Reactivity was higher in atopic dogs with cytological evidence of *Malassezia* dermatitis than in atopics without. These observations are analogous to the suggestion that IgE-mediated hypersensitivity to *Malassezia*-derived allergens may be important in the pathogenesis of the head–neck form of atopic dermatitis in humans (Kieffer *et al.*, 1990). Owners were invited to check for evidence of delayed reactivity but this was not reported, although delayed reactivity to flea allergen was described in some cases.

Eleven healthy laboratory beagles, seven healthy basset hounds and 18 basset hounds with *Malassezia* dermatitis were tested intradermally using extracts prepared from two *M. pachydermatis* isolates, namely CBS 1879, a type culture originally isolated from a dog with otitis externa, and an isolate from the author's collection (42/1192) obtained from a clinical case (Bond *et al.*, in press). Aliquots of each extract were diluted to concentrations of 200 and 20 μg protein/ml, in 0.5% phenol saline. Each dog was injected intradermally with 0.05 ml of 200 μg/ml and 20 μg/ml dilutions along with saline and histamine (1:100 000) controls. In addition, each beagle was injected with 2 μg/ml and 0.2 μg/ml dilutions.

When assessed 15 min after injection, all dogs except for one beagle showed strong reactions to histamine (10–17 mm weals) and none of the dogs reacted to the 0.5% phenol saline negative control. Two affected basset hounds showed strong immediate intradermal test reactivity (12–14 mm weals) to both extracts at 200 μg/ml dilution. One of these dogs also reacted strongly (12–13 mm weals) to both extracts at 20 μg/ml, whereas the remaining dog reacted (8.5 mm weal) only to 42/1192 at this concentration. None of the other dogs tested showed immediate test reactivity.

In contrast, examination of test sites at 24 h after-injection showed frequent lesions characterised by erythematous plaques in the healthy and affected basset hounds. Some beagles also showed 24 reactions but, where present, these tended to be less obvious.

A comparison of lesion diameters showed that the reactions to 200 and 20 μg/ml concentrations for both strains in laboratory beagles were significantly ($p < 0.01$) smaller that those seen in both groups of basset hounds. Differences between healthy and affected bassets were not significant.

Skin biopsy specimens were obtained from saline and test (42/1192, 200 μg/ml) sites in six affected basset hounds. Sections were examined by a histopathologist unaware of the origin of each specimen. Control sites showed either no abnormalities (three cases) or mild changes (three cases) characterised by mild acanthosis and mild superficial or interstitial infiltrates of neutrophils and lymphocytes. Test sites showed either moderate (two cases) or severe (four cases) inflammatory changes, principally characterised by perivascular, interstitial and or periadnexal infiltrates of neutrophils and lymphocytes.

It is clear that a spectrum of cutaneous reactivity to *M. pachydermatis* antigens can be seen following intradermal injection. Immediate responses suggest that an IgE-mediated process is involved in some individuals and it is reasonable to suggest that yeast hypersensitivity may contribute to the development of clinical signs in those individuals, especially, but not exclusively, in dogs with other features of atopic disease. However, *Malassezia* dermatitis occurs in dogs without immediate reactivity to the yeast and without evidence of atopic disease or other cutaneous hypersensitivity disorders (Mason & Evans, 1991; Bond *et al.*, 1996). Other dogs with *Malassezia* dermatitis show only delayed reactivity, a response frequently not seen in healthy laboratory dogs. The variable immune responsiveness seen among dogs suggests that any future immunomodulatory therapeutic or prophylactic approach may have to target different components of the skin immune system.

Conclusion

Since the publication of the first volume of *Advances in Veterinary Dermatology*, a great deal of information on the clinical aspects of *Malassezia* dermatitis has been elucidated. The clinical signs associated with the yeast have been well described and *Malassezia* dermatitis is now commonly diagnosed in many veterinary practices. The use of diagnostic techniques suitable for demonstrating the presence of the yeast, such as cytology, has become commonplace. In many countries, specific treatments licensed and registered for the therapy of *Malassezia* dermatitis have become available. These events have enhanced the abilities of veterinarians to improve the welfare of many of their patients with skin disease and, in this regard, the work of Dufait (1983) and Mason (Mason & Evans, 1991; Mason, 1992) deserves special mention.

Despite these advances, the interaction between *M. pachydermatis* in healthy dogs and dogs with skin disease remains incompletely understood and further work on the effects of the yeast on its canine host in different circumstances is required so that the factors that render dogs either susceptible or resistant to disease can be identified. Comparative studies involving lipid-dependent *Malassezia* species and other mammalian host species may also yield further information that will allow the development of novel therapeutic approaches for the treatment of mammalian skin disease associated with commensal micro-organisms.

Acknowledgements

The author gratefully acknowledges funding received from BSAVA Petsavers, ESVD Allerderm Award, Derm-Care Vet and Leo Animal Health. The author thanks David Lloyd, Anne Lamport, Clive Elwood, Rebecca Littler, Cathy Curtis, Ewan Ferguson, Anke Hendricks, Jane Rose, Jason Ellis and Janet Patterson-Kane for their valuable contributions to aspects of the work discussed here.

References

Aizawa, T., Kano, R., Nakamura, Y., Watanabe, S. & Hasegawa, A. (1999) Molecular heterogeneity in clinical isolates of *Malassezia pachydermatis* from dogs. *Veterinary Microbiology*, **70**, 67–75.

Anthony, R. M., Howell, S. A., Lloyd, D. H. & Pinter, L. (1994) Application of DNA typing methods to the study of the epidemiology of *Malassezia pachydermatis*. *Microbial Ecology in Health and Disease*, **7**, 161–168.

Bastide, J. M., Mallie, M. & Montes, B. (1988) Morphologie et physiologie des *Malassezia*. *Bulletin de la Societe Francaise de Mycologie Medicale*, **17**, 232–244.

Bergbrant, I. M. & Faergemann, J. (1994) Adherence of *Malassezia furfur* to human stratum corneum cells *in vitro*, a study of healthy individuals and patients with seborrhoeic dermatitis. *Mycoses*, **37**, 5–6.

Bergbrant, I. M., Andersson, B. & Faergemann, J. (1999) Cell-mediated immunity to *M. furfur* in patients with seborrhoeic dermatitis and pityriasis versicolor. *Clinical and Experimental Dermatology*, **24**, 402–406.

Bond, R. (1996) *Malassezia pachydermatis* colonisation and infection of canine skin. Royal Veterinary College. PhD Thesis, University of London.

Bond, R. & Lloyd, D. H. (1996) Factors affecting the adherence of *Malassezia pachydermatis* to canine corneocytes *in vitro*. *Veterinary Dermatology*, **7**, 49–56.

Bond, R. & Lloyd, D. H. (1997) Skin and mucosal populations of *Malassezia pachydermatis* in healthy and seborrhoeic basset hounds. *Veterinary Dermatology*, **8**, 101–106.

Bond, R. & Lloyd, D. H. (1998a) Studies on the role of carbohydrates in the adherence of *Malassezia pachydermatis* to canine corneocytes *in vitro*. *Veterinary Dermatology*, **9**, 105–109.

Bond, R. & Lloyd, D. (1998b) The relationship between population sizes of *Malassezia pachydermatis* in healthy dogs and in basset hounds with *M. pachydermatis*-associated seborrhoeic dermatitis and adherence to canine corneocytes *in vitro*. In: *Advances in Veterinary Dermatology*, Vol. 3 (Eds K. Kwochka, T. Willemse & C. von Tscharner), pp. 284–289. Butterworth Heinemann, Oxford.

Bond, R., Collin, N. S. & Lloyd, D. H. (1994) Use of contact plates for the quantitative culture of *Malassezia pachydermatis* from canine skin. *Journal of Small Animal Practice*, **35**, 68–72.

Bond, R., Rose, J. F., Ellis, J. W. & Lloyd, D. H. (1995a) Comparison of two shampoos for treatment of *Malassezia pachydermatis*-associated seborrhoeic dermatitis in Basset Hounds. *Journal of Small Animal Practice*, **36**, 99–104.

Bond, R., Saijonmaa-Koulumies, L. E. M. & Lloyd, D. H. (1995b) Population sizes and frequency of *Malassezia pachydermatis* at skin and mucosal sites on healthy dogs. *Journal of Small Animal Practice*, **36**, 147–150.

Bond, R., Ferguson, E. A., Curtis, C. F., Craig, J. M. & Lloyd, D. H. (1996) Factors associated with elevated cutaneous *Malassezia pachydermatis* populations in dogs with pruritic skin disease. *Journal of Small Animal Practice*, **37**, 103–107.

Bond, R., Elwood, C. M., Littler, R. M., Pinter, L. & Lloyd, D. H. (1998) Humoral and cell-mediated immune responses to *Malassezia pachydermatis* in healthy dogs and dogs with *Malassezia* dermatitis. *Veterinary Record*, **143**, 381–384.

Bond, R., Patterson-Kane, J. C. & Lloyd, D. N. (in press.) Intradermal test reactivity to *Malassezia pachydermatis* in healthy basset hounds and bassets with *Malassezia* dermatitis. *Veterinary Record*.

Coutinho, S. D. & Paula, C. R. (2000) Proteinase, phospholipase, hyaluronidase and chondroitin-sulphatase production by *Malassezia pachydermatis*. *Medical Mycology*, **38**, 73–76.

Coutinho, S. D., Souza, T. de & Paula, C. R. (1997) Protein profiles of *Malassezia pachydermatis* isolated from dogs. *Mycopathologia*, **139**, 129–135.

Dufait, R. (1983) Pityrosporon canis as the cause of canine chronic dermatitis. *Veterinary Medicine/Small Animal Clinician*, **78**, 1055–1057.

Guého, E., Midgley, G. & Guillot, J. (1996) The genus *Malassezia* with description of four new species. *Antonie van Leeuwenhoek*, **69**, 337–355.

Guillot, J. & Guého, E. (1995) The diversity of *Malassezia* yeasts confirmed by rRNA sequence and nuclear DNA comparisons. *Antonie van Leeuwenhoek*, **67**, 297–314.

Guillot, J., Gueho, E., Chevrier, G. & Chermette, R. (1997) Epidemiological analysis of *Malassezia pachydermatis* isolates by partial sequencing of the large subunit ribosomal RNA. *Research in Veterinary Science*, **62**, 22–25.

Gustafson, B. A. (1955) Otitis externa in the dog. A bacteriological and experimental study. Royal Veterinary College, Stockholm.

Hajsig, M., Tadic, V. & Lukman, P. (1985) *Malassezia pachydermatis* in dogs, significance of its location. *Veterinarski Arhiv*, **55**, 259–266.

Kennedy, M. J. (1988) Adhesion and association mechanisms of *Candida albicans*. In: *Current Topics in Medical Mycology*, Vol. 2 (Ed. M. R. McGinnis), pp. 73–169. Springer, New York.

Kennis, R. A., Rosser, E. J., Olivier, N. B. & Walker, R. W. (1996) Quantity and distribution of *Malassezia* organisms on the skin of clinically normal dogs. *Journal of the American Veterinary Medical Association*, **208**, 1048–1051.

Kesavan, S., Walters, C. E., Holland, K. T & Ingham, E. (1998) The effects of *Malassezia* on pro-inflammatory cytokine production by human peripheral blood mononuclear cells *in vitro*. *Medical Mycology*, **36**, 97–106.

Kesavan, S., Holland, K. T. & Ingham, E. (2000) The effects of lipid extraction on the immunomodulatory activity of *Malassezia* species *in vitro*. *Medical Mycology*, **38** 239–247.

Kieffer, M., Bergbrant, I. M., Faergemann, J., Jemec, G. B. E., Ottevanger, V., Skov, P. S. & Svejgaard, E. (1990) Immune reactions to *Pityrosporum ovale* in adult patients with atopic and seborrheic dermatitis. *Journal of the American Academy of Dermatology*, **22**, 739–742.

Lintu, P., Savolainen, J. & Kalimo, K. (1997) IgE antibodies to protein and mannan antigens of *Pityrosporum ovale* in atopic dermatitis patients. *Clincal and Experimental Allergy*, **27**, 87–95.

Mason, K. V. (1992) Seborrhoeic dermatitis – the aetiology rediscovered. *Veterinary Dermatology Newsletter*, pp. 6–12.

Mason, K. V. & Evans, A. G. (1991) Dermatitis associated with *Malassezia pachydermatis* in 11 dogs. *Journal of the American Animal Hospital Association*, **27**, 13–20.

Mason, K. V. & Stewart, L. J. (1993) Malassezia and canine dermatitis. In: *Advances in Veterinary Dermatology*, Vol. 2 (Eds P. J. Ihrke, I. S. Mason & S. D. White), pp. 399–402. Pergamon Press, Oxford.

Mathieson, I. (1998) Enzymatic activity of *Malassezia pachydermatis*. In: *Advances in Veterinary Dermatology*, Vol. 3 (Eds K. Kwochka, T. Willemse & C. von Tscharner), pp. 532–533. Butterworth Heinemann, Oxford.

Morris, D. O., Olivier, N. B. & Rosser, E. J. (1998) Type-1 hypersensitivity reactions to *Malassezia pachydermatis* extracts in atopic dogs. *American Journal of Veterinary Research*, **59**, 836–841.

Muhsin, T. M., Aubaid, A. H. & Duboon, A. H. (1997) Extracellular enzyme activities of dermatophytes and yeast isolates on solid media. *Mycoses*, **40**, 465–469.

Nissen, D., Petersen, L., Esch, R., Svejgaard, E., Skov, P. S., Poulsen, L. K. & Nolte, H. (1998) IgE sensitization to cellular and culture filtrates of fungal extracts in patients with atopic dermatitis. *Annals of Asthma Allergy and Immunology*, **81**, 247–255.

Reynaud, M. C. & Chauve, C. (1983) *Pityrosporum canis*, clinical observations and a contribution to the study of the enzyme system of the strains isolated. *Bulletin de la Societe Francaise de Mycologie Medicale*, **12**, 209–212.

Tengvall Linder, M., Johansson, C., Scheynius, A. & Wahlgren, C. (2000) Positive atopy patch test reactions to *Pityrosprum orbiculare* in atopic dermatitis patients. *Clinical and Experimental Allergy*, **30**, 122–131.

Weidman, F. D. (1925) Exfoliative dermatitis in the Indian rhinoceros (*Rhinoceros unicornis*) with description of a new yeast species, *Pityrosporum pachydermatis*. In: *Report of the Laboratory Museum Comparative Pathology Zoological Society*. Comparative Pathology Zoological Society, Philadelphia, PA.

White, S. D., Bourdeau, P., Blumstein, P., Ibish, K., Scott, K. V., Salman, N. D. & Chapman, P. L. (1998) Comparison via cytology and culture of carriage of *Malassezia pachydermatis* in atopic and healthy dogs. In: *Advances in Veterinary Dermatology*, Vol. 3 (Eds K. Kwochka, T. Willemse & C. von Tscharner), pp. 291–298. Butterworth Heinemann, Oxford.

2.3

Application of the skin xenograft–mouse model in veterinary dermatology research: modeling canine demodicosis

K.E. Linder DVM, PhD,[1] G.A. Kunkle DVM, DACVD,[3] W.M. Parker DVM[2] and J.A. Yager BVSc, PhD[1]

[1,2] Departments of Pathology and Clinical Studies, Ontario Veterinary College, University of Guelph, Guelph, Ontario, Canada

[3] Department of Small Animal Clinical Sciences, College of Veterinary Medicine, University of Florida, Gainesville, Florida, USA

Summary

Clinical observations and *in vitro* lymphocyte studies support the current hypothesis that cellular immunity is important for *Demodex canis* elimination and lesion development in canine demodicosis. Thus, dogs with generalized demodicosis are unable to control mite populations because of a genetic and/or an acquired defect in lymphocyte function. The objectives of this experimental study were: (1) to develop a reproducible mouse model of canine demodicosis; and (2) to test the hypothesis that lymphocytes affect *D. canis* populations *in vivo*.

Four strains of immunodeficient mice (scid/bg, ICR scid, tgε26 and *Rag2*) supported canine skin xenografts and could be reliably infected with *D. canis*. Only *Rag2* mice were suitable for the long-term experiments modeling demodicosis. Mites proliferated to high numbers on xenografts, directly confirming the importance of systemic dog factors in the control of mite populations. Heavy *D. canis* infestations did not induce hair loss in the absence of inflammation. Unexpectedly, intragraft inoculation of *in vitro* mitogen-stimulated autologous canine lymphocytes was associated with a significant increase in mite numbers on skin xenografts.

Introduction

Canine demodicosis is a multifactorial inflammatory skin disease associated with overgrowth of the skin commensal *Demodex canis* (Scott *et al.*, 1995). Scott and co-workers hypothesized that generalized demodicosis results from a T-cell function defect, due to either a genetic predisposition or acquired immunosuppression (Scott *et al.*, 1974, 1976). *Demodex canis* overgrowth and/or concomitant bacterial skin infection potentiates immunosuppression and disease progression (Barta *et al.*, 1983; Barriga *et al.*, 1992). Most studies have evaluated the cutaneous or peripheral blood lymphocyte (PBL) response to mitogens and not the immune response in relation to mite antigens. A specific T-cell function defect has not been demonstrated for demodicosis and the tacit hypothesis that normal lymphocytes limit *D. canis* proliferation has gone untested.

Investigations of demodicosis have been hampered by the lack of a suitable experimental test system. *Demodex canis* does not survive *in vitro* and generalized demodicosis cannot be re-created experimentally without severely immunosuppressing dogs, which complicates investigations of host immunity (Greve & Gaafar, 1966; Sheahan & Gaafar, 1970a; Healey & Gaafar, 1977). The authors' laboratory has taken a new approach based on the skin xenograft–mouse model, used extensively in human dermatology (Briggaman, 1980; Gilhar & Etzioni, 1994). In this model, immunodeficient mice support full-thickness canine skin xenografts, on which *D. canis* will survive after topical application (Caswell *et al.*, 1996).

The skin xenograft environment is immunodeficient and isolated from host systemic factors. For this reason, infection of grafts assesses local skin mechanisms of resistance to mite colonization and mite contributions to skin lesion development. After reintroduction of autologous lymphocytes to infected grafts, mites can be quantified to provide a direct measure of lymphocyte-mediated resistance to mite proliferation (Petzelbauer *et al.*, 1996; Gilhar *et al.*, 1999).

Materials and methods

Animals

Mice

Male scid/bg (C.B-*Igh-1*^{b}GbmsTac-*Prkdc*^{scid}-*lyst*^{bg}N7), ICR scid (Tac:Ucr:Ha(ICR)-*Prkdc*^{scid}) and *Rag2* knockout mice (129S6/SvEvTac-*Rag2*^{tm1}) were obtained from Taconic Labs (Germantown, NY, USA). Male tgε26 mice (B6;CBA-TgN(*CD3E*)26Cpt) were a kind gift from Dr Croy (University of Guelph, Ontario, Canada). Mice were housed as described previously (Greenwood *et al.*, 1997). Scid/bg and ICR scid mice were prescreened for endogenous immunoglobulin by enzyme-linked immunosorbent assay (ELISA) (see below). All procedures followed the Canadian Council on Animal Care guidelines and were approved by the University of Guelph Animal Care Committee.

Dogs

Adult, intact male dogs were purchased from and maintained by Animal Care Services (University of Guelph).

Skin xenografting

A full-thickness skin sample was excised from the anesthetized dog (dorsal back) and placed into transport medium (RPMI 1640, Life Technologies, Ontario, Canada) on ice, containing penicillin (200 IU/ml) (ICN Biomedicals Canada, Ontario) and streptomycin (80 μg/ml) (Life Technologies). Dogs received 1 g of cefazolin (Novopharm, Ontario, Canada) before surgery. Subcutaneous fat was removed from the excised sample before individual round skin grafts (10–16 mm in diameter) were trimmed using a no. 10 scalpel blade.

A circular graft bed, which retained the panniculus carnosus, was created on the shaved dorsolateral thorax of an anesthetized mouse with small curved Metzenbaum scissors. The skin graft was anchored at the epidermal margin at four to six points using tissue adhesive (Vetbond®; 3M Animal Care Products, Ontario, Canada) delivered with a 30 G needle. A bandage consisted of two layers of paraffin-impregnated gauze (15 × 15 mm) supported by a Band-Aid (Comfort Strips; 3M Canada, Ontario) and two layers of hospital tape (Renfrew Tape, Ontario). Bandages were stabilized with two or three stainless-steel skin staples (Auto Suture®, United States Surgical Corp., Norwalk, CT, USA) and trimmed to 5–10 mm ventrally. Mice were bandaged for 7–24 days. Grafting occurred 6–9.5 h after skin collection. The scid/bg and some tgε26 mice were grafted according to Caswell *et al.* (1996) (see Table 2.3.1).

Demodex *infection of skin grafts*

Demodex canis were collected from dogs with generalized squamous demodicosis by hair plucking and were transported in sterile containers. Each mite inoculum was standardized by intermixing mites on microscope slides in 100–150 μl of mineral oil and viable mites were quantified by microscopy. Grafts were infected by wiping the mite-coated slide over the graft surface while the graft was raised between the thumb and index finger. Table 2.3.1 lists the infective doses per graft. Grafts were bandaged for 5 days, as described above. Mite transfer efficiency was >90% and mites remaining on slides after transfer were viable. Graft infections were performed 2.5–7.5 h after mite collection.

Canine lymphocyte preparation

Canine peripheral blood mononuclear cells (PBMC) were isolated by discontinuous density gradient centrifugation (Barta & Barta, 1993). Lymphocytes were stimulated *in vitro* with phytohemagglutinin (PHA) and human recombinant interleukin-2 (hr-IL-2) (Somberg *et al.*, 1992; Barta & Barta, 1993; Mizuno *et al.*, 1993). PBMC were resuspended at 1 × 10^{6} cells/ml in supplemented RPMI before receiving 10 μg/ml PHA (Sigma Chemical Co., St Louis, MO, USA). Forty-eight hours later, hr-IL-2 (PharMingen, Ontario, Canada) was added at 1000 units/ml and cells were cultured for an additional 24 h. Lymphocytes were washed twice

Table 2.3.1. Comparison of skin xenografting results, *Demodex canis* infection rates and outcomes for the different strains of mice used to model canine demodicosis

Mouse strain	Skin donor	Graft quality[c]	Mite dose[d]	Infection (rate)	Usefulness	Outcome
Scid/bg	Dog 1[a]	+ (n = 25)	60	Yes (NA)	Poor	Became 'leaky'; developed GVHD
	Dog 2[a]	+/++ (n = 20)	300	Yes (NA)	Poor	Became 'leaky'
ICR scid	Dog 3[b]	++ (n = 25)	220[e]	Yes (18/20)	Poor	Became 'leaky'
Tgε26	Dog 4[a]	+ (n = 12)	300	Yes (12/12)	Fair	Low survivability
	Dog 5[b]	++ (n = 10)	100	Yes (9/10)	Fair	Low survivability; some graft rejection
Rag2	Dog 6[b]	+++ (n = 33)	200	Yes (25/25)	Good	No complications

[a] Skin grafting methods according to Caswell *et al.* (1996).
[b] Skin grafting methods according to Materials and methods.
[c] Graft quality score: + = hair growth at margin, extensive central scarring, wide variation; ++ = hair growth at margin and center, mild/moderate central scarring, wide variation; +++ = hair growth over entire graft, little or no scarring, uniform grafts.
[d] Average viable *D. canis* (adults and nymphs) dose applied to each graft. Each dose contained approximately 85% adults and 15% combined eggs, larvae and nymphs.
[e] Total mite dose given. Grafts were infected on three occasions.
NA: not available; GVHD: graft-versus-host disease.

with phosphate-buffered saline (PBS) before use. A stimulation index was calculated (Barta & Barta, 1993) and cell counts, leukocyte differentials and cell viability were determined by standard techniques.

Evaluation of skin xenografts and mouse tissues

Skin grafts were subjectively graded for hair growth, erythema, scaling, crusting or pigmentary changes before *D. canis* infection and lymphocyte transfer and at the end of the experiment. Hair growth was scored as 1 (>50% of surface) or 2 (<50% of surface).

At completion, mice were anesthetized (Greenwood *et al.*, 1997) for blood collection (Bivin & Smith, 1984) and euthanized. A packed cell volume was recorded. Canine and murine immunoglobulin G (IgG) in mouse sera was quantified by direct sandwich ELISA using methods adapted from the Diagnostic Immunology Laboratory (Ontario Veterinary College, Ontario, Canada). A 2 × 4 mm full-thickness graft sample was submitted to the Animal Health Laboratory (Ontario Veterinary College) for bacterial culture.

For histology, hematoxylin and eosin-stained sections were prepared by standard methods after tissues were fixed in 10% buffered formalin. Immunohistochemical detection of T-cells was performed by Prairie Diagnostic Services (Western College of Veterinary Medicine, Saskatchewan, Canada) on paraffin-embedded skin grafts as well as murine spleen, liver and lung using polyclonal rabbit anti-human CD3 antiserum (Dako, Carpentia, CA, USA) (Caswell *et al.*, 1997).

To enumerate *D. canis* on grafts, half of each skin graft was trimmed of hair and fat and digested in 3 ml of 4% NaOH for 25 min in a boiling water bath. After washing, pelleted mites were resuspended in a fixed volume of water and the total occurrence of eggs, larvae, nymphs and adults was recorded in sample aliquots.

Necropsies were performed at the time of euthanasia.

Protocol for modeling demodicosis using Rag2 mice

The timeline for the *Rag2* experiment is shown in Figure 2.3.1. Mice were bandaged for 24 days after grafting. Skin grafts were subjectively graded and allocated to four groups with comparable hair growth. At 52 days postgrafting, group I (n = 9), II (n = 8) and III (n = 8) grafts were infected with approximately 200 viable mites consisting of 80% adults and 20% nymphs, protonymphs, larvae and eggs. Skin grafts in group IV (n = 8) received only mineral oil. At 63 days after *D. canis* infection, 15 × 10^6 viable stimulated PBL were injected intradermally into grafts of groups I and IV. The inoculum contained 99% lymphocytes (viability = 81%). The stimulation index was 32.3. At 66 days after infection, PBMC were again isolated from the same donor dog and 25 × 10^6 viable unstimulated lymphocytes were injected into each graft of group II. This second inoculum contained 76% lymphocytes and 93% PBMC (viability = 98%). Skin grafts in group III received phosphate-buffered saline (PBS).

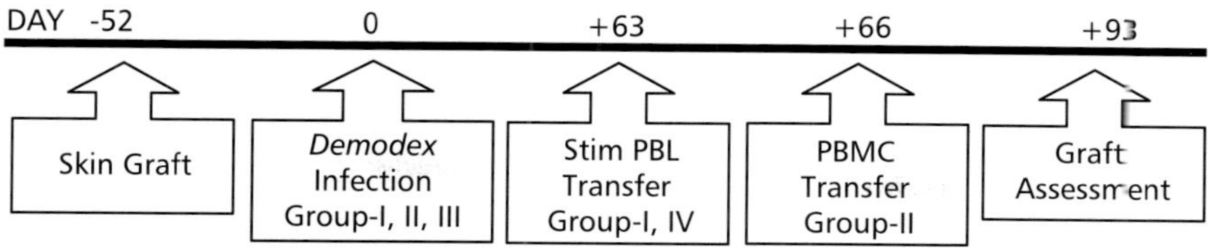

Figure 2.3.1. Experimental timeline for modeling demodicosis with *Rag2* null mice.

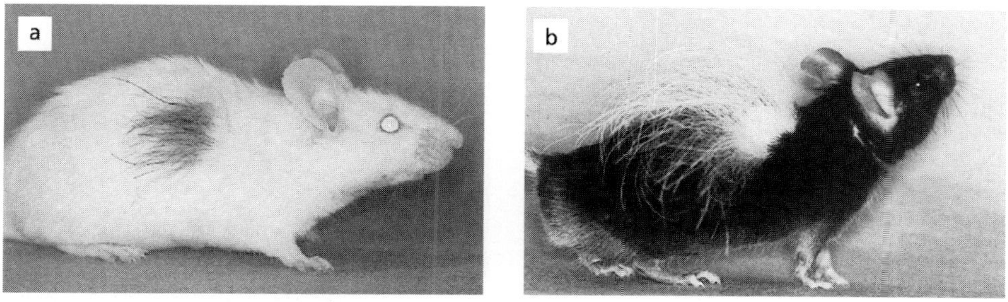

Figure 2.3.2. Gross appearance of representative full-thickness canine skin xenografts on (a) an ICR scid mouse and (b) a tgε26 mouse. Xenografts grew hair resembling that of the skin-donor dog and did not show hair loss after *Demodex canis* infection.

Statistical methods

Analysis of variance was performed with the SAS® computer software package, Version 6.12 for Windows (SAS Institute, Cary, NC, USA).

Results

Experiments on scid/bg, ICR scid and tgε26 mice

Skin grafts healed on all mice, survived for the duration of the experiments (4–5 months) and regrew variable amounts of hair (Figure 2.3.2). *Demodex canis* graft infection rates were high (Table 2.3.1) and large numbers were recovered (hundreds to over 6000), including all life-cycle stages. Mite numbers depended on the number of hair follicle units. Skin grafting procedures that eliminated the panniculus carnosus in the graft bed (Caswell *et al.*, 1996) or that used shorter bandaging times (7–9 days) led to slower graft healing, central scarring and reduced hair growth.

A high percentage (up to 60%) of scid/bg and ICR scid mice produced immunoglobulin and some had evidence of graft rejection, consistent with the 'leaky' phenotype (Bosma *et al.*, 1988). In addition, some scid/bg mice reconstituted with canine PBMC developed evidence of graft-versus-host disease (GVHD), including hemolytic anemia (Taylor, 1994). Up to 40% of tgε26 mice did not survive experiments and some developed functional lymphocytes with evidence of graft rejection.

Experiment on Rag2 *mice*

Skin grafts healed well after mild transient central crusting. Hair started to regrow 3–4 weeks after transplantation and was abundant on grafts at completion of the experiment. Three skin grafts grew very little hair. Grafts did not develop lesions after *D. canis* infection or after leukocyte injection and there was no difference between experimental groups (Figure 2.3.3).

Large numbers of *D. canis*, including all life-cycle stages, were recovered from grafts that were infected with mites (25/25) (Figure 2.3.4). The calculated mean total number of mites per NaOH digest sample (mean ± SEM) for groups I, II and III was 15 331 ± 3584, 6582 ± 1119 and 8931 ± 1717, respectively. Immature stages outnumbered adults (Figure 2.3.4). Mites were not recovered from group IV.

There were significantly more mites on grafts in group I than in group II (score = 1, $p = 0.016$; score = 2, $p < 0.001$) or group III (score = 1, $p = 0.049$; score = 2, $p < 0.001$) when bacteria (*Staphylococcus intermedius*) were not recovered. Similarly, when

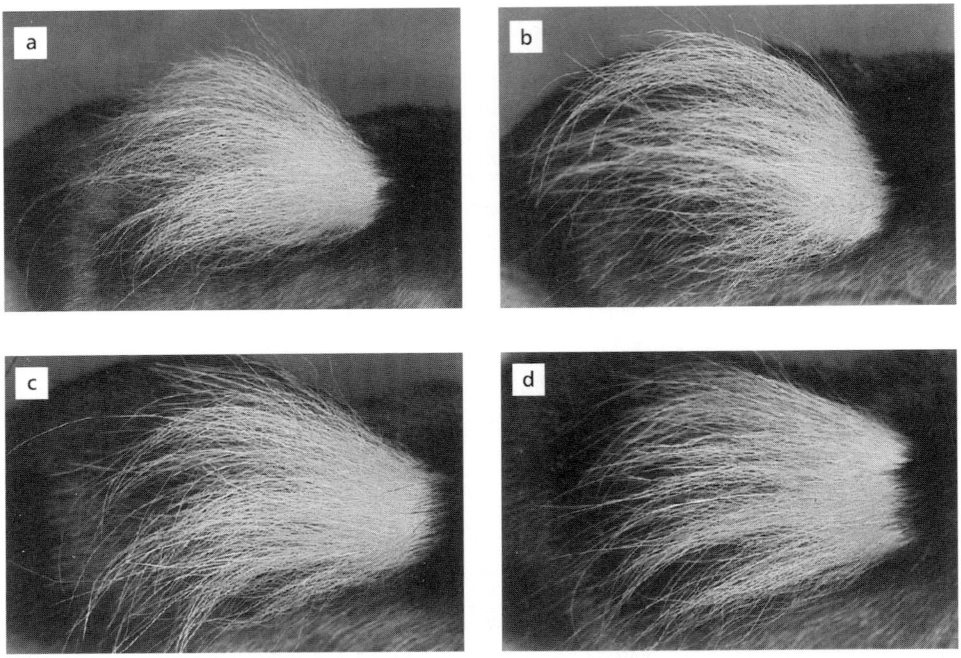

Figure 2.3.3. Gross appearance of representative full-thickness canine skin grafts on *Rag2* null mice at the end of the experiment, approximately 90 days after *Demodex canis* infection: (a) stimulated peripheral blood lymphocyte (PBL)-treated group (group I); (b) peripheral blood mononuclear cell (PBMC)-treated group (group II); and (c) phosphate-buffered saline (PBS) control group (group III). Skin grafts in group IV (d) received only stimulated PBL. Thick hair growth developed on grafts in all groups. Skin lesions did not develop after infection with *D. canis* or after injection with canine lymphocytes.

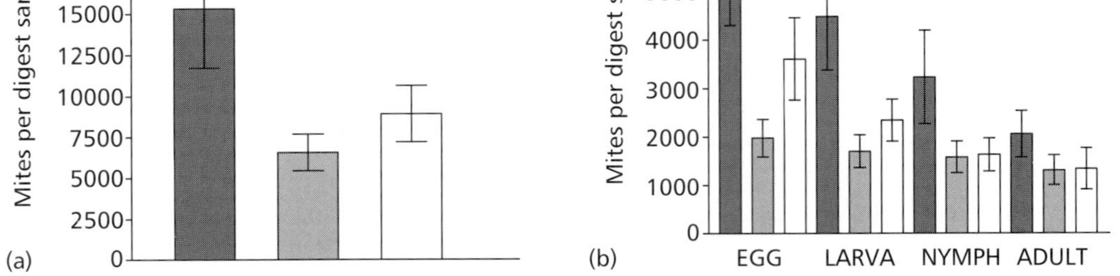

Figure 2.3.4. Bar graph showing the number of *Demodex canis* recovered from canine skin grafts on *Rag2* mice by NaOH digestion. (a) The calculated total number of *D. canis* mites per graft digest sample (mean ± SE) for the stimulated peripheral blood lymphocyte (PBL)-treated group (group I), the peripheral blood mononuclear cell (PBMC)-treated group (group II), and the phosphate-buffered saline (PBS) control group (group III). (b) The calculated total number of each *D. canis* life cycle stage per graft digest sample (mean ± SEM) recovered from canine skin grafts for groups I, II and III. Mites were not recovered from grafts in the group IV that received only stimulated PBL (not shown).

bacteria were present (score = 2), there were significantly more mites in group I than in group III ($p = 0.041$). In contrast, when bacteria were present (score = 1), there were fewer mites on grafts in group I than in group III ($p = 0.012$). Treatment effect depended on bacterial culture and hair growth score.

Histology confirmed *D. canis* infection but did not identify differences between groups. Mites were

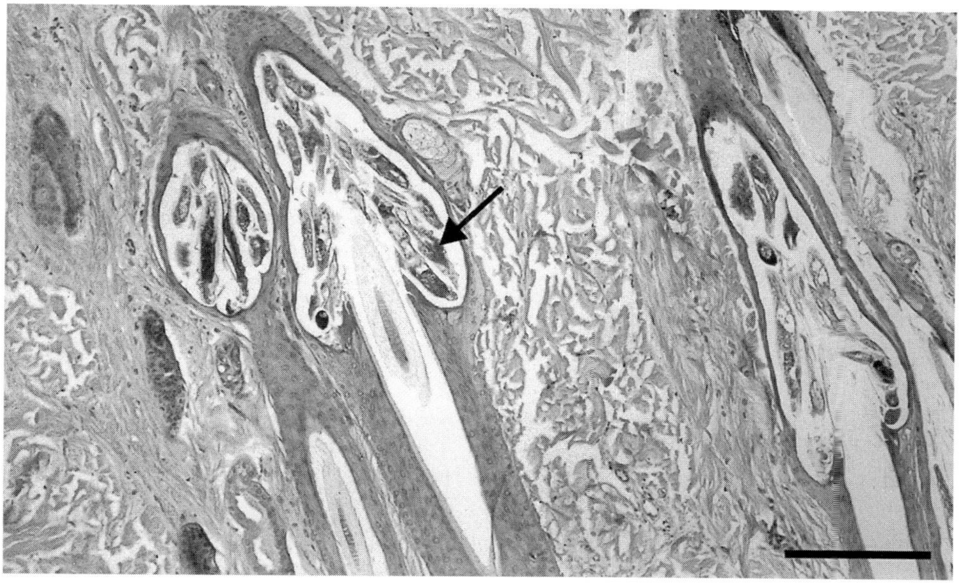

Figure 2.3.5. Photomicrograph of a representative full-thickness canine skin graft on a *Rag2* mouse from group I, approximately 90 days after *Demodex canis* infection. Numerous mites are present within hair follicles (arrow) and are associated with dilatation of the follicle lumen. Inflammation is not present. (Hematoxylin and eosin-stained, paraffin-embedded tissue sections.) Scale bar = 200 μm.

located in the lumen of primary and secondary hairs and occasionally sebaceous gland ducts (Figure 2.3.5). Minimal changes were associated with mite colonization and included follicular dilatation with thinning of the follicle wall. A keratinized layer always separated mites from viable external root sheath cells. Skin graft morphology, including hair follicles and skin glands, resembled pregrafted skin. Inflammation was absent in most grafts and did not target mite-infected hair follicles. In three out of 32 skin grafts, regional to diffuse perivascular infiltrates of granulocytes and mononuclear cells, predominantly histiocytes, were associated with *S. intermedius* infection.

Immunohistochemistry identified rare T-cells within skin grafts of all groups. Typically, one to three cells with positive CD3 membrane staining were present per tissue section (<1 cell per 20 high-power fields) and were found in the dermis, surface epidermis or follicular epithelium. An occasional CD3-positive cell was present in the spleen of mice from each group.

Canine IgG was detected in sera from all mice inoculated with canine leukocytes (24/24) (Figure 2.3.6). IgG levels in group I (mean ± SEM, 34.01 ± 4.91) were significantly higher than in either group II (1.07 ± 0.25; $p < 0.001$) or group IV (11.42 ± 5.42; $p = 0.002$). IgG levels in group IV were significantly higher than in group II ($p = 0.007$). Canine IgG was not detected in pre-experiment serum samples (all mice) or in serum from mice in group III. Anemia was not detected.

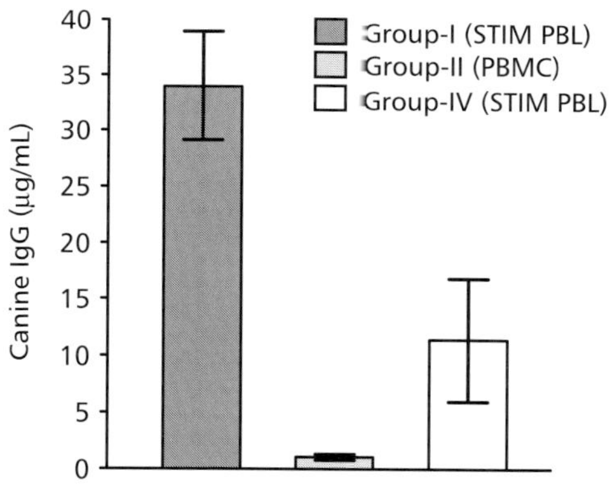

Figure 2.3.6. Bar graph depicting canine immunoglobulin G (IgG) concentration (μg/ml, mean ± SE) in sera from *Rag2* mice approximately 30 days after intragraft transfer of autologous canine leukocytes. Group I ($n = 9$) and group IV ($n = 8$) mice received *in vitro* stimulated peripheral blood lymphocytes (PBL) and group II ($n = 7$) received unstimulated peripheral blood mononuclear cells (PBMC). Canine IgG was not detected in sera from mice in group III ($n = 8$) that did not receive canine lymphocytes (not shown).

Staphylococcus intermedius was recovered at 1 to 4+ colony growth from nine grafts (two to four culture-positive grafts in groups I, II, and III).

Necropsy findings were insignificant for 32 *Rag2* mice completing the study. One sick mouse, removed 85 days after mite transfer, had evidence of systemic bacterial infection.

Discussion

This study successfully developed the skin xenograft mouse model as an *in vivo* experimental system for re-creating aspects of demodicosis. Canine skin was grafted to scid/bg mice and to ICR scid, tgε26 and *Rag2* mice for the first time (Rosenquist *et al.*, 1988; Caswell *et al.*, 1996). In contrast to human studies, the techniques finally adopted led to well-haired uniform canine grafts (Van Neste, 1996). To achieve good hair growth, it was essential to retain the panniculus carnosus in the graft bed and to bandage grafts for at least 4 weeks. These procedures ensure early successful graft revascularization and limit ischemic hair follicle damage.

Although the different murine strains supported canine skin grafts, only *Rag2* knockout mice were useful for long-term experiments modeling demodicosis. Large numbers of scid/bg mice and ICR scid mice developed the 'leaky' phenotype, i.e. generated functional lymphocytes, compared with results from human xenograft studies (Bosma *et al.*, 1988; Carroll & Bosma, 1988; Mosier *et al.*, 1993). The prolonged experiments, multiple procedures and/or exposure to *D. canis* and *S. intermedius* probably exacerbated this recognized complication of the scid mutation (Taylor, 1994). Some scid/bg mice also developed evidence of GVHD, including hemolytic anemia (Taylor, 1994). Tgε26 mice were not robust and suffered high mortality, and the immunodeficient phenotype was not stable in some mice.

The results extend Caswell's observation that *D. canis* would survive on canine skin xenografts (Caswell *et al.*, 1996). Grafts from several different normal adult dogs were reliably infected and large mite populations developed on grafts, similar in number to naturally occurring demodicosis (Unsworth, 1946). Because immature stages dominated, mite populations were still expanding 3 months after graft infection. These findings establish the xenograft model as a useful *in vivo* experimental system for studying canine demodicosis and as the first reliable means for culturing *D. canis* in the laboratory.

The relative role of systemic versus local skin defense mechanisms can be addressed with the xenograft model (Briggaman, 1980). *Demodex canis* readily colonized the isolated xenografts, thereby confirming the importance of systemic host factors for controlling mite numbers. Innate skin mechanisms of host resistance alone do not appear to limit mite colonization. Furthermore, a continued stimulus from the diseased host was not necessary for mite replication. This suggests that dogs with demodicosis do not preferentially stimulate mite proliferation. Because mites were collected from dogs with generalized demodicosis, it is possible that intrinsic differences in mite populations affected the level of skin colonization.

In order to address a central question in the pathogenesis of canine demodicosis, the hypothesis was tested that lymphocytes could limit mite colonization on infected xenografts (Scott *et al.*, 1974, 1976). Treatment with *in vitro* stimulated autologous lymphocytes was associated with a significant increase in mite numbers on skin grafts. Although a sustained lymphocytic tissue reaction was not observed, the levels of serum canine IgG were significantly higher in association with *D. canis* infection, confirming that lymphocytes interacted with mites in grafts. The paradoxical trophic effect of lymphocytes on mite fecundity may be an adaptive response of mites to increase survival in the face of an activated host defense system. Alternatively, experimental conditions may have selected for a lymphocyte population capable of stimulating mites. The relative balance of functional lymphocyte populations in demodicosis may affect mite proliferation and disease progression, similarly to murine and human Th-1 and Th-2 lymphocyte models of parasite resistance (Goldsby *et al.*, 2000). Nonetheless, the results support the possibility that lymphocytes interact with mites via diffusible chemical mediators. These results contrast with the frequently referenced hypothesis that lymphocytes play a protective role in demodicosis (Scott *et al.*, 1995) and highlight the need for further functional studies.

The observation that *S. intermedius*, detectable by culture, influenced the effect of lymphocytes on mite numbers is consistent with previous findings suggesting that bacterial infection alters lymphocyte function in demodicosis (Barta *et al.*, 1983). Further *in vivo* experiments are required to characterize this interaction.

Extensive *D. canis* colonization of grafts did not induce hair loss or significant follicular damage and therefore, in the absence of inflammation, mite activity does not contribute to skin lesion development in canine demodicosis. This finding contrasts with reports stating that mites induce non-specific histological changes in demodicosis (e.g. epidermal hyperplasia, hyperpigmentation, hair loss and follicle rupture), probably as a result of feeding (Nutting, 1976; Nutting *et al.*, 1989). Follicle-dwelling *Demodex* spp. are thought to feed by puncturing keratinocytes and/or by ingesting sebaceous secretions (Nutting *et al.*, 1989). The lack of follicle damage by mites in this study supports the latter possibility and is more consistent with the conclusion of others that *D. canis* does not puncture keratinocytes (Sheahan & Gaafar, 1970b). In the absence of mechanical damage by mites, attention should focus on the role of mite surface antigens or secretory products, such as salivary components, to identify mechanisms of mite recognition by the host immune system.

The skin xenograft–mouse model has received little attention in veterinary investigative dermatology. This study establishes its use with canine tissues and demonstrates its value in addressing basic questions of skin disease pathogenesis.

Acknowledgements

Support provided by Pet Trust, American College of Veterinary Dermatology, European Society of Veterinary Dermatology and the Morris Animal Foundation.

References

Barriga, O. O., Al Khalidi, N. W., Martin, S. & Wyman, M. (1992) Evidence of immunosuppression by *Demodex canis*. *Veterinary Immunology and Immunopathology*, **32**, 37–46.

Barta, O. & Barta, V. (1993) Immunological techniques evaluating cells and their functions. In: *Veterinary Clinical Immunology Laboratory*, Vol. 2 (Ed. O. Barta), pp. B1(1–7), B4(1–17). BAR-LAB, Blacksburg, VA.

Barta, O., Waltman, C., Oyekan, P. P., McGrath, R. K. & Hribernik, T. N. (1983) Lymphocyte transformation suppression caused by pyoderma – failure to demonstrate it in uncomplicated demodectic mange. *Comparative Immunology, Microbiology and Infectious Disease*, **6**, 9–18.

Bivin, S. & Smith, G. (1984) Techniques of experimentation. In: *Laboratory Animal Medicine* (Eds J. Fox, B. Cohen & F. Loew), pp. 565–567. Academic Press, San Diego, CA.

Bosma, G. C., Fried, M., Custer, R. P., Carroll, A., Gibson, D. M. & Bosma, M. J. (1988) Evidence of functional lymphocytes in some (leaky) scid mice. *Journal of Experimental Medicine*, **167**, 1016–1033.

Briggaman, R. A. (1980) Localization of the defect in skin diseases analyzed in the human skin graft–nude mouse model. *Current Problems in Dermatology*, **10**, 115–126

Carroll, A. M. & Bosma, M. J. (1988) Detection and characterization of functional T cells in mice with severe combined immune deficiency. *European Journal of Immunology*, **18**, 1965–1971.

Caswell, J. L., Yager, J. A., Barta, J. R. & Parker, W. (1996) Establishment of *Demodex canis* on canine skin engrafted onto scid–beige mice. *Journal of Parasitology*, **82**, 911–915.

Caswell, J. L., Yager, J. A., Parker W. M. & Moore P. F. (1997) A prospective study of the immunophenotype and temporal changes in the histologic lesions on canine demodicosis. *Veterinary Pathology*, **34**, 279–287.

Gilhar, A. & Etzioni, A. (1994) The nude mouse model for the study of human skin disorders. *Dermatology*, **189**, 5–8.

Gilhar, A., Shalaginov, R., Assy, B., Serafimovich, S. & Kalish, R. S. (1999) Alopecia areata is a T-lymphocyte medicated autoimmune disease: lesional human T-lymphocytes transfer alopecia areata to human skin grafts on SCID mice. *Journal of Investigative Dermatology Symposium Proceedings*, **4**, 207–210.

Goldsby, R. A., Kindt, T. J. & Osborne, B. A. (2000) *Kuby Immunology*, 4th edn, pp. 318–322. W. H. Freeman, New York.

Greenwood, J. D., Croy, B. A., Trout, D. R. & Wilcock, B. P. (1997) Xenogeneic (bovine) peripheral blood leukocytes engrafted into severe combined immunodeficient mice retain primary immune function. *Veterinary Immunology and Immunopathology*, **59**, 93–112.

Greve, J. H. & Gaafar, S. M. (1966) Natural transmission of *Demodex canis* in dogs. *Journal of the American Veterinary Medical Association*, **148**, 1043–1045.

Healey, M. C. & Gaafar, S. M. (1977) Immunodeficiency in canine demodectic mange. I. Experimental production of lesions using antilymphocyte serum. *Veterinary Parasitology*, **3**, 121–131.

Mizuno, S., Fujinaga, T. & Hagio, M. (1993) Characterization of dog interleukin-2 activity. *Journal of Veterinary Medical Science*, **55**, 925–930.

Mosier, D. E., Stell, K. L., Gulizia, R. J., Torbett, B. E. & Gilmore, G. L. (1993) Homozygous scid/scid;beige/beige mice have low levels of spontaneous or neonatal T cell-induced B cell generation. *Journal of Experimental Medicine*, **177**, 191–194.

Nutting, W. B. (1976) Pathogenesis associated with hair follicle mites (Acari:Demodicidae). *Acarologia*, **17**, 493–507.

Nutting, W. B., Firda, K. E., Desch, C. E., Jr, ChannaBasavanna, G. P. & Viraktamath, C. A. (1989) Topology and histopathology of hair follicle mites (Demodicidae) of man. *Progress in Acarology*, **1**, 113–121.

Petzelbauer, P., Groger, M., Kunstfeld, R., Petzelbauer, E. & Wolff, K. (1996) Human delayed-type hypersensitivity reaction in a SCID mouse engrafted with human T cells and autologous skin. *Journal of Investigative Dermatology*, **107**, 576–581.

Rosenquist, M. D., Cram, A. E. & Kealey, G. P. (1988) Skin preservation at 4 degrees C: a species comparison. *Cryobiology*, **25**, 31–37.

Scott, D. W., Miller, W. H. & Griffin, C. E. (1995) Parasitic skin diseases. In: *Muller and Kirk's Small Animal Dermatology*, 5th edn, pp. 417–434. W. B. Saunders, Philadelphia, PA.

Scott, D. W., Farrow, B. R. H. & Schultz, R. D. (1974) Studies on the therapeutic and immunologic aspects of generalized demodectic mange in the dog. *Journal of the American Animal Hospital Association*, **10**, 233–244.

Scott, D. W., Schultz, R. D. & Baker, E. B. (1976) Further studies on the therapeutic and immunologic aspects of generalized demodectic mange in the dog. *Journal of the American Animal Hospital Association*, **12**, 203–213.

Sheahan, B. J. & Gaafar, S. M. (1970a) Experimental production of the lesions of canine demodicidosis. *American Journal of Veterinary Research*, **31**, 1241–1243.

Sheahan, B. J. & Gaafar, S. M. (1970b) Histologic and histochemical changes in cutaneous lesions of experimentally induced and naturally occurring canine demodicidosis. *American Journal of Veterinary Research*, **31**, 1245–1254.

Somberg, R. L., Robinson, J. P. & Felsburg, P. J. (1992) Detection of canine interleukin-2 receptors by flow cytometry. *Veterinary Immunology and Immunopathology*, **33**, 17–24.

Taylor, P. C. (1994) *The Use of SCID Mice in the Investigation of Human Autoimmune Disease*, pp. 17–21, 107–113. R. G. Landes, Austin, TX.

Unsworth, K. (1946) Studies on the clinical and parasitological aspects of canine demodectic mange. *Journal of Comparative Pathology and Therapeutics*, **56**, 114–127.

Van Neste, D. (1996) The use of scalp grafts onto nude mice as a model for human hair growth: is there something new for hair growth drug screening programs? In: *Dermatologic Research Techniques* (Ed. H. I. Maibach), pp. 37–48. CRC Press, Boca Raton, FL.

2.4

Prevalence of feline staphylococci with special reference to *Staphylococcus felis* among domestic and feral cats in the south-east of England

A. Patel BVM, CertSAD, MRCVS, D.H. Lloyd BVetMed, PhD, FRCVS, DipECVD and A.I. Lamport BA, AIMBS

Dermatology Unit, Department of Small Animal Medicine and Surgery, Royal Veterinary College, Hatfield, UK

Summary

The prevalence of cutaneous staphylococci was studied in three groups of cats: feral cats, healthy pet cats and pet cats with skin lesions. Swab specimens and contact plate samples were obtained from a total of 13 sites on each cat and also from lesions where present. There was no significant difference ($p > 0.05$) in the isolation rates between the feral (49%) and the healthy pet cats (38%), or between the feral and the affected cats (54%). However, when affected pet cats were compared with healthy pets there was a significant difference ($p < 0.05$). Staphylococci were isolated from at least two sites from every cat and from every lesion sampled. Sixteen different species were identified from the samples obtained. *Staphylococcus felis* was isolated from all three populations and there was no significant difference between the three groups ($p > 0.05$), suggesting that this species may be a resident *Staphylococcus* of cats. *Staphylococcus intermedius* was the most common pathogenic species isolated and was derived mainly from multiple sites on lesional cats, suggesting that it may play a role in perpetuating skin disease in cats.

Introduction

The occurrence of staphylococci on the coat, skin and mucosae of dogs has often been reported (Allakar *et al.*, 1992a, b; Harvey & Lloyd, 1994; Saijonmaa-Koulumies & Lloyd, 1996) but there have been no recent studies on cats. In 1967 Hearst isolated *Staphylococcus aureus* from 98% of the cats sampled in a pet shop. In a later qualitative study (Krogh & Kristensen, 1976) *S. aureus* was isolated from 8% of the sites on 10 normal cats, whereas *S. epidermidis* was isolated from 12% of the sites. It has been suggested that the high isolation rate in the former study may have been due to environmental contamination.

Before the classification introduced by Kloos & Schleifer (1975a), three species of human staphylococci, *S. aureus*, *S. epidermidis* and *S. saprophyticus*, were recognised and classified according to the scheme proposed by Baird-Parker (1974). Since then several new coagulase-negative species have been identified (Kloos & Schleifer, 1975b; Schleifer & Kloos, 1975). In addition, Hajek (1976) described a new coagulase-positive species, *S. intermedius*, which had previously been recognised as biotypes E and F of *S. aureus*. In a semiquantitative study conducted by Cox *et al.* (1985), *S. intermedius* was the most commonly isolated coagulase-positive species and *S. simulans* the most common coagulase-negative species isolated from healthy cats. Neither Hearst (1967) nor Krogh & Kristensen (1976) biotyped their *S. aureus* isolates and hence the possibility of these including *S. intermedius* remains.

Staphylococcus simulans, which is frequently found on human skin, has been reported as having a resident status on cats (Devriese *et al.*, 1984; Cox *et al.*, 1985). Igimi *et al.* (1989) suggested that these feline isolates might have been the newly identified coagulase-negative species *S. felis*, as the two have similar biochemical properties but can be distinguished by differences in mannose fermentation, phosphatase reaction and bacitracin sensitivity (Igimi *et al.*, 1994). A more recent study by Espinola & Lilenbaum (1996) showed that coagulase-negative staphylococci, which they suggested may be *S. felis*, were present in the eyelid margins and conjunctival sacs of healthy cats, suggesting a resident status. However, they did not differentiate between *S. felis* and *S. simulans*.

The main purpose of the present study was to report on the prevalence of staphylococci on the coat and mucosae of three different groups of cats, with special reference to the resident status of *S. felis*.

Materials and methods

Cats

Ten feral cats, which had had no known contact with humans, 11 healthy pet cats and nine pet cats with skin lesions were sampled. All of the pet cats came from either single or multi-cat homes but only one cat per household was sampled. The healthy pets ranged between 7 months and 11 years (median age 3.4 years) and the affected pet cats ranged between 6 months and 13 years (median age 5.6 years) of age. The ages of the feral cats were unknown. Both males and females were sampled in each group and the study included four cats with a long coat (Table 2.4.1).

The feral cats were trapped by the Cats Protection League for neutering. They were anaesthetised using medetomidine/ketamine (Domitor; Pfizer Animal Health, Sandwich, UK; Ketaset, Willows Francis Veterinary, Crawley, UK) injected intramuscularly whilst still in their traps and were then handled wearing sterile gloves. Samples were obtained before proceeding with surgery. The healthy pet cats were those that had been admitted for routine clean surgery, had not received any form of medication for at least 2 weeks before sampling, and were free of skin disease. The pet cats with skin lesions admitted to the study had not received any antibacterial therapy in the previous 2 weeks; they underwent a full dermatological investigation and the underlying cause of the lesions was identified wherever possible. The samples were obtained at the first examination, under sedation.

Specimen collecting and processing

A swab sample was obtained from the oral cavity, both anterior nostrils, both external ear canals, the anus and the interdigital skin of the left forefoot and the right hindfoot. A mini-tipped swab (SW06; Microbiological Supply, Toddington, UK) moistened in sterile water (Water for injection; Braun Medical, Sheffield, UK) was rubbed vigorously on each site for 10 s. The forehead, left and right axillae, and the left and right groin were sampled by pressing one contact plate at each site for 10 s. The contact plates were made up in a manner described by Bond *et al.* (1994), using sterile lids from bijou bottles, but for this study they were filled with bovine blood agar (Oxoid Blood Agar Base CM271; 5% defibrinated bovine blood). The swabs were plated out, in overlapping streaks, onto bovine blood agar within 2 h of sampling. The plates were examined after being incubated aerobically at 37°C for 24 h. Catalase-positive colonies of Gram-positive bacteria with morphology consistent with staphylococci were counted and their numbers categorised as no growth, scanty growth (between one and 50 colonies), moderate growth (between 51 and 100 colonies) and overgrowth (>100 colonies).

Table 2.4.1. Characteristics of cats

Cat population	Age[a] (years)	Sex		Breed		
		Male	Female	DSH	DLH	Other
Feral ($n = 10$)	NK	7	3	10	–	–
Healthy pet cats ($n = 11$)	3.4 (7 months to 11 years)	4	7	8	2	1[b]
Affected pet cats ($n = 9$)	5.6 (6 months to 13 years)	3	6	8	1	–

[a] Median (range).
[b] Birman.
DLH: domestic long hair; DSH: domestic short hair; NK: not known.

Species identification

The colonies were subcultured onto blood agar plates to obtain pure isolates for further identification. The presence of deoxyribonuclease (DNase) was confirmed by the appearance of a clear zone after flooding a DNase agar (Oxoid CM321) plate, which had a stab inoculum of the isolate, with hydrochloric acid after 24 h of incubation at 37°C. The presence of coagulase was confirmed by the clumping of rabbit plasma in a slide coagulase test.

Species were identified using commercial API ID32 STAPH tests (API Biomerieux, Basingstoke, Hants, UK). This system uses the following miniaturised biochemical tests: production of urease, arginine dihydrolase, ornithine decarboxylase, acetoin, β-galactosidase, arginine arylamidase, alkaline phosphatase, pyrrolidonyl arylamidase and β-glucuronidase; hydrolysis of aesculin; reduction of nitrates; resistance to novobiocin; and fermentation of glucose, fructose, mannose, maltose, lactose, trehalose, mannitol, raffinose, ribose, cellobiose, sucrose, *N*-acetyl-glucosamine, turanose and arabinose. The biochemical tests were recorded as positive or negative and then used to derive a profile number that was compared with that from the API STAPH-IDENT profile register for species identification. *Staphylococcus felis* isolates were identified by comparing API profile numbers of the isolates obtained in this study with those obtained from *S. felis* type strains (ATCC 49168 and GD521) and from sucrose fermenting strains (S36 and S141) isolated by Igimi *et al.* (1989).

The isolates were tested for bacitracin sensitivity using the Kirby–Bauer disc diffusion method (Bauer *et al.*, 1966). Pure isolates were suspended in sterile water to make an inoculum with opacity equivalent to McFarland Standard 1, which was then spread uniformly on Mueller–Hinton agar (Oxoid337). Discs impregnated with 10 IU of bacitracin were placed on the plates and incubated aerobically at 37°C for 24 h. On the basis of the clear zone diameter the results were categorised as susceptible, moderately resistant or resistant (Barry & Thornsberry, 1985).

Statistical analysis

The data were analysed using Epi Info Version 5.0, which is public domain software produced by CDC Atlanta. Comparisons between groups were made using chi-squared and Fisher's exact tests. A *p*-value of <0.05 was considered to be significant.

Results

From 398 sites sampled, 187 staphylococcal isolates (47% of sites) were obtained. These isolates came from 49% of the sites in the feral cats, from 38% of the sites in healthy pet cats and from 54% of the sites in affected pet cats (Table 2.4.2). Chi-squared analysis showed significant differences in isolation rate ($p = 0.02$) among the three groups. Subanalysis (chi-squared test with Yates' correction) revealed that these significant differences existed only between the affected and unaffected pet cats ($p = 0.013$).

A staphylococcal species was isolated from at least two sites in each of the cats sampled. The rate of isolation from the different sites varied among individual animals and among groups. Overall, staphylococci were isolated from the forehead of 26 cats (87%) out of the 30 sampled. The remainder of the sites yielded isolates, with decreasing frequency, from the axillae (62%), anterior nostrils (60%), interdigital skin (40%), groin (36%), external ear canals (27%) and anal ring (13%) (Table 2.4.3). A staphylococcal species was isolated from every lesion sampled. There was no growth from 53% of the swabs; of the remainder, 30% showed scanty, 5% moderate and 12% confluent growth. Heavy growth of Gram-negative bacteria was obtained from the oral cavity of all cats.

Sixteen different staphylococcal species were identified using the API Staph ID32 identification system. The coagulase-positive isolates, in addition to being haemolytic, were DNase positive. With *S. felis*, the API STAPH-IDENT system produced a profile number of 3653 5640 for type strains ATCC 49168 and GD521, and the sucrose-fermenting strains S141 and S36

Table 2.4.2. Frequency of isolation of staphylococci in the three populations of cats

Group	No. of cats	No. of specimens[a]	No. of isolates	No. of positive sites[b]
Feral	10	130	64	6.2 (2–10)
Healthy pets	11	143	55**	5 (2–7)
Affected pets	9	125	68	7.42 (2–11)

[a] A total of 13 sites was sampled on each cat plus lesional sites in affected cats.
[b] Mean (range).
** $p = 0.013$ when isolation rates between healthy and affected pet cats were compared.

Table 2.4.3. Frequency of isolation of staphylococci from the different sites

Site	Total sites sampled	Feral (n = 10)	Healthy pets (n = 11)	Affected pets (n = 9)	Total isolates n (%)
Forehead	30	9	9	8	26 (87)
Axillae	60	11	13	13	37 (62)
Anterior nares	60	14	8	14	36 (60)
Groin	60	10	14	12	36 (60)
Interdigital skin	60	12	6	6	24 (40)
External ear canal	60	5	5	6	16 (27)
Anal ring	30	3	0	1	4 (13)
Lesional skin	9	–	–	9	9 (100)

Table 2.4.4. Biochemical tests of the *Staphylococcus felis* isolates showing similarities to and differences from the type strains (ATCC 49168 and GD521) and sucrose-fermenting strain S141, using the API STAPH-IDENT test

Biochemical test	API profile numbers			
	3653 5640 (ATCC 49168 and GD521)	3653 5660 (S141)	1653 5660	1653 5661
Urease	+	+	+	+
Arginine dehydrolase	+	+	–	–
Glucose	+	+	+	+
Fructose	+	+	+	+
Mannose	+	+	+	+
Maltose	–	–	–	–
Lactose	+	+	+	+
Trehalose	+	+	+	+
Alkaline phosphatase	+	+	+	+
Sucrose	–	+	+	+
Turanose	–	–	–	+

produced profile numbers 3653 5660 and 3651 5660, respectively. These profiles and the ability of isolates to produce alkaline phosphatase and to ferment mannose were used to identify *S. felis*. In addition, isolates with profile numbers 1653 5660 and 1653 5661 (Table 2.4.4) were identified as *S. felis* because they produced alkaline phosphatase and fermented mannose, trehalose and sucrose but not maltose. The remaining staphylococcal species were identified using the API STAPH-IDENT profile register and database. Isolates with profiles that did not match those held in the database were classified as unidentified.

The 64 *S. felis* isolates (35% of all staphylococcal isolates) were derived from all three groups of cats: seven feral and seven healthy pet cats and three cats with skin disease (Table 2.4.5). There was no significant difference in the isolation rate between the three groups (chi-squared test, $p = 0.65$). *Staphylococcus intermedius* was also isolated from all three groups (three isolates from one feral cat, single isolates from each of three healthy pets and 30 isolates from five affected cats) and made up 20% of the isolates. Of the 30 isolates from affected cats, 28 were from lesions and other sites on three cats. The remaining two isolates were from single non-lesional sites on the other two affected cats. The number of cats in each group was too small to allow meaningful analysis. *Staphylococcus aureus* (2% of isolates), *S. chromogenes* (4%), *S. cohnii* (3%), *S. epidermidis* (2%), *S. equorum* (1%), *S. hominis* (2%), *S. simulans* (7%), *S. warneri* (7%) and *S. xylosus* (4%) were also isolated from more than one cat. *Staphylococcus sciuri* (2%) was isolated

Table 2.4.5. API profiles and the origin of the *Staphylococcus felis* isolates

API profile	No. of *S. felis* isolates		
	Feral	Healthy	Lesional
3653 5640	1	7	0
3653 5660	13	7	9
1653 5660	12	8	6
1653 5661	0	0	1
Total	26	22	16

from three sites on the same cat, while the other species, *S. auricularis* (0.5%), *S. haemolyticus* (0.5%), *S. kloosii* (0.5%) and *S. saprophyticus* (0.5%), were isolated only once on different cats. The 25 unidentified isolates were all coagulase-negative.

Staphylococcus spp. were isolated from all the lesions sampled and five different species, *S. felis*, *S. sciuri*, *S. intermedius*, *S. xylosus* and *S. aureus*, were identified from the nine affected pet cats. In all but one case, the same species was isolated from the lesions and the nostrils of the affected cats. *Staphylococcus felis* and *S. intermedius* were isolated from three lesional cats, whereas *S. aureus*, *S. sciuri* and *S. xylosus* were each isolated from one lesional cat.

All isolates were susceptible to bacitracin, producing a clear zone of more than 0.5 cm from the outer edge of the disc to the beginning of bacterial growth.

Discussion

Devriese *et al.* (1984) reported that *S. simulans* was the most common coagulase-negative species and *S. aureus* the most common coagulase-positive species isolated from cats, and that these species were probably acquired from their owners. In a subsequent study (Cox *et al.*, 1985), *S. intermedius* was reported as being the most commonly isolated coagulase-positive species, while *S. simulans* was still the most commonly isolated coagulase-negative species. Cox *et al.* (1985) did not differentiate *S. felis* as it had not yet been described. Although *S. felis* was described by Igimi *et al.* in 1989, prior to the current work no published studies have reported the occurrence of *S. felis* in healthy cats or in clinically affected cats. A recent study (Espinola & Lilenbaum, 1996) showed that coagulase-negative staphylococci were present on the eyelid margins and the conjunctival sacs of healthy cats, but did not differentiate *S. simulans* from *S. felis*; both were classified as the former species.

The current study describes the use of a commercially available test to differentiate between *S. simulans* and *S. felis* using profile numbers for the type strains (ATCC 49168 and GD521) and for the sucrose-fermenting strain (S141). In agreement with Igimi *et al.* (1989), all of the isolates produced alkaline phosphatase and urease, reduced nitrate, and fermented mannose, trehalose and lactose. However, 27 strains of *S. felis* in this study did not produce arginine dehydrolase, compared with only three (7.7%) in the previous report (Igimi *et al.*, 1989). No isolates in the current study matched the profile of the second sucrose-fermenting strain, S36. Identification of staphylococcal species using the API STAPH-IDENT system has been shown to have a high congruence with other methods described in the literature (Kloos & Wolfshohl, 1982) and the results of the present study support the use of this system by commercial laboratories to recognise *S. felis*.

Staphylococcus felis can be differentiated from *S. simulans* by its susceptibility to bacitracin (Igimi *et al.*, 1989). However, the Kirby–Bauer method, as used in this study, was not helpful as all the staphylococcal isolates were sensitive to bacitracin including *S. simulans*, which was expected to be resistant. Igimi *et al.* (1989) used Eiken susceptibility test agar plates containing 2 U of bacitracin per millilitre, a technique that may have given a higher level of discrimination.

The observation that *S. felis* was present in all three groups of cats and that there was no significant difference between the groups suggests that *S. felis* is a normal resident on cats, both at mucosal sites and on the coat. It is possible that in previous studies (Devriese *et al.*, 1984) *S. felis* was mistaken for *S. simulans* and reported as being acquired from humans. In the present study, *S. felis* was isolated from feral cats which, to the best of the authors' knowledge, had not been handled, lending support to the concept of this organism being a component of the normal flora in cats. A larger quantitative study to evaluate the residency status of *S. felis* is now indicated to confirm this finding.

Although coagulase activity correlates well with virulence, coagulase-negative organisms are capable of producing enzymes and extracellular proteins that could contribute to disease (Gemmel, 1983; Noble, 1993), and are being increasingly recognised as human pathogens. Igimi *et al.* (1989) first isolated *S. felis* from clinical specimens obtained from cats and there have been reports (Higgins & Gottchalk, 1991; Aarestrup & Jacobeson, 1993) suggesting a pathogenic role for this species. In the current study *S. felis* was isolated from both lesions and other sites on cats with skin lesions, although it did not predominate on lesional animals. Further studies on its role in the pathogenesis of feline skin disease are warranted.

In accordance with Cox *et al.* (1985), the present study also found *S. intermedius* to be the second most common staphylococcal species isolated from healthy cats. However, in this study most of the isolates were from affected cats, suggesting that *S. intermedius* may play a role in perpetuating skin disease. Further investigation into the pathogenic role of *S. intermedius* in the cat is therefore needed. *Staphylococcus aureus* was not found to be the predominant coagulase-positive species isolated from cats, as has been suggested in the past (Krogh & Kristensen, 1976; Devriese *et al.*, 1984; Medleau & Blue, 1988).

Nasal carriage of staphylococci has been implicated as an important factor in introducing pathogenic staphylococci onto skin sites in people (Noble *et al.*, 1964) and in dogs (Harvey & Lloyd, 1994; Saijonmaa-Koulumies & Lloyd, 1996). In the present study some of the healthy cats and most of the affected cats were found to be carrying the same staphylococcal species and strain (profile number) in the anterior regions of one or both of nostril and on other sites on the same cat. It may be inferred that staphylococci were seeded onto the hair coat and onto lesions during grooming. However, the prevalence of staphylococci in the oral cavity could not be estimated in the current study owing to overgrowth by Gram-negative bacteria in cultures from oral swabs. Overall, the staphylococcal isolation rate was low and when isolated a high proportion of samples produced a scanty growth score, which implies a low carriage of staphylococci, as reported before (Baker, 1970; Cox *et al.*, 1985). It was suggested that this might be due to the fastidious grooming habits of cats (Baker, 1970; Muller *et al.*, 1989). However, in the present study, staphylococci were found on foreheads, in the axillae and on the groin, all of which are areas that are frequently groomed.

It is possible that other factors determining the carriage of bacteria in cats involve the immune status of the individual and ecological conditions affecting the skin surface (Noble, 1990). The availability of nutrients, the ability of the bacterium to adhere to the skin and the lipid composition at the skin surface are important in determining the skin flora in humans. Mason & Lloyd (1993) suggested that dogs were more prone to bacterial colonisation and subsequent infections owing to less intercellular lipid material in the stratum corneum compared with humans and cattle. Such studies on the lipid composition of the feline skin surface may help to explain the low carriage of bacteria on cats' skin.

Conclusion

This study indicates that *S. felis* is the most common coagulase-negative species found on cats and that it is a resident organism. Furthermore, it may play a role in the pathogenesis of skin disease. *Staphylococcus intermedius* was the most common coagulase-positive species found in the study and as most of the isolates were from cats with skin lesions, this species may be involved in perpetuating skin disease. However, this was a small study in a restricted geographical area and more extensive studies are needed to substantiate the findings.

Acknowledgements

The authors would like to thank Bayer plc for their financial support, Dr S. Igimi for providing the type strain GD521 and the sucrose-fermenting strains S141 and S36 used in this study and Biomerieux, UK, for supplying some of the API test kits.

References

Aarestrup, F. M. & Jacobeson, M. J. (1993) Bacterial paronychia caused by *Staphylococcus felis* in cats. *Dansk Veterinaertidsskrift*, **76**, 1066–1067.

Allaker, R. P., Lloyd, D. H. & Simpson, A. I. (1992a) Occurrence of *Staphylococcus intermedius* on the hair and skin of normal dogs. *Research in Veterinary Science*, **52**, 174–176.

Allaker, R. P., Lloyd, D. H. & Bailey, R. M. (1992b) Population sizes and the frequency of staphylococci at mucocutaneous sites on healthy dogs. *Veterinary Record*, **130**, 303–304.

Baird-Parker, A. C. (1974) *Staphylococcus*. In: *Bergey's Manual of Determinative Bacteriology*, 8th edn .(Eds R. E. Buchanan & N. E. Gibbons), pp. 483–489. Williams & Wilkins, Baltimore, MD.

Baker, K. P. (1970) Some aspects of feline dermatoses. *Veterinary Record*, **86**, 62–66.

Barry, A. L. & Thornsberry, C. (1985) Susceptibility tests: diffusion test procedures. In: *Manual of Clinical Microbiology*, 4th edn (Eds E. H. Lennette, A. Balows, W. J. Hausler & H. J. Shadomy), pp. 978–987. American Society of Microbiology, Washington, DC.

Bauer, A. W., Kirby, W. M., Sherris, J. C. & Turck, M. (1966) Antibiotic susceptibility testing by a standardized single disc method. *American Journal of Clinical Pathology*, **45**, 493–496.

Bond, R., Collin, N. S. & Lloyd, D. H. (1994) Use of contact plates for the quantitative culture of *Malassezia pachydermatis* from canine skin. *Journal of Small Animal Practice*, **35**, 68–72.

Cox, H. U., Hoskins, J. D., Newman, S. S., Turnwald, G. H., Foil, C. S., Roy, A. F. & Kearney, M. T. (1985) Distribution of staphylococcal species on clinically healthy cats. *American Journal of Veterinary Research*, **46**, 1824–1828.

Devriese, L. A., Nzuambe D. & Godard, C. (1984) Identification and characterization of staphylococci isolated from cats. *Veterinary Microbiology*, **9**, 279–285.

Espinola, M. B. & Lilenbaum, W. (1996) Prevalence of bacteria in the conjunctival sac and on the eyelid margin of clinically normal cats. *Journal of Small Animal Practice*, **37**, 364–366.

Gemmell, C. G. (1983) Extracellular toxins and enzymes of coagulase-negative staphylococci. In: *Staphylococci and Staphylococcal Infections*, Vol. 2 (Eds C. S. F. Easmon & C. Adlam), pp. 809–827. Academic Press, London.

Hajek, V. (1976) *Staphylococcus intermedius*, a new species isolated from animals. *International Journal of Systematic Bacteriology*, **26**, 401–408.

Harvey, R. G. & Lloyd, D. H. (1994) The distribution of *Staphylococcus intermedius* and coagulase-negative staphylococci on the hair, skin surface, within the hair follicles and on the mucous membranes of dogs. *Veterinary Dermatology*, **5**, 75–81.

Hearst, B. R. (1967) Low incidence of staphylococcal dermatitides in animals with high incidence of *Staphylococcus aureus*. *Veterinary Medicine/Small Animal Clinician*, **62**, 475–477.

Higgins, R. & Gottchalk, M. (1991) Isolation of *Staphylococcus felis* from cases of external otitis in cats. *Canadian Veterinary Journal*, **32**, 312–313.

Igimi, S., Kawamura, S., Takahashi, E. & Mmitsuoka, A. J. (1989) *Staphylococcus felis*, a new species from clinical specimens from cats. *International Journal of Systematic Bacteriology*, **39**, 373–377.

Igimi, S., Atobe, H., Tohya, Y., Inoue, A., Takahashi, E. & Konishi, S. (1994) Characterisation of the most frequently encountered staphylococcal species in cats. *Veterinary Microbiology*, **39**, 255–260.

Kloos, W. E. & Schleifer, K. H. (1975a) Simplified scheme for routine identification of human *Staphylococcus* species. *Journal of Clinical Microbiology*, **1**, 82–88.

Kloos, W. E. & Schleifer, K. H. (1975b) Isolation and characterization of staphylococci from human skin. II. Description of four new species: *Staphylococcus warneri, Staphylococcus capitis, Staphylococcus hominis* and *Staphylococcus simulans. International Journal of Systematic Bacteriology*, **25**, 62–79.

Kloos, W. E. & Wolfshohl, J. F. (1982) Identification of *Staphylococcus* species with the API staph-ident system. *Journal of Clinical Microbiology*, **16**, 506–516.

Krogh, H. V. & Kristensen, S. (1976) A study of skin diseases in dogs and cats: II. Microflora of the normal skin of dogs and cats. *Nordisk Veterinaermedicin*, **28**, 459–463.

Mason, I. S. & Lloyd, D. H. (1993) Scanning electron microscopical studies of the living epidermis and stratum corneum in dogs. In: *Advances in Veterinary Dermatology*, Vol. 2 (Eds P. J. Ihrke, I. S. Mason & S. W. White), pp. 131–139. Pergamon Press, Oxford.

Medleau, L. & Blue, J. L. (1988) Frequency and antimicrobial susceptibility of *Staphylococcus* spp. isolated from feline skin lesion. *Journal of the American Veterinary Medical Association*, **193**, 1080–1081.

Muller, G. H., Kirk, R. W. & Scott, D. W. (1989) Bacterial skin diseases. In: *Small Animal Dermatology*, 4th edn, pp. 244–287. W. B. Saunders, Philadelphia, PA.

Noble, W. C. (1993) Staphylococci as pathogens. In: *The Skin Microflora and Microbial Skin Disease* (Ed. W. C. Noble), pp. 153–167. Cambridge University Press, Cambridge.

Noble, W. C. (1990) Systematics and the natural history of staphylococci 2. *Journal of Applied Bacteriology Symposium* (Suppl.), 39S–48S.

Noble, W. C., Williams, R. E. O., Patricia-Jevons, M. & Shooter, R. A. (1964) Some aspects of nasal carriage of staphylococci. *Journal of Clinical Pathology*, **17**, 79–83.

Saijonmaa-Koulumies, L. E. & Lloyd, D. H. (1996) Colonization of canine skin with bacteria. *Veterinary Dermatology*, **7**, 153–162.

Schleifer, K. H. & Kloos, W. E. (1975) Isolation and characterization of staphylococci from human skin. I. Amended description of *Staphylococcus epidermidis* and *Staphylococcus saprophyticus* and description of three new species: *Staphylococcus cohnii, Staphylococcus haemolyticus*, and *Staphylococcus xylosus. International Journal of Systematic Bacteriology*, **25**, 50–61.

2.5

Evaluation of the specific immune response in dogs infected by *Leishmania infantum*

L. Ferrer DVM, PhD,[1] L. Solano-Gallego DVM,[2] M. Arboix PhD[2] and J. Alberola DVM, PhD[2]

Departments of [1]Animal Medicine and Surgery, and [2]Pharmacology and Therapeutics, Universitat Autònoma de Barcelona, Barcelona, Spain

Summary

The immune system plays a key role in *Leishmania* infection. Dogs that show clinically patent leishmaniosis have a predominantly humoral, non-protective immune response (Th_2-like). In contrast, infected dogs that do not develop the disease display a predominantly cellular, protective immune response (Th_1-like). This research aimed to assess the usefulness of immunological techniques in the evaluation of dogs infected by *Leishmania* and also to define the immune profiles of this population of dogs. The following parameters were studied: anti-*Leishmania* immunoglobulin G-1 (IgG_1), IgG_2, total IgG antibodies, delayed type hypersensitivity (DTH) to leishmanin, lymphocyte proliferation assay and production of cytokines (γ-interferon [IFN-γ] and tumour necrosis factor-α [TNF-α]). Three groups of dogs were investigated: (1) healthy, non-infected; (2) infected without patent disease; and (3) infected with clinically patent leishmaniosis (before and after treatment). Healthy, non-infected dogs were consistently negative for all assays performed. Infected animals without clinically patent disease showed two different immune profiles. The majority showed low titres of anti-*Leishmania* antibodies with a positive DTH test and a high production of IFN-γ. The remainder showed positive titres of anti-*Leishmania* antibodies with a negative or a weakly positive DTH. Before treatment, ill dogs had a high level of anti-*Leishmania* antibodies (mainly IgG_2), negative DTH, no production of IFN-γ but production of TNF-α. Clinical recovery was associated with a decrease in the titre of antibodies (initially, IgG_1 titres were reduced, followed by IgG_2/total IgG) and also an increase in the diameter on the DTH test. The combination of serology, DTH test and measurement of cytokines constitutes a useful, clinically relevant method to evaluate the immune response to *Leishmania*.

Introduction

In the past few years there has been revision and reformulation of some of the main paradigms of infectious diseases. First, the line that has historically existed between infectious and non-infectious diseases has become somewhat blurred. Infectious agents are now considered as the cause of many diseases that previously had been considered non-infectious. The role of *Helicobacter pylori* in the pathogenesis of gastric ulcers is a good example (Maconi *et al.*, 1999). Secondly, the relationship between infection and disease has become more complex. The simple scheme consisting of contagion, infection and disease has been demonstrated to be false in most diseases, at least in part. As an example, it has been shown that not all dogs infected by *Borrelia* spp. develop Lyme disease and that many remain asymptomatic (Greene, 1990). Finally, it seems that in most cases clinical healing is not associated with complete elimination of the infection. When techniques of high sensitivity, e.g. polymerase chain reaction (PCR) are used to investigate the presence of infectious agents, most patients remain infected for a long period after treatment and clinical improvement. The huge advances in molecular diagnostic techniques and immunology are responsible for these radical changes in the conception of infectious diseases of humans and other animals.

Canine leishmaniosis serves as an excellent example for describing the conceptual changes discussed previously. As in many other infectious diseases, we must alter or replace the old paradigm and begin to discuss and to spread the new paradigm. The major change is the difference between infection and disease. Various authors have demonstrated that the rate of infection in the dog population is much higher than the prevalence of the disease. One communication presented at the 4th World Congress of Veterinary Dermatology (Solano-Gallego *et al.*, 2000b) demonstrates that, similarly to the situation in humans, only a small proportion of dogs infected by *Leishmania* develop the disease leishmaniosis.

Extensive research in experimental rodent models suggests that the immune system plays a key role in *Leishmania* infection (Solbach & Laskay, 2000). Dogs showing clinically patent leishmaniosis have a predominantly humoral, non-protective immune response (Th_2-like). In contrast, dogs that are infected but do not develop the disease have a predominantly cellular, protective immune response (Th_1-like) (Cabral *et al.*, 1992; Pinelli *et al.*, 1994). Therefore, the evaluation of the type of immune response in a single patient appears to be a key prognostic parameter. This research aimed to evaluate the usefulness of immunological techniques in the evaluation of dogs infected by *Leishmania* and also to define the immune profiles of these animals.

Materials and methods

Animals

Three groups of dogs were studied: group 1: 28 healthy non-infected dogs (negative by PCR and serology for *Leishmania*); group 2: 30 clinically healthy infected dogs (positive PCR for *Leishmania* or serology); group 3: 25 infected dogs with clinically patent leishmaniosis (direct observation of parasite or positive PCR for *Leishmania* or serology) and treated with Glucantime® (Rhone-Merieux) and/or allopurinol for at least 1 year. All dogs included in the study lived in endemic areas in Spain and were of different breeds, sexes and ages.

Serology

Enzyme-linked immunosorbent assay (ELISA) was performed as described by Solano-Gallego *et al.* (2000a). In brief, microtitre plates were coated with 20 μg/ml of *Leishmania infantum* antigen (WHO code MHOM/FR/78/LEM 75) in 0.1 ml of 0.1 M carbonate–bicarbonate buffer, pH 9.6, and incubated overnight at 4°C. Dog sera, 100 μl/well, diluted 1:400 in phosphate-buffered saline–0.05% Tween 20 (PBST)–1% dried skimmed milk, were incubated for 1 h at 37°C. After washing, 100 μl/well of anti-dog immunoglobulin G (IgG) (1:20 000), anti-dog IgG_2 (1:5000) and anti-dog IgG_1 (1:2000) conjugated to horseradish peroxidase (Bethyl Laboratories, Montgomery, TX, USA) were added and incubated for 1 h at 37°C. The substrate solution was ortho-phenylene-diamine. The reaction was stopped with 3 M H_2SO_4. Absorbance values were read at 490 nm in an automatic ELISA reader (Bio-tek Instruments EL 312e microplate). The reaction was quantified as units (U) related to a positive serum used as a calibrator and arbitrarily set at 100 U. The cut-off, above which was considered positive, was established at 20 U for IgG, 22 U for IgG_1 and 11 U for IgG_2 (mean + 4 SD of 32 dogs from non-endemic areas).

Delayed type hypersensitivity to leishmanin

Leishmanin reagent was an inactivated suspension of 3×10^8 *L. infantum* (WHO code MHOM/FR/78/LEM 75) promastigotes per millilitre in 0.4% phenol–saline (kindly provided by Dr Alvar, Instituto de Salud Carlos III, Madrid, Spain). The solution (100 μl) was intradermally injected into the skin of the groin. Skin reactions were recorded after 72 h and an induration or erythematous area >5 mm in diameter was considered positive, as described by Pinelli *et al.* (1994) and Cardoso *et al.* (1998). Purified protein derivative (2500 TU/ml) (Central Veterinary Institute Lelystad, The Netherlands) and leishmanin diluent as well as saline solution (0.1 ml of each) served as controls.

Isolation of peripheral blood mononuclear cells

Peripheral blood mononuclear cells (PBMC) were isolated from heparinized venous blood samples from the different groups of dogs by standard ficoll-hypaque (Histopaque 1.077; Sigma, St Louis, MO, USA) density gradient centrifugation, as described by Böyum (1968). The isolated cells were washed three times in phospate-buffered saline (PBS) and resuspended at a final concentration of 1×10^7 cells/ml in supplemented RPMI-1640 (Gibco, Paisley, UK) before use in experiments.

Lymphoycte proliferation assay

PBMC were cultured in a flat-bottomed 96-well-microtitre plate, at a density of 10^5 cells/well in RPMI supplemented with 10% v/v heat-inactivated foetal calf serum, 2 mM sodium pyruvate, 2 mM L-glutamine, 10 mM HEPES buffer, penicillin (100 U/ml), and streptomicin (100 μg/ml). The cells were incubated (37°C, 5% CO_2) for 5 days with either 5 μg/ml of phytohaemagglutinin (PHA), 10 μg/ml of leishmanial soluble antigen (LSA) or without antigen and pulsed during the last 8 h with 10 μM of 5-bromodeoxyuridine (BrdU). Optimal concentrations of antigens and mitogens were determined in kinetic experiments performed before the present study. The cell proliferation was determined using a non-radioactive ELISA technique, according to the manufacturer's instructions [Cell proliferation ELISA, BrdU (colorimetric); Boehringer Mannheim, Germany]. The data are reported as the mean of optical density (OD) (450 nm) of triplicate cultures.

Measurement of cytokine production by PBMC after stimulation

PBMC at 1×10^6 cells/ml in complete medium were cultured and incubated with 5 μg/ml PHA, 10 μg/ml LSA and with medium alone. Supernatants were collected after 48 or 72 h, centrifuged and stored at −80°C until tested.

Tumour necrosis factor alpha (TNF-α) activity was assessed in cell supernatants using a cytotoxicity bioassay (Brazis *et al.*, 2000) using the TNF-α-sensitive L929 cell line. In brief, 50 μl/well of 1×10^6 L929 cells/ml were seeded into flat-bottomed plates and cultured overnight in supplemented RPMI medium. The medium was then replaced with 50 μl/well of fresh medium containing 5 μg/ml of cycloheximide and 100 μg/ml of soybean trypsin inhibitor (STI). Mouse recombinant TNF-α was used to construct a standard curve ranging from 2 to 2000 pg/ml. Samples and standards were added (50 μl/well), and plates were incubated for 18 h at 37°C. Then, 10 μl/well of 3-(4,5-dimethylthiazol-2-yl)-2,5-diphenyltetrazolium bromide (MTT) (5 mg/ml) was added, and after a 4 h incubation, 50 μl of a solution of 50% *N,N*-dimethylformamide and 20% sodium dodecyl sulfate (SDS) was incubated overnight. The plates were read in an ELISA reader at 570 nm, and results were extrapolated from the standard curve constructed using recombinant murine TNF-α.

γ-Interferon (IFN-γ) activity was assessed in cell supernatants using a bioassay based on the inhibition of the cytopathic effect caused by vesicular stomatitis virus (VSV) on Madin–Darby canine kidney cells, ATCC CCL 34 (MDCK2), as described by Pinelli *et al.* (1995). In a 96-well flat-bottomed plate 50 μl of the test supernatant was added in two-fold dilutions. The MDCK2 cells, at a density of 1×10^5 cells/well in supplemented RPMI-1640 medium, were added and incubated overnight at 37°C and 5% CO_2. On the following day the supernatants were removed and 50 μl of VSV at 10^5 pfu/ml was added to the attached cells in each well. After 24 h, when untreated infected cells showed complete cytopathic effect, all cells were stained with 50 μl 0.75% crystal violet in 0.9% formaldehyde for 15 min. The IFN-γ activity was expressed as standard units/ml, which represents the reciprocal of the maximum dilution protecting 50% of the cell monolayer as estimated visually.

PCR Leishmania

PCR was used to detect the infection by *Leishmania* of all dogs studied. Samples of bone marrow and skin were used. *Leishmania*-specific oligonucleotide primers SP176 (5′-TCTTGCGGGGAGGGGGTG-3′) and SP17 (5′-TTGACCCCCAACCACATTTTA-3′), as described by Rodgers *et al.* (1990), were used to amplify a 120-base-pair fragment of *Leishmania* kinetoplast DNA minicircles. PCR was conducted as described elsewhere (Roura *et al.*, 1999).

Statistical analysis

Differences between groups were evaluated by one-way analysis of variance (ANOVA) using a post-hoc Bonferroni test. A *p*-value of <0.05 was considered significant. All calculations were done using the SPSS statistical analysis package.

Results

*Determination of specific anti-*Leishmania *antibodies*

Results are presented in Table 2.5.1 and Figure 2.5.1. Group 1 animals were negative to specific anti-*Leishmania* antibodies. The majority of group 2 dogs (infected but asymptomatic) were positive to specific anti-*Leishmania* antibodies, but with low levels. The average absorbance for IgG, IgG_1 and IgG_2 was 56.2, 29.8 and 51.3, respectively. The number of positive animals for IgG, IgG_1 and IgG_2 was 23, 13 and 25, respectively. Dogs in group 3 (sick dogs before treatment) were clearly positive with all techniques. Titres of total IgG and IgG_2 were consistently high in all patients, but IgG_1 titres were highly variable. IgG_1 titres decreased

Table 2.5.1. Enzyme-linked immunosorbent assay results for immunoglobulin G (IgG), IgG_1 and IgG_2 in the three groups studied

Group of dogs	*n*	IgG	IgG_2	IgG_1
1. Non-infected	28	9.9 ± 4.5	6.2 ± 2.2	9 ± 4.4
2. Healthy but infected	30	56.2 ± 62.8	51.3 ± 65.8	29.8 ± 23.7
3. Sick, before treatment	25	164 ± 35	156 ± 14	76 ± 77
3. Sick, after treatment	25	111 ± 41	121 ± 40	22 ± 18

Data are means ± SD.

rapidly, with the majority of dogs being negative 1 year after the diagnosis. IgG_2 and IgG decreased in parallel during the period of the treatment. Differences between groups were statistically significant for all immunoglobulins ($p = 0.001$).

DTH to leishmanin

The majority of group 2 dogs were positive for delayed type hypersensitivity (DTH) to leishmanin (21 out of 30). By contrast, dogs affected by leishmaniosis were negative, but six out of seven patients became positive after the end of the treatment (see Table 2.5.2). Differences between groups 2 and 3 before treatment were statistically significant ($p < 0.001$). The clinical improvement in the treated group ran parallel to the increase in the intradermal reaction to leishmanin.

Lymphocyte proliferation assay

Asymptomatic infected dogs displayed good proliferative responses that were comparable for both PHA and LSA. Dogs with clinically patent leishmaniosis did not have a significant proliferative response to LSA and also showed a lower proliferative response to PHA which was, however, not signficantly different from groups 1 ($p = 0.349$) and 2 ($p = 0.061$) (Table 2.5.3.). The proliferative responses to PHA of dogs from groups 1 and 2 were similar ($p = 1.000$). The differences in proliferative responses to LSA between groups were statistically significant ($p = 0.003$).

Measurement of IFN-γ produced by PBMC after stimulation

PBMC from dogs in group 2 showed a high production of IFN-γ after stimulation with either PHA or

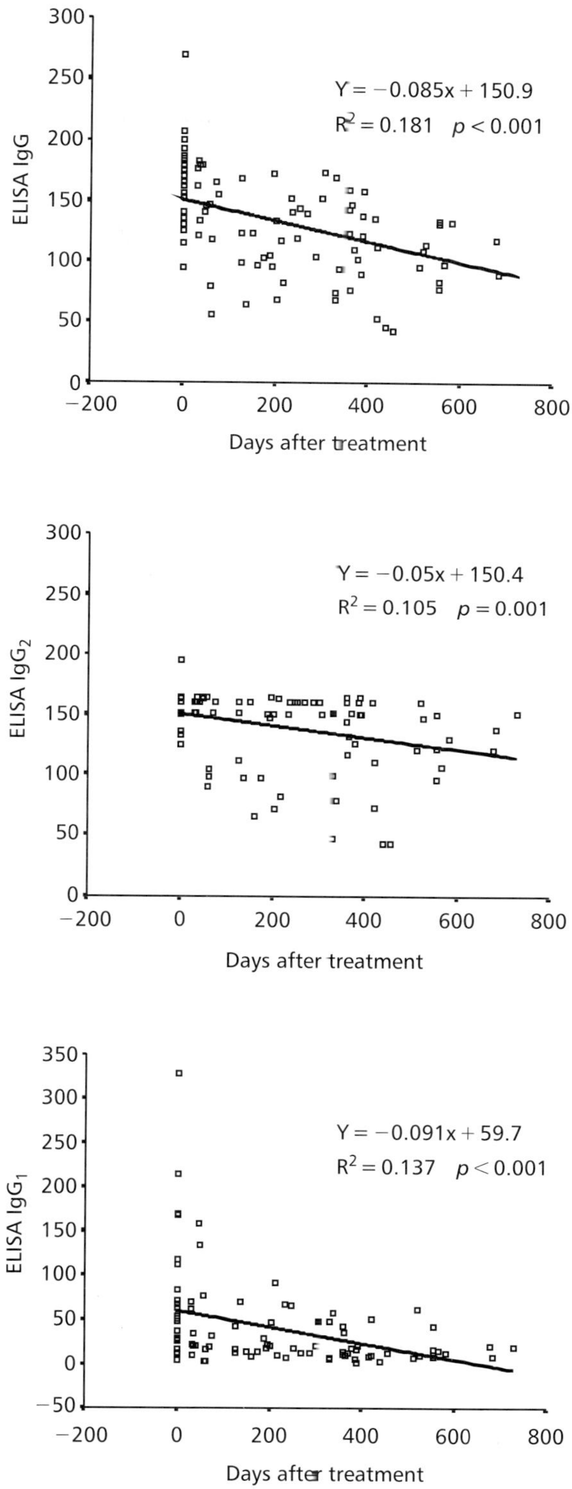

Figure 2.5.1. Anti-*Leishmania* specific immunoglobulin G (IgG), IgG_1 and IgG_2 antibodies in 25 treated dogs.

LSA. In contrast, PBMC from dogs in group 3 showed a lower production of IFN-γ after stimulation either with PHA or LSA compared with group 2 ($p = 0.042$, $p = 0.029$, respectively). Differences between groups for PHA and LSA were statistically significant ($p = 0.043$, $p = 0.012$, respectively) (see Table 2.5.4).

Table 2.5.2. Delayed type hypersensitivity (DTH) to leishmanin in the three groups studied

Group of dogs	*n*	DTH to leishmanin (mm)
1. Non-infected	15	0
2. Healthy but infected	30	13.3 ± 9.4
3. Sick, before treatment	14	1.1 ± 1.9
4. Sick, after treatment	17	10.1 ± 7.4

Data are means ± SD.

Measurement of TNF-α produced by PBMC after stimulation

PBMC from all groups showed a similar production of TNF-α after stimulation with PHA ($p = 0.258$). However, the production of TNF-α after stimulation with LSA was significantly higher in group 3 (ill dogs) than in groups 1 and 2 ($p = 0.001, p = 0.006$, respectively) (see Table 2.5.5).

Discussion

Based on the results obtained using these techniques, it was possible to define the pattern of immune response of a single canine patient. This study combined techniques that assess the humoral response (serology) with techniques that evaluate the specific cellular immunity (Cabral *et al.*, 1998; Rhalem *et al.*, 1999a), i.e. DTH or the production of IFN-γ by PBMC. In practice, DTH

Table 2.5.3. Lymphocyte proliferation assay results in the three groups studied

Group of dogs	*n*	Unstimulated	PHA	LSA
1. Non-infected	7	0.098 ± 0.034	0.852 ± 0.383	0.070 ± 0.043
2. Healthy but infected	7	0.102 ± 0.086	1.015 ± 0.270	0.756 ± 0.603
3. Sick, before treatment	8	0.110 ± 0.056	0.554 ± 0.352	0.108 ± 0.075

Data are means ± SD.
PHA: phytohaemagglutinin; LSA: leishmanial soluble antigen.

Table 2.5.4. Production of γ-interferon (IU/ml) in the three groups studied

Group of dogs	*n*	Unstimulated	PHA	LSA
1. Non-infected	9	28.9 ± 24.7	137.8 ± 107.9	26.7 ± 26.5
2. Healthy but infected	12	23.3 ± 29.3	176.7 ± 163.1	196.7 ± 221.4
3. Sick, before treatment	7	2.9 ± 8	20 ± 20	0
4. Sick, after treatment	4	10 ± 11.5	60 ± 23	10 ± 20

Data are means ± SD.
PHA: phytohaemagglutinin; LSA: leishmanial soluble antigen.

Table 2.5.5. Production of tumour necrosis factor-α (pg/ml) in the three groups studied

Group of dogs	*n*	Unstimulated	PHA	LSA
1. Non-infected	9	0	1.4 ± 1.3	0
2. Healthy but infected	12	0.2 ± 0.5	4.7 ± 4	1.6 ± 1.5
3. Sick, before treatment	7	0.9 ± 1.2	4 ± 3.8	5.6 ± 3.1

Data are means ± SD.
PHA: phytohaemagglutinin; LSA: leishmanial soluble antigen.

is possibly more accommodating because of the complexity of current techniques available to measure the production of IFN-γ. In the near future, the development of better techniques to measure the production of canine cytokines (i.e. interleukin-4 and IFN-γ) based on ELISA may allow for easier evaluation of the type of immunity against *Leishmania* occurring in a patient undergoing examination.

Dogs living in an endemic area of leishmaniosis can be grouped into various categories. First, dogs can be classified as asymptomatic healthy or ill dogs. Dogs with clinically patent leishmaniosis are infected animals that have an inefficient immune response against *Leishmania* (Pinelli *et al.*, 1994). Asymptomatic dogs, however, are a heterogeneous group of animals (Cabral *et al.*, 1998). This group includes healthy, non-infected animals (PCR negative, seronegative, DTH negative, no production of IFN-γ), infected dogs that control the parasite by means of a cellular immune response (PCR positive, low titre of specific IgG antibodies and DTH/IFN-γ positive) and infected dogs that are incubating the disease and will probably be symptomatic in the future (PCR positive, seropositive, low DTH and low production of IFN-γ). It is necessary, as stated before, to use several techniques to classify a single patient correctly into one of the four groups.

Dogs affected by canine leishmaniosis show severe immunological abnormalities. They have a predominantly humoral immune response characterised by the production of high amounts of specific anti-*Leishmania* IgG_2 antibodies and a variable production of IgG_1 antibodies. These results are in agreement with the ELISA reagents, because the Bethyl antidog antisera IgG_1 and IgG_2 are not subclass specific. Canine IgG is composed of four fractions, which have been termed γw, γx, γy and γz (Mazza *et al.*, 1993). The Bethyl anti-dog antisera specific to IgG_2 reacts with the four fractions of IgG and the Bethyl anti-dog antisera specific to IgG_1 reacts with IgG fraction γz (Mazza *et al.*, 1993). Accordingly, the specific anti-*Leishmania* total IgG antibodies are highly correlated with the specific anti-*Leishmania* IgG_2 antibodies. However, the correlation between the specific anti-*Leishmania* IgG_1 and the specific anti-*Leishmania* IgG_2 or total IgG antibodies is low (Solano-Gallego *et al.*, 2001). Increasing numbers of papers in the field of canine leishmaniosis are using these reagents, and the serological data are becoming confusing. This information has to be taken into account with the results obtained from Bethyl reagents.

The cellular immune response against *Leishmania*, however, is very weak or absent in patients with patent leishmaniosis, as demonstrated by the low DTH, the low production of IFN-γ and the lack of proliferative responses of PBMC. These results are similar to those described by Pinelli *et al.* (1994) in dogs infected experimentally and indicate that these animals have a Th_2-like immune response (non-protective and permitting a wide dissemination of the parasite). The production of TNF-α by PBMC in these patients was elevated and highly variable. It is difficult to give a unique interpretation to this finding. TNF-α is a proinflammatory cytokine that provides a rapid form of host defence against infection (Nacy *et al.*, 1991) but also has many undesirable effects on the host (Blackwell, 1999). High production of TNF-α could play a role in the protection against *Leishmania* but could also be responsible for some of the clinical signs and lesions of leishmaniosis, such as cachexia, fever or weight loss, as also reported in humans (Pearson *et al.*, 1992; Morsy *et al.*, 1995; Da-Cruz *et al.*, 1996; Ribeiro-de-Jesus *et al.*, 1998). However, such results must be interpreted with caution because these dogs appear to be immunosuppressed, as demonstrated by the low proliferative responses of PBMC when stimulated by PHA. Some authors have previously described the anergic state to mitogens of dogs suffering from leishmaniosis (De Luna *et al.*, 1999; Moreno *et al.*, 1999) and have also found low numbers of blood $CD4^+$ cells (Moreno *et al.*, 1999)

Drug treatment for leishmaniosis has a noticeable effect on the immune response of ill dogs. However, the effect is highly variable and difficult to predict. Some patients show a decrease in the IgG titre which runs parallel to the recovery of cellular immunity and to the clinical recovery (Rhalem *et al.*, 1999b). Other dogs, however, retain the humoral immune response and fail to recover cellular immunity; these are the patients with the worst prognosis. It is likely, as has been demonstrated in *Leishmania major* infection in mice (Nabors & Farrell, 1996), that the treatment causes a reduction in the parasite burden and could be the inducer for a switch from a Th_2 to Th_1-like immune response. Many factors influence this evolution of the immune response during treatment, such as type and duration of the treatment, concomitant infections or diseases, reinfections and the status of the cellular immune response at the beginning of the treatment.

As expected, non-infected dogs were completely negative by all techniques performed. However, they were immunocompetent, as their PBMC responded with an intense proliferation when stimulated with mitogens (PHA).

Healthy, infected dogs can also be divided into two groups: (1) dogs that clearly have specific *Leishmania* cellular immunity demonstrated by a positive DTH, proliferation and production of IFN-γ and low specific *Leishmania* humoral immunity; and (2) dogs that fail to have a specific *Leishmania* cellular immunity and instead show only humoral immunity. The appearance of 'resistant' dogs was reported in the 1990s, demonstrating cellular immunity in natural and experimental infection and determining this cellular immunity as a Th_1-like immune response (Cabral *et al.*, 1992; Pinelli *et al.*, 1994). However, the term resistant must be interpreted with caution as the parasites probably remain in these individuals in equilibrium without producing pathology. This is not an unchangeable situation and several factors can break the equilibrium and lead to clinical disease. This situation is similar to that in humans (Schubach *et al.*, 1998a, b) and other animals (de Rossell *et al.*, 1992; Aebischer *et al.*, 1993; Belkaid *et al.*, 2000) after healing, which are persistently infected but clinically healthy for long periods. The mechanisms of persistence of the parasite are currently being investigated (Bogdan *et al.*, 1996; Bogdan & Rollinghoff, 1998). Some authors have hypothesised that *Leishmania* could persist in low nitric oxide-producing cells such as fibroblasts (Bogdan *et al.*, 2000).

The integration of data obtained in broad epidemiological and immunological studies (Berrahal *et al.*, 1996; Cabral *et al.*, 1998; Solano-Gallego *et al.*, 2000a, b) is changing the understanding of canine leishmaniosis. Infection and disease are no longer synonymous and the diagnosis has to be established by combining several techniques. Diagnosis and prognosis can be more accurately established if, together with the detection of the parasite, the type of immune response of the patient, humoral versus cellular, is evaluated.

Acknowledgements

The authors are grateful for the valuable contribution in the performance of the IFN-γ bioassay by Dr Victor Rutten and co-workers from the Department of Immunology, Institute of Infectious Diseases and Immunology, Faculty of Veterinary Medicine, Utrecht University.

References

Aebischer, T., Moody, S. F. & Handman, E. (1993) Persistence of virulent *Leishmania major* in murine cutaneous leishmaniasis: a possible hazard for the host. *Infection and Immunity*, **61**, 220–226.

Belkaid, Y., Mendez, S., Lira, R., Kadambi, N., Milon, G. & Sacks, D. (2000) A natural model of *Leishmania major* infection reveals a prolonged 'silent' phase of parasite amplification in the skin before the onset of lesion formation and immunity. *Journal of Immunology*, **165**, 969–977.

Berrahal, F., Mary, C., Roze, M., Berenger, A., Escoffier, K., Lamoroux, D. & Dunan, S. (1996) Canine leishmaniasis: identification of asymptomatic carriers by polymerase chain reaction and immunoblotting. *American Journal of Tropical Medicine and Hygiene*, **55**, 273–277.

Blackwell, J. M. (1999) Tumour necrosis factor alpha and mucocutaneous leishmaniasis. *Parasitology Today*, **15**, 73–75.

Bogdan, C. & Rollinghoff, M. (1998) The immune response to *Leishmania*: mechanisms of parasite control and evasion. *International Journal of Parasitology*, **28**, 121–134.

Bogdan, C., Gessner, A., Solbach, W. & Rollinghoff, M. (1996) Invasion, control and persistence of *Leishmania* parasites. *Current Opinion in Immunology*, **8**, 517–525.

Bogdan, C., Donhauser, N., Doring, R., Rollinghoff, M., Diefenbach, A. & Rittig, M. G. (2000) Fibroblasts as host cells in latent leishmaniosis. *Journal of Experimental Medicine*, **191**, 2121–2130.

Böyum, A. (1968) Isolation of mononuclear cells and granulocytes from human blood. *Scandinavian Journal of Clinical Laboratory Investigation*, **21**, 77–89.

Brazis, P., Queralt, M., Mora, F. de, Ferrer, L. & Puigdemont, A. (2000) Stem cell factor enhances IgE-mediated histamine and TNF-alpha release from dispersed canine cutaneous mast cells. *Veterinary Immunology and Immunopathology*, **75**, 97–108.

Cabral, M., O'Grady, J. & Alexander, J. (1992) Demonstration of *Leishmania* specific cell mediated and humoral immunity in asymptomatic dogs. *Parasite Immunology*, **14**, 531–539.

Cabral, M., O'Grady, J. E., Gomes, S., Sousa, J. C., Thompson, H. & Alexander, J. (1998) The immunology of canine leishmaniosis: strong evidence for a developing disease spectrum from asymptomatic dogs. *Veterinary Parasitology*, **76**, 173–180.

Cardoso, L., Neto, F., Sousa, J. C., Rodrigues, M. & Cabral, M. (1998) Use of a leishmanin skin test in the detection of canine *Leishmania*-specific cellular immunity. *Veterinary Parasitology*, **79**, 213–220.

Da-Cruz, A. M., Oliveira, M. P. de, De Luca, P. M., Mendonca, S. C. & Coutinho, S. G. (1996) Tumor necrosis factor-alpha in human american tegumentary leishmaniasis. *Memorias Instituto Oswaldo Cruz*, **91**, 225–229.

De Luna, R., Vuotto, M. L., Ielpo, M. T., Ambrosio, R., Piantedosi, D., Moscatiello, V. *et al.* (1999) Early suppression of lymphoproliferative response in dogs with natural infection by *Leishmania infantum*. *Veterinary Immunology and Immunopathology*, **70**, 95–103.

Greene, R.T. (1990) An update on the serodiagnosis of canine Lyme borreliosis. *Journal of Veterinary Internal Medicine*, **4**, 167–171.

Maconi, G., Kurihara, H., Tascheri, A. M. & Bianchi Porro, G. (1999) Management of *Helicobacter* pylori infection: gastroenterological and surgical perspectives. *Journal of Chemotherapy*, **11**, 581–590.

Mazza, G., Duffus, W. P .H., Elson, C. J., Stokes, C. R., Wilson, A. D. & Whiting, A. H. (1993) The separation and identification by monoclonal antibodies of dog IgG fractions. *Journal of Immunological Methods*, **161**, 193–203.

Moreno, J., Nieto, J., Chamizo, C., Gonzalez, F., Blanco, F., Barker, D. C. & Alvar, J. (1999) The immune response and PBMC subsets in canine visceral leishmaniasis before, and after, chemotherapy. *Veterinary Immunology and Immunopathology*, **71**, 181–195.

Morsy, T. A., el Missiry, A. G., Sarwat, M. A., el Rassed, M. M., Habib, F. S. & Abou Gamra, M. M. (1995) Tumour necrosis factor-alpha (cachectin) in human visceral leishmaniasis. *Journal of the Egyptian Society of Parasitology*, **25**, 31–51.

Nabors, G. S. & Farrell, J. P. (1996) Successful chemotherapy in experimental leishmaniasis is influenced by the polarity of the T cell response before treatment. *Journal of Infectious Disease*, **173**, 979–986.

Nacy, C. A., Meierovics, A. I., Belosevic, M. & Green, S. J. (1991) Tumor necrosis factor-alpha: central regulatory cytokine in the induction of macrophage antimicrobial activities. *Pathobiology*, **59**, 182–184.

Pearson, R. D., Cox, G., Jeronimo, S. M., Castracane, J., Drew, J. S., Evans, T. & Alencar, J. E. de (1992) Visceral leishmaniasis: a model for infection-induced cachexia. *American Journal of Tropical Medicine and Hygiene*, **47**, 8–15.

Pinelli, E., Killick-Kendrick, R., Wagenaar, J., Bernardina, W., Real, G. del & Ruitenberg, J. (1994) Cellular and humoral immune response in dogs experimentally and naturally infected with *Leishmania infantum*. *Infection and Immunity*, **62**, 229–235.

Pinelli, E., Gonzalo, R. M., Boog, C. J., Rutten, V. P., Gebhard, D., Real, G. del & Ruitenberg, E. J. (1995) *Leishmania infantum*-specific T cell lines derived from asymptomatic dogs that lyse infected macrophages in a major histocompatibility complex-restricted manner. *European Journal of Immunology*, **25**, 1594–1600.

Ribeiro-de-Jesus, A., Almeida, R. P., Lessa, H., Bacellar, O. & Carvalho, E. M. (1998) Cytokine profile and pathology in human leishmaniasis. *Brazilian Journal of Medicine and Biology Research*, **31**, 143–148.

Rhalem, A., Sahibi, H., Guessous-Idrissi, N., Lasri, S., Natami, A., Riyad, M. & Berrag, B. (1999a) Immune response against *Leishmania* antigens in dogs naturally and experimentally infected with *Leishmania infantum*. *Veterinary Parasitology*, **81**, 173–184.

Rhalem, A., Sahibi, H., Lasri, S. & Jaffe, C. L. (1999b) Analysis of immune responses in dogs with canine visceral leishmaniasis before, and after, drug treatment. *Veterinary Immunology and Immunopathology*, **71**, 69–76.

Rodgers, M. R., Stephen, J. & Wirth, D. F. (1990) Amplification and diagnosis of *Leishmania*. *Experimental Parasitology*, **71**, 267–275.

Rossell, R. A. de, Duran, R. J. de, Rossell O. & Rodriguez, A. M. (1992) Is leishmaniasis ever cured? *Transactions of the Royal Society of Tropical Medicine and Hygiene*, **86**, 251–253.

Roura, X., Sanchez, A. & Ferrer, L. (1999) Diagnosis of canine leishmaniasis by a polymerase chain reaction technique. *Veterinary Record*, **144**, 262–264.

Schubach, A., Marzochi, M. C., Cuzzi-Maya, T., Oliveira, A. V., Araujo, M. L., Oliveira, A. L. *et al.* (1998a) Cutaneous scars in American tegumentary leishmaniasis patients: a site of *Leishmania (Viannia) braziliensis* persistence and viability eleven years after antimonial therapy and clinical cure. *American Journal of Tropical Medicine and Hygiene*, **58**, 824–827.

Schubach, A., Haddad, F., Oliveira-Neto, M. P., Degrave, W., Pirmez, C., Grimaldi, G. Jr. & Fernandes, O. (1998b) Detection of *Leishmania* DNA by polymerase chain reaction in scars of treated human patients. *Journal of Infectious Diseases*, **178**, 911–914.

Solano-Gallego, L., Llull, J., Ramos, G., Riera, C., Arboix, M., Alberola, J. & Ferrer, L. (2000a) The ibizian hound presents a predominantly cellular immune response against natural *Leishmania* infection. *Veterinary Parasitology*, **90**, 37–45.

Solano-Gallego, L., Morell, P., Arboix, M., Alberola, J. & Ferrer, L. (2000b) Prevalence of *Leishmania* infection in endemic regions. In: *Scientific Abstracts of the Fourth World Congress of Veterinary Dermatology*, San Francisco, CA, August–September 2000, p. 22.

Solano-Gallego, L., Riera, C., Roura, X., Iniesta, L., Gállego, M., Valladares, J. E. *et al.* (2001) *Leishmania infantum*-specific IgG, IgG_1 and IgG_2 antibody responses in healthy and ill dogs from endemic areas. Evolution in the course of infection and after treatment. *Veterinary Parasitology*, **96**, 265–276.

Solbach, W. & Laskay, T. (2000) The host response to *Leishmania* infection. *Advances in Immunology*, **74**, 275–317.

2.6

Local cell recruitment and cytokine production following intradermal injection with *Microsporum canis* antigen in cats

A. Robinson BA, BVSc (Hons), CertSAD, MRCVS,[1] A.H. Sparkes BVetMed, PhD, DipECVIM, MRCVS[1] and M.J. Day BSc BVMS (Hons), PhD, FASM, DipECVP, MRCPath, FRCVS[2]

Departments of [1]Clinical Veterinary Science and [2]Pathology and Microbiology, University of Bristol, Langford, UK

Summary

Eight cats that had recovered from experimental *Microsporum canis* infection were injected intradermally with a soluble *M. canis* antigen preparation (SMCA) and saline (control). All cats received both SMCA and saline injections. Injection sites were scored for gross inflammation at 30 min, 24, 48 and 72 h after injection and skin biopsy specimens from these sites were taken at 48 h (four cats) and 72 h (the other four cats) after injection. Tissue sections were stained using haematoxylin and eosin (H&E) or labelled immunohistochemically using antibodies specific for: major histocompatibility complex (MHC) class II, macrophages and polymorphonuclear leucocytes, B-cells, plasma cells (immunoglobulin G [IgG], IgM, IgA), T-cells and T-cell subsets (CD4, CD8). The number of labelled cells of each type in the inflammatory infiltrate was graded. Tissue biopsies were assayed using semiquantitative reverse transcription–polymerase chain reaction to detect mRNA for γ-interferon (IFN-γ), interleukin-4 (IL-4), IL-10 and IL-12p40.

All of the SMCA injection sites had evidence of gross inflammation at all time points after 30 min, whereas the control sites did not. At 48 h after injection, eosinophils and mast cells predominated in the infiltrate, whereas at 72 h after injection, lymphocytes and macrophages predominated. There were very few plasma or B-cells in any sections. Peak numbers of macrophages were seen 48 h after injection, whereas peak numbers of cells expressing MHC class II or CD3 were seen 72 h after injection. mRNA for IFN-γ, IL-10 and IL-12p40 was detected in both SMCA and control skin biopsy specimens. mRNA for IL-4 was not detected.

This study showed that intradermal injection of SMCA induces a delayed-type hypersensitivity response in cats that have recovered from *M. canis* infection.

Introduction

In cats dermatophytosis is a cutaneous infection, most frequently caused by *Microsporum canis*. Following resolution of infection, many cats become resistant to cutaneous challenge with dermatophytes (Sparkes *et al.*, 1996). Local cutaneous immune responses at the site of dermatophyte infection are likely to be very important in the resolution of lesions and the development of resistance to subsequent challenge. Cell-mediated immunity (CMI) is thought to be of major importance in the resolution of dermatophytosis (Calderon & Hay, 1984) and the development of resistance to reinfection (Hay, 1994). The use of intradermal testing using dermatophyte antigens and analysis of the delayed type hypersensitivity (DTH) response have been widely used as a measure of cutaneous CMI in many species (DeLamater, 1941; Cruickshank *et al.*, 1960; Grappel & Blank, 1972; Lepper, 1972; Jones *et al.*, 1973, 1974a–c; Hanifin *et al.*, 1974; Abraham *et al.*, 1975; Sorensen & Jones, 1976; Hay & Brostoff, 1977; Kerbs *et al.*, 1977; Hunjan *et al.*, 1981), including cats (DeBoer *et al.*, 1991).

Intradermal testing with dermatophyte antigen is a commonly used investigative tool in human medicine. It has been used to investigate immune responses in several animal species, including cats (DeBoer *et al.*, 1991). In guinea-pigs immunised with *Trichophyton mentagrophytes*, both immediate and delayed reactions develop (Cruickshank *et al.*, 1960; Kaaman *et al.*, 1976). Immediate reactions reflect reaginic antibody-mediated hypersensitivity (Cruickshank *et al.*, 1960), whereas delayed reactions reflect the presence of cell-mediated immunity and correlate well with immunity to reinfection (Hanifin *et al.*, 1974). In human patients who have recovered from acute dermatophytosis and are resistant to reinfection, strong DTH reactions to dermatophyte antigens can be demonstrated (Jones *et al.*, 1973), but positive immediate reactions are variable. In contrast, patients with chronic non-resolving or relapsing dermatophytosis typically develop strong immediate reactions, but negative DTH reactions to intradermal injection with dermatophyte antigens (Jones *et al.*, 1974c; Hay, 1982).

Previous studies in the cat of the immune response to dermatophyte infection have focused on systemic immunity. Cats recovered from *M. canis* infection develop a protective immunity to reinfection, associated with a specific systemic cell-mediated, but not humoral immunity (Sparkes *et al.*, 1996). However, systemic responses may not be a good indicator of local, cutaneous responses. Studies in cats have demonstrated that cutaneous infection may still develop in the face of vaccine-induced, specific systemic cell-mediated immune responses (DeBoer & Moriello, 1994, 1995). There is, therefore, clearly a need to examine the cutaneous immune response in feline dermatophytosis.

The aim of this study was to characterise the cellular infiltrate and cytokine mRNA profile at the site of intradermal injection of a soluble *M. canis* crude antigen preparation (SMCA) in cats that had recovered from *M. canis* infection, using histology, immunohistochemistry and semiquantitative reverse transcription–polymerase chain reaction (RT–PCR) to measure cytokine mRNA.

Materials and methods

Animals

Eight domestic short-haired, specific pathogen-free (SPF) adult cats, barrier maintained at the School of Veterinary Science, University of Bristol, UK, were used in this study. The cats had *M. canis* infection experimentally induced in the skin, as described by Sparkes *et al.* (1995), over the left lateral thorax, 26 weeks previously. At the time of this study all cats had completely recovered, were fungal culture negative and had no skin lesions.

Preparation of antigen

A strain of *M. canis*, derived from infected cat hairs submitted to the Feline Diagnostic Service, University of Bristol, was grown in liquid Sabouraud's medium at room temperature (20–22°C) with constant stirring for 14 days. Mycelial mats were harvested and washed with sterile distilled water. SMCA was prepared following the method of Sparkes *et al.* (1993). Mycelia were suspended in sterile phosphate-buffered saline (PBS, pH 7.4) and macerated using glass beads in a rotary homogeniser. The supernatant was recovered and centrifuged at 20 000 *g* for 60 min. It was filtered through a 0.45 μm filter and then dialysed against sterile distilled water. The SMCA preparation was lyophilised and stored at −70°C until used.

Intradermal testing

Lyophilised SMCA was reconstituted with sterile saline (0.9%) to a concentration of 1 mg/ml (total protein content measured by the bicinchoninic acid method, Smith *et al.*, 1985). The reconstituted SMCA was non-irritant in SPF barrier-maintained adult cats that had not previously been exposed to dermatophytes or dermatophyte antigens. Cats were sedated using meditomidine hydrochloride (100 μg/kg, Domitor®; Pfizer Animal Health, Sandwich, UK). Hair was clipped from the right lateral thorax (contralateral to the site of previous infection). SMCA or saline (negative control) was injected intradermally into sites on the prepared area, so that each of the eight cats had three injections of SMCA and three of saline. The volume of solution or saline injected at each site was 100 μl. Each injection site was separated from the adjacent one by at least 1.5 cm to minimise the possibility of spillover from one site to the next. No positive control was used. Injection sites were examined for gross signs of inflammation 30 min, 24, 48 and 72 h after injection. The degree of inflammation was scored subjectively by evaluating erythema, induration (by palpation of the skin) and, at 30 min after injection only, weal formation. A score of 0–3 was assigned (0 = no change, 1 = mild, 2 = moderate, 3 = marked inflammatory change).

All injection sites were examined by the same veterinarian (A. R.), who was experienced in the interpretation of feline intradermal tests.

Skin biopsy

At each of two time points after intradermal injection (48 and 72 h), 6 mm punch skin biopsy specimens were taken from the cats at the sites of intradermal injections (three SMCA and three control sites per cat, i.e. a total of six biopsies per cat). Four of the cats were sampled 48 h after intradermal injection and the other four cats 72 h after intradermal injection. One of the triplicate repeat skin biopsies for each cat was processed for routine histopathology, the second was frozen for immunohistochemistry and the third was snap-frozen for RT–PCR assay. Skin biopsy specimens for routine histopathology and fixed tissue immunohistochemistry were fixed in 10% neutral buffered formalin solution for 24 h and embedded in paraffin wax. Sections (4 μm) were stained routinely with haematoxylin and eosin (H&E) or labelled with specific antibodies (see below). For immunohistochemistry using frozen tissue, tissues were embedded in OCT medium (Sakura Tissue-Tek OCT compound; Raymond A Lamb, Eastbourne, UK) and dropped into isopentane cooled over liquid nitrogen. Tissue for RT–PCR assay was placed into a cryovial and snap-frozen in liquid nitrogen. Frozen tissue was stored at −70°C.

Immunohistochemical labelling of formalin-fixed sections

A panel of monoclonal and polyclonal antibodies was used to evaluate the cells present in the skin biopsies (Table 2.6.1). As negative controls isotype-matched antibodies of irrelevant specificities were used in place of specific monoclonal antisera and normal serum from the same species was used in place of the polyclonal antibodies. The optimal concentration of each of the antibodies used was determined by chequerboard titration. After each stage of the method, sections were washed in PBS. Epitope retrieval was performed by trypsin digestion, or by heating in citrate buffer, pH 6.0, for the major histocompatibility complex (MHC) class II and B-cell antibodies. Endogenous peroxidase was blocked by incubating sections in a solution of 50% methanol and 50% PBS with 0.5 v/v of hydrogen peroxide for 30 min at room temperature. To reduce non-specific binding, sections were incubated with a 1:10 dilution of rabbit serum (obtained from a 3-month-old SPF-derived barrier-maintained rabbit) in PBS (or for the CD3 antibody 20% goat serum; Sigma Chemical Co., Poole, UK) and 2.5% cat serum (from a 6-month-old SPF-derived barrier-maintained cat) for 30 min at room temperature. Primary antibody or control antibody or serum was then applied, diluted in PBS (Table 2.6.1). All monoclonal antibodies were incubated overnight at 4°C. Incubations with polyclonal antibodies were for shorter periods at room temperature (Table 2.6.1). Sections were incubated at room temperature with secondary antibody in PBS at an optimal dilution (Table 2.6.1). When a biotinylated secondary antibody was used, sections were then incubated with the conjugate, streptavidin/biotin horseradish peroxidase complexes (Dako), for 30 min at room temperature before washing and developing. Slides were developed using

Table 2.6.1. Antibodies used for the characterisation of cells by immunohistochemistry in formalin-fixed skin biopsies

Specificity	Primary antibody		Secondary antibody		
	Description	Dilution (time)	Isotype	Description	Dilution (time)
Macro/gran	Mouse α-human L1[a] (Mac387)	1000 (overnight)	IgG_1	Rabbit α-mouse Ig (B)[a]	500 (30 min)
MHC class II	Mouse α-HLA-DR (αchain)[a]	25 (overnight)	IgG_1	Rabbit α-mouse Ig (B)[a]	100 (30 min)
B-cells	Mouse α-human CD79a[a]	20 (overnight)	IgG_1	Rabbit α-mouse Ig (B)[a]	100 (30 min)
IgG	Goat α-cat IgG (Fc)[b]	500 (90 min)	PC	Rabbit α-goat (HRP)[a]	500 (60 min)
IgA	Goat α-cat IgA (Fc)[c]	400 (90 min)	PC	Rabbit α-goat (HRP)[a]	500 (60 min)
IgM	Goat α-cat IgM (Fc)[c]	400 (90 min)	PC	Rabbit α-goat (HRP)[a]	500 (60 min)
T-cells	Rabbit α-human CD3[a]	200 (30 min)[d]	PC	Goat α-rabbit IgG (B)[b]	800 (30 min)[d]

[a]Dako (High Wycombe, UK); [b]Jackson Immunoresearch Labs (Pennsylvania, PA, USA); [c]Nordic Laboratories (Tilburg, The Netherlands).
[d]In 2.5% cat serum.
Macro/gran: macrophage/granulocyte; MHC: major histocompatibility complex; Ig: immunoglobulin; HLA: human leucocyte antigen; B: biotinylated; HRP: horseradish peroxidase conjugated.

3,3′-diaminobenzidine (DAB) as the substrate and stopped by washing in PBS. Sections were counter-stained with Mayer's haematoxylin for 1 min and then washed in tap water. Following dehydration sections were mounted under DPX.

Preparation and immunohistochemical staining of frozen sections

Frozen sections (5–8 μm thick on poly-L-lysine-coated slides) were air-dried at room temperature, then fixed by immersion in ice-cold acetone for 10 min. They were allowed to air-dry before being stored at −20°C. Stored sections were rehydrated in PBS for 10 min. Endogenous peroxidase was blocked using a 0.2% (w/v) solution of periodic acid in normal saline for 25 s. To reduce non-specific binding, sections were incubated with 10% rabbit serum, obtained from a 3-month-old SPF-derived barrier-maintained rabbit (with the addition of 25% cat serum, from a 6-month-old SPF-derived barrier-maintained cat, and 5% bovine serum albumin [Sigma Chemical Co., UK] for the CD4 antibody) for 30 min before washing again with PBS. The primary antibodies (Table 2.6.2) were diluted to the optimal concentration in 2.5% cat serum in PBS and incubated with the tissue biopsies overnight at 4°C. Incubation with the secondary antibody (Table 2.6.2) and streptavidin/biotinylated horseradish peroxidase conjugate, and development and counterstaining were as described above.

Scoring of stained and labelled sections

Sections were examined by an experienced veterinary pathologist (M. J. D.). To prevent bias, all sections were encoded. For the H&E-stained slides the whole slide was examined under medium- and high-power magnification; the epidermis and dermis were examined for the distribution and type of cellular infiltrates. For each section the predominant cells types were noted. In addition, each section was given a subjective score reflecting the severity of the inflammatory infiltrate: 0 = no infiltrate, 1 = mild infiltrate, 2 = moderate infiltrate, 3 = severe infiltrate. The numerical grade assigned to a particular biopsy reflected the intensity of inflammatory infiltration (i.e. the area of tissue occupied by an inflammatory infiltrate) taking into account each of the affected dermal sites. Slides stained using each immunohistochemical marker were scored separately using a subjective scoring system. Sections were examined under high-power magnification. The whole of each section was evaluated. Four different anatomical compartments of the skin were examined and separately scored (epidermis and interface area, the hair follicles and perifollicular area, the superficial dermis and the deep dermis). The score was based on subjective assessment of the number of positively stained cells in the compartment: 0 = none, 1 = 1–5 cells; 2 = 5–15 cells; 3 = >15 cells. A total score for each biopsy was obtained by adding together the scores for each of the four anatomical compartments.

RT–PCR for cytokine mRNA

Each biopsy in a cryotube was placed in liquid nitrogen. It was chopped into small pieces using sterile scalpel blades and placed in lysis buffer in a Ribolyser tube (Hybaid, Ashford, Middlesex, UK) for complete disruption in a Ribolyser (Hybaid). The mixture of lysis buffer and macerated skin was used for RNA isolation and purification using the SV Total RNA Isolation System (Promega, Southampton, UK), following the manufacturer's instructions. To check for contamination with genomic DNA before reverse transcription, a PCR for glyceraldehyde-3-phosphate dehydrogenase was performed on all RNA samples. Contaminated samples were rejected. The PCR assays and primer pairs used for cytokine mRNA detection and the method used for semiquantification have been

Table 2.6.2. Antibodies used for the characterisation of cells by immunohistochemistry in frozen skin biopsies

Specificity	Primary antibody		Secondary antibody	
	Description	Dilution	Description	Dilution and time
CD4	Mouse α-cat CD4[a]	10	Rabbit α-mouse Ig (B)[b]	400 (30 min)
CD8	Mouse α-cat CD8[a]	50	Rabbit α-mouse Ig (B)[b]	400 (30 min)

[a]N Gengozian (University of Tennessee, USA); [b]Dako (High Wycombe, UK).
B: Biotinylated.

reported previously (Harley *et al.*, 1999) (Table 2.6.3). Each PCR run included a positive control, the appropriate cDNA standard, and a negative control, RNAse and DNAse free purified water (Sigma Chemical Co., UK). The final result for each sample was expressed as the amount of cDNA template for each cytokine relative to the sample glyceraldehyde-3-phosphate dehydrogenase cDNA concentration.

Interpretation of data and statistics

The small sample sizes and nature of the data analysed necessitated the use of non-parametric tests, including the Kruskal–Wallis test (with Dunn's multiple comparison post test), the Wilcoxon signed rank test and Spearman's rank correlation coefficient as appropriate. The level of significance was set at $p < 0.05$.

Table 2.6.3. Primers used for polymerase chain reaction for feline cytokines

Target gene		Primer sequence 5′ → 3′	Product size (bp)
G3PDH	Forward	ACTTTCCAGGAGCGAGATCC	
	Reverse	TGCCGAAGTGGTCATGGATG	282
IL-4	Forward	TTGAACATCCTCACAGCGAG	
	Reverse	TTCATTCACAGAACAGGTCCTG	218
IL-10	Forward	GACTTTCTTTCAAACCAAGGACG	
	Reverse	AGGGTCTTCAGCTTTTCTCC	201
IL-12 p40	Forward	GGAAGATGGAATTTGGTCCAC	
	Reverse	TGAGCTTGTGAATAGCGTCC	340
IFN-γ	Forward	CAAAGCCAAATTGTCTCCTTC	
	Reverse	CTTGGTGAGAGATCATTCATCAC	237

IL: interleukin; IFN: interferon.

Results

Intradermal testing

For every cat similar reactions were seen at each of the three replicate sites of intradermal injection. Scores of sites of intradermal injection with saline were zero in all eight cats at all time points. At the SMCA injection sites an erythematous weal was seen 30 min after injection in two of the eight cats, while in the remaining cats no reaction was evident. Positive reactions (i.e. score > 0) at SMCA sites were seen in all eight cats at 24 h after injection and all later times. These were characterised by areas of firm induration, sometimes with mild erythema (Table 2.6.4). Scores at SMCA injection sites were significantly higher than at control sites at the same time after injection (Kruskal–Wallis test, with Dunn's multiple comparison test, $p < 0.01$, 24 and 48 h; $p < 0.05$, 72 h). Scores at SMCA injection sites at 24 and 48 h after injection were significantly higher than at 30 min after injection (Kruskal–Wallis test, with Dunn's multiple comparison test, $p < 0.01$).

Histopathology

On histological examination all biopsies from sites of intradermal injection with SMCA showed evidence of an inflammatory infiltrate (median score [range]: 48 h biopsies = 1.5 [0.5–2.5], 72 h biopsies = 2.25 [2.0–2.5]), whereas no control biopsies showed any evidence of an inflammatory infiltrate (score = 0) (significant difference between scores for SMCA and control biopsies, $p < 0.05$, Wilcoxon signed rank test). There was a significant correlation between intradermal test score and histological inflammatory infiltrate

Table 2.6.4. Number of cats with positive reactions (score > 0) and the median score (and range) for all intradermal injection sites

	No. of cats with positive reactions and median score							
	30 min		24 h		48 h		72 h	
	n	Score	*n*	Score	*n*	Score	*n*	Score
Control	0	0	0	0	0	0	0	0
SMCA	2	0 (0–1)	8	1.5 (1–2)[ab]	8	1.5 (1–3)[ab]	4 of 4	1 (1–2)[a]

n: number of cats with positive reactions, out of eight (unless otherwise shown). Similar reactions were seen at all three repeat injection sites in all cats for both SMCA and control. Control: intradermal injection with saline; SMCA: soluble *Microsporum canis* antigen.
Significant differences (Kruskal–Wallis test, with Dunn's multiple comparison test): [a] from control site at the same time ($p < 0.01$, 24 and 48 h, $p < 0.05$, 72 h); [b] from SMCA, 30 min ($p < 0.05$).

score (Spearman's rank correlation coefficient $r_s = 0.8248$, $p < 0.001$). In the SMCA biopsies inflammatory change was observed in the superficial dermis (superficial perivascular dermatitis), associated with superficial to mid-level hair follicles (mural interface folliculitis) or with the deep dermis (perivascular inflammation) to panniculus (Plate 5). In three out of the four biopsies taken 48 h after SMCA injection, eosinophils and mast cells either predominated or were present in similar numbers to macrophages and lymphocytes (based on a subjective assessment). In all biopsies taken 72 h after SMCA injection, macrophages and lymphocytes predominated.

Immunohistochemistry

The immunohistochemical markers for B-cells and immunoglobulin G (IgG), IgA or IgM plasma cells labelled very few cells in any of the skin biopsy specimen. Total scores (i.e. the sum of the scores for the four anatomical compartments assessed) for the markers for MHC class II, macrophages and granulocytes, and CD3 were significantly higher for the SMCA biopsies than for the control biopsies (Table 2.6.5, Wilcoxon's rank sum test, $p = 0.0078$). For the CD3 and MHC class II markers, more cells were labelled in the 72 h biopsies than in the 48 h biopsies. For the SMCA biopsies, MHC class II-labelled cells were present in all compartments examined (Table 2.6.6) and included the majority of cells comprising the inflammatory infiltrate, and cells in the epidermis with a dendritic morphology. Cells labelled with macrophage/granulocyte marker were present in all compartments except for the epidermis. CD3, CD4 and CD8-labelled cells showed a similar distribution, with relatively few labelled cells in the epidermis. The number of $CD4^+$ and $CD8^+$ cells appeared similar. CD3, CD4 and CD8-labelled cells in the perifollicular compartment appeared to be homing towards the follicular epithelium.

Table 2.6.5. Subjective scoring of cells labelled with immunohistochemical markers in skin biopsy specimens

	Median total immunohistochemistry score[a] (range)									
	MHC class II		Macro/gran		CD3		CD4		CD8	
	SMCA*	Control	SMCA*	Control	SMCA*	Control	SMCA*	Control	SMCA*	Control
48 h	9 (8–10)	2.5 (0–3)	8 (8)	0 (0)	5.5 (4–7)	0 (0–2)	4.5 (3–8)	0 (0–1)	5.5 (3–8)	0 (0–1)
72 h	10 (9–10)	1.5 (0–5)	5 (4–6)	0 (0)	7.5 (6–8)	0 (0–1)	5.5 (4–8)	0 (0–1)	5.5 (4–7)	0 (0–1)

[a] The total immunohistochemistry score for each biopsy is derived by summating the scores for four anatomical compartments which were scored. MHC: major histocompatibility complex; Macro/gran: macrophages/granulocytes; SMCA: soluble *Microsporum canis* antigen; Control: intradermal injection of saline.
*Scores for SMCA biopsies were significantly higher than for control biopsies (Wilcoxon's signed rank test, $p = 0.0078$).

Table 2.6.6. Subjective scoring of cells labelled with immunohistochemical markers in different cutaneous compartments in skin biopsy specimens collected after intradermal injection of soluble *Microsporum canis* antigen

	Median immunohistochemistry score (range)									
	MHC class II		Macro/gran		CD3		CD4		CD8	
	48 h	72 h	48 h	72 h	48 h	72 h	48 h	72 h	48 h	72 h
Perifollicular	3 (3)	3 (3)	3 (3)	2 (2)	2 (1–2)[a]	3 (2–3)[a]	1.5 (1–2)[a]	2 (2–3)[a]	1.5 (1–2)[a]	2 (2–3)[a]
Sup. dermis	3 (3)	3 (3)	3 (3)	2 (1–2)	2 (1–3)	2 (2–3)	1.5 (1–2)	1 (1–2)	1.5 (1–2)	2 (1–2)
Epidermis	1 (0–2)	2 (1–2)	0 (0)	0 (0)	0 (0)	0.5 (0–1)	0 (0–1)	0 (0)	0 (0)	0 (0–1)
Deep dermis	2 (2)	2 (2)	2 (2)	1.5 (0–2)	2 (1–2)	2 (1–2)	1 (0–2)	1 (1–2)	1.5 (1–2)	1.5 (1–2)

[a]Labelled cells appeared to be homing to the follicular epithelium.
MHC: major histocompatibility complex; Macro/gran: macrophages/granulocytes; Sup. dermis: superficial dermis.

Cytokine RT–PCR assays

mRNA for interleukin-4 (IL-4) was not detected in any biopsy. There was no significant difference between levels of cytokine mRNA in control and SMCA biopsies for any of the other cytokines measured (γ-interferon [IFN-γ], IL-10, IL-12p40); however, marked variation in cytokine levels was seen between cats (Table 2.6.7). There was no correlation between cytokine mRNA levels and histological inflammatory cell scores or total immunohistochemistry score for any of the cytokines measured or markers used.

Discussion

In the present study, injection of the dermatophyte antigen into recovered cats produced clear reactions, both immediate and delayed, which were easily distinguished from the control, saline-injected. The intradermal test scores were highly consistent in every cat at all triplicate repeat sites of intradermal injection for both SMCA and saline at all time points. A high degree of correlation between the intradermal test score and histological inflammatory infiltrate score of individual skin biopsies was demonstrated. Interpretation of feline intradermal test reactions is notoriously difficult (McCusker & Aitken, 1967; Aitken & McCusker, 1969; Kunkle, 1984; Pedersen, 1987) but this may be less of a problem with DTH responses than immediate-type reactions. Intradermal testing has been successfully used to evaluate cell-mediated immunity in cats (Otto *et al.*, 1993).

In this study only two out of eight cats demonstrated positive immediate-type hypersensitivity reactions to SMCA antigen at 30 min after injection, characterised by an erythematous weal. Biopsies were not taken at this time so the histological characteristics of these reactions are not known. All eight cats demonstrated positive DTH reactions to SMCA, at 24, 48 and 72 h after injection, characterised by induration. These results are similar to previously reported studies in recovered cats (DeBoer *et al.*, 1991).

In the present study, inflammation at the SMCA injection sites, 48 and 72 h after injection, was characterised by superficial perivascular dermatitis with folliculitis, perifolliculitis and mural folliculitis. The infiltrate comprised varying numbers of mast cells, eosinophils, neutrophils, lymphocytes and macrophages. The predominant cells in the infiltrate changed over time from eosinophils and mast cells at 48 h to lymphocytes and macrophages at 72 h. The lymphocytic mural interface folliculitis seen in the 72 h biopsies was very similar to that seen in lesions of clinical feline dermatophytosis (Gross *et al.*, 1997), lesions sampled during the recovery phase of experimentally induced feline dermatophytosis and at the site of

Table 2.6.7. Levels of cytokine mRNA (relative to G3PDH) in skin biopsy specimens

	Cat	IFN-γ		IL-10		IL-12	
		SMCA	Control	SMCA	Control	SMCA	Control
48 h	1	0.75	nd	0.75	nd	15.84	31.06
	2	1.83	0.53	0.68	0.59	16.76	7.13
	3	4.14	nd	0.47	0.26	10.67	0.13
	4	4.87	5.65	1.08	1.42	2.41	7.07
Median		2.99	0.26	0.72	0.43	13.25	7.10
72 h	5	nd	nd	0.05	nd	26.86	0.01
	6	nd	2.20	50.97	2.29	16.35	17.04
	7	1191.46	0.55	3.34	13.69	88.20	40.09
	8	1.01	nd	17.65	25.16	39.18	54.36
Median		0.51	0.27	10.49	7.99	33.02	28.56

mRNA for IL-4 was not detected in any biopsy.
G3PDH: glyceraldehyde 3-phosphate dehydrogenase, a constitutively expressed housekeeping gene which serves as an internal standard for comparison; IFN: interferon; IL: interleukin; SMCA: skin biopsies from sites of intradermal injection of soluble *Microsporum canis* antigen; Control: skin biopsies from sites of intradermal injection of saline; nd: not detectable.

rechallenge of recovered cats (A. Robinson *et al.*, unpublished data, University of Bristol, UK, 1999). The characteristics of the DTH reactions in this study are similar to those previously reported in cats, including a change in the cellular composition of the infiltrate over time, due to increasing numbers of lymphocytes and macrophages in 48 h biopsies compared with 24 h biopsies (DeBoer *et al.*, 1991). A predominantly lymphohistiocytic infiltrate is also reported for positive DTH reactions to dermatophyte antigens in humans (Rajka, 1963; Szepes *et al.*, 1993).

Investigation of the phenotype of cells in the inflammatory infiltrate in intradermal reactions to dermatophyte antigen using immunohistochemistry has not previously been reported in cats. The lymphocytes seen in these infiltrates were almost exclusively $CD3^+$ T-cells (with similar numbers of $CD4^+$ and $CD8^+$ cells) which appeared to be homing to the follicular epithelium, and there were few, if any, B-cells or plasma cells. Similar findings have been reported in humans following intradermal injection with dermatophyte antigen (Szepes *et al.*, 1993). The observed tropism of T-cells for the follicular epithelium is of note and has parallels in other diseases involving follicular pathogens, such as canine demodicosis (Day, 1997).

MHC class II-labelled cells included the majority of the cells in the inflammatory infiltrate and dendritic cells in the follicular epithelium. The morphological characteristics and location of these MHC class II-labelled dentritic cells suggest that they may be Langerhans' cells. More specific markers could be used to investigate this possibility. The number of MHC class II-labelled cells increased over the period 48–72 h after antigen injection, probably reflecting the increasing numbers of infiltrating inflammatory cells over this period and suggesting increasing antigen presentation. In contrast, numbers of Mac 387-labelled cells declined over the same period. This may be a reflection of increasing numbers of tissue macrophages, as the marker recognised by this antibody is expressed by newly differentiated macrophages, not mature tissue macrophages (Brandtzaeg, 1988).

Using RT–PCR assays, mRNA coding for IFN-γ, IL-12p40 and IL-10 was detected in the majority of both the SMCA and control (saline injection) biopsies, although large variations were apparent between cats. mRNA for IL-4 was not detected in any biopsy. The cytokine profile of IFN-γ, IL-12p40 and IL-10 in the cat is consistent with a Th_1-type response (Pedersen *et al.*, 1998). Since histological examination of the control biopsies demonstrated no infiltrate, this raises questions about the source of the cytokine mRNA. Cells normally present in the epidermis such as keratinocytes, Langerhans' cells and melanocytes have the ability to produce these cytokines and many others (Luger & Schwarz, 1990). It is possible that the damage induced by injection of saline is sufficient to induce cells present in normal skin to transcribe these cytokine mRNAs. Comparable levels of these cytokine mRNAs were seen in the SMCA biopsies. It is impossible to tell whether the cytokines seen in the SMCA biopsies represent a similar non-specific response to injection or a specific immune response to the antigen. The histological and immunohistochemical data strongly suggest that a specific immune response to SMCA occurs. A major problem in investigating cytokine mRNA levels in tissue homogenates is that no information is provided about which cells are producing the mRNA. Moreover, measurement of mRNA rather than protein does not necessarily indicate release of functionally active cytokine.

This experiment was performed to characterise the immune response to intradermal injection of dermatophyte antigen in recovered cats using the techniques of histology, immunohistochemistry and RT–PCR for cytokine mRNA. The use of this combination of techniques has not previously been reported in the cat. Detailed characterisation of the cutaneous immune response to intradermal testing with *M. canis* antigens in immune cats may offer an alternative to challenge models for the assessment of putative vaccines. Intradermal testing using purified antigens from *M. canis* could be used to investigate the role played in the immune response by component antigens in crude antigen mixtures and thereby provide a rational basis for the selection of antigens as potential vaccine candidates.

Acknowledgements

A. Robinson was supported by the Cat Welfare Trust. A. H. Sparkes was supported by the Feline Advisory Bureau.

References

Abraham, S., Pandhi, R. K., Kumar, R., Mohapatrra, L. N. & Bhutani, L. K. (1975) A study of the immunological status of patients with dermatophytosis. *Dermatologica*, **151**, 281–287.

Aitken, I. D. & McCusker, H. B. (1969) Immunological studies in the cat. III. Attempts to induce delayed hypersensitivity. *Research in Veterinary Science*, **10**, 208–213.

Brandtzaeg, P., Jones, D. B., Flavell, D. J. & Fagerhol, M. K. (1988) Mac 387 antibody and detection of formalin resistant myelomonocytic L1 antigen. *Journal of Clinical Pathology*, **41**, 963–970.

Calderon, R. A. & Hay, R. J. (1984) Cell mediated immunity in experimental murine dermatophytosis. II: Adoptive transfer of immunity to dermatophyte infections by lymphoid cells from donors with acute or chronic infections. *Immunology*, **53**, 465–472.

Cruickshank, C. N. D., Trotter, M. D. & Wood, S. R. (1960) Studies on trichophyton sensitivity. *Journal of Investigative Dermatology*, **35**, 219–223.

Day, M. J. (1997) An immunohistochemical study of the lesions of demodicosis in the dog. *Journal of Comparative Pathology*, **116**, 203–216.

DeBoer, D. J. & Moriello, K. A. (1994) The immune response to *Microsporum canis* induced by a fungal cell wall vaccine. *Veterinary Dermatology*, **5**, 47–55.

DeBoer, D. J. & Moriello, K. A. (1995) Investigation of a killed dermatophyte cell-wall vaccine against infection with *Microsporum canis* in cats. *Research in Veterinary Science*, **59**, 110–113.

DeBoer, D. J., Moriello, K. A. & Cooley, A. J. (1991) Immunological reactivity to intradermal dermatophyte antigens in cats with dermatophytosis. *Veterinary Dermatology*, **2**, 59–67.

DeLamater, E. D. (1941) Experimental studies with the dermatophytes. III. Development and duration of immunity and hypersensitivity in guinea pigs. *Journal of Investigative Dermatology*, **4**, 143–158.

Grappel, S. F. & Blank, F. (1972) Role of keratinases in dermatophytosis. I. Immune responses of guinea pigs immunised with keratinases. *Dermatologica*, **45**, 245–255.

Gross, T. L., Stannard, A. H. & Yager, J. A. (1997) An anatomical classification of folliculitis. *Veterinary Dermatology*, **8**, 147–156.

Hanifin, J. M., Ray, L. F. & Lobitz, W. C. (1974) Immunological reactivity in dermatophytosis. *British Journal of Dermatology*, **90**, 1–8.

Harley, R., Helps, C. R., Harbour, D. A., Gruffydd-Jones, T. J. & Day, M. J. (1999) Cytokine mRNA expression in lesions in cats with chronic gingivostomatitis. *Clinical and Diagnostic Laboratory Immunology*, **6**, 471–478.

Hay, R. J. (1982) Chronic dermatophyte infections. I: Clinical and mycological features. *British Journal of Dermatology*, **106**, 1–9.

Hay, R. J. (1994) Immunology of dermatophytosis. *Japanese Journal of Medical Mycology*, **35**, 1–8.

Hay, R. J. & Brostoff, J. (1977) Immune responses in patients with chronic *Trichophyton rubrum* infections. *Clinical and Experimental Dermatology*, **2**, 37–80.

Hunjan, B. S., Silverman, I. H., Curlovic, K. M., Osuamkpe, C. O., Melvin, J. R. & Cronholm, L. S. (1981) A simplified *in vitro* assay of delayed hypersensitivity in diagnosis of dermatomycoses. *Journal of Allergy and Clinical Immunology*, **67**, 485–494.

Jones, H. E., Reinhardt, J. H. & Rinaldi, M. G. (1973) A clinical, mycological and immunological survey of dermatophytosis. *Archives of Dermatology*, **108**, 61–65.

Jones, H. E., Reinhardt, J. H. & Rinaldi, M. G. (1974a) Acquired immunity to dermatophytosis. *Archives of Dermatology*, **109**, 840–848.

Jones, H. E., Reinhardt, J. H. & Rinaldi, M. G. (1974b) Model dermatophytosis in naturally infected subjects. *Archives of Dermatology*, **110**, 369–374.

Jones, H. E., Reinhardt, J. H. & Rinaldi, M. G. (1974c) Immunological susceptibility to chronic dermatophytosis. *Archives of Dermatology*, **110**, 213–220.

Kaaman, T., Von Stedingk, L. V. & Wasserman, J. (1976) An evaluation of delayed hypersensitivity in guinea pigs to various trichophytin preparations. *Acta Dermato-Venereologica (Stockholm)*, **56**, 283–287.

Kerbs, S., Greenberg, J. & Jesrani, K. (1977) Temporal correlation of lymphocyte blastogenesis, skin test responses and erythema during dermatophyte infections. *Clinical Experimental Immunology*, **27**, 526–530.

Kunkle, G. A. (1984) Feline Dermatology. *Veterinary Clinics of North America: Small Animal Practice*, **14**, 1065–1087.

Lepper, A. W. D. (1972) Experimental bovine *Trichophyton verrucosum* infection. Preliminary clinical, immunological and histological observations in primarily infected and reinoculated cattle. *Research in Veterinary Science*, **13**, 105–115.

Luger, T. A. & Schwarz, T. (1990) Evidence for an epidermal cytokine network. *Journal of Investigative Dermatology*, **95**, 100S–104S.

McCusker, H. B. & Aitken, I. D. (1967) Immunological studies in the cat. II. Experimental induction of skin reactivity to foreign proteins. *Research in Veterinary Science*, **8**, 265–271.

Otto, C. M., Brown, C. A., Linol, P. A. & Dane, D. L. (1993) Delayed hypersensitivity testing as a clinical measure of cell-mediated immunity in the cat. *Veterinary Immunology and Immunopathology*, **38**, 91–102.

Pedersen, N. C. (1987) Basic and clinical immunology. In: *Diseases of the Cat: Medicine and Surgery*, Vol. 1 (Ed. J. Holtzworth), pp. 146–181. W. B. Saunders, Philadelphia, PA.

Pedersen, N. C., Dean, G. A., Bernales, J., Sukura, A. & Higgins, J. (1998) *Listeria monocytogenes* and *Serratia marcenscens* infections as models for Th1/Th2 immunity in laboratory cats. *Veterinary Immunolology and Immunopathology*, **63**, 83–103.

Rajka, G. (1963) Studies in hypersensitivity to moulds and staphylococci in prurigo besnier (atopic dermatitis). *Acta Dermato-Venereologica*, **43** (Suppl. 54), 43–101.

Smith, P. K., Krohn, R. I., Hermanson, G. T., Mallian, A. K., Gartner, F. H., Provenzano, M. D. *et al.* (1985) Measurement of protein using bicinchoninic acid. *Analytical Biochemistry*, **150**, 76–85.

Sorensen, G. W. & Jones, H. E. (1976) Immediate and delayed hypersensitivity in chronic dermatophytosis. *Archives of Dermatology*, **112**, 40–42.

Sparkes, A. H., Stokes, C. R. & Gruffydd-Jones, T. J. (1993) Humoral immune responses in cats with dermatophytosis. *American Journal of Veterinary Research*, **54**, 1869–1873.

Sparkes, A. H., Stokes, C. R. & Gruffydd-Jones, T. J. (1995) Experimental *Microsporum canis* infection in cats: correlation between immunological and clinical observations. *Journal of Medical and Veterinary Mycology*, **33**, 177–184.

Sparkes, A. H., Gruffydd-Jones, T. J. & Stokes, C. R. (1996) Acquired immunity in experimental feline *Microsporum canis* infection. *Research in Veterinary Science*, **61**, 165–168.

Szepes, E., Magyarlaki, M., Battyani, Z. & Schneider, I. (1993) Immunohistochemical characterisation of the cellular infiltrate in dermatophytosis. *Mycoses*, **36**, 203–206.

Part 3

Dysplasia and neoplasia

3.1

Histiocytes in skin disease

V.K. Affolter Dr med vet, DipECVP, PhD and P.F. Moore BVSc, DipACVP, PhD

School of Veterinary Medicine, Department of Pathology, Microbiology, Immunology, University of California, Davis, California, USA

Summary

The original term 'histiocytes' includes three leukocyte subpopulations: the peripheral blood monocytes, tissue macrophages and myeloid dendritic cells. They derive from a common bone marrow precursor. Upon differentiation tissue macrophages and myeloid dendritic cells develop phenotypic and functional differences and are considered separate cell lineages with partially overlapping functions. Macrophages are effector cells of the innate immune system. Their primary function consists of phagocytosis and digestion of infectious pathogens and foreign material. Myeloid dendritic cells are a heterogeneous group of professional antigen-presenting cells, which play a key function in the activation of the adaptive immune system by initiating the development of an antigen-specific primary immune response. Most inflammations associated with infectious pathogens harbor both cell types. Diseases characterized by a marked prevalence of either macrophages or dendritic cells are uncommon.

Macrophages and dendritic cells have identical morphological features when evaluated by light microscopy. Immunophenotyping is therefore required to differentiate between these two cell types. Access to immunophenotyping has also clearly demonstrated that a variety of cells, including large lymphocytes and non-leukocytic cells, can mimic the morphological features of histiocytes. This is particularly obvious with cutaneous round-cell tumors of different cell origin. Hence, the morphological term 'histiocytes' is often used inappropriately as it includes cells other than macrophages or dendritic cells. An accurate identification of lesional cells, however, is fundamental to the understanding of a disease process and may ultimately result in the development of specific and more successful therapies.

Introduction

In 1887 Metchnikoff characterized the macrophage by documenting its ability for phagocytosis and amoeboid locomotion (Metchnikoff, 1887). Later, Aschoff introduced the term histiocyte and classified the cell as a component of the reticuloendothelial or reticulohistiocytic system (Aschoff, 1924). The reticuloendothelial system was considered to be a system composed of scattered and fixed macrophages and specialized endothelial cells that contribute to the natural resistance of mammals to pathogens (Aschoff, 1924). The term histiocyte was chosen as an abbreviation for 'histiogenic wandering cell', to describe its potential to move within the tissue and to indicate its putative derivation from mesenchymal precursors in various tissues. Subsequently, the histiocytes were identified as bone marrow-derived cells and classified as cells of the mononuclear phagocyte system and the dendritic cell system (van Furth *et al.*, 1975; Tew *et al.*, 1982). Tissue histiocytes include macrophages and myeloid dendritic cells which differ in their primary functions and fulfill different functional aspects of the immune system (Banchereau *et al.*, 2000; Kimber *et al.*, 2000).

Other leukocytes and non-leukocytic cells can mimic morphological features of histiocytes. The access to immunohistochemistry using monoclonal antibodies (Moore *et al.*, 1998) specific for numerous surface antigens on leukocytes and non-leukocytic cells demonstrated that the morphological terms 'histiocytes' or 'histiocytic cells' have been used for cells other than tissue macrophages and dendritic cells. Histological terms such as 'histiocytic lymphoma', 'malignant fibrous histiocytoma' and 'histiocytic mast cell tumor' clearly demonstrate this unfortunate situation (Wilcock *et al.*, 1986; Chastain *et al.*, 1988; Thoolen *et al.*, 1992; Kerlin & Hendrick, 1996; Soslow *et al.*, 1996; Seo *et al.*, 1999). Hence, mononuclear cell populations of uncertain origin must be evaluated by immunohistochemistry to allow accurate identification and the term histiocytes should be limited to the morphological description of tissue macrophages and dendritic cells (Favara & Jaffe, 1994; Favara *et al.*, 1997).

This review focuses on the ontogeny of histiocytes and their distribution and functions in the different compartments of the skin and its skin-associated lymphoid tissue. It further describes the involvement of histiocytes in cutaneous infectious diseases, cutaneous deposition disorders, immune-mediated skin lesions, immune-dysregulatory processes and cutaneous neoplasia. A correct identification of lesional cells is crucial to a complete characterization and understanding of a disease process and provides the basis of subsequent development of more specific and successful therapies (Yamaguchi & Ogawa, 1999).

Ontogeny of histiocytic cell lineages

Peripheral blood monocytes, tissue macrophages and myeloid dendritic cells arise from a common precursor in the bone marrow (Figure 3.1.1) (Reid *et al.*, 1992). This has been documented in cultures of $CD34^+$ bone marrow progenitor cells in semisolid methylcellulose colony-forming assays (Young, 1999). The developing colonies consist of a mixture of monocytes, macrophages and dendritic cells. A disruption of myeloid dendritic cell differentiation leads to enhanced production of macrophages, which supports the concept of a common progenitor cell and shared intermediate stages (Yamaguchi & Ogawa, 1999). As differentiated cells in the periphery, macrophages and dendritic cells are characterized by morphological, phenotypic and functional differences. Although they are closely related cells, the interconversion of differentiated myeloid dendritic cells and macrophages has not been clearly demonstrated (Janeway, 1992; Yamaguchi & Ogawa, 1999). Therefore, differentiated dendritic cells and macrophages are specified polar representatives of one common regulatory system and are best considered to represent different cell sublineages. The myeloid dendritic cell system itself consists of phenotypically and functionally diverse subpopulations (Maraskovsky *et al.*, 1999). Most studies of dendritic cell ontogeny and differentiation have been conducted in mice and humans. Currently, there is evidence of three separate pathways giving rise to three subpopulations of myeloid dendritic cells (Figure 3.1.1) (Olweus *et al.*, 1997; Caux *et al.*, 1999; Shortman & Wu, 1999).

In addition to the myeloid dendritic cells, a separate lymphoid dendritic cell system has been documented in mice (Figure 3.1.1) (Shortman & Caux, 1997; Shortman & Wu, 1999). Murine lymphoid dendritic cells evolve from a lymphoid-committed bone marrow progenitor cell (Caux *et al.*, 1999; Maraskovsky *et al.*, 1999; Shortman & Wu, 1999). As differentiated cells, they express CD8αα, major histocompatibility complex (MHC) classes I and II, and CD2. Thymic murine lymphoid dendritic cells are involved in the thymic negative selection of potentially self-reactive T-cells (Steinman *et al.*, 1997). Peripheral murine lymphoid dendritic cells may regulate inappropriate or chronic expansions of Th_1-cells and help to maintain self-tolerance (Steinman *et al.*, 1997; Maraskovsky *et al.*, 1999). A few observations suggest the existence of a lymphoid dendritic cell population in humans, but no evidence thereof has been documented in other species (Shortman & Caux, 1997; Caux *et al.*, 1999; Maraskovsky *et al.*, 1999).

Ontogeny of macrophages

Macrophages were first described by Metchnikoff, who documented their marked ability for phagocytosis and amoeboid locomotion (Metchnikoff, 1887). Stem cell factors (c-kit, flt-3L) and cytokines [granulocyte–monocyte–colony-stimulating factor (GM-CSF), monocyte–colony-stimulating factor (M-CSF) and interleukin-6 (IL-6)] induce the development of a $CD14^+$, $CD1^-$ bipotent intermediate cell from the $CD34^+$ bone marrow precursor or from peripheral blood monocytes *in vitro* (Young, 1999). Subsequently, M-CSF, IL-6, IL-10, IL-1 and platelet-derived growth factor (PDGF) guide these intermediate $CD14^+$ bipotent cells to differentiate into $CD16^+$, $CD14^+$, $CD68^+$, $CD1^-$ macrophages (Santiago-Schwarz *et al.*, 1992; De Smedt *et al.*, 1997; Caux *et al.*, 1999). IL-4 interferes with this differentiation (Santiago-Schwarz *et al.*, 1992). Differentiated macrophages express a variety of surface receptors including mannose-fucosyl receptors, receptors for immunoglobulins (FcγR: CD16, CD32) and complement factors (CR: CD11b, CD35) (Seljelid & Eskeland, 1993). Upon occupation of these receptors the macrophages become activated and produce numerous

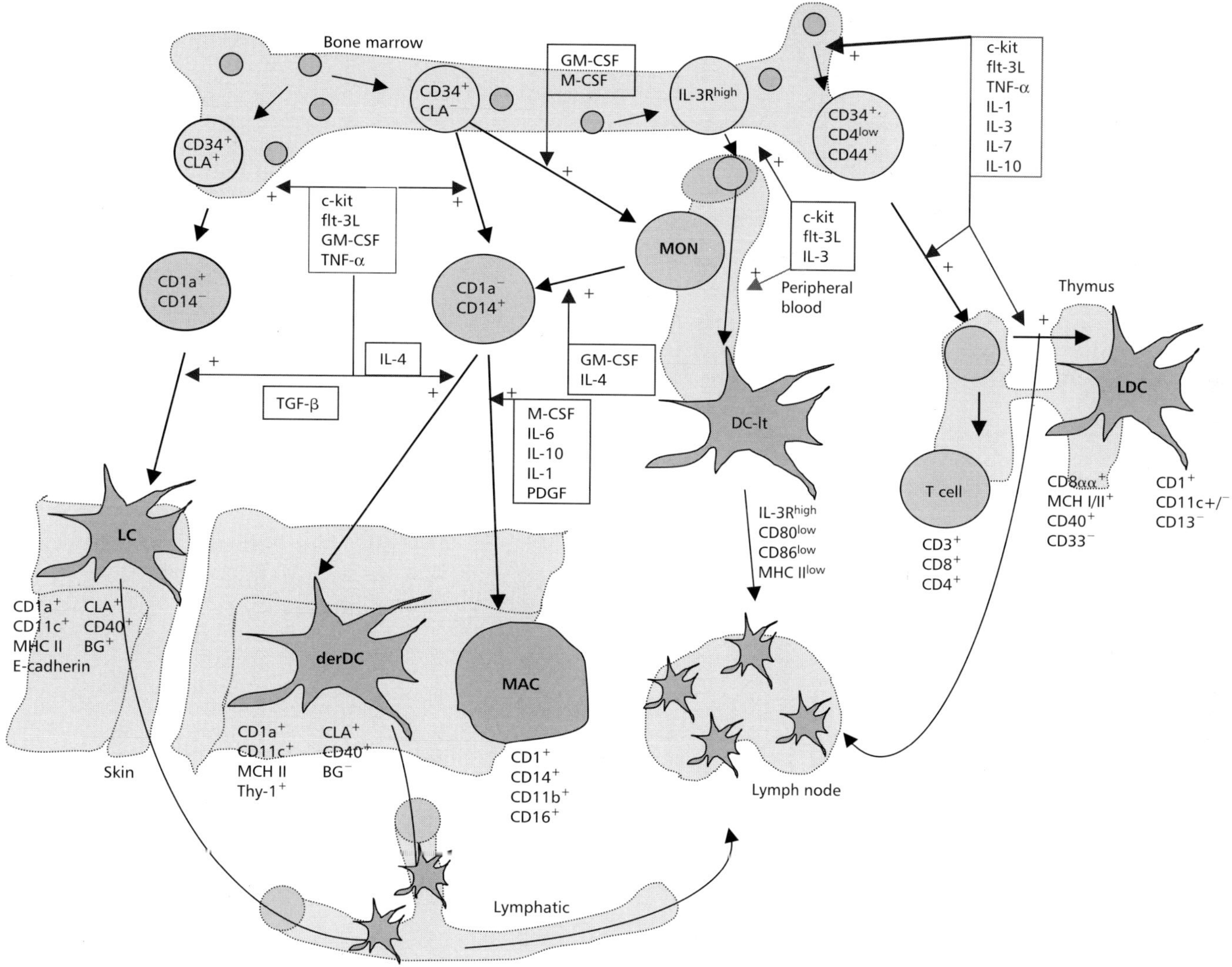

Figure 3.1.1. Ontogeny of dendritic cells (DC). The development of DC of the skin-associated lymphoid tissue is guided by a variety of stem cell factors and cytokines. Myeloid DC include Langerhans' cells (LC), dermal DC (derDR) and myeloid DC of lymphoid tissues (CD-lt). Macrophages (MAC) and derDC evolve from a common intermediate bipotent $CD1a^-$, $CD14^+$ cell which can be recruited from the bone marrow precursor or peripheral blood monocytes (MON). LC and derDC migrate to the lymph node following antigen exposure and activation. CD-lt migrate to the lymph node as immature cells. Mice have a separate lymphoid DC population (LDC).

cytokines [IL-1, -6, -8, -10 and -12, tumor necrosis factor-α (TNF-α), α-interferon (IFN-α), IFN-γ, M-CSF, GM-CSF, granulocyte–colony-stimulating factor (G-CSF) and transforming growth factor-β (TGF-β)] and chemokines [monocyte chemotactic protein-1 (MCP-1), MCP-3, migration inhibitory factor (MIF), macrophage inflammatory protein-1 (MIP-1), MIP-2, leukemia inhibitory factor (LIF) and oncostatin M (OsM)]. Moreover, they release a variety of digestive proteases from their lysosomal compartment (Unanue & Allen, 1987; Seljelid & Eskeland, 1993; Cavaillon, 1994). As effector cells of the innate immune system, macrophages are dispersed throughout the different organ systems and predominantly reside in close proximity to the microvasculature (van Furth, 1981).

Ontogeny of myeloid dendritic cells

Myeloid dendritic cells develop from $CD34^+$ hematopoietic progenitor cells, which also give origin to monocytes and macrophages (Figure 3.1.1) (Young, 1999). These dendritic cells express CD33 and CD13, which confirms their myeloid origin (Wu *et al.*, 1995; Ardavin, 1997; Galy *et al.*, 1999). Three major developmental pathways (Figure 3.1.1) of myeloid dendritic cells have been documented in humans (Olweus *et al.*, 1997; Caux *et al.*, 1999; Young, 1999). Stem cell factors (c-kit and flt-3L), GM-CSF and TNF-α induce the development of two separate intermediate MHC II^+ populations (Figure 3.1.1) which can be differentiated based on their expression of surface proteins such as CD14, CD1 and the cutaneous lymphoid-associated antigen (CLA) (Szabolcs *et al.*, 1995; Caux *et al.*, 1996, 1999). These intermediate cells give raise to the intraepithelial dendritic cells called Langerhans' cells and the interstitial dendritic cells (Figure 3.1.1). The latter include the population of dermal dendritic cells. IL-3 initiates the development of a third distinct myeloid dendritic cell subpopulation (Figure 3.1.1), which constitutes the major dendritic cell population of peripheral lymphoid organs in humans (Olweus *et al.*, 1997).

Dendritic cells of Langerhans' cell type

Langerhans' cells develop from $CD34^+$, CLA^+ progenitor cells (Figure 3.1.1), which start to express CD1 at an intermediate stage (Strunk *et al.*, 1997). TGF-β is responsible for their expression of E-cadherin and it is required to induce formation of Birbeck granules observed in Langerhans' cells in some species (Figure 3.1.2) (Birbeck *et al.*, 1961; Geissmann *et al.*, 1998; Caux *et al.*, 1999). Langerhans' cells coexpress the chemokine receptor CCR10, which binds the chemokines CCL27 and CCL28 (Dieu-Nosjean *et al.*, 1999; Morales *et al.*, 1999; Homey *et al.*, 2000; Wang *et al.*, 2000). Moreover, Langerhans' cells express CCR6, which binds to the chemokine MIP-3α (Dieu-Nosjean *et al.*, 1999). All three chemokines are constitutively expressed by keratinocytes (Figure 3.1.2) (Dieu-Nosjean *et al.*, 1999; Morales *et al.*, 1999; Homey *et al.*, 2000; Wang *et al.*, 2000). Homing of Langerhans' cells into the epidermis and epithelia of mucous membranes is therefore induced by the following mechanisms (Figure 3.1.2) (Hart, 1997; Maurer & Stingle, 1999): (1) CLA expression of Langerhans' cells guides their homing into the skin by ligation to E-selectin on cutaneous postcapillary venules (Alon *et al.*, 1994); (2) interaction of CCL27 or CCL28 with CCR10 as well as MIP-3α with CCR6 guides their migration into the epidermis; and (3) homeotypic ligation of E-cadherin tethers Langerhans' cells to the neighboring keratinocytes (Tang *et al.*, 1993; Banchereau *et al.*, 2000). In contrast to macrophages, Langerhans' cells lack mannose receptors, but express the C-type lectin langerin instead (Mommaas *et al.*, 1999; Valladeau *et al.*, 1999, 2000). Langerin is also involved in the formation of Birbeck granules (Valladeau *et al.*, 1999, 2000). Expression of FcεRI (CD23) and FcγRII (CD32) enables Langerhans' cells to bind the Fc portions of immunoglobulins (IgE and IgG) (Maurer & Stingle, 1999; Banchereau *et al.*, 2000). The phenotype of differentiated Langerhans' cells is characterized by expression of CD1, CD11c, MHC II and CD40 (Young, 1999). Upon activation and up-regulation of the accessory molecules (CD86 and CD80), Langerhans' cells become professional antigen-presenting cells (APC). Langerhans' cells are considered poor stimulators of antigen-specific $CD4^+$ T-cells and may predominantly be involved in the priming of $CD8^+$ T-cells (Mommaas *et al.*, 1999).

Interstitial dendritic cells and dermal dendritic cells

The bipotential $CD1^-$, $CD14^+$ intermediate cell pool evolves from $CD34^+$, CLA^- bone marrow precursors or can be developed *in vitro* from $CD14^+$ peripheral blood monocytes (Sallusto & Lanzavecchia, 1994; Caux *et al.*, 1996; Romani *et al.*, 1996; Strunk *et al.*, 1997). The bipotential intermediate cells have receptors for M-CSF as well as GM-CSF and TNF-α and, hence, can

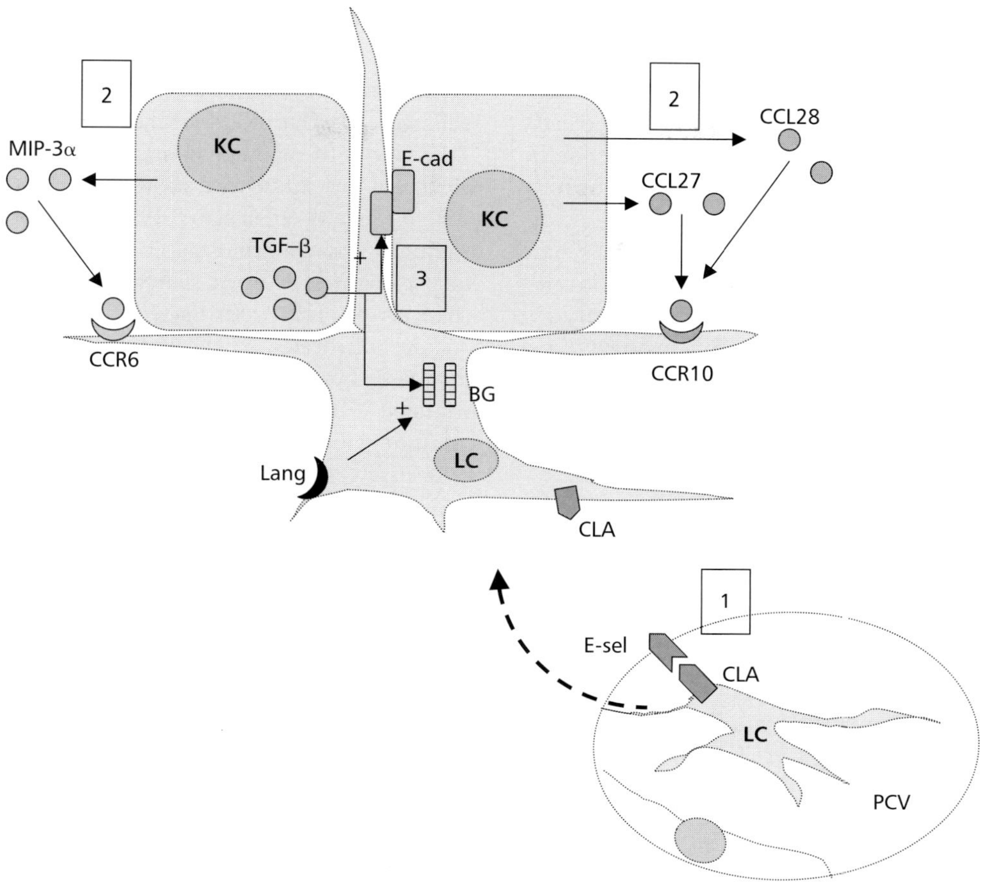

Figure 3.1.2. Homing of Langerhans' cells (LC). Several mechanisms induce homing of LC to the skin. (1) Expression of cutaneous lymphoid-associated antigen (CLA) enables LC to ligate E-selectin (E-Sel) on cutaneous postcapillary venules (PCV). (2) Keratinocytes (KC) secrete the chemokines CCL27, CCL28 and MIP-3α. LC have receptors (CCR10 and CCR6) for these chemokines and, hence, migrate into the epidermis. (3) Transforming growth factor-β (TGF-β) and langerin (Lang) induce the formation of Birbeck granules (BG) and TGF-β induces E-cadherin (E-cad) expression on DC. The homeotypic ligation of E-cad tethers LC to the KC.

mature into $CD1^-$, $CD14^+$ macrophages (as described above) or into $CD1^+$, $CD14^-$ dendritic cells (Caux *et al.*, 1999). GM-CSF and TNF-α initiate the differentiation into dendritic cells and IL-4 supports this differentiation by blocking the development of macrophages. These myeloid dendritic cells migrate into a variety of peripheral tissues where they reside as interstitial dendritic cells in close proximity to the microvasculature (Meunier *et al.*, 1993; McWilliam *et al.*, 1999; Maurer & Stingle, 1999; Steptoe & Thomas, 1999). A subpopulation of interstitial dendritic cell precursors up-regulates CLA and migrates as dermal dendritic cells into the perivascular areas of the dermis (Meunier *et al.*, 1993; Caux *et al.*, 1999; Maurer & Stingle, 1999). Dermal dendritic cells lack Birbeck granules and expression of E-cadherin, but express $CD90^+$ (Thy-1) instead (Meunier *et al.*, 1993; Shortman & Caux, 1997; Caux *et al.*, 1999; Young, 1999). The phenotype of dermal dendritic cells is therefore characterized by expression of CD1, CD11b, CD11c, MHC II, CD54 [intercellular adhesion molecule-1 (ICAM-1)], and CD90 (Thy-1) (Meunier *et al.*, 1993; Shortman & Caux, 1997; Caux *et al.*, 1999; Young, 1999). Their coexpression of FcεR1 (CD23), FcγR1 (CD64) and FcγR2 (CD32) allows ligation of IgE and IgG (Fanger *et al.*, 1996; Maurer & Stingle, 1999; Banchereau *et al.*, 2000), an important step in internalizing antigens previously captured by immunoglobulins. Upon stimulation, dermal dendritic cells up-regulate CD4 and the accessory molecules CD80 and CD86 (Meunier *et al.*, 1993; Caux *et al.*, 1999; Young, 1999). In contrast to Langerhans' cells, dermal dendritic cells are capable of inducing IL-2-driven differentiation of B-cells and they secrete IL-10, which regulates excessive dendritic cell activation by blocking their further differentiation and function (Caux *et al.*, 1997; de Saint-Vis *et al.*, 1998a).

Dermal factor XIIIa$^+$ dendritic-shaped cells were originally described as dermal dendrocytes (Cerio *et al.*, 1989). However, factor XIIIa positivity is not limited to myeloid dermal dendritic cells; it can also be expressed by dendritic-shaped, non-leukocytic cells such as perivascular fibroblast (Nestle *et al.*, 1993; Narvaez *et al.*, 1996). Factor XIIIa expression is therefore not a reliable marker to identify myeloid dermal dendritic cells.

Primary dendritic cells of lymphoid organs

A large subset of dendritic cells in T-cell-dependent areas of human lymphoid organs belongs to a separate lineage (Olweus *et al.*, 1997). These cells were first referred to as 'plasmacytoid' cells (Grouard *et al.*, 1997) and, despite their myeloid origin, are sometimes inappropriately referred to as human 'lymphoid dendritic cells'. Primary dendritic cells of lymphoid tissues develop from IL-3Rα^{high} (CD123), CD34$^+$ myeloid progenitor cells (Figure 3.1.1) and their differentiation is mainly guided by IL-3. They migrate as morphologically and functionally immature dendritic cells through the vascular system and enter the lymph organs independently from previous stimulation, up-regulation of MHC II or accessory molecules (Olweus *et al.*, 1997). Primary dendritic cells of lymphoid tissues express an IL-3Rα^{high}, CD45RA$^+$, CD4$^+$, CD11c$^-$, MHC II^{low} phenotype and constitute the major dendritic cell subpopulation of interdigitating cells in T-cell-rich areas in lymph nodes. Upon binding of GM-CSF, IL-3Rα^{high} dendritic cells develop into morphologically and functionally differentiated dendritic APC (Olweus *et al.*, 1997). They up-regulate expression of the antigen-presenting molecules MHC II, CD1 and accessory molecules (CD80 and CD86) and, hence, become potent stimulators of allogenic CD4$^+$ T-cells (Olweus *et al.*, 1997).

Function of histiocytic cells

Function and activation of macrophages

Macrophages are important effector cells of the innate immune system (Seljelid & Eskeland, 1993). They are dispersed throughout the different organ systems and their primary function involves phagocytosis and subsequent lysis of engulfed particles and pathogens (van Furth, 1981; Seljelid & Eskeland, 1993). The activity of macrophages as effector cells can be enhanced by influences of the adaptive immune system (Seljelid & Eskeland, 1993). Macrophages are equipped with pattern recognition receptors by which they recognize patterns shared between pathogens (Banchereau *et al.*, 2000). Bacterial lipopolysaccharides and carbohydrates are recognized by the mannose-fucosyl receptor. Other receptors recognize double-stranded viral RNA or proteins. Receptors for immunoglobulins and complement (FcR and CR, respectively) enable the macrophages to bind particles and organisms opsonized by immunoglobulins or complement factors (Seljelid & Eskeland, 1993). Receptor-bound pathogens are internalized by phagocytosis and endocytosis (Unanue & Allen, 1987). Phagosomes fuse with intracytoplasmic lysosomes and the content of phagosomes is subsequently subjected to intracellular metabolic changes within the phagolysosomes (Unanue & Allen, 1987). During this process the macrophages secrete and produce a myriad of factors which are important contributors to the development of inflammation (Seljelid & Eskeland, 1993). These factors include proteases, complement factors, cytokines (TNF-α, IL-1, IL-6), chemokines [MIP-1, -2, -3, IL-8, macrophage-derived chemokine (MDC)], arachidonate derivatives, toxic oxygen metabolites (O_2^-, OH^-) and nitrogen metabolites (NO_2^-). Chemokines such as MDC attract natural killer (NK) cells, which act as potent effector cells of the innate immune system (Chantry *et al.*, 1998).

Several factors released by effector cells of the innate immune system support the activation of the adaptive immune system. Moreover, the involvement of the adaptive immune system enhances the effectiveness of the innate effector cells such as macrophages and NK cells. The MDC provides such a link to the adaptive immune system by attracting dendritic cells and T-cells (Chantry *et al.*, 1998). Macrophages activated by IFN-γ, IL-3 and GM-CSF increase their microbicidal and tumoricidal activity by increasing their nitric oxide production and by initiating a 'respiratory burst', whereby increased cellular oxygen uptake results in production of potent oxygen radicals (Mackaness, 1964; Knight, 2000). Moreover, cytokine-activated macrophages increase their release of cytokines

(IL-1, -6, -8, -10 and -12, TNF-α, IFN-α and-γ, M-CSF, G-CSF and GM-CSF) and chemokines (MCP-1, -3, MIF, MIP-1, -2, LIF and OsM) (Cavaillon, 1994). Many of these cytokines and chemokines are capable of enhancing activation of macrophages in an autocrine and a paracrine fashion. In addition to their phagocytic function, macrophages are able to act as professional APC by presenting processed antigens in context with MHC class I and II molecules (Unanue & Allen, 1987; Seljelid & Eskeland, 1993).

Function and activation of myeloid dendritic cells

Myeloid dendritic cells are considered professional APC and are primarily involved in capturing an antigen, processing it and subsequently presenting it to lymphocytes to trigger a primary antigen-specific immune response. Dendritic cells are essential to maintain the survival of naive and memory T-cells (Brocker, 1997; Ludewig *et al.*, 1999).

Antigen uptake

Dendritic cells screen their environment for the presence of foreign antigens, which they internalize by receptor-mediated endocytosis, phagocytosis or macropinocytosis (Hanau *et al.*, 1987; Sallusto *et al.*, 1995; Matsuno *et al.*, 1996). C-type lectin receptors, such as the mannose receptors on dermal dendritic cells or langerin on Langerhans' cells, recognize the bacterial glycosylation patterns, which are different from mammalian cells (Sallusto *et al.*, 1995; Valladeau *et al.*, 1999, 2000). Immunoglobulin-opsonized pathogens are ligated by FcR on Langerhans' cells (FcεR1 and FcγR2) and dermal dendritic cells (FcεR1, FcγR1 and FcγR2), and this interaction initiates the internalization of the entire complex (Fanger *et al.*, 1996; Maurer *et al.*, 1998; Banchereau *et al.*, 2000). During the phase of active antigen uptake, the immature $CD1^+$ dendritic cells have low expression of accessory molecules (CD80, CD86) and MHC II, while some monocyte markers, such as CD68, may still be expressed (Caux *et al.*, 1999).

Antigen processing

As professional APC, dendritic cells exhibit different pathways of antigen processing. Cytosolic proteins are conjugated with ubiquitin and directed to the proteasomes for degradation into peptides by an ATP-dependent proteolytic system (Banchereau *et al.*, 2000). The peptides are translocated to the endoplasmatic reticulum and accommodated into the binding-groove of MHC I molecules (class I pathway). Subsequently, the MHC I–peptide complex moves to the cell surface. Dendritic cells may also use heat-shock proteins such as hsp96 to deliver antigens via the class I pathway (Arnold-Schild *et al.*, 1999).

Alternatively, captured extracellular antigens are transported into the lysosome-related intracellular MHC II-rich compartments, where catalytic removal of the MHC II-associated invariant chain renders MCH II molecules available for binding of antigenic peptides (class II pathway) (Jensen, 1999; Banchereau *et al.*, 2000). Phagocytosed extracellular antigens may also be released into the cytosole, conjugated with ubiquitin, directed to the proteasomes and eventually presented in the context of MHC I molecules (Banchereau *et al.*, 2000; Fong & Engleman, 2000). The latter process is referred to as cross-priming and has been documented with transplantation antigens, particular antigens, tumors and viruses (Banchereau *et al.*, 2000; Fong & Engleman, 2000).

The third group of antigen-presenting molecules is the family of CD1 molecules. CD1a, b, c and d are heterogeneous in their tissue distribution (Porcelli *et al.*, 1998; Banchereau *et al.*, 2000). They are efficient presenters of endogenous and exogenous lipids (such as microbial lipids) and glycolipid-containing antigens (Porcelli *et al.*, 1998; Banchereau *et al.*, 2000). CD1-restricted presentation appears to regulate γδ-T-cells (Porcelli *et al.*, 1998).

Dendritic cell migration, activation and maturation

Cytokines (GM-CSF, IL-1β and TNF-α) and chemokines guide the process of dendritic cell migration, maturation and activation, which are best documented in Langerhans' cells (Figure 3.1.3) (Kimber *et al.*, 2000). Initiation of migration requires previous detachment of the Langerhans' cells from the neighboring keratinocytes. Subsequent to any injury to the epidermis, keratinocytes secrete TNF-α, which binds to the TNF-R2 receptor on the Langerhans' cells (Koch *et al.*, 1990). IL-1β, produced by Langerhans' cells and keratinocytes, further enhances the release of TNF-α, and ligation of IL-1β to IL-1RI on the Langerhans' cells supports the following effects of TNF-α (Cumberbatch *et al.*, 1999). First, the Langerhans' cells down-regulate E-cadherin and, hence, are released from their binding to E-cadherin on keratinocytes (Tang *et al.*, 1993;

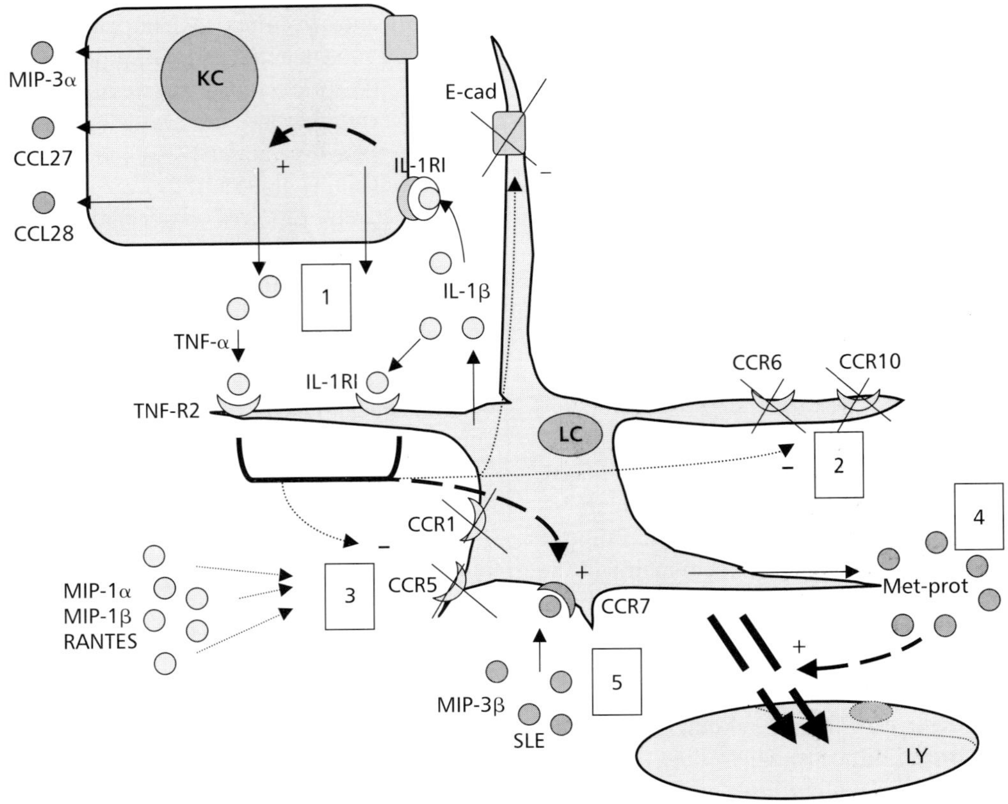

Figure 3.1.3. Migration of Langerhans' cells (LC). After antigen uptake, the LC detach from the keratinocytes (KC) and injured KC release tumor necrosis factor-α (TNF-α). Binding of KC-derived TNF-α and interleukin-1 (IL-1) initiates (1) DC detachment by down-regulation of E-cadherin (E-cad); (2) down-regulation of chemokine receptors CCR6 and CCR10 on LC, which abrogates binding of the chemokines CCL27, CCL28 and MIP-3α; and (3) down-regulation of CCR1 and CCR5 on DC, which interferes with their retention in the site of injury. LC-derived IL-1β enhances these effects by increasing production of KC-derived TNF-α. (4) LC enhance their migration by digesting the extracellular matrix with metalloproteinases. (5) As the DC up-regulate CCR7, they will be attracted by the chemokines MIP-3β and SLC. Both chemokines support their migration into afferent lymphatics (LY).

Borkowski *et al.*, 1994; Dieu *et al.*, 1998; Sallusto *et al.*, 1998; Sozzani *et al.*, 1999). Secondly, the Langerhans' cells down-regulate the expression of CCR6 and therefore are no longer attracted to keratinocyte-derived MIP-3α (Borkowski *et al.*, 1994; Dieu *et al.*, 1998; Sallusto *et al.*, 1998; Sozzani *et al.*, 1999). Sites of injury and inflammation have high levels of the chemokines MIP-1α, MIP-1β and RANTES (regulated on activation, normal T-cell expressed and secreted) (Kimber *et al.*, 2000). While immature Langerhans' cells are attracted to these chemokines, mature activated Langerhans' cells lose their expression of CCR1 and CCR5 and are no longer capable of binding these chemokines (Sozzani *et al.*, 1998). The release from their neighboring keratinocytes and the non-responsiveness to local chemoattractants are crucial steps in allowing Langerhans' cells to migrate away from the primary site of inflammation (Forster *et al.*, 1999; Kimber *et al.*, 2000).

After a successful release, the Langerhans' cells up-regulate CCR7, a ligand for MIP-3β and secondary lymphoid tissue cytokine (SLC) (Sozzani *et al.*, 1995; Morelli *et al.*, 1996; Forster *et al.*, 1999; Vecchi *et al.*, 1999). Both chemokines attract Langerhans' cells to the paracortical area of the draining lymphoid nodes (Dieu *et al.*, 1998; Gunn *et al.*, 1998; Yanagihara *et al.*, 1998). Activated Langerhans' cells support their migration by the secretion of metalloproteinases and by changing their expression of adhesion molecules (Caux *et al.*, 1999; Kimber *et al.*, 2000). Collagenases, stromlysin-1 and -2 and macrophage elastase induce degradation of extracellular matrix proteins. Expression of the integrin $\alpha_6\beta_1$ (VLA-6) initiates the binding to laminin and up-regulated CD44 binds to hyaluronic acid components of the extracellular matrix (Caux *et al.*, 1999; Kimber *et al.*, 2000). As 'veiled cells', the migrating Langerhans' cells enter the lymph nodes via afferent lymphatics, where they are primarily found in the paracortex and give rise to interdigitating cells in the lymph node (Austyn, 1999).

During their migration, Langerhans' cells differentiate into potent APC (Caux *et al.*, 1999; Banchereau *et al.*, 2000; Kimber *et al.*, 2000). Differentiated APC are characterized by an increased transport of peptide-occupied or glycolipid-occupied antigen-presenting molecules (MHC I, MHC II and CD1) to the cell surface. Moreover, they up-regulate the expression of adhesion molecules (ICAM, β-integrins) and accessory molecules (CD80, CD86). At the same time, the dendritic cells lose their capability for antigen uptake by down-regulating the appropriate receptors.

There are several mechanism to counter-regulate these activating effects on Langerhans' cells (Enk & Katz, 1992; de Saint-Vis *et al.*, 1998b). Keratinocytes and dermal dendritic cells are capable of releasing IL-10, which has counter-regulatory effects on TNF-α and IL-1β. IL-10 also inhibits translocation of peptide-bound MHC II complexes to the cell surface (Koppelman *et al.*, 1997). IL-10 and certain neuropeptides (calcitonin gene-related peptide [CGRP] and α-melanocyte-stimulating hormone [α-MSH]) are known to convert immature dendritic cells into inefficient APC, which induce tolerance of T-cells and may have an inductive effect on suppressor T-cells (Maurer & Stingle, 1999). These mechanisms ensure temporary activation of Langerhans' cells and inhibit an excessive response.

Migration, maturation and activation of dermal dendritic cells have not been studied thoroughly. However, perivascular mast cells release preformed and newly synthesized factors in response to a variety of stimuli (Welle, 1997; Kube *et al.*, 1998). Mast cell-derived TNF-α could certainly initiate similar events in dermal dendritic cells. Once the migration is initiated, dermal dendritic cells enter the lymph nodes by afferent lymphatics and become interdigitating cells in the T-cell-rich areas of the lymph node.

Antigen presentation to T-cells

The most common assessment of dendritic cell function relates to their remarkable ability to stimulate T-cells, as documented in allogenic mixed lymphocyte reactions (Crow & Kunkel, 1982; Van Voorhis *et al.*, 1983). *In vivo* primary lymphocyte activation occurs in the lymph node and is initiated by an interaction between the interdigitating dendritic cells and lymphocytes in the paracortical area. Myeloid dendritic cells express MHC I, MHC II and CD1 and by presenting antigens in the context of these molecules they initiate the stimulation of T-cells (Figure 3.1.4) (Inaba *et al.*, 1987; Porcelli *et al.*, 1998; Jensen, 1999). *In vitro*, Langerhans' cells are less efficient stimulators of antigen-specific $CD4^+$ T-cells than are dermal dendritic cells (Mommaas *et al.*, 1999). They seem predominantly involved in priming $CD8^+$ T-cells (Banchereau *et al.*, 2000).

The primary antigen-specific lymphocyte activation (MHC II–peptide complex binding TCR–CD3 complex) is followed by a cascade of multiple events (Figure 3.1.4) provided by ligation of adhesion molecules (β_2 integrins, ICAM-1, ICAM-3, CD2, CD58) and accessory molecules (CD80, CD86, CD28). Early interaction of MHC II–peptide complexes on dendritic cells with TCR–CD3 complex on $CD4^+$ lymphocytes (Figure 3.1.4) induces up-regulation of CD40 ligand (CD40L) in the lymphocyte. The subsequent ligation of CD40 on dendritic cells with CD40L on lymphocytes enhances changes in the cell morphology, phenotype and function of both cells (Romani *et al.*, 1989; Larsen *et al.*, 1990; Caux *et al.*, 1994). Dendritic cells start to secrete cytokines (IL-1 and TNF-α) and chemokines [IL-8, MIP-1α, MIP-1β, MDC, T-cell-associated chemokine receptor (Tarc) and DC-chemokine-1 (DC-CK1)], further enhance their translocation of cytoplasmic MHC molecules to the cell surface and up-regulate CD58 and the accessory molecules CD80 and CD86 (Figure 3.1.4). The release of dendritic cell-specific chemokines (MDC, Tarc, DC-CK1) attracts an increasing number of T-cells (Adema *et al.*, 1997; Godiska *et al.*, 1997; Caux *et al.*, 1999).

The response of T-lymphocytes to CD40–CD40L ligation is characterized by increased expression of CD28 and subsequent induction of CTLA-4 expression (Figure 3.1.4) (Caux *et al.*, 1994; McLellan *et al.*, 1996; Van Gool *et al.*, 1996). The interaction of CD80 or CD86 with CD28 provides the second signal necessary for the development of an immune response (Greenfield *et al.*, 1998; Chambers & Allison, 1999; Slavik *et al.*, 1999). With increasing expression of CTLA-4 the dendritic cell accessory molecules (CD80 and CD86) will

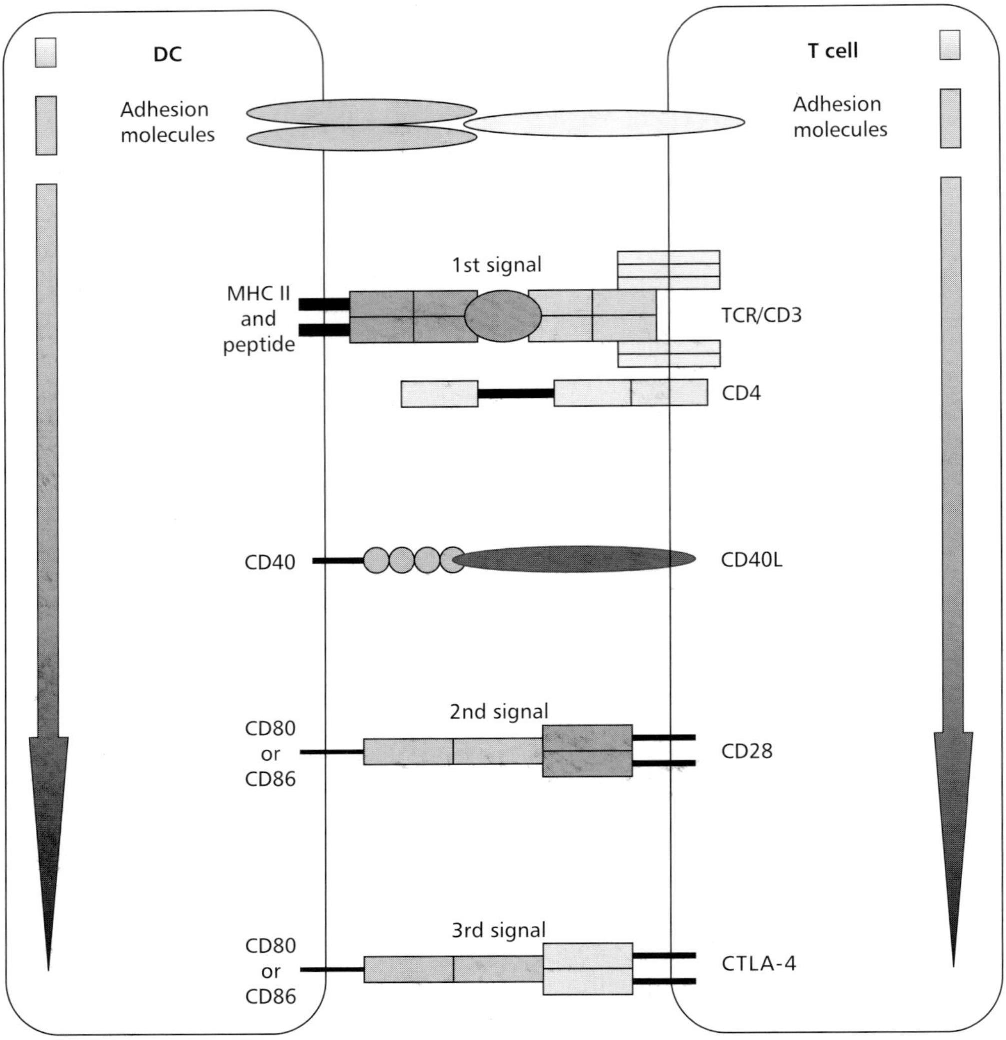

Figure 3.1.4. Interaction of mature dendritic cells with T-lymphocytes. A specific immune response against exogenous antigens is induced by two major separate activating signals. The first signal consists of presentation of processed antigen-peptides by major histocompatibility complex (MHC) class II molecules by the dendritic cells (DC). The peptide–MHC II complex binds to the T-cell receptor (TCR)–CD3 complex on the $CD4^+$ T-cell. Simultaneous interactions of different adhesion molecules keep DC and T-cells close together, which supports further interactions between the cells. In response to the antigen-specific first signal, T-cells up-regulate CD40L, which then can bind to CD40 on DC. T-cells also start to secrete cytokines and up-regulate expression of CD28 and subsequently CTLA-4. CD40–CD40L ligation induces up-regulation of CD80 and CD86 on DC. CD80 and CD86 binding to CD28 on lymphocytes induces the important second signal for lymphocyte activation. As the expression of CTLA-4 in T-cells increases, CTLA-4 molecules capture the majority of CD80 and CD86 on the DC. This interaction triggers a third signal, which will induce the down-regulation of the immune response.

preferentially bind to CTLA-4. This initiates the down-regulation of the immune response (June *et al.*, 1994; Gribben *et al.*, 1995; Greenfield *et al.*, 1998; Chambers & Allison, 1999; Slavik *et al.*, 1999).

Dendritic cells can elicit distinct T-helper cell responses. $CD11c^+$ dendritic cells (including Langerhans' cells and dermal dendritic cells) polarize naive T-cells predominantly towards a Th_1 response (Rissoan *et al.*, 1999). CD40 activation in dendritic cells induces their secretion of IL-12 (Macatonia *et al.*, 1993). As a result, the primed T-cells produce IFN-γ, which supports a Th_1 response (Macatonia *et al.*, 1993). There is also some evidence that a predominance of CD80–CD28 ligation induces a Th_1 response (Kuchroo *et al.*, 1995).

IL-3Rα^{high}, CD11c$^-$ dendritic cells of lymphoid tissues and a predominance of CD86–CD28 interactions tend to favor a Th_2 response (Kuchroo *et al.*, 1995; Rissoan *et al.*, 1999). Moreover, the presence of IL-10, steroids and prostglandin E_2 can convert a Th_1 response into a Th_2 response (Piemonti *et al.*, 1999; Banchereau *et al.*, 2000).

Dendritic cells are equally important in priming cytotoxic CD8$^+$ T-cells. Presentation of peptide–MHC I complexes to the TCR–CD3 complex can activate CD8$^+$ lymphocytes directly in the absence of CD4$^+$ helper cells (Young & Steinman, 1990). However, CD4$^+$ T-cell help is often required and a conditioned dendritic cell is considered to act as a bridge between the CD4$^+$ T-cell and the CD8$^+$ T-cell (Young & Steinman, 1990; Banchereau *et al.*, 2000).

Interaction of myeloid dendritic cells and B-lymphocytes

Little information is currently available regarding direct interactions between dendritic cells and B-lymphocytes. T-cell-dependent primary B-cell activation requires dendritic cell involvement (Inaba *et al.*, 1983a, b; Sornasse *et al.*, 1992). It appears that CD40–CD40L ligations are a key factor in this interaction, as *in vitro* studies have shown that dendritic cells can directly modulate B-cell growth and differentiation in the presence of soluble CD40L (Dubois *et al.*, 1997). Alternatively, dendritic cells can transfer captured antigens to naive B-cells, which will proceed in processing the antigen and subsequently presenting the peptides to T-cells. This pathway initiates a Th_2-associated antibody response (Wykes *et al.*, 1998).

Dendritic cell interaction with the innate immune system

Dendritic cells can directly influence effector cells of the innate immune system, such as macrophages and natural killer (NK) cells (Banchereau *et al.*, 2000). Differentiated dendritic cells release IL-12, IL-15 and IL-18, which regulate the activity of NK cells (Banchereau *et al.*, 2000). In response, stimulated NK cells release IFN-γ, which enhances the microbicidal and tumoricidal activity of macrophages (Mackaness, 1964).

Histiocytes in skin diseases

As the primary functions of macrophages and myeloid dendritic cells differ, it can be expected that their predominance varies in different diseases. The primary function of macrophages involves phagocytosis and digestion of pathogens. Myeloid dendritic cells provide a link to the adaptive immune system and with it they initiate the diversity and memory associated with an antigen-specific immune response. Macrophages and dendritic cells cannot be differentiated based on morphological features provided by conventional light microscopy and often it is impossible to delineate them from other large, cytoplasm-rich cells. The latter is especially difficult in tumors characterized by poorly differentiated round cells or spindle cells.

Reactive histiocytic infiltrate

Reactive histiocytic infiltrates with infectious diseases

Pleocellular inflammatory infiltrates as a result of infectious diseases are characterized by variable numbers of histiocytes. Macrophages and dendritic cells are observed. The two populations play a decisive role in the interaction between the infectious agents (parasites, bacteria and fungi) and the host's immune system. This has been clearly demonstrated with cutaneous leishmaniasis (Moll, 1997). Chemokines such as MCP-1, -2 and -3, RANTES, MIP-1α and MIP-1β attract macrophages and immature dendritic cells to the location of the pathogens and tissue damage (Cavaillon, 1994; Moll, 1997). Macrophages remain in the primary site of tissue damage and as effector cells, they initiate leishmanicidal activity (Moll, 1997). Antigen exposure and uptake initiate migration and differentiation of lesional dendritic cells. This process provides the transport of parasite antigens to the paracortical area of the draining lymph node, where the interaction of interdigitating cells with T-cells triggers the antigen-specific primary immune response (Moll, 1997). Activated antigen-specific T-cells will home back to the site of inflammation (Barker & MacDonald, 1992; Robert & Kupper, 1999; Campbell & Butcher, 2000). Their production of IFN-γ supports and increases the effectiveness of the leishmanicidal activity of lesional macrophages. Parasite antigens can persist in interdigitating dendritic cells in the lymph node, a process considered to contribute to the maintenance of specific immunity (Moll, 1997). Reactive lesional dendritic cell infiltrates will regress as the inducing pathogens are removed and primary disease is controlled (McClain & Weiss, 1994; Favara *et al.*, 1997).

Dendritic cells are a key factor in the induction of a specific immune response. Current research is therefore focusing more and more on their use in therapeutic or preventive approaches to different diseases. Treatment with antigen-pulsed dendritic cells can result in protective immunity (Yamaguchi & Ogawa, 1999), as shown in mice treated with *Leishmania* antigen-pulsed Langerhans' cells (Moll, 1997). These mice developed a specific immunity and were no longer susceptible to infections of cutaneous leishmaniasis (Moll, 1997).

Reactive histiocytic infiltrates with deposition disorders

Metabolic diseases are often associated with the deposition of glycoproteins or lipids (Feingold *et al.*, 1989; Touart & Sau, 1998). Hypertriglyceremia and hypercholesteremia may result in nodular cutaneous depositions of lipids and cholesterol (Wisselink *et al.*, 1994; Furue *et al.*, 1995; Matsushima *et al.*, 1999). Cats tend to develop these xanthomatous nodules around their eyes or in the preauricular area (Vitale *et al.*, 1998). Xanthomas are characterized by a fairly monomorphic population of lipid-laden CD68$^+$ macrophages, as shown in humans (Furue *et al.*, 1995). Metabolite overload and secondary trauma may result in tissue disruption characterized by a more pleocellular inflammation composed of macrophages, neutrophils, some dendritic cells and lymphocytes.

Cutaneous deposition of amyloid derived from immunoglobulin lambda-light chain occurs with cutaneous plasmacytomas and cutaneous B-cell lymphomas, and secondary to B-cell lymphomas located in other organ systems (Linke *et al.*, 1991; Rowland *et al.*, 1991; Gliatto & Alroy, 1995; Hagari *et al.*, 1996). Amyloid accumulates between the dermal collagen bundles, as well as around and within vascular walls. Minor trauma induces hemorrhage and tissue damage, which provoke an inflammatory response with numerous macrophages.

Reactive histiocytic infiltrates secondary to foreign bodies

Trauma is often associated with the implantation of foreign bodies such as plant material. Alternatively, tissue degeneration may result in alteration and displacement of the host's own tissues, which will act as an endogenous foreign body. Common examples are ruptured follicular cysts with the release of keratin and hair shafts, sebaceous hyperplasia with the release of sebum or foci of eosinophilic degranulation. Foreign-body reactions are predominantly composed of macrophages, histiocytic multinucleated giant cells and neutrophils (Gross *et al.*, 1992; Yager & Wilcock, 1994).

Immune-dysregulatory and immune-mediated reactive histiocytosis

Canine reactive dendritic cell histiocytosis includes a cutaneous and a systemic form (Affolter & Moore, 2000). Both diseases target the skin and subcutaneous tissue, with nodular lesions predominantly on the head, neck, extremities and scrotum (Moore, 1984; Mays & Bergeron, 1986; Scott *et al.*, 1987; Affolter & Moore, 2000). With systemic histiocytosis, additional lesions develop in other organ systems, including the lymph nodes, eye-lids, sclera, nasal cavity, lungs, spleen and bone marrow. Canine reactive histiocytosis can develop in any breed. The systemic form, however, is predominantly seen in Bernese mountain dogs, rottweilers, Irish wolfhounds and golden retrievers, which supports the hypothesis of a genetic predisposition in these breeds (Moore, 1984; Scott *et al.*, 1987; Affolter & Moore, 2000). In canine reactive histiocytosis, the nodular cutaneous lesions are characterized by angiocentric and vasoinvasive accumulations of CD1a, b, c$^+$, CD4$^+$, CD11b, c$^+$, MHC II$^+$, ICAM-1, -3$^+$, CD80$^+$, CD86$^+$, CD90$^+$ activated dermal dendritic cells, CD8$^+$, TCR-$\alpha\beta^+$ T-cells and neutrophils (Affolter & Moore, 2000). The disorder is probably an antigen-driven process. However, the identity and characteristics of possible antigens remain unknown. The waxing and waning clinical course and the successful treatment with immunomodulatory drugs suggest an immunoregulatory disorder (Affolter & Moore, 2000). Disrupted proliferation, activation and function of T-lymphocytes or dendritic cells, disturbed interactions between T-cells and dendritic cells, altered local cytokine milieu, involvement of superantigens, or a combination thereof, are mechanisms to consider for the development of this immune dysregulation (Affolter & Moore, 2000). Older lesions of Langerhans' cell histiocytosis in humans may be characterized by an increasing number of macrophages and, hence, are no longer diagnostic for a primary Langerhans' cell histiocytosis (Favara & Jaffe, 1994). Similar features have been seen in cases of canine reactive histiocytosis (personal observation).

Nodular pleocellular dermal accumulations of CD1a, c$^+$, CD11b$^+$, MHC II$^+$ dendritic cells, with admixed CD8$^+$ lymphocytes and fewer neutrophils, have been identified in two cats (personal observation).

The dendritic cells do not exhibit epitheliotropism, which suggests an accumulation of dermal dendritic cells similar to canine reactive dendritic cell histiocytosis. However, angiocentric behavior is not as prominent. The small number of cases evaluated to date does not allow any reliable conclusions to be drawn at this point.

Other immune-mediated processes, such as granulomatous drug reactions, may present as sterile, pleocellular panniculitis and dermatitis composed of macrophages, numerous dendritic cells and lymphocytes (Magro *et al.*, 1998; Magro & Crowson, 2000). These lesions lack angiocentric and vasoinvasive behavior. They may contain numerous plasma cells and eosinophils (personal observations). Currently poorly understood, sterile, immune-mediated granulomatous lesions may be associated with other histological changes observed with immune-mediated diseases, including interface dermatitis, prominent keratinocyte apoptosis and vasculitis.

Reactive histiocytic infiltrates with cutaneous neoplasia

Secondary dendritic cell accumulations within tumor tissue have been documented in patients with various malignancies (Pimpinelli *et al.*, 1988; Chaux, 1995; Shurin, 1996; Favara *et al.*, 1997; Stoppacciaro *et al.*, 1997). The dendritic APC are attracted by cytokines and chemokines produced by the degenerating tumor-invaded tissues or the tumor cells themselves. Secondary dendritic cell infiltrations and expansions are considered important for the development of a tumor-specific immune response (Chaux, 1995; Stoppacciaro *et al.*, 1997; Fong & Engleman, 2000). The presence of numerous reactive dendritic cells within a neoplasm indicates a more favorable prognosis (Lotze & Jaffe, 1999). The initial hypothesis suggested that dendritic cells pick up tumor antigens and present them to T-cells in the draining lymph node, whereby a specific anti-tumor immune response develops. The efficiency of this mechanism is somewhat questionable, as tumor-derived dendritic cells often lack appropriate expression of accessory molecules and, hence, are incapable of inducing the secondary activating signal for lymphocytes (Chaux *et al.*, 1997).

An alternative hypothesis suggests that lesional dendritic cells support the survival of infiltrating T-cells (Lotze & Jaffe, 1999). Tumor cells often express the surface molecule FasL and therefore can eliminate infiltrating T-cells by Fas–FasL-induced T-cell apoptosis (Lotze & Jaffe, 1999). The infiltrating dendritic cells may provide enough stimulatory signals and cytokines to rescue the infiltrating T-cells from apoptosis (Lotze & Jaffe, 1999). Moreover, dendritic cells express Fas-L and hence can bind Fas on tumor cells, whereby apoptosis of the tumor cells is induced (Lotze & Jaffe, 1999). Secondary reactive dendritic cell infiltrates may outnumber the tumor cell population and their long cytoplasmic processes can enclose solitary tumor cells completely (personal observation). Immunophenotypic evaluation of these neoplastic processes is challenging, as entrapped tumor cells can mimic expression of dendritic cell surface molecules and, hence, may be misdiagnosed as primary dendritic cell tumors.

In vitro manipulated dendritic cells are currently undergoing major investigation as possible anti-tumor immunotherapy (Fong & Engleman, 2000). Dendritic cells are pulsed with tumor-derived antigens or tumor-derived RNA *in vitro*. Subsequent reinjection of pulsed dendritic cells induces regression of the tumor tissue (Yamaguchi & Ogawa, 1999). Immunotherapy carries the risk of undesired reactions, such as the induction of an immune response to self-antigens as self-reactive T-cells to cryptic epitopes may escape thymic negative selection (Fong & Engleman, 2000). Alternatively, if tumor-antigen pulsed dendritic cells do not have adequate expression of accessory molecules or fail to secrete IL-12, inappropriate costimulation will result in T-cell anergy (Yamaguchi & Ogawa, 1999). Although specific tumor antigens exist, they remain unidentified in most neoplasms (Yamaguchi & Ogawa, 1999). Moreover, tumor antigens may vary between individuals with an identical tumor type (Fong & Engleman, 2000). The development of a routine anti-tumor immunotherapy with manipulated dendritic cells is therefore very difficult and further studies are required before this method can be used as a reliable therapeutic tool.

Involvement of dendritic cells in autoimmune diseases

Potentially autoreactive T-cells are eliminated in the thymus during the process of negative selection (Drexhage *et al.*, 1999). However, similarly to the development of a specific immune response, thymic negative selection of autoreactive T-cells predominantly develops against dominant antigen determinants, and T-cells specific for cryptic antigens may escape this elimination (Sercarz *et al.*, 1993; Drakesmith *et al.*, 2000). A similar process of negative selection probably exists for self-reacting B-cells in the bone marrow. However, a certain fraction of circulating self-reactive B-cells, which produce anti-self low-affinity IgM called natural autoantibodies, can be found in healthy individuals. In the absence of appropriate T-cell support these antibodies do not induce disease.

The pathogenesis of organ-specific and systemic autoimmune diseases is described as a multistep process which can be separated in three major phases (Drexhage *et al.*, 1999). Dendritic cells are critically involved in each phase (Drexhage *et al.*, 1999). The first step is characterized by a genetic or an acquired loss of recognizing 'self'. Acquired loss of tolerance to self-antigens occurs with tissue damage and subsequent exposure of 'cryptic antigen determinants', which are sampled and presented by dendritic cells. Cross-reactivity is an alternative pathway of breaking the self-tolerance. Cytokine imbalances or gene defects can induce dysfunctional dendritic cells with altered processing and presentation of antigens (Drakesmith *et al.*, 2000). During the second phase, the migrating dendritic cells induce the activation and expansion of autoreactive T-cells (Drexhage *et al.*, 1999). The terminal phase is predominantly characterized by tissue damage induced by either autoantibodies or autoreactive $CD8^+$ T-cells (Drexhage *et al.*, 1999). Local interactions between dendritic cells and autoreactive T-cells in the vicinity of the target tissue may increase the tissue damage by enhancing the effector functions of tissue macrophages (Drexhage *et al.*, 1999).

Neoplastic histiocytic diseases

Canine cutaneous histiocytoma

Canine cutaneous histiocytoma is a common, mostly benign neoplasm predominantly seen in young dogs (Moore *et al.*, 1996). The incidence drops markedly after the age of 3 years. The majority of cases are characterized by a solitary skin nodule that tends to ulcerate. The cutaneous nodules consist of a proliferation of monomorphic CD1a, b, c^+, $CD4^-$, $CD11c^+$, MHC II^+, $CD90^-$ Langerhans' cells (Moore *et al.*, 1996), which display epidermotropic behavior and coexpress E-cadherin (personal observation). Infiltration of $CD8^+$ cytotoxic T-cells is observed with initiation of spontaneous regression of the tumor nodule, a phenomenon observed in most solitary cutaneous histiocytomas. Occasionally, the neoplastic Langerhans' cells migrate from the cutaneous histiocytoma into the draining lymph node (Moore *et al.*, 1996). The lymphadenopathy tends to resolve simultaneously with the regression of the skin nodule.

Solitary nodules in young dogs seldom represent a diagnostic challenge. However, histiocytomas may develop in older dogs. Moreover, some dogs develop multiple cutaneous histiocytomas, which can persist for a long time. The nodules fail to regress and there is marked migration of Langerhans' cells into draining lymph nodes (personal observation). These skin nodules usually lack infiltration of $CD8^+$ T-cells, which would indicate the initiation of regression, but have an infiltrate of plasma cells instead. Multiple cutaneous histiocytomas in young and middle-aged dogs may persist over months and may evolve into a malignant neoplastic process with internal metastases (personal observation). The latter clinical presentation resembles disseminated Langerhans' cell histiocytosis in humans (Broadbent *et al.*, 1994; Favara *et al.*, 1997).

Histiocytomas and other cutaneous round-cell tumors may present with almost identical morphological features. Cutaneous histiocytomas in older dogs, recurrent and persistent histiocytomas as well as multiple cutaneous histiocytomas, therefore, require immunophenotypic evaluation to be differentiated from other cutaneous round-cell tumors, in particular epitheliotropic and non-epitheliotropic cutaneous lymphomas or poorly differentiated melanomas (Bender & Muller, 1989; Moore *et al.*, 1996). The use of immunohistochemistry will help to avoid the use of unfortunate morphological terms such as 'histiocytic lymphoma', as such cells do not exist (Chastain *et al.*, 1988; Thoolen *et al.*, 1992; Kerlin & Hendrick, 1996; Soslow *et al.*, 1996; Seo *et al.*, 1999). An accurate identification of the proliferating cells is required to provide a more specific prognosis for the patient and to initiate appropriate therapies.

Epitheliotropic histiocytosis in cats

A few cases of cutaneous proliferations of moderately to marked pleomorphic large round cells with abundant cytoplasm, irregular oval and indented nuclei, and epidermal tropism have been recognized in cats (personal observations). The proliferating cells were identified as CD1a, c^+, $CD4^-$, $CD11b^+$, MHC II^+ dendritic cells. The phenotype of the dendritic cells associated with the presence of intraepithelial cell aggregates suggests a proliferation of Langerhans' cells. However, in the limited number of cases evaluated, the proliferating cells did not express E-cadherin. Moreover, electron-microscopic evaluation of skin lesions in one cat failed to provide evidence of Birbeck's granules. Therefore, the exact origin of the proliferating dendritic cells remains to be determined.

The cats present with multiple cutaneous nodules, often located on the head and neck. The lesions have a progressive clinical course and internal lesions have been observed. The morphological features and clinical behavior of epitheliotropic histiocytosis of cats most closely resemble canine histiocytomas with malignant behavior (personal observation) and Langerhans' cell histiocytosis in humans (Broadbent *et al.*, 1994; Moore *et al.*, 1996; Favara *et al.*, 1997). Feline epitheliotropic histiocytosis must be differentiated from cutaneous epitheliotropic and non-epitheliotropic lymphomas and poorly granulated mast cell tumors, previously documented as 'histiocytic mast cell tumors' and feline cutaneous xanthomas (Wilcock *et al.*, 1986; Vitale *et al.*, 1998). Both can be characterized by histiocytes with marked foamy cytoplasm (personal observation).

Histiocytic sarcoma of dendritic cell origin

Canine disseminated histiocytic sarcoma or malignant histiocytosis predominantly affects internal organs, but may be characterized by concurrent subcutaneous and cutaneous non-epitheliotropic tumor masses (Gross & Affolter, 1998; Affolter, 1999; Affolter & Moore, 2002). Canine localized histiocytic sarcomas occur as solitary invasive tumors that tend to metastasize into draining lymph nodes (Gross & Affolter, 1998; Affolter, 1999). They often develop in the deep dermal and subcutaneous tissue, with a predilection for the extremities and proximity to joints (Affolter & Moore, 2002). A subgroup of localized histiocytic sarcomas arises from synovial tissues. These tumors subsequently may infiltrate into the overlying subcutis and deep dermis. Localized and disseminated canine histiocytic sarcomas are composed of dense proliferations of either plump spindle cells or large individualized round cells with abundant cytoplasm. Often the tumors are characterized by a mixture of both cell types and multinucleated giant tumor cells are common. Independent from their morphological features, the tumor cells consistently express CD1a, b, c^+, $CD11c^+$, $CD11b^+$, MHC II^+, a phenotype characteristic of myeloid dendritic cells (Gross & Affolter, 1998; Affolter, 1999; Affolter & Moore, 2002). They consistently lack expression of CD4 cells (Affolter, 1999; Affolter & Moore, 2002) and E-cadherin (personal observation) and a subpopulation of the tumor cells occasionally expresses CD90 (Thy-1) (Affolter, 1999).

The exact dendritic cell sublineage of canine histiocytic sarcomas has not been determined. Histiocytic sarcomas of non-lymphoid tissues probably arise from peripheral interstitial dendritic cells (Meunier *et al.*, 1993; Maurer & Stingle, 1999; McWilliam *et al.*, 1999; Steptoe & Thomas, 1999). Histiocytic sarcomas of lymphoid organs are likely to arise from the interdigitating cells within the lymphoid tissues. In humans, interdigitating cells consist of migrating Langerhans' cells, migrating interstitial dendritic cells and IL-3Rα^{high}, $CD45RA^+$, $CD4^+$ dendritic cells. The existence of the latter subpopulation has not been shown in dogs as appropriate tools to recognize canine IL-3Rα expression are not available. However, all tumor samples were consistently negative for CD4 and only a few canine histiocytic sarcomas coexpressed CD45RA.

Based on their morphology, localized histiocytic sarcomas were previously documented as 'malignant fibrous histiocytomas' (Hendrick *et al.*, 1992; Kerlin & Hendrick, 1996). Immunophenotypic evaluation clearly demonstrated that malignant fibrous histiocytoma does not represent a specific entity, but rather describes a collection of sarcomas with similar histological features but of different cellular origin, including poorly differentiated fibrosarcomas, leiomyosarcomas, rhabdomyosarcomas, liposarcomas, synovial cell sarcomas and histiocytic sarcomas (Thoolen *et al.*, 1992; Kerlin & Hendrick, 1996). A correct cell identification, however, is fundamental to providing a more accurate prognosis as histiocytic sarcomas, for example, tend to behave more aggressively than fibrosarcomas (personal observation).

Histiocytic sarcomas composed of CD1a, c^+, $CD4^-$, $CD11b^+$, MHC II^+ DC have also been recognized in cats (personal observation). Similarly to the lesions in dogs, histiocytic sarcomas in cats develop as solitary cutaneous and subcutaneous masses or as more disseminated disease processes.

Conclusion

Tissue histiocytes include macrophages or members of the heterogeneous group of dendritic cells. Both cell types originate from a common $CD34^+$ bone marrow precursor. The development, activation and maturation of macrophages and dendritic cells are orchestrated by the influence of stem cell factors, cytokines, chemokines and direct interactions with neighboring cells and the extracellular matrix. The primary function and phenotype of macrophages and dendritic cells differ and interconversion between the fully differentiated cells has not been documented. Macrophages and myeloid dendritic cells are therefore best considered separate sublineages within a common regulatory system. Macrophages are important effector cells of the innate immune system and as such are predominantly involved in phagocytosis and lysis of pathogens. They are numerous in infectious skin lesions, deposition disorders and foreign-body reactions. Myeloid dendritic cells are professional APC and, hence, provide an important link to the adaptive immune system. Dendritic cells are present in infectious skin lesions, cutaneous neoplasia and several still poorly understood, sterile pleocellular cutaneous and subcutaneous disorders. The latter are likely to be induced by immune-mediated processes. Reactive dermal dendritic cells are the predominant cells in the immune-regulatory disorder of canine and feline reactive dendritic cell histiocytosis. Differentiation between macrophages and dendritic cells, as well as a delineation of histiocytes from morphologically similar non-histiocytic cells, requires immunophenotypic evaluation of a tissue sample. The terms 'histiocytes' and 'histiocytic cells' should be limited to the morphological description of tissue macrophages and dendritic cells. To avoid the use of these terms as inaccurate descriptive terms, undifferentiated spindle-shaped mesenchymal cell populations and mononuclear cell populations of uncertain origin should be identified as such, while awaiting a more accurate identification by immunophenotypic evaluations. An accurate characterization of lesional cells provides the basis to understand a disease process and it may offer new insights into the possible development of more specific and successful therapies.

References

Adema, G. J., Hartgers, F., Verstraten, R., Vries, E. de, Marland, G., Menon, S. *et al.* (1997) A dendritic-cell-derived C-C chemokine that preferentially attracts naive T cells. *Nature*, **387**, 713–717.

Affolter, V. K. (1999) Histiocytic proliferative diseases in the dog. D Phil Thesis, University of California, Davis, CA.

Affolter, V. K. & Moore, P. F. (1995) Immunohistological phenotyping of proliferative histiocytic disorders of the dog. Abstract. *Proceedings of the Annual Meeting of the AAVD and ACVD*, Santa Fe, New Mexico.

Affolter, V. K. & Moore, P. F. (2000) Canine cutaneous and systemic histiocytosis: reactive histiocytosis of dermal dendritic cells. *American Journal of Dermatopathology*, **22**, 40–48.

Affolter, V. K. & Moore, P. F. (2002) Localized and disseminated histocytic sarcoma of dendritic cell origins in dogs. *Veterinary Pathology*, 39, 74–82.

Alon, R., Rossiter, H., Wang, X., Springer, T. A. & Kupper, T. S. (1994) Distinct cell surface ligands mediate T lymphocyte attachment and rolling on P and E selectin under physiological flow. *Journal of Cell Biology*, **127**, 1485–1495.

Ardavin, C. (1997) Thymic dendritic cells. *Immunology Today*, **18**, 350–361.

Arnold-Schild, D., Hanau, D., Spehner, D., Schmid, C., Rammensee, H. G., Salle, H. de la & Schild, H. (1999) Cutting edge: receptor-mediated endocytosis of heat shock proteins by professional antigen-presenting cells. *Journal of Immunology*, **162**, 3757–3760.

Aschoff, L. I. (1924) Das Reticulo-Endotheliale System. *Ergebnisse der inneren Medizin*, **26**, 1–118.

Austyn, J. M. (1999) Dendritic cells in the spleen and lymph node. In: *Dendritic Cells* (Eds M. T. Lotz & A. W. Thomson), pp. 179–204. Academic Press, San Diego, CA.

Banchereau, J., Briere, F., Caux, C., Davoust, J., Lebecque, S., Liu, Y. J. *et al.* (2000) Immunobiology of dendritic cells. *Annual Review of Immunology*, **18**, 767–811.

Barker, J. N. & MacDonald, D. M. (1992) Cutaneous lymphocyte trafficking in the inflammatory dermatoses. *British Journal of Dermatology*, **126**, 211–215.

Bender, W. M. & Muller, G. H. (1989) Multiple, resolving, cutaneous histiocytoma in a dog. *Journal of the American Veterinary Medical Association*, **194**, 535–537.

Birbeck, M. S. C., Breathnach, A. S. & Everall, J. D. (1961) An electron microscopic study of basal melanocytes and high level dendritic cells (Langerhans cells) in vitiligo. *Journal of Investigative Dermatology*, **37**, 51–76.

Borkowski, T. A., Van Dyke, B. J., Schwarzenberger, K., McFarland, V. W., Farr, A. G. & Udey, M. C. (1994) Expression of E-cadherin by murine dendritic cells: E-cadherin as a dendritic cell differentiation antigen characteristic of epidermal Langerhans cells and related cells. *European Journal of Immunology*, **24**, 2767–2774.

Broadbent, V., Egeler, R. M. & Nesbit, M. E., Jr (1994) Langerhans cell histiocytosis–clinical and epidemiological aspects. *British Journal of Cancer*, **23** (Suppl.), S11–S16.

Brocker, T. (1997) Survival of mature CD4 T lymphocytes is dependent on major histocompatibility complex class II-expressing dendritic cells. *Journal of Experimental Medicine*, **186**, 1223–1232.

Campbell, J. J. & Butcher, E. C. (2000) Chemokines in tissue-specific and micro-environment-specific lymphocyte homing. *Current Opinion in Immunology*, **12**, 336–341.

Caux, C., Massacrier, C., Vanbervliet, B., Dubois, B., Van Kooten, C., Durand, I. & Banchereau, J. (1994) Activation of human dendritic cells through CD40 cross-linking. *Journal of Experimental Medicine*, **180**, 1263–1272.

Caux, C., Vanbervliet, B., Massacrier, C., Dezutter-Dambuyant, C., Saint-Vis, B. de, Jacquet, C. *et al.* (1996) $CD34^+$ hematopoietic progenitors from human cord blood differentiate along two independent dendritic cell pathways in response to $GM\text{-}CSF^+TNF$ alpha. *Journal of Experimental Medicine*, **184**, 695–706.

Caux, C., Massacrier, C., Vanbervliet, B., Dubois, B., Durand, I., Cella, M. *et al.* (1997) $CD34^+$ hematopoietic progenitors from human cord blood differentiate along two independent dendritic cell pathways in response to granulocyte-macrophage colony-stimulating factor plus tumor necrosis factor alpha: II. Functional analysis. *Blood*, **90**, 1458–1470.

Caux, C., Lebecque, S., Liu, Y.-J. & Banchereau, J. (1999) Developmental pathway of human myeloid dendritic cells. In: *Dendritic Cells* (Eds T. M. Lotz & A. W. Thomson), pp. 63–92. Academic Press, San Diego, CA.

Cavaillon, J. M. (1994) Cytokines and macrophages. *Biomedicine and Pharmacotherapy*, **48**, 445–453.

Cerio, R., Griffiths, C. E., Cooper, K. D., Nickoloff, B. J. & Headington, J. T. (1989) Characterization of factor XIIIa positive dermal dendritic cells in normal and inflamed skin. *British Journal of Dermatology*, **121**, 421–431.

Chambers, C. A. & Allison, J. P. (1999) Costimulatory regulation of T cell function. *Current Opinion in Cell Biology*, **11**, 203–210.

Chantry, D., DeMaggio, A. J., Brammer, H., Raport, C. J., Wood, C. L., Schweickart, V. L. *et al.* (1998) Profile of human macrophage transcripts: insights into macrophage biology and identification of novel chemokines. *Journal of Leukocyte Biology*, **64**, 49–54.

Chastain, C. B., Turk, M. A. & O'Brien, D. (1988) Benign cutaneous mastocytomas in two litters of Siamese kittens. *Journal of the American Veterinary Medical Association*, **193**, 959–960.

Chaux, P. (1995) [Dendritic cells and immune function in cancer]. *Pathologie Biologie (Paris)*, **43**, 897–903.

Chaux, P., Favre, N., Bonnotte, B., Moutet, M., Martin, M. & Martin, F. (1997) Tumor-infiltrating dendritic cells are defective in their antigen-presenting function and inducible B7 expression. A role in the immune tolerance to antigenic tumors. *Advances in Experimental Medicine and Biology*, **417**, 525–528.

Crow, M. K. & Kunkel, H. G. (1982) Human dendritic cells: major stimulators of the autologous and allogeneic mixed leucocyte reactions. *Clinical and Experimental Immunology*, **49**, 338–346.

Cumberbatch, M., Dearman, R. J. & Kimber, I. (1999) Langerhans cell migration in mice requires intact type I interleukin 1 receptor (IL-1RI) function. *Archives of Dermatological Research*, **291**, 357–361.

De Smedt, T., Van Mechelen, M., De Becker, G., Urbain, J., Leo, O. & Moser, M. (1997) Effect of interleukin-10 on dendritic cell maturation and function. *European Journal of Immunology*, **27**, 1229–1235.

Dieu, M. C., Vanbervliet, B., Vicari, A., Bridon, J. M., Oldham, E., Ait-Yahia, S. *et al.* (1998) Selective recruitment of immature and mature dendritic cells by distinct chemokines expressed in different anatomic sites. *Journal of Experimental Medicine*, **188**, 373–386.

Dieu-Nosjean, M. C., Vicari, A., Lebecque, S. & Caux, C. (1999) Regulation of dendritic cell trafficking: a process that involves the participation of selective chemokines. *Journal of Leukocyte Biology*, **66**, 252–262.

Drakesmith, H., Chain, B. & Beverley, P. (2000) How can dendritic cells cause autoimmune disease? *Immunology Today*, **21**, 214–217.

Drexhage, H. A., Delemarre, F. G. A., Radosevic, K. & Leenen, P. J. M. (1999) Dendritic cells and autoimmunity. In: *Dendritic Cells* (Eds M. T. Lotz & A. W. Thomson), pp. 361–401. Academic Press, San Diego, CA.

Dubois, B., Vanbervliet, B., Fayette, J., Massacrier, C., Van Kooten, C., Briere, F. *et al.* (1997) Dendritic cells enhance growth and differentiation of CD40-activated B lymphocytes. *Journal of Experimental Medicine*, **185**, 941–951.

Enk, A. H. & Katz, S. I. (1992) Identification and induction of keratinocyte-derived IL-10. *Journal of Immunology*, **149**, 92–95.

Fanger, N. A., Wardwell, K., Shen, L., Tedder, T. F. & Guyre, P. M. (1996) Type I (CD64) and type II (CD32) Fc gamma receptor-mediated phagocytosis by human blood dendritic cells. *Journal of Immunology*, **157**, 541–548.

Favara, B. E. & Jaffe, R. (1994) The histopathology of Langerhans cell histiocytosis. *British Journal of Cancer*, **23** Suppl., S17–S23.

Favara, B. E., Feller, A. C., Pauli, M., Jaffe, E. S., Weiss, L. M., Arico, M. *et al.* (1997) Contemporary classification of histiocytic disorders. The WHO Committee on Histiocytic/Reticulum Cell Proliferations. Reclassification Working Group of the Histiocyte Society. *Medical and Pediatric Oncology*, **29**, 157–166.

Feingold, K. R., Castro, G. R., Ishikawa, Y., Fielding, P. E. & Fielding, C. J. (1989) Cutaneous xanthoma in association with paraproteinemia in the absence of hyperlipidemia. *Journal of Clinical Investigation*, **83**, 796–802.

Fong, L. & Engleman, E. G. (2000) Dendritic cells in cancer immunotherapy. *Annual Review of Immunology*, **18**, 245–273.

Forster, R., Schubel, A., Breitfeld, D., Kremmer, E., Renner-Muller, I., Wolf, E. & Lipp, M. (1999) CCR7 coordinates the primary immune response by establishing functional microenvironments in secondary lymphoid organs. *Cell*, **99**, 23–33.

Furth, R. van (1981) Current view of the mononuclear phagocyte system. *Hamatologie und Bluttransfusion*, **27**, 3–10.

Furth, R. van, Lamgevoort, H. L. & Schaberg, A. (1975) Mononuclear phagocytes in human pathology – a proposal for an approach to improved classification. In: *Mononuclear Phagocytes in Immunity, Infection, and Pathology* (Ed. R. van Furth), pp. 1–15. Blackwell Scientific, Oxford.

Furue, M., Suzuki, H., Kodama, T., Hiramoto, T., Sugiyama, H. & Tamaki, K. (1995) Colocalization of scavenger receptor in CD68 positive foam cells in verruciform xanthoma. *Journal of Dermatological Science*, **10**, 213–219.

Galy, A., Georgopoulos, K. & Wu, L. (1999) Hematopoietic cell fate and the development of dendritic cells. In: *Dendritic Cells* (Eds T. M. Lotz & A. W. Thomson), pp. 3–14. Academic Press, San Diego, CA.

Geissmann, F., Prost, C., Monnet, J. P., Dy, M., Brousse, N. & Hermine, O. (1998) Transforming growth factor beta1, in the presence of granulocyte/macrophage colony-stimulating factor and interleukin 4, induces differentiation of human peripheral blood monocytes into dendritic Langerhans cells. *Journal of Experimental Medicine*, **187**, 961–966.

Gliatto, J. M. & Alroy, J. (1995) Cutaneous amyloidosis in a horse with lymphoma. *Veterinary Record*, **137**, 68–69.

Godiska, R., Chantry, D., Raport, C. J., Sozzani, S., Allavena, P., Leviten, D. *et al.* (1997) Human macrophage-derived chemokine (MDC), a novel chemoattractant for monocytes, monocyte-derived dendritic cells, and natural killer cells. *Journal of Experimental Medicine*, **185**, 1595–1604.

Greenfield, E. A., Nguyen, K. A. & Kuchroo, V. K. (1998) CD28/B7 costimulation: a review. *Critical Reviews in Immunology*, **18**, 389–418.

Gribben, J. G., Freeman, G. J., Boussiotis, V. A., Rennert, P., Jellis, C. L., Greenfield, E. *et al.* (1995) CTLA4 mediates antigen-specific apoptosis of human T cells. *Proceedings of the National Academy of Sciences of the United States of America*, **92**, 811–815.

Gross, T. L. & Affolter, V. K. (1998) Advances in skin oncology. In: *Advances in Veterinary Dermatology*, Vol. 3 (Eds K. W. Kwochka, T. Willemse & C. von Tscharner), pp. 382–385. Butterworth-Heinemann, Oxford.

Gross, T. L., Ihrke, P. J. & Walder, E. J. (1992) *Veterinary Dermatopathology; A Macroscopic Evaluation of Canine and Feline Skin Diseases*, p. 520. Mosby Year Book, St Louis, MO.

Grouard, G., Rissoan, M. C., Filgueira, L., Durand, I., Banchereau, J. & Liu, Y. J. (1997) The enigmatic plasmacytoid T cells develop into dendritic cells with interleukin (IL)-3 and CD40-ligand. *Journal of Experimental Medicine*, **185**, 1101–1111.

Gunn, M. D., Tangemann, K., Tam, C., Cyster, J. G., Rosen, S. D. & Williams, L. T. (1998) A chemokine expressed in lymphoid high endothelial venules promotes the adhesion and chemotaxis of naive T lymphocytes. *Proceedings of the National Academy of Sciences of the United States of America*, **95**, 258–263.

Hagari, Y., Mihara, M. & Hagari, S. (1996) Nodular localized cutaneous amyloidosis: detection of monoclonality of infiltrating plasma cells by polymerase chain reaction. *British Journal of Dermatology*, **135**, 630–633.

Hanau, D., Fabre, M., Schmitt, D. A., Stampf, J. L., Garaud, J. C., Bieber, T. *et al.* (1987) Human epidermal Langerhans cells internalize by receptor-mediated endocytosis T6 (CD1 'NA1/34') surface antigen. Birbeck granules are involved in the intracellular traffic of the T6 antigen. *Journal of Investigative Dermatology*, **89**, 172–177.

Hart, D. N. (1997) Dendritic cells: unique leukocyte populations which control the primary immune response. *Blood*, **90**, 3245–3287.

Hendrick, M. J., Brooks, J. J. & Bruce, E. H. (1992) Six cases of malignant fibrous histiocytoma of the canine spleen. *Veterinary Pathology*, **29**, 351–354.

Homey, B., Wang, W., Soto, H., Buchanan, M. E., Wiesenborn, A., Catron, D. *et al.* (2000) Cutting edge: the orphan chemokine receptor G protein-coupled receptor-2 (GPR-2, CCR10) binds the skin-associated chemokine CCL27 (CTACK/ALP/ILC). *Journal of Immunology*, **164**, 3465–3470.

Inaba, K., Granelli-Piperno, A. & Steinman, R. M. (1983a) Dendritic cells induce T lymphocytes to release B cell-stimulating factors by an interleukin 2-dependent mechanism. *Journal of Experimental Medicine*, **158**, 2040–2057.

Inaba, K., Steinman, R. M., Van Voorhis, W. C. & Muramatsu, S. (1983b) Dendritic cells are critical accessory cells for thymus-dependent antibody responses in mouse and in man. *Proceedings of the National Academy of Sciences of the United States of America*, **80**, 6041–6045.

Inaba, K., Young, J. W. & Steinman, R. M. (1987) Direct activation of $CD8^+$ cytotoxic T lymphocytes by dendritic cells. *Journal of Experimental Medicine*, **166**, 182–194.

Janeway, C. A., Jr (1992) The immune system evolved to discriminate infectious nonself from noninfectious self. *Immunology Today*, **13**, 11–16.

Jensen, P. E. (1999) Mechanisms of antigen presentation. *Clinical Chemistry and Laboratory Medicine*, **37**, 179–186.

June, C. H., Bluestone, J. A., Nadler, L. M. & Thompson, C. B. (1994) The B7 and CD28 receptor families. *Immunology Today*, **15**, 321–331.

Kerlin, R. L. & Hendrick, M. J. (1996) Malignant fibrous histiocytoma and malignant histiocytosis in the dog – convergent or divergent phenotypic differentiation? *Veterinary Pathology*, **33**, 713–716.

Kimber, I., Cumberbatch, M., Dearman, R. J., Bhushan, M. & Griffiths, C. E. (2000) Cytokines and chemokines in the initiation and regulation of epidermal Langerhans cell mobilization. *British Journal of Dermatology*, **142**, 401–412.

Knight, J. A. (2000) Review: Free radicals, antioxidants, and the immune system. *Annals of Clinical and Laboratory Science*, **30**, 145–158.

Koch, F., Heufler, C., Kampgen, E., Schneeweiss, D., Bock, G. & Schuler, G. (1990) Tumor necrosis factor alpha maintains the viability of murine epidermal Langerhans cells in culture, but in contrast to granulocyte/macrophage colony-stimulating factor, without inducing their functional maturation. *Journal of Experimental Medicine*, **171**, 159–171.

Koppelman, B., Neefjes, J. J., Vries, J. E. de & Waal Malefyt, R. de (1997) Interleukin-10 down-regulates MHC class II alphabeta peptide complexes at the plasma membrane of monocytes by affecting arrival and recycling. *Immunity*, **7**, 861–871.

Kube, P., Audige, L., Kuther, K. & Welle, M. (1998) Distribution, density and heterogeneity of canine mast cells and influence of fixation techniques. *Histochemistry and Cell Biology*, **110**, 129–135.

Kuchroo, V. K., Das, M. P., Brown, J. A., Ranger, A. M., Zamvil, S. S., Sobel, R. A. *et al.* (1995) B7-1 and B7-2 costimulatory molecules activate differentially the Th1/Th2 developmental pathways: application to autoimmune disease therapy. *Cell*, **80**, 707–718.

Larsen, C. P., Steinman, R. M., Witmer-Pack, M., Hankins, D. F., Morris, P. J. & Austyn, J. M. (1990) Migration and maturation of Langerhans cells in skin transplants and explants. *Journal of Experimental Medicine*, **172**, 1483–1493.

Linke, R. P., Geisel, O. & Mann, K. (1991) Equine cutaneous amyloidosis derived from an immunoglobulin lambda-light chain. Immunohistochemical, immunochemical and chemical results. *Biology and Chemistry Hoppe Seyler*, **372**, 835–843.

Lotze, M. T. & Jaffe, R. (1999) Cancer. In: *Dendritic Cells* (Eds T. M. Lotz & A. W. Thomson), pp. 326–338. Academic Press, San Diego, CA.

Ludewig, B., Oehen, S., Barchiesi, F., Schwendener, R. A., Hengartner, H. & Zinkernagel, R. M. (1999) Protective antiviral cytotoxic T cell memory is most efficiently maintained by restimulation via dendritic cells. *Journal of Immunology*, **163**, 1839–1844.

Macatonia, S. E., Hsieh, C. S., Murphy, K. M. & O'Garra, A. (1993) Dendritic cells and macrophages are required for Th1 development of $CD4^+$ T cells from alpha beta TCR transgenic mice: IL-12 substitution for macrophages to stimulate IFN-gamma production is IFN-gamma-dependent. *International Immunology*, **5**, 1119–1128.

McClain, K. & Weiss, R. A. (1994) Viruses and Langerhans cell histiocytosis: is there a link? *British Journal of Cancer*, **23** Suppl., S34–S36.

Mackaness, G. B. (1964) The immunologic basis of acquired cellular resistance. *Journal of Experimental Medicine*, **120**, 105–120.

McLellan, A. D., Sorg, R. V., Williams, L. A. & Hart, D. N. (1996) Human dendritic cells activate T lymphocytes via a CD40:CD40 ligand-dependent pathway. *European Journal of Immunology*, **26**, 1204–1210.

McWilliam, A. S., Stumbles, P. A. & Holt, P. G. (1999) Dendritic cells in the lung. In: *Dendritic Cells* (Eds T. M. Lotz & A. W. Thomson), pp. 123–140. Academic Press, San Diego, CA.

Magro, C. M. & Crowson, A. N. (2000) Lichenoid and granulomatous dermatitis. *International Journal of Dermatology*, **39**, 126–133.

Magro, C. M., Crowson, A. N. & Schapiro, B. L. (1998) The interstitial granulomatous drug reaction: a distinctive clinical and pathological entity. *Journal of Cutaneous Pathology*, **25**, 72–78.

Maraskovsky, E., Pulendran, B. & Shortman, K. (1999) Lymphoid-related dendritic cells. In: *Dendritic Cells* (Eds T. M. Lotz & A. W. Thomson), pp. 93–107. Academic Press, San Diego, CA.

Matsuno, K., Ezaki, T., Kudo, S. & Uehara, Y. (1996) A life stage of particle-laden rat dendritic cells *in vivo*: their terminal division, active phagocytosis, and translocation from the liver to the draining lymph. *Journal of Experimental Medicine*, **183**, 1865–1878.

Matsushima, Y., Hayashi, S. & Tachibana, M. (1999) Spontaneously hyperlipidemic (SHL) mice: Japanese wild mice with apolipoprotein E deficiency. *Mammalian Genome*, **10**, 352–357.

Maurer, D. & Stingle, G. (1999) Dendritic cells in the context of skin immunity. In: *Dendritic Cells* (Eds T. M. Lotz & A. W. Thomson), pp. 111–122. Academic Press, San Diego, CA.

Maurer, D., Fiebiger, E., Reininger, B., Ebner, C., Petzelbauer, P., Shi, G. P. *et al.* (1998) Fc epsilon receptor I on dendritic cells delivers IgE-bound multivalent antigens into a cathepsin S-dependent pathway of MHC class II presentation. *Journal of Immunology*, **161**, 2731–2739.

Mays, M. B. & Bergeron, J. A. (1986) Cutaneous histiocytosis in dogs. *Journal of the American Veterinary Medicine Association*, **188**, 377–381.

Metchnikoff, E. (1887) Ueber den Kampf der Zellen gegen Erysipelkokken. Ein Beitrag zur Phagozytenlehre. *Virchow's Archives*, **107**, 209.

Meunier, L., Gonzalez-Ramos, A. & Cooper, K. D. (1993) Heterogeneous populations of class II MHC+ cells in human dermal cell suspensions. Identification of a small subset responsible for potent dermal antigen-presenting cell activity with features analogous to Langerhans cells. *Journal of Immunology*, **151**, 4067–4080.

Moll, H. (1997) The role of chemokines and accessory cells in the immunoregulation of cutaneous leishmaniasis. *Behring Institute Mitteilungen*, **99**, 73–78.

Mommaas, A. M., Mulder, A. A., Jordens, R., Out, C., Tan, M. C., Cresswell, P. *et al.* (1999) Human epidermal Langerhans cells lack functional mannose receptors and a fully developed endosomal/lysosomal compartment for loading of HLA class II molecules. *European Journal of Immunology*, **29**, 571–580.

Moore, P. F. (1984) Systemic histiocytosis of Bernese mountain dogs. *Veterinary Pathology*, **21**, 554–563.

Moore, P. F., Schrenzel, M. D., Affolter, V. K., Olivry, T. & Naydan, D. (1996) Canine cutaneous histiocytoma is an epidermotropic Langerhans cell histiocytosis that expresses CD1 and specific beta 2-integrin molecules. *American Journal of Pathology*, **148**, 1699–1708.

Moore, P. F., Affolter, V. K., Olivry, T. & Schrenzel, M. D. (1998) The use of immunological reagents in defining the pathogenesis of canine skin diseases involving proliferation of leukocytes. In: *Advances in Veterinary Dermatology*, Vol. 3 (Eds K. W. Kwochka, T. Willemse & C. von Tscharner), pp. 77–94. Butterworth-Heinemann, Oxford.

Morales, J., Homey, B., Vicari, A. P., Hudak, S., Oldham, E., Hedrick, J. *et al.* (1999) CTACK, a skin-associated chemokine that preferentially attracts skin-homing memory T cells. *Proceedings of the National Academy of Sciences of the United States of America*, **96**, 14470–14475.

Morelli, A., Larregina, A., Chuluyan, I., Kolkowski, E. & Fainboim, L. (1996) Expression and modulation of C5a receptor (CD88) on skin dendritic cells. Chemotactic effect of C5a on skin migratory dendritic cells. *Immunology*, **89**, 126–134.

Narvaez, D., Kanitakis, J., Faure, M. & Claudy, A. (1996) Immunohistochemical study of CD34-positive dendritic cells of human dermis. *American Journal of Dermatopathology*, **18**, 283–288.

Nestle, F. O., Zheng, X. G., Thompson, C. B., Turka, L. A. & Nickoloff, B. J. (1993) Characterization of dermal dendritic cells obtained from normal human skin reveals phenotypic and functionally distinctive subsets [published erratum appears in *Journal of Immunology* 1994; **152**, 376]. *Journal of Immunology*, **151**, 6535–6545.

Olweus, J., BitMansour, A., Warnke, R., Thompson, P. A., Carballido, J., Picker, L. J. & Lund-Johansen, F. (1997) Dendritic cell ontogeny: a human dendritic cell lineage of myeloid origin. *Proceedings of the National Academy of Sciences of the United States of America*, **94**, 12551–12556.

Piemonti, L., Monti, P., Allavena, P., Sironi, M., Soldini, L., Leone, B. E. *et al.* (1999) Glucocorticoids affect human dendritic cell differentiation and maturation. *Journal of Immunology*, **162**, 6473–6481.

Pimpinelli, N., Romagnoli, P., Moretti, S. & Giannotti, B. (1988) Non-lymphoid accessory cells in the cutaneous infiltrate of B cell lymphomas. An immunohistochemical and ultrastructural study. *British Journal of Dermatology*, **118**, 353–362.

Porcelli, S. A., Segelke, B. W., Sugita, M., Wilson, I. A. & Brenner, M. B. (1998) The CD1 family of lipid antigen-presenting molecules. *Immunology Today*, **19**, 362–368.

Reid, C. D., Stackpoole, A., Meager, A. & Tikerpae, J. (1992) Interactions of tumor necrosis factor with granulocyte–macrophage colony-stimulating factor and other cytokines in the regulation of dendritic cell growth *in vitro* from early bipotent CD34+ progenitors in human bone marrow. *Journal of Immunology*, **149**, 2681–2688.

Rissoan, M. C., Soumelis, V., Kadowaki, N., Grouard, G., Briere, F., Waal Malefyt, R. de & Liu, Y. J. (1999) Reciprocal control of T helper cell and dendritic cell. *Science*, **283**, 1183–1186.

Robert, C. & Kupper, T. S. (1999) Inflammatory skin diseases, T cells, and immune surveillance. *New England Journal of Medicine*, **341**, 1817–1828.

Romani, N., Lenz, A., Glassel, H., Stossel, H., Stanzl, U., Majdic, O. *et al.* (1989) Cultured human Langerhans cells resemble lymphoid dendritic cells in phenotype and function. *Journal of Investigative Dermatology*, **93**, 600–609.

Romani, N., Reider, D., Heuer, M., Ebner, S., Kampgen, E., Eibl, B. *et al.* (1996) Generation of mature dendritic cells from human blood. An improved method with special regard to clinical applicability. *Journal of Immunologic Methods*, **196**, 137–151.

Rowland, P. H., Valentine, B. A., Stebbins, K. E. & Smith, C. A. (1991) Cutaneous plasmacytomas with amyloid in six dogs. *Veterinary Pathology*, **28**, 125–130.

Saint-Vis, B. de, Fugier-Vivier, I., Massacrier, C., Gaillard, C., Vanbervliet, B., Ait-Yahia, S. *et al.* (1998a) The cytokine profile expressed by human dendritic cells is dependent on cell subtype and mode of activation. *Journal of Immunology*, **160**, 1666–1676.

Saint-Vis, B. de, Fugier-Vivier, I., Massacrier, C., Gaillard, C., Vanbervliet, B., Ait-Yahia, S. *et al.* (1998b) The cytokine profile expressed by human dendritic cells is dependent on cell subtype and mode of activation. *Journal of Immunology*, **160**, 1666–1676.

Sallusto, F. & Lanzavecchia, A. (1994) Efficient presentation of soluble antigen by cultured human dendritic cells is maintained by granulocyte/macrophage colony-stimulating factor plus interleukin 4 and downregulated by tumor necrosis factor alpha. *Journal of Experimental Medicine*, **179**, 1109–1118.

Sallusto, F., Cella, M., Danieli, C. & Lanzavecchia, A. (1995) Dendritic cells use macropinocytosis and the mannose receptor to concentrate macromolecules in the major histocompatibility complex class II compartment: downregulation by cytokines and bacterial products. *Journal of Experimental Medicine*, **182**, 389–400.

Sallusto, F., Schaerli, P., Loetscher, P., Schaniel, C., Lenig, D., Mackay, C. R. *et al.* (1998) Rapid and coordinated switch in chemokine receptor expression during dendritic cell maturation. *European Journal of Immunology*, **28**, 2760–2769.

Santiago-Schwarz, F., Belilos, E., Diamond, B. & Carsons, S. E. (1992) TNF in combination with GM-CSF enhances the differentiation of neonatal cord blood stem cells into dendritic cells and macrophages. *Journal of Leukocyte Biology*, **52**, 274–281.

Scott, D. W., Angarano, D. K. & Suter M. M. (1987) Systemic histiocytosis in two dogs. *Canine Practice*, **14**, 7–12.

Seljelid, R. & Eskeland, T. (1993) The biology of macrophages: I. General principles and properties. *European Journal of Haematology*, **51**, 267–275.

Seo, I. S., Henley, J. D., Min, K. W. & Yum, M. N. (1999) True histiocytic lymphoma of the esophagus in an HIV-positive patient: an ultrastructural study. *Ultrastructural Pathology*, **23**, 333–339.

Sercarz, E. E., Lehmann, P. V., Ametani, A., Benichou, G., Miller, A. & Moudgil, K. (1993) Dominance and crypticity of T cell antigenic determinants. *Annual Review of Immunology*, **11**, 729–766.

Shortman, K. & Caux, C. (1997) Dendritic cell development: multiple pathways to nature's adjuvants. *Stem Cells*, **15**, 409–419.

Shortman, K. & Wu, L. (1999) Thymic dendritic cells. In: *Dendritic Cells* (Eds T. M. Lotz & A. W. Thomson), pp. 15–28. Academic Press, San Diego, CA.

Shurin, M. R. (1996) Dendritic cells presenting tumor antigen. *Cancer Immunology Immunotherapy*, **43**, 158–164.

Slavik, J. M., Hutchcroft, J. E. & Bierer, B. E. (1999) CD28/CTLA-4 and CD80/CD86 families: signaling and function. *Immunological Research*, **19**, 1–24.

Sornasse, T., Flamand, V., De Becker, G., Bazin, H., Tielemans, F., Thielemans, K. *et al.* (1992) Antigen-pulsed dendritic cells can efficiently induce an antibody response *in vivo*. *Journal of Experimental Medicine*, **175**, 15–21.

Soslow, R. A., Davis, R. E., Warnke, R. A., Cleary, M. L. & Kamel, O. W. (1996) True histiocytic lymphoma following therapy for lymphoblastic neoplasms. *Blood*, **87**, 5207–5212.

Sozzani, S., Sallusto, F., Luini, W., Zhou, D., Piemonti, L., Allavena, P. *et al.* (1995) Migration of dendritic cells in response to formyl peptides, C5a, and a distinct set of chemokines. *Journal of Immunology*, **155**, 3292–3295.

Sozzani, S., Allavena, P., D'Amico, G., Luini, W., Bianchi, G., Kataura, M. *et al.* (1998) Differential regulation of chemokine receptors during dendritic cell maturation: a model for their trafficking properties. *Journal of Immunology*, **161**, 1083–1086.

Sozzani, S., Allavena, P., Vecchi, A. & Mantovani, A. (1999) The role of chemokines in the regulation of dendritic cell trafficking. *Journal of Leukocyte Biology*, **66**, 1–9.

Steinman, R. M., Pack, M. & Inaba, K. (1997) Dendritic cells in the T-cell areas of lymphoid organs. *Immunological Review*, **156**, 25–37.

Steptoe, R. & Thomas, A. W. (1999) Dendritic cells in the liver, kidney, heart and pancreas. In: *Dendritic Cells* (Eds T. M. Lotz & A. W. Thomson), pp. 153–178. Academic Press, San Diego, CA.

Stoppacciaro, A., Paglia, P., Lombardi, L., Parmiani, G., Baroni, C. & Colombo, M. P. (1997) Genetic modification of a carcinoma with the IL-4 gene increases the influx of dendritic cells relative to other cytokines. *European Journal of Immunology*, **27**, 2375–2382.

Strunk, D., Egger, C., Leitner, G., Hanau, D. & Stingl, G. (1997) A skin homing molecule defines the Langerhans cell progenitor in human peripheral blood. *Journal of Experimental Medicine*, **185**, 1131–1136.

Szabolcs, P., Moore, M. A. & Young, J. W. (1995) Expansion of immunostimulatory dendritic cells among the myeloid progeny of human $CD34^+$ bone marrow precursors cultured with c-kit ligand, granulocyte-macrophage colony-stimulating factor, and TNF-alpha. *Journal of Immunology*, **154**, 5851–5861.

Tang, A., Amagai, M., Granger, L. G., Stanley, J. R. & Udey, M. C. (1993) Adhesion of epidermal Langerhans cells to keratinocytes mediated by E-cadherin. *Nature*, **361**, 82–85.

Tew, J. G., Thorbecke, G. J. & Steinman, R. M. (1982) Dendritic cells in the immune response: characteristics and recommended nomenclature. (A report from the Reticuloendothelial Society Committee on Nomenclature.) *Journal of the Reticuloendothelial Society*, **31**, 371–380.

Thoolen, R. J., Vos, J. H., Linde-Sipman, J. S. van der, Weger, R. A. de, Unnik, J. A. van, Misdorp, W. & Dijk, J. E. van (1992) Malignant fibrous histiocytomas in dogs and cats: an immunohistochemical study. *Research in Veterinary Sciences*, **53**, 198–204.

Touart, D. M. & Sau, P. (1998) Cutaneous deposition diseases. Part I [published erratum appears in *Journal of the American Academy of Dermatology* 1998; **39**, 1042]. *Journal of the American Academy of Dermatology*, **39**, 149–171.

Unanue, E. R. & Allen, P. M. (1987) The basis for the immunoregulatory role of macrophages and other accessory cells. *Science*, **236**, 551–557.

Valladeau, J., Duvert-Frances, V., Pin, J. J., Dezutter-Dambuyant, C., Vincent, C., Massacrier, C. *et al.* (1999) The monoclonal antibody DCGM4 recognizes Langerin, a protein specific of Langerhans cells, and is rapidly internalized from the cell surface. *European Journal of Immunology*, **29**, 2695–2704.

Valladeau, J., Ravel, O., Dezutter-Dambyuant, C., Moore, K., Kleijmeer, M., Duvert-France, V. *et al.* (2000) Langerin, a novel C-type lectin specific of Langerhans cells, is an endocytic receptor that induces the formation of Birbeck granules. *Immunity*, **12**, 71–81.

Van Gool, S. W., Vandenberghe, P., Boer, M. de & Ceuppens, J. L. (1996) CD80, CD86, and CD40 provide accessory signals in a multiple-step T cell activation model. *Immunological Review*, **153**, 47–83.

Van Voorhis, W. C., Valinsky, J., Hoffman, E., Luban, J., Hair, L. S. & Steinman, R. M. (1983) Relative efficacy of human monocytes and dendritic cells as accessory cells for T cell replication. *Journal of Experimental Medicine*, **158**, 174–191.

Vecchi, A., Massimiliano, L., Ramponi, S., Luini, W., Bernasconi, S., Bonecchi, R. *et al.* (1999) Differential responsiveness to constitutive vs. inducible chemokines of immature and mature mouse dendritic cells. *Journal of Leukocyte Biology*, **66**, 489–494.

Vitale, C. B., Ihrke, P. J. & Gross, T. L. (1998) Diet-induced alterations in lipid metabolism and associated cutaneous xanthoma formation in 5 cats. In: *Advances in Veterinary Dermatology*, Vol. 3 (Eds K. W. Kwochka, T. Willemse & C. von Tscharner), pp. 243–249. Butterworth-Heinemann, Oxford.

Wang, W., Soto, H., Oldham, E. R., Buchanan, M. E., Homey, B., Catron, D. *et al.* (2000) Identification of a novel CC chemokine (CCL28) which binds CCR10 (GPR2). *Journal of Biological Chemistry*, **274**, 22313–22323.

Welle, M. (1997) Development, significance, and heterogeneity of mast cells with particular regard to the mast cell-specific proteases chymase and tryptase. *Journal of Leukocyte Biology*, **61**, 233–245.

Wilcock, B. P., Yager, J. A. & Zink, M. C. (1986) The morphology and behavior of feline cutaneous mastocytomas. *Veterinary Pathology*, **23**, 320–324.

Wisselink, M. A., Koeman, J. P., Wensing, T., Bruijne, J. de & Willemse, T. (1994) Hyperlipoproteinaemia associated with atherosclerosis and cutaneous xanthomatosis in a cat. *Veterinary Quarterly*, **16**, 199–202.

Wu, L., Vremec, D., Ardavin, C., Winkel, K., Suss, G., Georgiou, H. *et al.* (1995) Mouse thymus dendritic cells: kinetics of development and changes in surface markers during maturation. *European Journal of Immunology*, **25**, 418–425.

Wykes, M., Pombo, A., Jenkins, C. & MacPherson, G. G. (1998) Dendritic cells interact directly with naive B lymphocytes to transfer antigen and initiate class switching in a primary T-dependent response. *Journal of Immunology*, **161**, 1313–1319.

Yager, J. A. & Wilcock, B. P. (1994) *Color Atlas and Text of Surgical Pathology of the Dog and Cat; Dermatopathology and Skin Tumors*, Vol. 1, p. 320. M. Wolfe, London.

Yamaguchi, Y. & Ogawa, M. (1999) Dendritic cells and cells of the monocyte/macrophage lineage. In: *Dendritic Cells* (Eds T. M. Lotz & A. W. Thomson), pp. 281–293. Academic Press, San Diego, CA.

Yanagihara, S., Komura, E., Nagafune, J., Watarai, H. & Yamaguchi, Y. (1998) EBI1/CCR7 is a new member of dendritic cell chemokine receptor that is up-regulated upon maturation. *Journal of Immunology*, **161**, 3096–3102.

Young, J. W. (1999) Cell fate development in the myeloid system. In: *Dendritic Cells* (Eds T. M. Lotz & A. W. Thomson), pp. 29–50. Academic Press, San Diego, CA.

Young, J. W. & Steinman, R. M. (1990) Dendritic cells stimulate primary human cytolytic lymphocyte responses in the absence of $CD4^+$ helper T cells. *Journal of Experimental Medicine*, **171**, 1315–1332.

3.2

Maturation states of dendritic cells in canine cutaneous histiocytoma

S.J. Baines MA, VetMB, CertVR, CertSAS, MRCVS,[1] R. Bujdoso BSc, PhD,[1] B.A. Blacklaws BSc, PhD,[1] E. McInnes BVSc, PhD, MRCPath, MRCVS,[1] P.F. Moore, BVSc, PhD[2] and I. McConnell BVM&S, MA, PhD, FRCPath, FRSE, MRCVS[1]

[1] Centre for Veterinary Science, Department of Clinical Veterinary Medicine, University of Cambridge, Cambridge, UK

[2] Department of Pathology, Microbiology and Immunology, School of Veterinary Medicine, University of California, Davis, California, USA

Summary

Canine cutaneous histiocytoma is a common, benign tumour of Langerhans' cells. This tumour undergoes an early period of rapid growth followed by spontaneous regression.

Immunophenotyping of tumour cells obtained from excised tumours by flow cytometry revealed expression of CD1a, CD1c, CD11c, major histocompatibility complex class I (MHC I), MHC II and E-cadherin, confirming their Langerhans' cell origin. In addition, the cells also showed uniform staining with CD1b, and expressed CD11b, CD44, CD49d and intercellular adhesion molecule-1 (ICAM-1), consistent with an activated Langerhans' cell phenotype. Tumour cells isolated from lesions in the regressing phase had higher expression of MHC I, MHC II and ICAM-1 compared with cells isolated from lesions in the early proliferative phase.

Tumour cells induced a strong proliferative response in allogenic and autologous peripheral blood mononuclear cells, consistent with a dendritic cell origin. Tumour cells isolated from lesions undergoing regression induced a greater proliferative response than those isolated from lesions in the early growth phase. Tumour cells exhibited a high rate of macropinocytosis, as expected for cells of the myeloid/dendritic lineage. Tumour cells from later lesions showed a significantly higher rate of macropinocytosis than those from earlier lesions.

These data show that the neoplastic Langerhans' cells in canine cutaneous histiocytoma are present at different stages of maturation depending on the clinical stage of the tumour. Tumour cells isolated from early lesions are analogous to immature dendritic cells and those isolated from lesions undergoing regression are analogous to mature dendritic cells.

Introduction

Canine cutaneous histiocytoma (CCH) is a common, generally benign skin tumour of Langerhans' cells. Its biological behaviour is characterised by a period of rapid growth over 1–4 weeks, followed by spontaneous regression, in most cases, over the next 1–3 months (Conroy, 1983; Pulley & Stannard, 1990). Immunohistochemical staining of these tumours reveals that the cells express CD1, CD11c, major histocompatibility complex class I (MHC I) and MHC II (Moore & Schrenzel, 1991; Moore *et al.*, 1996). Histological examination of specimens from the early phase of growth reveals uniform sheets of large, histiocytic cells, with numerous mitotic figures, in the dermis and epidermis (Taylor *et al.*, 1969; Kelly, 1970). Sections from the later regression phase show fewer mitotic figures and infiltration by $CD8^{+}$ T-lymphocytes, suggesting that immunological recognition of the neoplastic Langerhans' cells plays a part in the regression of these tumours (Cockerell & Slauson, 1979; Moore *et al.*, 1996).

Langerhans' cells are the peripheral sentinels of the dendritic cell family of antigen-presenting cells.

Dendritic cells play a pivotal role in the induction of immune responses *in vivo* (Steinman, 1991). They exist in two states of maturation which can be defined in terms of their immunophenotype and function. As immature cells, dendritic cells are present throughout the body in non-lymphoid organs. Following uptake and processing of antigen, they undergo maturation and migrate to the T-dependent areas of secondary lymphoid organs, where they activate naive T-cells recirculating through these areas (Austyn, 1992; Romani & Schuler, 1992).

Immature Langerhans' cells express relatively high levels of CD1 molecules and E-cadherin and relatively low levels of MHC I and II. Upon maturation there is a reciprocal down-regulation of CD1 and E-cadherin expression and up-regulation of MHC I and II expression, as befits their antigen-presenting phenotype (Schuler & Steinman, 1985). Mature Langerhans' cells also up-regulate the expression of intercellular adhesion molecule-1 (ICAM-1) (Schuler & Steinman, 1985). Immature dendritic cells are concerned with antigen acquisition and constitutively exhibit high levels of macropinocytosis, which is down-regulated on maturation (Sallusto *et al.*, 1995).

This study investigated the phenotypic and functional characteristics of the cells obtained from clinical cases of CCH to examine whether these characteristics were consistent with a dendritic cell origin. In addition, the presence of phenotypic and functional differences between CCH cells isolated from tumours at different clinical stages was investigated to assess whether variation in these parameters might explain the pathogenesis of the disease. This study reports that dendritic cells isolated from CCH lesions at different clinical stages are present at different stages of maturation, and that the biological behaviour of the tumour can be explained in the context of normal development and differentiation of Langerhans' cells *in vivo* and *in vitro* (Winzler *et al.*, 1997).

Materials and methods

Media and reagents

The medium used throughout was RPMI 1640 supplemented with 20 mM HEPES, 200 U/ml penicillin, 10 μg/ml streptomycin, 2 mM L-glutamine and 5×10^{-5} 2-mercaptoethanol (complete RPMI) with 2% or 10% foetal calf serum (FCS). Lucifer yellow, potassium salt (Sigma, Dorset, UK), was reconstituted in phosphate-buffered saline (PBS) and spun in a microfuge before use to eliminate any aggregates.

Tissue specimens

Tumours and blood samples from clinical cases of dogs suspecting of having a cutaneous histiocytoma were collected from neighbouring veterinary practices within a 100 km radius of the Department of Clinical Veterinary Medicine, Cambridge. Blood was obtained from experimental dogs held in the department. A portion of each tumour was retained for histological diagnosis and immunohistochemistry and fixed in 10% buffered formalin.

Isolation of canine cutaneous histiocytoma cells

Excised tumours were harvested into sterile, ice-cold complete RPMI supplemented with 10% FCS and incubated in complete RPMI, supplemented with 200 U/ml collagenase type 1A (Sigma, Dorset, UK), 0.05% $CaCl_2$ and 10% FCS for 2 h at 37°C. The single-cell suspension was harvested, passed through a 70 μm cell strainer (Falcon, Becton Dickenson Labware, Oxford, UK) and centrifuged at 1500 rpm for 5 min. The cell pellet was resuspended in complete RPMI supplemented with 2% FCS. The CCH cells were enriched by density gradient sedimentation (400 *g*, 10 min) over 62.5% Percoll (Sigma, UK). The cells at the interface were removed and washed three times, and viable cells counted after staining with trypan blue. Peripheral blood mononuclear cells (PBMC) were isolated from heparinised blood by density gradient centrifugation (400 *g*, 45 min) over 62.5% Percoll and washed three times as above.

FACS analysis

Indirect immunofluorescence staining was performed using mouse or rat monoclonal antibodies (mAb) followed by fluorescein isothiocyanate (FITC)-conjugated $F(ab)_2$ rabbit anti-mouse immunoglobulin G (IgG) (Serotec, Oxford, UK) or FITC-conjugated sheep anti-rat IgG (Serotec) antibodies. Appropriate controls consisting of unstained cells and cells incubated with either normal serum or an isotype-specific irrelevant mAb were included in each analysis. The mAbs used are indicated in Tables 3.2.1 and 3.2.2. The samples were analysed on a FACScan® (Becton Dickinson, Oxford, UK) using propidium iodide (20 μg/ml) to exclude dead cells. All events were acquired and cells with

Table 3.2.1. Monoclonal antibodies against cell-surface antigens

Specificity	Clone	Isotype	Form	Source	Reference
CD1a	CA9.AG5	mu IgG_1	TCSN	P.F.M.	Moore *et al.* (1996)
CD1b	CC20	mu IgG_{2a}	Purified	C.H.	Moore *et al.* (1996)
CD1c	CA13.9H11	mu IgG_1	TCSN	P.F.M.	Moore *et al.* (1996)
CD3ε	CD3-12	rat IgG_1	Purified	Serotec	Ferrer *et al.* (1992)
CD4	YKIX 302.9.3.7	rat IgG_{2a}	Ascites	S.C.	Cobbold & Metcalfe (1994)
CD5	YKIX 322.3.2	rat IgG_{2a}	Ascites	S.C.	Cobbold & Metcalfe (1994)
CD8α	YCATE.55	rat IgG_1	Ascites	S.C.	Cobbold & Metcalfe (1994)
CD11a	CA11.4D3	mu IgG_1	TCSN	P.F.M.	Danilenko *et al.* (1992)
CD11b	CA16.3E10	mu IgG_1	TCSN	P.F.M.	Moore *et al.* (1996)
CD11c	CA11.6A1	mu IgG_1	TCSN	P.F.M.	Danilenko *et al.* (1992)
$\alpha D\beta_2$	CA11.8H2	mu IgG_1	TCSN	P.F.M.	Danilenko *et al.* (1995)
CD18	CA1.4E9	mu IgG_1	TCSN	P.F.M.	Moore *et al.* (1990)
CD21	CA2.1D6	mu IgG_1	TCSN	P.F.M.	Moore *et al.* (1996)
CD44	YKIX 337.8.7	rat IgG_{2a}	Ascites	S.C.	Cobbold & Metcalfe (1994)
CD45	YKIX 334.2.1	rat IgG_{2b}	Ascites	S.C.	Cobbold & Metcalfe (1994)
CD45R	YKIX 337.217.7	rat IgG_{2b}	Ascites	S.C.	Cobbold & Metcalfe (1994)
CD45RA	CA4.1D3	mu IgG_1	TCSN	P.F.M.	Moore *et al.* (1996)
CD49d	CA4.5B3	mu IgG_1	TCSN	P.F.M.	Moore *et al.* (1996)
CD54	155D	mu IgG_1	Purified	C.W.S.	Smith *et al.* (1991)
CD90 (Thy-1)	753.22.21	rat IgG_{2b}	Ascites	S.C.	Cobbold & Metcalfe (1994)
MHC I	H58A	mu IgG_{2a}	Purified	V.M.R.D.	Davis *et al.* (1987)
MHC II	YKIX 334.2.1	rat IgG_{2a}	Ascites	S.C.	Cobbold & Metcalfe (1994)
MHC II	CVS 20	mu IgG_1	TCSN	M.H.	Cobbold & Metcalfe (1994)
Ig	K992E3	mu IgG_1	Purified	Serotec	None available
E-cadherin	DECMA-1	rat IgG_1	Purified	Sigma	Restucci *et al.* (1997)

MHC: major histocompatibility complex; Ig: immunoglobulin; TCSN: tissue culture supernatant; P.F.M.: Professor P. F. Moore, UC Davis, California, USA; C.H.: Dr C. Howard, BBSRC Institute for Animal Health, Compton, UK; S.C.: Dr S. Cobbold, University of Oxford, UK; C.W.S.: Dr C. Wayne Smith, Baylor College of Medicine, Texas, USA; M.H.: Dr M. Holmes, University of Cambridge, UK.

Table 3.2.2. Isotype-matched negative control antibodies

Control antibodies	Source
Purified mouse IgG_1 (MOPC 31C)	Sigma
Purified mouse IgG_{2a} (UPC-10)	Sigma
Purified rat IgG_1 (IR27)	Serotec
Purified rat IgG_{2a} (IR418)	Serotec
Purified rat IgG_{2b} (IR863)	Serotec
Purified rat IgG_{2c} (IR22)	Serotec

IgG: immunoglobulin G.

defined forward and side scatter profiles were gated on the forward scatter/side scatter dot plot to generate data for fluorescence histograms of this population. The fluorescence profile of a gated population of cells was displayed as a histogram of fluorescence intensity versus relative cell number. Positive fluorescence was established in comparison to background fluorescence obtained with cells stained with an isotype-matched control antibody.

Immunohistochemistry

Formalin-fixed, paraffin-embedded sections from the tumours were stained with a mAb recognising CD3ε using a standard indirect immunoperoxidase technique (Vectastain ABC®; Vector Laboratories, Peterborough, UK) and diaminobenzidine (DAB) as a chromogen. Sections were examined for the presence of CD3-positive cells.

Allogenic mixed lymphocyte reaction

Allogenic PBMC (10^5) were cultured in 96-well round-bottomed microplates (Falcon, Becton Dickenson Labware, Oxford, UK) with different numbers of irradiated (4000 rads from an orthovoltage source) stimulator cells (CCH cells or PBMC). Control triplicates of cells incubated with medium alone or with 10 μg/ml concanavalin A (ConA) were included. Thymidine incorporation was measured on day 5 after a 5 h pulse with [^{3}H]thymidine (1 μCi/well, specific activity 5 Ci/mmol; Amersham Life Science, Buckingham, UK).

The cells were harvested onto glass-fibre filter mats, using a Tomtec Harvester 99, allowed to dry at 56°C for 30 min and sealed in sample bags containing 4 ml scintillation fluid (Betaplate Scint). Filter mats were analysed on a Microbeta 1450™ (Wallac, Turku, Finland) liquid scintillation counter to determine tritiated thymidine uptake by the cells. The results were expressed as the arithmetic mean of triplicates. The stimulation index was calculated as the thymidine uptake in the test wells divided by the thymidine uptake in the negative control wells.

Autologous mixed lymphocyte reaction

Autologous PBMC (10^5) were cultured in 96-well round-bottomed microplates with different numbers of irradiated stimulator cells, either CCH cells or autologous PBMC. Proliferation was measured by [^{3}H]thymidine incorporation as above.

Quantitation of macropinocytosis in single cells

Cells were resuspended in RPMI/10% FCS at 37°C. Lucifer yellow was added at a final concentration of 1 mg/ml for various times. The cells were washed four times with ice-cold PBS containing 0.1% bovine serum albumin and 0.01% NaN_3 and analysed on a FACScan using propidium iodide to exclude dead cells.

Statistical analysis

Differences in measured variables between groups were analysed using the Mann–Whitney *U*-test and Kruskal–Wallis non-parametric tests (significance was set at $p < 0.05$).

Results

Immunohistochemistry

Early lesions were defined as those containing no or very few $CD3^+$ T-cells, and later lesions were defined as those with an appreciable infiltrate of $CD3^+$ T-cells, according to a modification of a previously described classification (Cockerell & Slauson, 1979) (Plate 6).

Isolation of CCH cells

Collagenase digestion yielded on average 2.3×10^7 cells (range 1.8×10^6 to 6.3×10^8), with a viability of more than 90%. The cells were large with a typical histiocytic morphology, with voluminous cytoplasm and a large, round or indented nucleus (Plate 7).

Tumour cells exhibit an activated Langerhans' cell phenotype

The forward scatter/side scatter dot plot from a representative tumour is illustrated in Figure 3.2.1a. All CCH cells expressed CD1a, CD1c, CD11a, CD11c, CD18, CD45, CD45R, MHC I, MHC II and E-cadherin, confirming their Langerhans' cell origin (Figure 3.2.1b). In addition, the cells expressed CD1b, CD11b, CD44, CD49d and ICAM-1, which are not expressed by resting canine Langerhans' cells or, in the case of CD1b, is only expressed by a subpopulation (Moore *et al.*, 1996). The CCH cells did not express CD4, CD5, CD8, $\alpha D\beta_2$, CD21, CD45RA, Thy-1 on surface immunoglobulin, thus ruling out T-cell, B-cell and dermal dendritic cell origin for these cells.

When analysed according to histological stage, CCH cells isolated from lesions with a lymphocytic infiltrate had significantly higher expression of MHC I ($p = 0.045$), MHC II ($p = 0.035$) and ICAM-1 ($p = 0.030$) compared with those cells isolated from earlier lesions without lymphocytic infiltrate (Figure 3.2.2).

CCH cells are potent stimulators in the allogenic mixed lymphocyte reaction

CCH cells were compared with PBMC for their capacity to stimulate alloreactive PBMC. CCH cells from all tumour samples induced a proliferative response in allogenic PBMC, which was greater than the response induced by autologous PBMC in all cases (Figure 3.2.3a).

When compared according to the clinical stage of the lesion, CCH cells isolated from later lesions resulted in a significantly greater proliferative response for a given number of stimulator cells than CCH cells isolated from early lesions (Figure 3.2.3b). The median thymidine uptake seen when 5000 CCH cells were incubated with 10^5 responders was 9237 (range 6806–15 500) counts per minute (cpm) for cells isolated from late lesions compared with 3119 (range 3083–3133) cpm for cells isolated from early lesions ($p = 0.049$) (Figure 3.2.3c).

CCH cells from lesions undergoing regression induce a strong proliferative response in autologous PBMC

CCH cells were compared with PBMC for their capacity to induce a proliferative response in autologous

PBMC. CCH cells induced a proliferative response in autologous PBMC, whereas autologous PBMC failed to do so (Figure 3.2.4a).

When compared according to clinical stage of the lesion, CCH cells isolated from later lesions resulted in a significantly greater proliferative response for a given number of stimulator cells than CCH cells isolated from early lesions (Figure 3.2.4b). The median thymidine uptake seen when 10^5 CCH cells were incubated with 10^5 responders was 13 419 (range 10 668–25 522) cpm for cells isolated from late lesions compared with 1934 (range 636–8266) cpm for cells isolated from early lesions ($p = 0.034$) (Figure 3.2.4c).

CCH cells from lesions undergoing regression exhibit high levels of macropinocytosis

The capacity of CCH cells and autologous PBMC for macropinocytosis was examined using uptake of the non-specific fluid-phase marker lucifer yellow. All cells exhibited macropinocytosis, showing a linear increase in fluorescence with time. When analysed according to the clinical stage of the lesion, CCH cells from later lesions showed a significantly higher rate of macropinocytosis than those from earlier lesions at time points from 8 to 64 min ($p = 0.0001$–0.0113) (Figure 3.2.5). The rate of macropinocytosis in cells

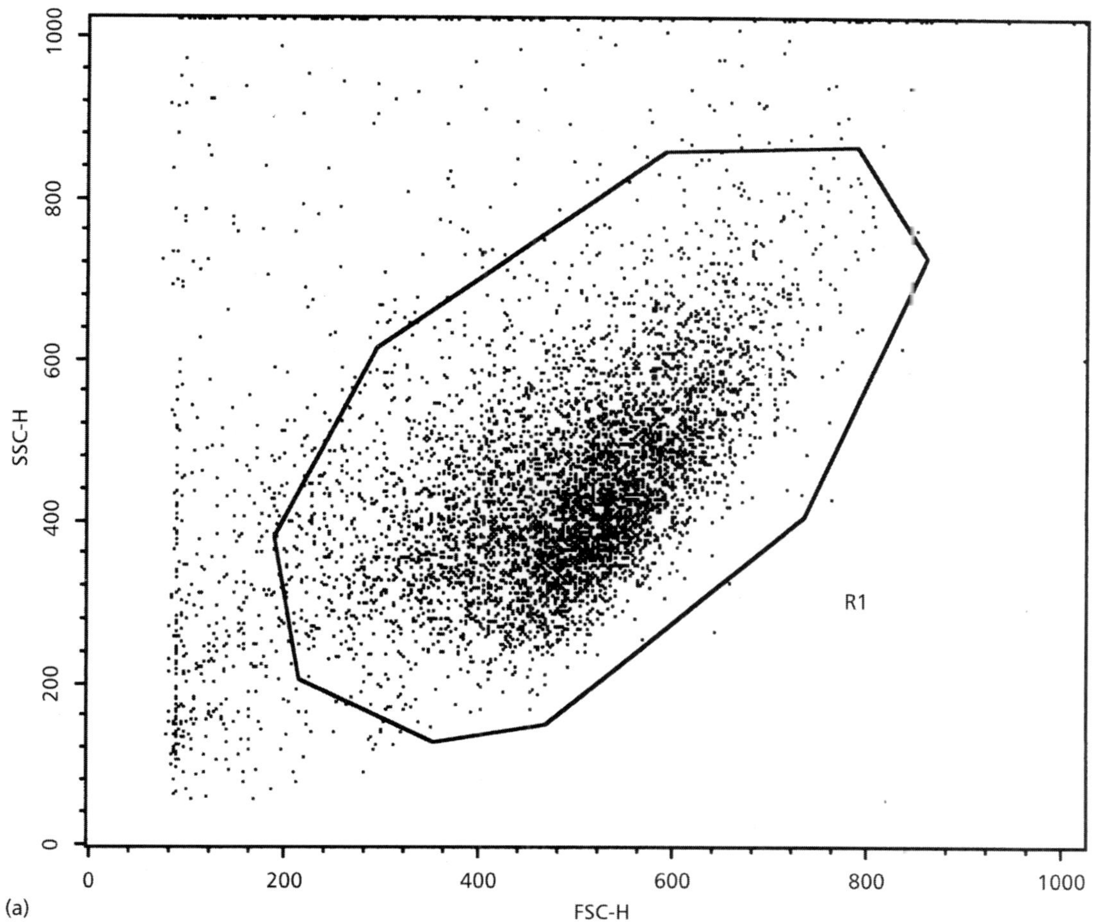

(a)

Figure 3.2.1. (a) Immunophenotype of canine cutaneous histiocytoma (CCH) cells. Scatterplot of forward scatter (FSC-H) versus side scatter (SSC-H) showing a single population of relatively large cells enclosed in the polygonal gate R1.

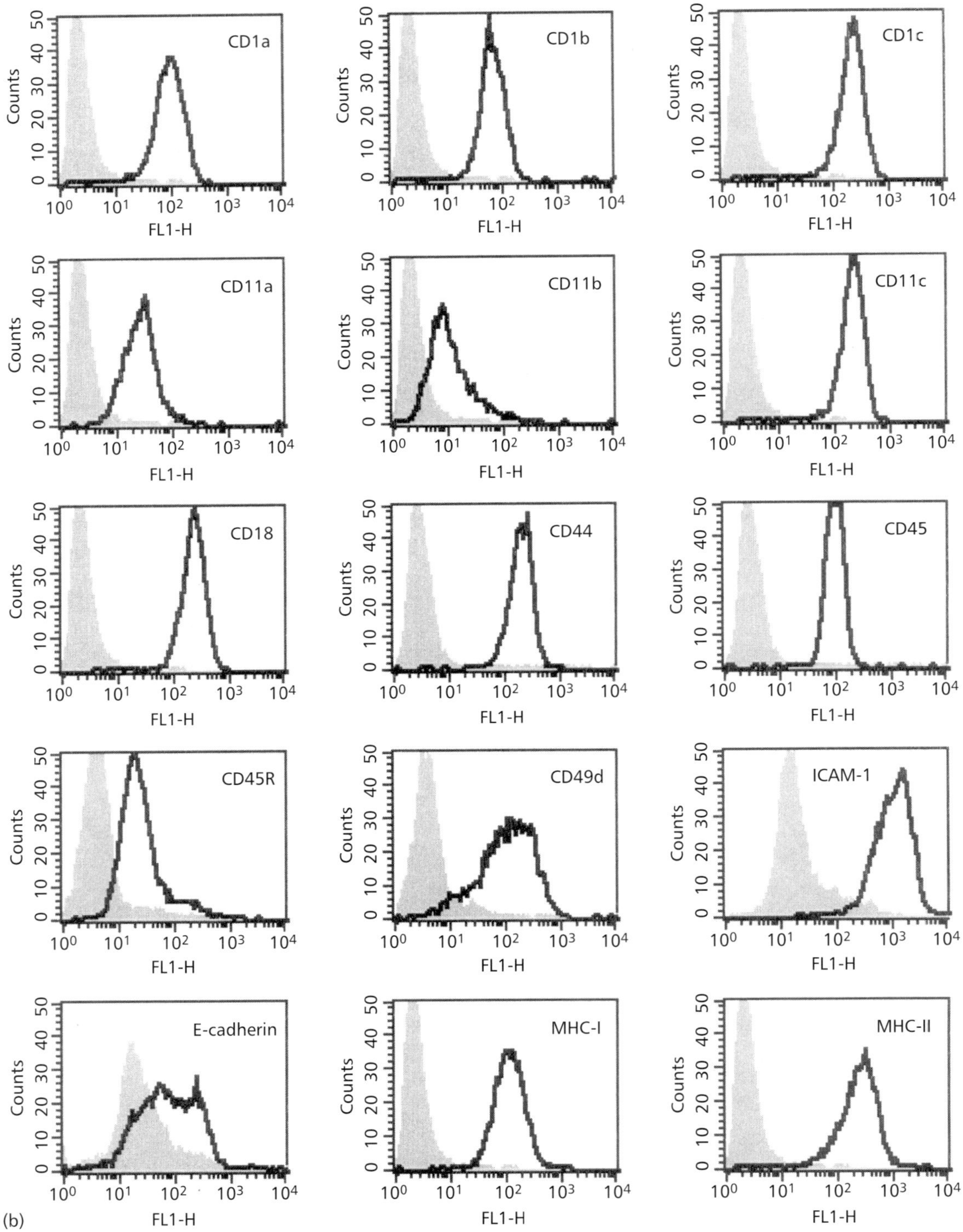

(b)

Figure 3.2.1. (b) Immunophenotypes of canine cutaneous histiocytoma (CCH) cells. Histograms showing fluorescence (FL1-H) on gated cells. Staining with the antibody indicated is shown as a thick line and with the isotype-matched control by a shaded histogram. The CCH cells expressed CD1a, CD1b, CD1c, CD11a, CD11c, CD18, CD45, CD45R, major histocompatibility complex class I (MHC I), MHC II and E-cadherin. In addition, they expressed CD11b, CD44, CD49d and intercellular adhesion molecule-1 (ICAM-1), which are not normally expressed on immature epidermal Langerhans' cells *in situ*.

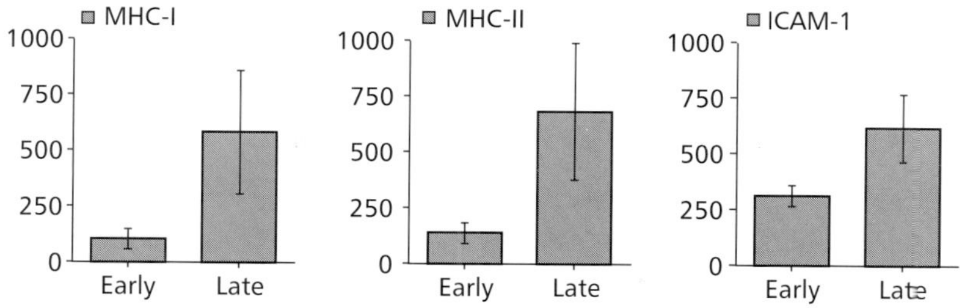

Figure 3.2.2. Immunophenotype of canine cutaneous histiocytoma (CCH) cells according to clinical stage. The graphs show the average mean channel fluorescence from at least 10 experiments; error bars represent the standard error of the mean (SEM). CCH cells isolated from lesions undergoing regression showed increased expression of major histocompatibility complex class I (MHC I), MHC II and intercellular adhesion molecule-1 (ICAM-1) compared with those in the early phase.

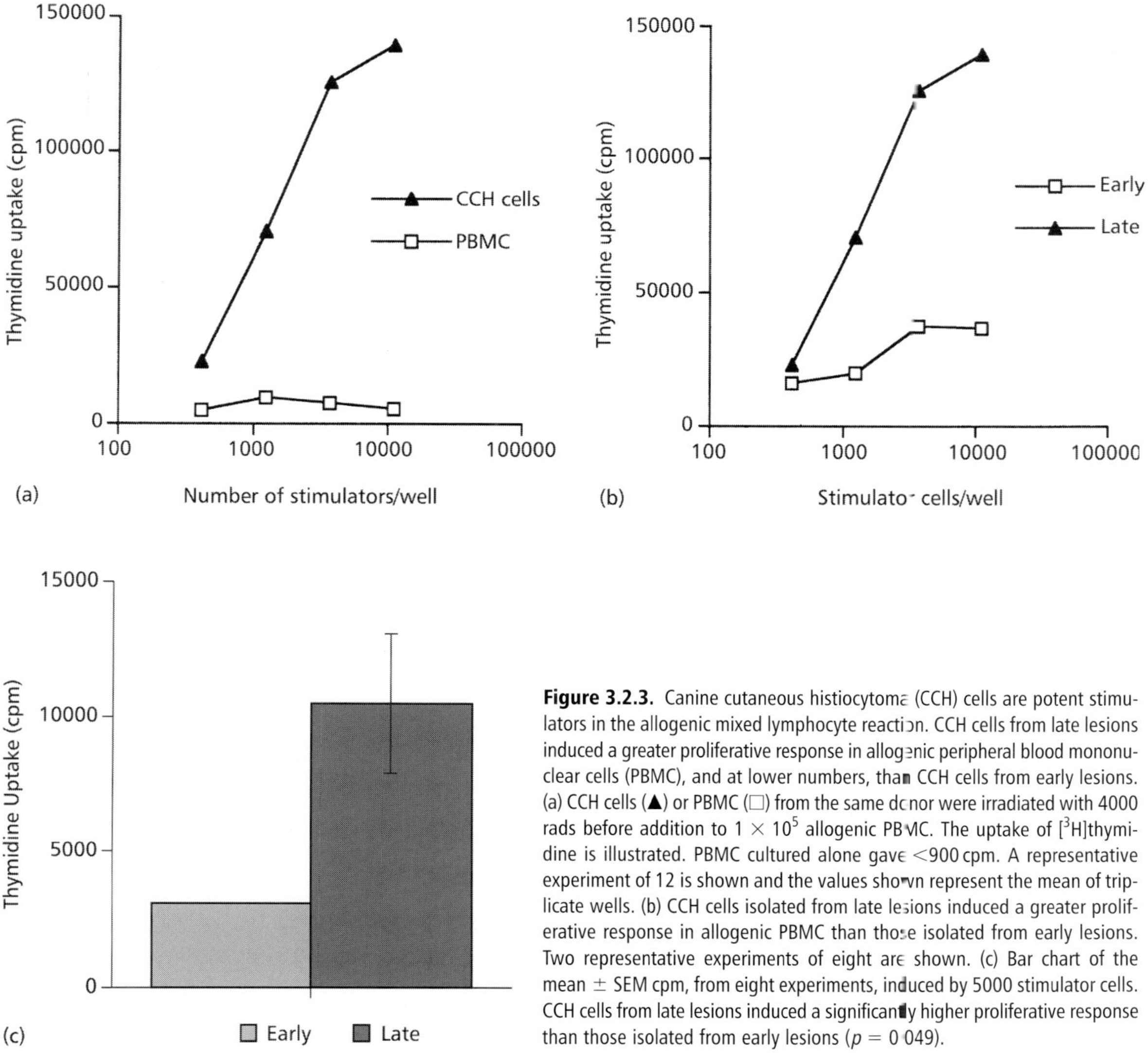

Figure 3.2.3. Canine cutaneous histiocytoma (CCH) cells are potent stimulators in the allogenic mixed lymphocyte reaction. CCH cells from late lesions induced a greater proliferative response in allogenic peripheral blood mononuclear cells (PBMC), and at lower numbers, than CCH cells from early lesions. (a) CCH cells (▲) or PBMC (□) from the same donor were irradiated with 4000 rads before addition to 1×10^5 allogenic PBMC. The uptake of [^{3}H]thymidine is illustrated. PBMC cultured alone gave <900 cpm. A representative experiment of 12 is shown and the values shown represent the mean of triplicate wells. (b) CCH cells isolated from late lesions induced a greater proliferative response in allogenic PBMC than those isolated from early lesions. Two representative experiments of eight are shown. (c) Bar chart of the mean ± SEM cpm, from eight experiments, induced by 5000 stimulator cells. CCH cells from late lesions induced a significantly higher proliferative response than those isolated from early lesions ($p = 0.049$).

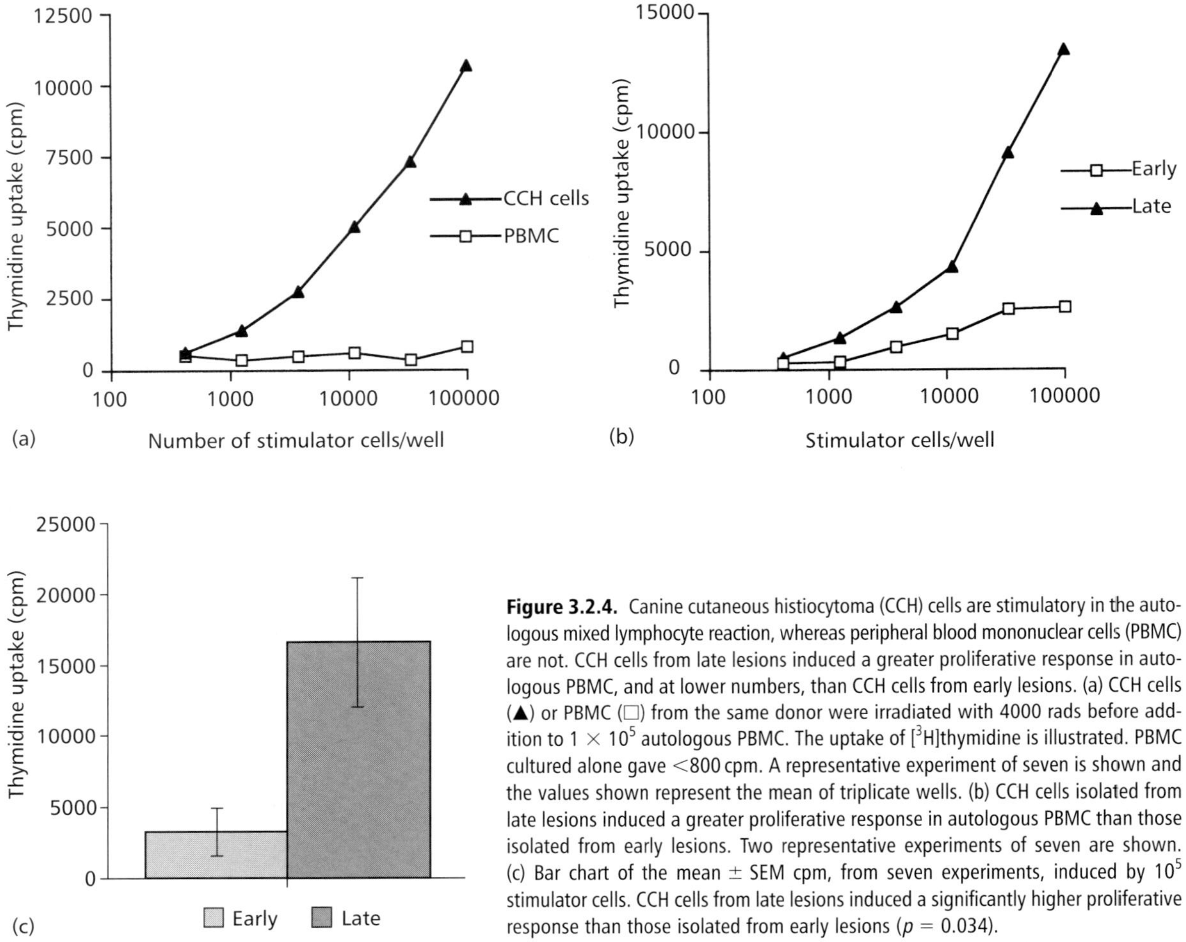

Figure 3.2.4. Canine cutaneous histiocytoma (CCH) cells are stimulatory in the autologous mixed lymphocyte reaction, whereas peripheral blood mononuclear cells (PBMC) are not. CCH cells from late lesions induced a greater proliferative response in autologous PBMC, and at lower numbers, than CCH cells from early lesions. (a) CCH cells (▲) or PBMC (□) from the same donor were irradiated with 4000 rads before addition to 1×10^5 autologous PBMC. The uptake of [^{3}H]thymidine is illustrated. PBMC cultured alone gave <800 cpm. A representative experiment of seven is shown and the values shown represent the mean of triplicate wells. (b) CCH cells isolated from late lesions induced a greater proliferative response in autologous PBMC than those isolated from early lesions. Two representative experiments of seven are shown. (c) Bar chart of the mean ± SEM cpm, from seven experiments, induced by 10^5 stimulator cells. CCH cells from late lesions induced a significantly higher proliferative response than those isolated from early lesions ($p = 0.034$).

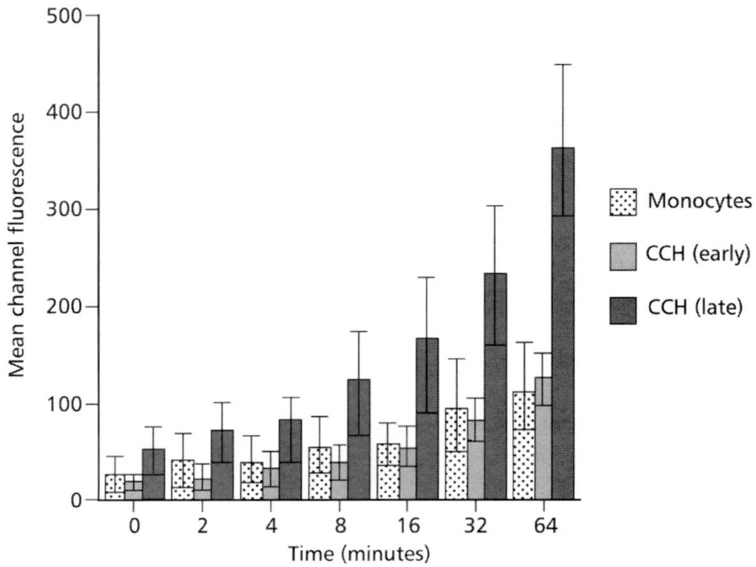

Figure 3.2.5. Canine cutaneous histiocytoma (CCH) cells exhibit high levels of macropinocytosis. CCH cells from late lesions showed a higher rate of macropinocytosis than those isolated from early lesions. CCH cells or peripheral blood mononuclear cells (PBMC) were incubated in medium containing 1 mg/ml lucifer yellow (LY) at 37°C for various times, washed with cold phosphate-buffered saline, and the amount of LY accumulated by the cells was measured by analysis on a FACScan®. The bar chart illustrates the difference in uptake of LY between monocytes and between CCH cells from early and late lesions. The mean ± SEM of eight experiments is shown. CCH cells from late lesions showed a significantly higher rate of macropinocytosis than early lesions ($p = 0.0001$–0.0113) at certain time points. CCH cells from early lesions did not show a significantly different rate of macropinocytosis from monocytes at any time point.

from early lesions was not significantly different from that shown by peripheral monocytes at all time points.

Discussion

It has been demonstrated previously that CCH is a proliferative disorder of Langerhans' cells and that CCH cells exhibit an activated phenotype (Moore & Schrenzel, 1991; Moore *et al.*, 1998). The present study shows that CCH cells isolated from the tumours display this activated Langerhans' cell phenotype and exhibit functional characteristics associated with dendritic cells *in vitro*, namely the induction of proliferative responses in allogenic and autologous PBMC and the presence of high levels of macropinocytosis.

The surface phenotype of the CCH cells isolated as single cells from the lesions is in accordance with that previously reported using immunohistochemistry on cryostat sections (Moore *et al.*, 1996). In addition, we have shown that CCH cells express E-cadherin, which identifies them as Langerhans' cells (Blauvelt *et al.*, 1995).

Langerhans' cells originate from the bone marrow (Katz *et al.*, 1979), enter the bloodstream as progenitors, and colonise lymphoid and non-lymphoid tissues (Strunk & Stingl, 1995). Upon receipt of appropriate stimuli, Langerhans' cells undergo maturation and migrate in the afferent lymph to the T-cell areas of the regional lymph node, where they present antigens acquired in the periphery to T-cells (Teunissen, 1992). Defined changes in phenotype and function can be measured at various points along this differentiation pathway, although the signals responsible for controlling these checkpoints are not fully elucidated (Steinman *et al.*, 1995).

The strong stimulatory activity of dendritic cells in the primary mixed lymphocyte reaction (MLR) is well established (Steinman & Inaba, 1985; Steinman, 1991). Freshly isolated murine Langerhans' cells do not stimulate a response in the MLR, but do so after 1–3 days in culture, and granulocyte–macrophage colony-stimulating factor (GM-CSF) plays a key role in this (Schuler & Steinman, 1985; Witmer-Pack *et al.*, 1987). Dendritic cells also have the unique ability to stimulate autologous T-cells in the autologous MLR (Scheinecker *et al.*, 1998). It has been shown that mature peripheral blood dendritic cells are potent stimulators of autologous T-cells, whereas immature blood dendritic cells or monocytes are not (Scheinecker *et al.*, 1998). In addition, this improvement in the proliferative response is dependent on the up-regulation of the costimulatory molecules B7-1 and B7-2 (Scheinecker *et al.*, 1998).

Macropinocytosis is a cytoskeleton-dependent mechanism of fluid uptake limited to dendritic cells, macrophages and epithelial cells (Racoosin & Swanson, 1989; Sallusto *et al.*, 1995). Macropinocytosis is present only for a few minutes after growth factor stimulation in macrophages or epithelial cells, but is constitutive in dendritic cells (Sallusto *et al.*, 1995). Immature dendritic cells exhibit very high levels of macropinocytosis, but this is rapidly down-regulated when maturation is induced with exogenous stimuli such as tumour necrosis factor-α (TNF-α), interleukin-1 (IL-1), CD40 ligand and lipopolysaccharide (Sallusto *et al.*, 1995).

This study has shown that CCH cells are strong stimulators in the allogenic and autologous MLR, consistent with their dendritic cell origin, and exhibit high levels of macropinocytosis as expected for cells of this lineage.

Differences between the phenotypic and functional properties of CCH cells isolated from lesions at different clinical stages were identified. The up-regulation of MHC I, MHC II and ICAM-1 is similar to the phenotypic changes that occur during maturation and migration of Langerhans' cells from the epidermis to the regional lymph node (Schuler & Steinman, 1985). This finding is consistent with the hypothesis that CCH cells isolated from early lesions have a similar phenotype to immature Langerhans' cells and those isolated from lesions undergoing regression have a similar phenotype to mature Langerhans' cells.

In addition, the enhanced stimulatory function in the allogenic MLR seen in CCH cells isolated from tumours undergoing regression supports the hypothesis that CCH tumours undergoing regression are composed of cells analogous to mature dendritic cells.

Similar findings are present in the autologous MLR. Cells from tumours in the early phase have a similar stimulatory capacity to monocytes or immature dendritic cells, and cells isolated from lesions undergoing regression exhibit the stimulatory capacity associated with mature dendritic cells. Appropriate reagents are not available to identify whether this improvement in stimulatory capacity is due to up-regulation of the costimulatory molecules B7-1 and B7-2.

$CD1a^{+}$ cells isolated from lesions of human Langerhans' cell histiocytosis stimulate a weak response in the primary allogenic MLR, but this response is considerably lower on a per cell basis than the response obtained with normal Langerhans' cells (Yu *et al.*, 1992, 1995). The addition of IL-1β, a potent maturation-inducing cytokine, did not reverse this diminished activity (Yu *et al.*, 1995); however, the maturation state of the normal or lesional Langerhans' cells was not assessed. The lack of a control population of normal canine dendritic cells prevents such a comparison being made in this study.

The level of macropinocytosis exhibited by the CCH cells is that expected from myeloid cells. However, the increased rate of macropinocytosis seen in cells isolated from lesions undergoing regression is interesting. These data are not in keeping with a simple progression of functionally normal cells from an immature dendritic cell to a mature dendritic cell phenotype. This may indicate that the maturation phenomenon suggested by the immunophenotyping data and other functional data represents the transition from a Langerhans' cell precursor to an immature Langerhans' cell, or from an immature Langerhans' cell to an intermediate transitional form. A transient increase in antigen acquisition, as measured by uptake of FITC–dextran, has been noted in transitional dendritic cells (Granucci *et al.*, 1998).

This apparent discordance may be explained in terms of the cytokine microenvironment. IL-10 is a cytokine produced by lymphoid and myeloid cells, including dendritic cells, and keratinocytes, which has an inhibitory effect on dendritic cell maturation (Morel *et al.*, 1997; Allavena *et al.*, 1998). Dendritic cells incubated in the presence of IL-10 show an increase in expression of MHC I, MHC II and ICAM-1 and show a small increase in their stimulatory capacity in the allogenic MLR. However, IL-10 results in an increase, rather than a decrease, in macropinocytosis (Allavena *et al.*, 1998). Further work is being carried out to examine the cytokine microenvironment of these tumours, particularly with respect to the inhibitory cytokine IL-10 and the proinflammatory, maturation-inducing cytokines IL-1β and TNF-α.

CCH cells isolated from lesions at different clinical stages differ with respect to phenotype and function. These differences are analogous to those changes that occur during maturation of dendritic cells (Schuler & Steinman, 1985; Sallusto *et al.*, 1995). Studying this tumour allows a dissection of the mechanisms involved in dendritic cell maturation *in vivo*.

Conclusion

This study provides further evidence that CCH is a tumour of Langerhans' cells. The CCH cells isolated from the lesions at different clinical stages have distinctly different phenotype and function, and these differences reflect different stages of dendritic cell maturation. Further studies are ongoing to examine the reasons for the accumulation of Langerhans' cells and to determine why this maturation phenomenon is not associated with migration of the neoplastic Langerhans' cell in the majority of cases. The influence of the cytokine microenvironment of the tumour in this context will be examined.

Acknowledgements

This work was supported by a grant from The Wellcome Trust. The authors would like to thank Jane Dobson and Phil Nicholls for their initial work on this project and to local veterinary surgeons for making the clinical material available.

References

Allavena, P., Piemonti, L., Longoni, D., Bernasconi, S., Stoppacciaro, A., Rucco, L. & Mantovani, A. (1998) IL-10 prevents the differentiation of monocytes to dendritic cells but promotes their maturation to macrophages. *European Journal of Immunology*, **28**, 359–369.

Austyn, J. M. (1992) Antigen uptake and presentation by dendritic leucocytes. *Seminars in Immunology*, **4**, 227–236.

Blauvelt, A., Katz, S. I. & Udey, M.C. (1995) Human Langerhans cells express E-cadherin. *Journal of Investigative Dermatology*, **104**, 293–296.

Cobbold, S. C. & Metcalfe, S. (1994) Monoclonal antibodies that define canine homologues of human CD antigens: summary of the First International Canine Leucocyte Antigen Workshop (CLAW). *Tissue Antigens*, **43**, 137–154.

Cockerell, G. L. & Slauson, D. O. (1979) Patterns of lymphoid infiltrate in the canine cutaneous histiocytoma. *Journal of Comparative Pathology*, **89**, 193–203.

Conroy, J. D. (1983) Canine skin tumours. *Journal of the American Animal Hospital Association*, **19**, 91–114.

Danilenko, D. M., Moore, P. F. & Rossitto, P. V. (1992) Canine leucocyte cell adhesion molecules (LeuCAMs): characterisation of the CD11/18 family. *Tissue Antigens*, **40**, 13–21.

Danilenko, D. M., Rossitto, P. V., Van der Vieren, M., Trong, H. L., McDonough, S. P., Affolter, V. K. & Moore, P. F. (1995) A novel leukointegrin, Alpha-d Beta-2, is expressed by specific macrophage subpopulations in tissue and a minor CD8+ lymphocyte subpopulation in peripheral blood. *Journal of Immunology*, **155**, 35–44.

Davis, W. C., Marusic S., Lewin H. A., Splitter, G. A., Perryman, L. E., McGuire, T. C. & Gorham, J. R. (1987) The development and analysis of species-specific and cross-reactive monoclonal antibodies to leucocyte differentiation antigens and antigens of the major histocompatibility complex for use in the study of the immune system in cattle and other species. *Veterinary Immunology and Immunopathology*, **15**, 337–376.

Ferrer, L., Fondevila, D., Rabanal, R. & Ramis, A. (1992) Detection of T lymphocytes in canine tissue embedded in paraffin wax by means of antibody to CD3 antigen. *Journal of Comparative Pathology*, **106**, 311–314.

Granucci, F., Foti, M., Ferrero, E., Aggujaro, D. & Ricciardi-Castagnoli, P. (1998) Transitional stages during dendritic cell maturation. *Journal of Leukocyte Biology*, Suppl. 2, Abstract B58, 43.

Katz, S. I., Tamaki, K. & Sachs, D. H. (1979) Epidermal Langerhans cells are derived from cells originating in bone marrow. *Nature*, **282**, 324–326.

Kelly, D. F. (1970) Canine cutaneous histiocytoma: a light and electron microscopic study. *Veterinary Pathology*, **7**, 12–27.

Moore, P. F. & Schrenzel, M. D. (1991) Canine cutaneous histiocytoma represents a Langerhans cell proliferative disorder based on an immunophenotypic analysis. *Proceedings of the American College of Veterinary Pathologists*, 119.

Moore, P. F., Rossitto, P. V. & Danilenko, D. M. (1990) Canine leukocyte integrins: characterisation of a CD18 homologue. *Tissue Antigens*, **36**, 211–220.

Moore, P. F., Schrenzel, M. D., Affolter, V. K., Olivry, T. & Naydan, D. (1996) Canine cutaneous histiocytoma is an epidermotropic Langerhans cell histiocytosis that expresses CD1 and specific Beta-2 integrin molecules. *American Journal of Pathology*, **148**, 1699–1708.

Moore, P. F., Affolter, V. K., Olivry, T. & Schrenzel, M. D. (1998) The use of immunological reagents in defining the pathogenesis of skin diseases. *Advances in Veterinary Dermatology*, **3**, 77–94.

Morel, A.-S., Quarantino, S., Douek, D. C. & Londei, M. (1997) Split activity of interleukin-10 on antigen capture and antigen presentation by human dendritic cells: definition of a maturative step. *European Journal of Immunology*, **27**, 26–34.

Pulley, L. T. & Stannard, A. A. (1990) Tumors of the skin and soft tissue. In: *Tumors in Domestic Animals* (Ed. J. E. Moulton), pp. 23–87. University of California Press, Berkeley, CA.

Racoosin, E. L. & Swanson, J. A. (1989) Macrophage colony-stimulating factor (M-CSF) stimulates pinocytosis in bone marrow-derived macrophages. *Journal of Experimental Medicine*, **170**, 1635–1648.

Restucci, B., Papparella, S., De Vico, G. & Maiolino, P. (1997) E cadherin expression in normal and neoplastic canine mammary gland. *Journal of Comparative Pathology*, **116**, 191–202.

Romani, N. & Schuler, G. (1992) The immunologic properties of epidermal Langerhans cells as part of the dendritic cell system. *Springer Seminars in Immunopathology*, **13**, 265–279.

Sallusto, F., Cella, M., Danieli, C. & Lanzavecchia, A. (1995) Dendritic cells use macropinocytosis and the mannose receptor to concentrate macromolecules in the major histocompatability complex class II compartment: downregulation by cytokines and bacterial products. *Journal of Experimental Medicine*, **182**, 389–400.

Scheinecker, C., Machold, K. P., Majdic, O., Hocker, P., Knapp, W. & Smolen, J. (1998) Initiation of the autologous mixed lymphocyte reaction requires the expression of costimulatory molecules B7-1 and B7-2 on human peripheral blood dendritic cells. *Journal of Immunology*, **161**, 3966–3973.

Schuler, G. & Steinman, R. M. (1985) Murine epidermal Langerhans cells mature into potent immunostimulatory dendritic cells *in vitro*. *Journal of Experimental Medicine*, **161**, 526–546.

Smith, C. W., Entman, M. L., Lane, C. L., Beaudet, A. L., Ty, T. I., Youker, K. *et al.* (1991) Adherence of neutrophils to canine cardiac myocytes *in vitro* is dependent on intercellular adhesion molecule-1. *Journal of Clinical Investigation*, **88**, 1216–1223.

Steinman, R., Hoffman, L. & Pope, M. (1995) Maturation and migration of cutaneous dendritic cells. *Journal of Investigative Dermatology*, **105**, 2S–7S.

Steinman, R. M. (1991) The dendritic cell and its role in immunogenicity. *Annual Reviews of Immunology*, **9**, 271–296.

Steinman, R. M. & Inaba, K. (1985) Stimulation of the primary mixed leukocyte reaction. *CRC Critical Reviews in Immunology*, **5**, 331–348.

Strunk, D. & Stingl, G. (1995) Human Langerhans cells derived from CD34+ blood precursors: mode of generation, phenotypic and functional analysis, and experimental and clinical applicability. In: *The Immune Functions of Epidermal Langerhans Cells* (Ed. H. Moll), pp. 21–36. R. G. Landes, New York.

Taylor, D. O. N., Dorn, C. R. & Luis, O. H. (1969) Morphologic and biologic characteristics of the canine cutaneous histiocytoma. *Cancer Research*, **29**, 83–92.

Teunissen, M. B. M. (1992) Dynamic nature and function of epidermal Langerhans cells *in vivo* and *in vitro*: a review, with emphasis on human Langerhans cells. *Histochemical Journal*, **24**, 697–716.

Winzler, C., Rovere, P., Rescigno, M., Granucci, F., Penna, G., Adorini, L. *et al.* (1997) Maturation stages of mouse dendritic cells in growth factor-dependent long-term cultures. *Journal of Experimental Medicine*, **185**, 317–328.

Witmer-Pack, M. D., Olivier, W., Valinsky, J., Schuler, G. & Steinman, R. M. (1987) Granulocyte/macrophage colony-stimulating factor is essential for the viability and function of cultured murine epidermal Langerhans cells. *Journal of Experimental Medicine*, **166**, 1484–1498.

Yu, R. C., Alaibac M. & Chu, A. C. (1995) Functional defect in cells involved in Langerhans cell histiocytosis. *Archives of Dermatological Research*, **287**, 627–631.

Yu, R. C. H., Morris, J. F., Pritchard, J. & Chu, T. C. (1992) Defective alloantigen-presenting capacity of Langerhans cell histiocytosis cells. *Archives of Diseases in Childhood*, **67**, 1370–1372.

3.3

Use of monoclonal antibodies as an adjunct to the diagnosis of epithelial skin tumors of the dog and cat using the EnVision Plus® system for the immunohistochemical detection of tissue antigens

M.H. Goldschmidt MSc, BVMS, MRCVS, DipACVP, A.C. Schneider DVM and J.D. Ferracone BS

Laboratory of Pathology and Toxicology, Department of Pathobiology, University of Pennsylvania, School of Veterinary Medicine, Philadelphia, Pennsylvania, USA

Summary

Cytokeratins are the intermediate filaments that form the cytoskeleton of epithelial cells. Cytokeratins are classified according to their molecular weight and isoelectric point, and are numbered from 1 to 20. The cytokeratins expressed by various epithelia are useful markers for evaluating epithelial cell differentiation. The Histological Classification of Epithelial and Melanocytic Tumors of the Skin of Domestic Animals defines the specific histopathological criteria required for the diagnosis of these neoplasms. This study evaluates the immunohistochemical staining of normal and neoplastic canine and feline epithelium and adnexa using cytokeratin-specific and other monoclonal antibodies.

Immunohistochemical evaluation was performed using the EnVision Plus® and Labeled-Streptavidin-Biotin-2 (LSAB2)® system and a Dako Autostainer®, to standardize procedures and reduce technical errors. Primary antibodies used were AE1, AE3, AE1/3, CAM5.2, cytokeratins 10, 15, 17, 19 and 20, a cytokeratin cocktail (Multi-CK), antibodies specific for human lymphocytes and for smooth muscle actin. Antibody detection methods used were the avidin–biotin complex, EnVision Plus or LSAB2 system.

AE1, AE3, Multi-CK, CK10 and CAM5.2 were the most useful antibodies to categorize and identify feline epithelial neoplasms. Cd79a and the above antibodies were most useful to identify canine neoplasms. CAM5.2 identifies neoplasms with atrichial and epitrichial differentiation, CD79a sebaceous and modified sebaceous glands in the dog, and CK10 trichogenic differentiation.

Introduction

Keratin is an intermediate-sized intracytoplasmic filament present in all true epithelia. Moll *et al.* (1982) identified 19 keratins in humans. The keratin composition of epithelia varies and is dependent on the cell type, the growth environment and the stage of development and differentiation (Cooper *et al.*, 1985). All epithelial keratins can be divided into an acidic (type I) and a basic (type II) subfamily, which react specifically with two monoclonal antikeratin antibodies prepared against human epidermal keratins, referred to as AE1 (acidic) and AE3 (basic) (Table 3.3.1). One member of the two subfamilies is found in all epithelia (Table 3.3.2). Cooper *et al.* (1985) established a number of rules governing cytokeratin expression: (1) 'keratin pairs' consist of an acidic and a basic member; (2) within each pair, the two keratins have identical 'size rank' in their respective subfamilies and

Table 3.3.1. Classification of epithelial cytokeratins

Basic (type II)			Acidic (type I)		
Keratin	Mol. wt (kDa)	AE3 staining	Keratin	Mol. wt (kDa)	AE1 staining
K1, 2	65–67	+	K10	56.5	+
K3	64	+	K12	55	−
K4	59	+	K13	51	−
K5	58	+	K14, 15	50	+
K6	56	+	K16	48	+
K7	54	+	K17	46	−
K8	52	+	K18	45	−
			K19	40	+
			K20	46	+

Table 3.3.2. Expression of cytokeratins by epithelia

Keratin type (K)	Differentiation
K1/2 and 10	Skin type
K3 and 12	Corneal type
K4 and 13	Esophageal, lingual, exocervix type
K5 and 14/15	All keratinocytes
K6 and 16	Hyperproliferative keratinocytes
K7 and 17	Simple and stratified epithelia
K8 and 18	Simple epithelia
K19	Simple epithelia
K20	Simple epithelia and Merkel cells

appear to follow similar rules for expression; and (3) within each keratin pair (Table 3.3.2) the basic member is always approximately 8 kDa larger than the acidic member (Table 3.3.1).

Cytokeratin 20, previously referred to as protein IT, is related to the acidic (type I) cytokeratins, has a molecular weight of 46 kDa, stains only with AE1, and is only present in Merkel cells in the epidermis and adnexa (Moll *et al.*, 1990).

In 1998, the second series of the Histological Classification of Epithelial and Melanocytic Tumors of the Skin of Domestic Animals was published by the World Health Organization in conjunction with the Armed Forces Institute of Pathology (Goldschmidt *et al.*, 1998). The classification system named the benign and malignant neoplasms according to either the type of neoplastic cell that constitutes them or the differentiation of the neoplastic cells. Repeatable and reliable criteria for the histopathological diagnosis of these neoplasms were established. This histological classification of the epithelial neoplasms is summarized below.

1. Neoplasms without squamous or adnexal differentiation
   Basal cell neoplasms
2. Neoplasms of the epidermis
   Papilloma, squamous cell carcinoma, basosquamous carcinoma
3. Neoplasms with adnexal differentiation
   a. Follicular neoplasms
      Infundibular keratinizing acanthoma, trichoblastoma, tricholemmoma, trichoepithelioma, pilomatricoma
   b. Nailbed neoplasms
      Keratoacanthoma, squamous cell carcinoma
   c. Sebaceous and modified sebaceous gland neoplasms
      Sebaceous, Meibomian and hepatoid gland – adenoma, ductal adenoma, epithelioma and carcinoma
   d. Apocrine (epitrichial) and modified apocrine gland neoplasms
      Apocrine, ceruminous and anal sac gland – adenoma, ductal adenoma, carcinoma and ductal carcinoma
   e. Eccrine (atrichial) gland neoplasms
      Adenoma and carcinoma.

The aim of this study was to use commercially available antibodies to specific cytokeratins for the immunohistochemical diagnosis of epithelial skin neoplasms, as an adjunct to the routine examination of hematoxylin and eosin (H&E)-stained sections. It must be stressed that in most cases when epithelial skin neoplasms are submitted for histopathology, a definitive diagnosis can be made using H&E-stained sections.

Materials and methods

Normal skin tissue was obtained from dogs and cats submitted to the necropsy service and the neoplasms to the surgical pathology service of the Laboratory of Pathology and Toxicology. Tissues were fixed in 10% neutral buffered formalin, routinely processed and embedded, and sections cut at 5 μm and mounted on ProbeOn Plus® microscope slides (Fisher Scientific, Pittsburgh, PA, USA). Slides were placed in a 60°C oven for 30 min, cooled to room temperature and deparaffinized. The Dako Autostainer® (Dako, Carpenteria, CA, USA), which is capable of simultaneously immunostaining 48 slides, was used, thereby reducing technical errors.

Table 3.3.3. Antibodies, enzyme predigestion procedures and detection systems used in the study

Antibody	Antibody source	Specificity[a]	Enzyme predigestion	Detection system
AE1	Boehringer	K[b] 10, 14, 15, 16, 19	Proteinase K	EnVision Plus
AE3	Boehringer	K1–8	Trypsin	EnVision Plus
AE1/3	Boehringer	K1–8, 10, 14, 15, 16, 19	Proteinase K	EnVision Plus
LP 34 34βE12 35βH11	Dako[c]	K1, 5, 6, 8, 10, 14, 18	Proteinase K	EnVision Plus
CAM5.2	Becton Dickinson	K8, 18	Proteinase K Trypsin	EnVision Plus
DE-K10	Dako	K10		EnVision Plus
Ks 20.8	Dako	K20	Proteinase K	EnVision Plus
Cd79a	Dako	B-cells	Trypsin	LSAB2
CALP	Dako	Myoepithelium	Proteinase K, 37°C	EnVision Plus

[a] Specificity described according to the manufacturer's information.
[b] K: cytokeratin numbers of Moll catalog.
[c] Hereafter referred to as Multi-CK.

Table 3.3.4. Antibodies, enzyme predigestion procedures and detection systems evaluated but not used in the study

Antibody	Antibody source	Specificity	Enzyme predigestion	Detection system
E3	Dako	K17	Trypsin Proteinase K Target retrieval solution	EnVision Plus
RCK 108	Dako	K19	Trypsin Proteinase K	EnVision Plus
–[a]		K15	Citrate buffer/ microwave	ABC
C8/144B	Dako	T-cells	Target retrieval solution	ABC

[a] Antibody provided and slides stained courtesy of Drs D. Jih and G. Cotsarelis, University of Pennsylvania, School of Medicine, Department of Dermatology.
ABC: avidin–biotin complex.

The primary antibodies, the source of these antibodies, their specificity, the enzyme predigestion and the detection system used are summarized in Tables 3.3.3 and 3.3.4. The EnVision Plus® (Dako) and Labeled-Streptavidin-Biotin-2 (LSAB2)® (Dako) detection systems replace the two-step biotinylated secondary antibody and streptavidin peroxidase conjugate method with a one-step method. 3,3′-Diaminobenzidene (DAB) was used for chromogenic development and the slides were counterstained with hematoxylin for 30 s. Controls consisted of omission of the primary antibody, detection system and the application of DAB alone. When available, a minimum of five cases of each of the epithelial neoplasms, except for eccrine neoplasms, was included in the study to ensure that consistent results were obtained with the immunohistochemical staining. Because these neoplasms were located in the dermis, the adjacent normal epidermis and adnexa served as internal controls in most cases.

C8/144B, a marker for human T-cells, was included as this antibody had been shown to cross-react with follicular stem cells in humans. Similarly, CD79a, a marker for B-cells, was included as it was previously observed that this antibody specifically stained canine sebaceous and modified sebaceous glands.

Results

Optimal staining was obtained using the enzyme predigestion methods, antibodies and detection systems listed in Table 3.3.3. Those listed in Table 3.3.4 were found to be suboptimal in their staining ability or did not stain normal skin. Microwave pretreatment was evaluated but produced marked tissue disintegration and was not used.

Normal skin and adnexa

The immunohistochemical staining of normal and hyperplastic canine and feline epidermis is summarized in Table 3.3.5. In dogs and cats AE3 and Multi-CK stained all four layers of normal and hyperplastic epidermis, while CK10, a cytokeratin specific for epidermal differentiation, stained the suprabasal cells of normal and hyperplastic epidermis. AE1/AE3, a commonly used antibody, did not stain normal epidermis but did stain hyperplastic epidermis. Merkel cells in the epidermis stained with AE1, AE1/3 and CK20.

Canine and feline adnexa

Hair follicles

The infundibulum had an identical staining pattern to the epidermis, the outer cells representing the basal cells and the inner cells the suprabasal cells (Table 3.3.6). The upper part of the external root sheath (ERS) stained with AE1, AE3, AE1/3 and Multi-CK, whereas the glycogen-rich cells of the inferior region of the external root did not stain with AE1 and AE1/3. The cells found in the lowest inferior segment of the external root sheath stained lightly with AE1 and AE1/3. The inner root sheath (IRS) cells only stained with CAM5.2. Follicular germinal cells did not stain with any of the cytokeratin markers, but some suprabasal follicular matrical cells stained with CK10, indicating that there is cross-reactivity between epidermal and follicular matrical cytokeratins.

Sebaceous glands

At the periphery of the sebaceous lobules the undifferentiated cells that have small, hyperchromatic nuclei and little cytoplasm did not stain with any of the immunohistochemical markers. Immature sebocytes with a small amount of cytoplasm stained with CD79a in the dog but not the cat, and stained with AE3 and Multi-CK in the dog and cat. Mature sebocytes with pyknotic nuclei and abundant vacuolated cytoplasm stained lightly with CD79a in the dog and with Multi-CK in the dog and cat. The sebaceous duct did not stain with CD79a but had the same staining pattern as the inner infundibulum (Table 3.3.7).

Apocrine and eccrine glands

The secretory epithelium of the canine and feline apocrine and eccrine glands stained with CAM5.2 but not Multi-CK. The myoepithelium stained with Multi-CK and calponin. The inner cells of the apocrine and eccrine ducts stain could be differentiated from the basal cells, as the basal cells only stained with AE3 and Multi-CK. The inner cells of the ducts in close proximity to the secretory epithelium stained with CAM5.2, but as the duct approached the infundibulum and the cells cornified, the staining affinity was lost. The eccrine acrosyringium stained with AE1, AE3, AE1/3 and CK10 (Table 3.3.8).

Neoplasms

The staining of normal and neoplastic epithelial cells with AE1 and AE1/3 is identical, so only the staining with AE1 will be reported for the neoplasms.

Table 3.3.5. Immunohistochemistry of canine and feline epidermis

	AE1	AE3	AE1/3	Multi-CK	CK10	CK20
Canine and feline						
Normal						
Cornified	±[a]	+	±[a]	+	+	−
Granular	−	+	−	+	+	−
Spinous	−	+	−	+	+	−
Basal	−	+	−	+	−	−
Hyperplastic						
Cornified	+	+	+	+	+	−
Granular	+	+	+	+	+	−
Spinous	+	+	+	+	+	−
Basal	−	+	−	+	−	−
Merkel cells	+	−	+	−	−	+

[a] Non-specific.

Table 3.3.6. Immunohistochemical staining of the hair follicle

		AE1	AE3	AE1/3	Multi-CK	CK10	CAM5.2	CK20	CD79a	CALP
Infundibulum	Outer cells	−	+	−	+	−	−	−	−	−
	Inner cells	±	+	±	+	+	−	−	−	−
Isthmus/inferior	OS/outer cells	±	+	±	+	−	−	−	−	−
	OS/inner cells	+	+	+	+	−	−	−	−	−
	IS	−	−	−	−	−	+	−	−	−
Bulb		−	−	−	−	−	−	−	−	−

IS: Inner root sheath; OS: outer root sheath.

Table 3.3.7. Immunohistochemical staining of the sebaceous gland

		AE1	AE3	AE1/3	Multi-CK	CK10	CAM5.2	CK20	CD79a	CALP
Canine										
Sebaceous gland	Basal cells	−	−	−	−	−	−	−	−	−
	Immature sebocytes	−	+	−	+	−	−	−	+	−
	Mature sebocytes	−	−	−	+	−	−	−	+	−
Duct		+	+	+	+	−	−	−	−	−
Feline										
Sebaceous gland	Basal cells	+	−	+	−	−	−	−	−	−
	Immature sebocytes	−	+	−	+	−	−	−	−	−
	Mature sebocytes	−	−	−	+	−	−	−	−	−
Duct		+	+	+	+	−	−	−	−	−

Table 3.3.8. Immunohistochemical staining of apocrine (epitrichial) and eccrine (atrichial) glands

		AE1	AE3	AE1/3	Multi-CK	CK10	CAM5.2	CK20	CD79a	CALP
Apocrine gland										
Secretory segment	Epithelium	+	+	+	−	−	+	−	−	−
	Myoepithelium	−	−	−	+	−	−	−	−	+
Ductal segment	Inner cells	+	+	+	+	−	±	−	−	−
	Basal cells	−	+	−	+	−	−	−	−	−
Eccrine gland										
Secretory segment	Epithelium	+	+	+	−	−	+	−	−	−
	Myoepithelium	−	−	−	+	−	−	−	−	+
Ductal segment	Inner cells	+	+	+	+	−	±	−	−	−
	Basal cells	−	+	−	+	−	−	−	−	−
Acrosyringium		+	+	+	+	+	−	−	−	−

Feline basal cell tumor

Composed of lobules of oval basaloid cells with a scant amount of cytoplasm, those neoplastic cells with little cytoplasm did not stain with AE1 and Multi-CK, whereas cells with a more abundant cytoplasm stained with AE1 and Multi-CK. All neoplastic cells stained with AE3, did not stain with CK10 and stained focally with CAM5.2. This is an indication of apocrine ductal differentiation in which the inner ductal cells stain with AE1, AE3 and Multi-CK. Thus, feline basal cell tumors should be classified as poorly differentiated apocrine ductal adenomas and not basal cell tumors of the epidermis.

Infiltrative feline basal cell carcinoma

All cells stained with AE3 and Multi-CK and there was focal staining with AE1, but no staining with CK10 and CAM5.2. In the clear-cell variant of feline basal cell carcinoma, all cells stained with AE3 and Multi-CK, but did not stain with AE1, CK10 and CAM5.2. The clear-cell variant represents a true basal cell carcinoma, while the presence of occasional cells that stained AE1 positive in the infiltrative variant is indicative of focal cytokeratin expression mimicking that found in the hyperplastic epidermis and the inner cells of the ERS of the hair follicle.

Canine papilloma and inverted papilloma

These had an identical staining pattern to hyperplastic epidermis. The keratinocytes, which on H&E staining have a basophilic cytoplasm, stained only faintly with AE3 and did not stain with AE1, Multi-CK or CK10, indicating that viral infection of these cells prevents the production of normally expressed cytokeratins by these cells.

Squamous cell carcinoma *in situ* in the feline and invasive squamous cell carcinoma in the canine and feline

These stained with AE3 and Multi-CK, but not with AE1 and CK10, the epidermal differentiation marker.

Invasive squamous cell carcinomas in the canine and feline did stain with AE1, AE3 and Multi-CK. The staining intensity was variable, with less differentiated cells at the periphery of the invasive cords and more anaplastic cells staining lightly with AE1, AE3 and Multi-CK. The staining of the *in situ* tumors resembled epidermal basal cells, and the staining of the invasive tumors resembled hyperplastic epidermis.

Basosquamous carcinoma in the canine

The peripheral basaloid cells stained lightly with AE3 and Multi-CK, while the central keratinized cells stained with AE1, AE3 and Multi-CK and focally with CK10. The staining pattern most resembled that of the hyperplastic epidermis and follicular infundibulum, although follicular matrical cells also stain with CK10.

Infundibular keratinizing acanthoma

The peripheral cords of epithelial cells stained with AE3 and Multi-CK, but not with AE1 and CK10. The central cells with the lightly eosinophilic cytoplasm stained with AE1, AE3 and Multi-CK and focally with CK10. As the name implies, this is a neoplasm with infundibular differentiation.

Canine trichoblastoma

The immunohistochemical staining varied depending on the subtype. In the ribbon subtype of trichoblastoma, neoplastic cells stained with AE3 and Multi-CK and did not stain with AE1 and CK10. In the medusa head pattern, the central cells of the head stained with AE1, whereas the cells radiating from the head were AE1 negative. All cells stained with AE3 and Multi-CK, but not with CK10. In the granular cell subtype, all cells stained with AE3 and Multi-CK, and multifocally with AE1, primarily in the center of the lobules, but not with CK10. The staining pattern resembled that of the isthmic portion of the ERS of the follicle.

Feline trichoblastoma

In the trabecular subtype, all cells stained with AE3 and Multi-CK, but not with AE1 and CK10. In the spindle cell subtype, all cells stained with AE3 and Multi-CK. Cells in the center of the lobules, with a more extensive eosinophilic cytoplasm, stained with AE1, while the peripheral cells did not stain. The staining pattern of the feline trichoblastomas also resembled that of the isthmic portion of the ERS of the follicle.

Tricholemmoma

In the isthmic variant, the cells at the periphery of the tumor stained with AE3 and Multi-CK. The central foci of tricholemmal keratinization stained with AE1, AE3 and Multi-CK. The neoplastic cells did not stain with CK10. In the inferior variant, the cells stained with AE1, AE3 and Multi-CK. CK10 stained the cells in the center of the lobules, indicating focal matrical differentiation by this tumor which shows differentiation to the lower inferior region of the follicle.

Trichoepitheliomas

These varied considerably in their histopathological appearance and immunohistochemical staining. The small basaloid cells analogous to those of the bulb and many of the larger basaloid cells did not stain with AE1, AE3, Multi-CK or CK10. There were foci of positive staining with AE1, AE3, Multi-CK, CK10 and CAM5.2, representing differentiation to the infundiulum, outer and inner root sheath and hair matrix. This is identical to the case described for the normal canine and feline follicle. Canine malignant trichoepithelioma cells stained positive with AE1, AE3, Multi-CK and CK10 where the neoplastic cells showed matrical differentiation.

Pilomatricoma

Many of the basaloid cells did not stain with AE1 and very lightly with AE3 and CK10. A single row of cells at the periphery of the lobules stained with Multi-CK, but the central cells did not. The 'ghost' cells stained with AE1 and AE3 but not with Multi-CK, CK10 or CAM5.2. Columns of cells, extending from the periphery to the center of the lobules, stained with AE1, AE3, Multi-CK and focally with CK10 and CAM5.2, which represents an abortive attempt to form a hair follicle. Individual cells within the foci of osseous metaplasia stained with AE1, AE3 and Multi-CK. Similar staining was found with malignant pilomatricoma.

Canine subungual keratoacanthoma

All neoplastic cells stained with AE1 and AE3 and the peripheral cells stained with Multi-CK but not with CK10. Subungual squamous cell carcinoma had the staining properties described above for epidermal squamous cell carcinoma.

Sebaceous and modified sebaceous glands

The immunohistochemical staining of canine and feline sebaceous and modified sebaceous gland neoplasms (Meibomian and hepatoid) is shown in Table 3.3.9.

Table 3.3.9. Immunohistochemical identification of apocrine and sebaceous neoplasms

	Canine				Feline				
	AE1	Multi-CK	CAM5.2	CD79a	AE1	AE3	Multi-CK	CK10	CAM5.2
Sebaceous glandular neoplasm	−	+	−	+	−	±	+	−	−
Sebaceous ductal neoplasm	+	+	−	−	+	+	+	+	−
Apocrine secretory neoplasm	+	−	+	−	+	+	−	−	+
Apocrine ductal neoplasm	+	+	+	−	+	+	+	−	+

Canine sebaceous, Meibomian and hepatoid gland tumors

Cells showing sebaceous (intracytoplasmic lipid vacuoles) and hepatoid cell (eosinophilic cytoplasm) differentiation stained with CD79a, AE3 and Multi-CK, but not with AE1 or CK10, while areas of ductal differentiation only stained with AE1, AE3 and Multi-CK. Reserve cells, which are the predominant cells in sebaceous and Meibomian gland epitheliomas, did not stain with any of the antibodies, but in hepatoid gland epitheliomas the reserve cells stained lightly with AE3 and Multi-CK.

Feline sebaceous and Meibomian tumor

Cells with sebaceous differentiation stained with Multi-CK and very lightly with AE3. Foci of ductal differentiation stained with AE1, AE3 and Multi-CK and lightly with CK10.

Apocrine and modified apocrine gland tumors

The immunohistochemical staining of canine and feline neoplasms of apocrine, ceruminous or anal sac gland (epitrichial glands) of secretory and ductal origin is shown in Table 3.3.9. Neoplasms showing differentiation to the secretory segment of epitrichial gland did not stain with Multi-CK, but the myoepithelial cells stained with Multi-CK. Those neoplasms showing differentiation to the ductal segment, the inner and outer cell, stained with Multi-CK. Apocrine carcinomas stained with AE1, AE3 and Multi-CK, indicating that they show inner ductal differentiation, whereas ceruminous carcinomas did not stain with Multi-CK, indicating that they show secretory epithelial differentiation.

Anal sac gland carcinoma

Cells stained Multi-CK negative in the dog, indicating secretory differentiation, and Multi-CK positive in the cat, indicating ductal differentiation. The few cases of eccrine carcinoma available for evaluation stained with AE1, AE3, Multi-CK and CAM5.2.

Discussion

One of the dilemmas faced by veterinary pathologists is making a definitive diagnosis on poorly differentiated or undifferentiated epithelial skin neoplasms. Malignant epithelial skin neoplasms exhibit differences in biological behavior that are directly related to the differentiation of these neoplasms. For example, apocrine carcinomas are more likely to metastasize than sebaceous carcinomas, while carcinomas showing ductal differentiation have a better prognosis than those of glandular origin. By establishing the staining pattern of epithelial neoplasms with specific monoclonal antibodies that are commercially available, a method is presented for achieving this in some but not all instances.

Using the methods described above, the AE1/3 combination of antibodies has the same staining affinity as AE1. Previous work by A.C. Schneider (personal communication) using AE1/3 with trypsin pretreatment rather than proteinase K pretreatment showed significantly less intense staining with AE1/3 than AE1 alone, indicating that the concentration of AE1 antibody in the cocktail is too low to stain the epidermal cells adequately. By using the EnVision system, the present group was also able to improve the staining intensity of the positively staining cells compared with the two-step biotinylated secondary antibody and streptavidin peroxidase conjugated method used previously. However, optimal staining was not achieved in all cases, which was attributed to the large size of some of the tumors, with poor fixation resulting in suboptimal staining, or to the length of time that the tumor had been in formalin before processing.

Feline basal cell tumors are not basal cell tumors but poorly differentiated apocrine ductal tumors, which confirms the findings previously reported by

Walder (1998). However, the staining pattern and intimate association of basal cell carcinoma with the epidermis suggest that they are epidermal basal cell carcinomas.

Although most squamous cell carcinomas can be identified on routine histopathology, poorly differentiated tumors should be stained with AE1, AE3 and Multi-CK as the neoplastic cells stain very lightly with these antibodies. Using all three antibodies increases the likelihood of obtaining positive staining. Squamous cell carcinoma *in situ* does not stain with CK10, the marker for epidermal differention, indicating that the proliferating neoplastic cells present in the basal and spinous layer and ERS of the hair follicles are not differentiated squamous epithelial cells but basal epidermal cells with an extensive amount of eosinophilic cytoplasm, in contrast to the normal basal keratinocyte which has scant amphophilic cytoplasm. Basosquamous carcinomas are best categorized as a neoplasm showing epidermal/infundibular differentiation.

CAM5.2 identifies all neoplasms with epitrichial and atrichial differentiation, and Multi-CK is a marker for ductal differentiation and myoepithelial cells in these neoplasms. CD79a is a marker for sebaceous differentiation in the dog but not the cat. The cross-reactivity of canine sebaceous cells and CD79a, a monoclonal antibody to human B-lymphocytes, is unusual, but probably analogous with the positive staining of follicular stem cells by anti-CD8 monoclonal antibody in humans (Lyle *et al.*, 1998). It is therefore possible, using immunohistochemistry, to differentiate apocrine from sebaceous neoplasms and ductal from secretory neoplasms in the dog and cat (Table 3.3.9).

The staining pattern of the follicular neoplasms, except for trichoblastomas, is analogous to the histological appearance of these neoplasms. CK10 is a useful marker for early trichogenic differentiation. Merkel cells stain with AE1 and CK20, but the authors have been unable to identify any Merkel cell tumors, although it was possible to identify normal Merkel cells within the epidermis and follicular bulbs of normal skin at the periphery of the neoplasms.

One of the dilemmas that remained unresolved is how to classify those carcinomas made up of sheets of small basophilic cells. This study was unable to determine whether these were epidermal, follicular, apocrine or sebaceous neoplasms. The undifferentiated cells that are found in the follicular bulb and sebaceous gland in normal skin did not stain with any of the cytokeratin markers used here This may be an indication that these neoplasms do not express any of the cytokeratins that could be identified with these antibodies, or that they are expressed at such low levels as to be undetectable by this method. Perhaps these are neoplasms resembling the germinative cells found in the developing skin during embrogenesis.

Conclusion

Five cytokeratin-specific antibodies, AE1, AE3, Multi-CK, CK10 and CAM5.2, were the most helpful in categorizing and identifying feline epithelial neoplasms, with the addition of CD79a to the canine panel to identify sebaceous or modified sebaceous glandular epithelial neoplasms, and CK20 to stain Merkel cells.

References

Cooper, D., Schermer, A. & Sun, T.-T. (1985) Classification of human epithelia and their neoplasms using monoclonal antibodies to keratins: strategies, applications and limitations. *Laboratory Investigation*, **52**, 243–256.

Goldschmidt, M. H., Dunstan, R. W., Stannard, A. A., Tscharner, C. von, Walder, E. J. & Yager, J. A. (1998) *Histological Classification of Epithelial and Melanocytic Tumors of the Skin of Domestic Animals*, 2nd Series, Vol. III. Armed Forces Institute of Pathology, Washington, DC.

Lyle, S., Christofidou-Solomidou, M., Liu, Y., Elder, D. E., Albelda, S. & Cotsarelis, G. (1998) The C8/144B monoclonal antibody recognizes cytokeratin 15 and defines the location of human hair follicle stem cells. *Journal of Cell Science*, **111**, 3179–3188.

Moll, R., Franke, W. W., Schiller, D. L., Geiger, B. & Krepler, R. (1982) The catalog of human cytokeratins patterns of expression in normal epithelia, tumors and cultured cells. *Cell*, **31**, 11–24.

Moll, R., Schiller, D. L. & Franke, W. W. (1990) Identification of protein IT of the intestinal cytoskeleton as a novel type I cytokeratin with unusual properties and expression patterns. *Journal of Cell Biology*, **111**, 567–580.

Walder, E. J. (1998) Immunohistochemical staining patterns in canine and feline basal cell carcinomas, trichoblastomas and trichoepitheliomas. In: *Advances in Veterinary Dermatology*, Vol. 3 (Eds K. W. Kwochka, T. Willemse & C. von Tscharner), pp. 384–385. Butterworth Heinemann, Oxford.

Part 4

Immunological Diseases

4.1

Atopic dermatitis: basic and comparative observations

J.M. Hanifin MD

Department of Dermatology, Oregon Health Sciences University, Portland, Oregon, USA

Summary

Atopic dermatitis (AD) is a highly pruritic, inflammatory skin disease that usually begins during infancy and follows a chronically relapsing course. AD is characterized by erythema, papulation and often weeping lesions due to the spongiotic microvesiculation within the epidermis. Secondary lesions include excoriation and lichenification, reflecting the severe pruritus and scratching. Hair loss, while not typical of human disease, does occur, secondary to scratching. AD is exacerbated by infection, stress, seasonal and climatic changes, irritants and allergens, but is basically a constitutional condition which can be transferred by bone marrow transplantation, giving the recipient abnormal immune and inflammatory cells that circulate and infiltrate the skin with $CD4^+$ T-cells, macrophages and eosinophils.

Patients with AD manifest a variety of physiological, pharmacological and immunological abnormalities that are caused by cyclic nucleotide dysregulation. Studies have demonstrated hyperfunctional phosphodiesterase isoforms and consequently deficient cyclic AMP modulation of the immune and inflammatory cells that infiltrate, causing hyperreactivity in skin and respiratory tissues. Immunological consequences include increased serum immunoglobulin E antibodies against airborne and food allergens, and disordered cellular immune responses. While it cannot be proven whether AD is caused primarily by allergens, new topical immunosuppressive therapies are able to correct disordered responses and bring stability to otherwise unrestrained inflammation.

Newer insights into the multiple points and pathways of dysregulation in atopic disease are providing an increasing variety of therapeutic approaches. New knowledge is also opening the way for the development of new murine models of AD which should further expand our understanding of AD.

Introduction

Atopic dermatitis (AD) is a highly pruritic, inflammatory skin disease that begins early in life and follows a chronic or chronically relapsing course. The disease usually moderates with age, but patients carry a lifelong sensitivity to irritants and a tendency towards dry skin problems. AD is eczematous, characterized by erythema, papulation, edema and often weeping lesions, reflecting the spongiotic microvesiculation within the epidermis. Secondary lesions may include excoriation and lichenification, reflecting the scratching and rubbing that arise from the intense itching associated with the disease. Hair loss, while not typically considered prominent in the human disease, definitely does occur, secondary to scratching, on the scalp and eyebrows. Diagnosis is usually clinically evident and based on the presence of a constellation of features (Hanifin & Lobitz, 1977). Four of the following features must be present for a diagnosis of AD:

- highly pruritic eczematous eruption
- typical morphology and distribution
  - face and extensors during infancy/childhood
  - elbow/knee flexors later
- chronic or chronically relapsing course
- early age of onset
- personal or family history of atopy.

While AD may be exacerbated by infection, psychological stress, seasonal and climatic changes, irritants and allergens, it is basically a constitutional, intrinsic inflammatory propensity to intense flaring in the absence of any discernible environmental triggers. This intrinsic trait has been shown to be transferred by bone marrow transplantation (Agosti *et al.*, 1988), conferring the recipient with abnormal immune and inflammatory cells that act as vectors, circulating through the blood and infiltrating the skin to bring the clinical disease.

This article is a review of the immunological and physiological features of AD, along with a discussion of pathogenic concepts that have emerged in recent years. The ongoing extensions of these theories are being translated into interesting and new novel directions for therapy of AD.

Basic abnormalities

Histologically, AD is characterized by epidermal spongiosis and varying degrees of epidermal proliferation (reflecting clinical lichenification), along with lymphocytic infiltration of predominantly $CD4^+$ T-cells into the dermis and epidermis, and increased numbers of dermal macrophages and eosinophils (Thepen *et al.*, 1996).

T-cells

T-helper ($CD4^+$) lymphocytes predominate in the dermal infiltrate of lesional AD. Histology closely resembles that of allergic contact dermatitis. Immunocytochemistry studies have demonstrated increased numbers of T-cells bearing the cutaneous lymphocyte-associated antigen (CLA), similar to other inflammatory skin diseases (Santamaria Babi *et al.*, 1995). Reflections from cytokine studies suggest that type 2 (Th_2) T-cells may predominate in the circulation and lesions of AD, but this surmise remains speculative (Thepen *et al.*, 1996), as will be discussed below.

Mononuclear phagocytes and dendritic cells

In recent years, considerable interest has focused on the role of Langerhans' cells in the pathogenesis of AD. The author has previously demonstrated increased numbers of these cells in chronic AD lesions (Uno & Hanifin, 1980), and Bruijnzeel-Koomen *et al.* (1986) subsequently showed that increased numbers of these cells bear cytophilic immunoglobulin E (IgE) antibodies, observations which led to the finding of increased FcεR2 (CD23) expression and the presence of FcεR1 high-affinity IgE receptors on Langerhans' cells and monocytes from patients with AD (Bieber *et al.*, 1989).

Eosinophils

The presence of eosinophils in AD lesions, while only sporadically evident on routine histology, was highlighted through the use of immunocytochemistry by Leiferman *et al.* (1985). They detected the presence of these cells, often in a degradative state, through the use of labeled polyclonal antibodies against eosinophil-specific major basic protein (MBP). Toxic eosinophil proteins such as MBP and eosinophil cationic protein (ECP) may be effector molecules which create an inflammatory milieu that leads to the clinical expression of AD.

Pharmacophysiological abnormalities

Patients with AD manifest a variety of physiological and pharmacological abnormalities including vasoconstriction in the fingers, a positive cold-pressor test and white dermographism (Hanifin, 1986). A delayed blanching response after intradermal injection of acetylcholine and methacholine is seen (Hanifin, 1986), similar to the hyperreactivity bronchoconstriction that asthma patients manifest after inhalation of methacholine (Barker *et al.*, 1991).

Observations from such clinical responses, along with information from animal models, led Szentivanyi (1968) to suggest that atopic patients appeared to have a blockade of β-adrenergic receptors, allowing the cholinergic overreactivity. He proposed that increased pharmacological reactivity is a basic characteristic of atopic disease and that allergic reactions are only one of a group of factors, along with infections, emotional stress, chemical and physical stimuli, that trigger the pathological reactions in asthma, AD and allergic rhinitis.

This work stimulated creative new research efforts using *in vitro* studies of leukocytes, and demonstrated deficient cyclic AMP (cAMP) responses to β-adrenergic agents in AD cells (Parker & Eisen, 1972). Subsequent studies showed that this defect was not limited to the β-adrenergic receptor, because similarly deficient cAMP responses occurred when cells were stimulated by other adenyl cyclase agonists such as prostaglandin E_2 (PGE_2) and histamine (Safko *et al.*, 1981). This forced the conclusion that a defect must therefore be further down the stimulatory pathway, leading to the demonstration of hyperfunctional phosphodiesterase (PDE) isoforms in atopic leukocytes causing increased cAMP hydrolysis (Grewe *et al.*, 1982; Chan *et al.*, 1993a). The resulting deficiency in intracellular cAMP modulation results in overactive responses of the immune and inflammatory cells that circulate and infiltrate skin and respiratory tissues in atopic disease.

Immunological associations

IgE reactivity

Individuals with AD usually have increased serum IgE antibodies against airborne or ingested protein antigens and a personal or family history of allergic rhinitis or asthma. Some of the earliest investigations of AD centered on the striking incidence and numbers of type I immediate skin-test responses to foods and aeroallergens. Then, with the later discovery of IgE, came quantitative evidence that this immunoglobulin was greatly increased in the serum of most patients with AD. This very consistent association has stimulated 80 years of research efforts aimed at finding a pathogenic role for the skin-sensitizing, reaginic, IgE-type antibodies in producing the eczematous lesions of AD.

In the years since identifying IgE, however, considerable doubt has evolved over the role of IgE in AD pathogenesis. Serum IgE is elevated in a wide variety of skin diseases other than AD and, conversely, 20% of patients with AD have neither elevated serum IgE nor allergen reactivity (Ohman & Johansson, 1974; Jones *et al.*, 1975). Typical flexural AD occurs in agammaglobulinemic children completely lacking IgE (Peterson *et al.*, 1966). In a study of patients treated with recombinant γ-interferon (IFN-γ), improvement occurred despite escalating serum IgE levels (Hanifin *et al.*, 1993). Clinical observations have long noted that AD usually improves in the spring and summer hayfever season, in spite of maximal aeroallergen levels.

While there is no disputing the role of IgE in causing the respiratory and acute urticarial conditions that accompany AD, there is little direct evidence for an IgE effector function in producing the eczematous cutaneous disease that is AD. Studies in recent years have shown a possible mechanism by which IgE may contribute to the abnormal cellular immune and eczematous responses seen in AD. As noted above, Langerhans' cells are increased in AD lesions. Lesional Langerhans' cells can be hyperstimulatory for autologous T-cells *in vitro* (Taylor *et al.*, 1991), suggesting that aeroallergen-specific IgE may have an antigen-focusing effect, increasing the antigen-presenting function of Langerhans' cells in patients with AD (Mudde *et al.*, 1990). This is difficult to demonstrate clinically, however; in fact, cellular immune responses are usually depressed in the skin of patients with AD (Hanifin & Lobitz, 1977). Recent studies in mice have shown amplification of IgE production when protein antigen is inoculated through skin compared with the nasal route (Herrick *et al.*, 2000). These results suggest the alternative conclusion that the increased IgE in patients with AD may simply result from excessive transcutaneous allergen exposure through damaged AD skin, i.e. elevated IgE may be an epiphenomenon that follows, rather than precedes, eczema.

Cellular immune responses

For over 100 years clinicians have surmised immune incompetence in patients with AD, as reflected in susceptibility to widespread herpes simplex infections and reduced sensitization to poison ivy and other contact allergens (Hanifin & Lobitz, 1977). The immunohistochemical similarities between AD and allergic contact dermatitis (ACD) seem paradoxical in this context (Zachary *et al.*, 1985), but some clarification has occurred in recent years through the conceptualization of the Th_1/Th_2 immunological dichotomy.

Investigators in the early 1990s demonstrated reduced IFN-γ production in cultured peripheral blood mononuclear cells of patients with AD (Reinhold *et al.*, 1990) and subsequent studies showed increased T-cell interleukin-4 (IL-4) production (Jujo *et al.*, 1992; Chan *et al.*, 1993b), although direct analysis of lesional cells was less clear. Immunocytochemical studies have suggested a two-phase process, with a predominance of Th_2 cells expressing IL-4 in acute lesions and later influx of IFN-γ-expressing Th_1 cells (Grewe *et al.*, 1995). The original prediction of distinct IL-4/IFN-γ polarity between AD and ACD was not borne out in studies of cytokine profiles: IFN-γ expression was equally prominent to IL-4 in the AD lesions and, conversely, IL-4 expression was evident in some cases of ACD (Ohmen *et al.*, 1995).

These various and conflicting studies indicate that the *in vivo* cellular expression of cytokines varies greatly within the complex milieu of inflammation and inflammatory mediators. One consistent finding from cytokine profile studies was the increased lesional expression of IL-10, and this was confirmed by the demonstration of increased spontaneous IL-10 production in cultured AD monocytes (Ohmen *et al.*, 1995). This finding of increased monocyte IL-10 production helps to explain the paradox of both increased and reduced cellular immune responsiveness in AD. IL-10 is known to have a suppressive effect on IFN-γ production and on Th_1 cell proliferation, and *in vitro* studies indicated that monocytes may be the cause of decreased IFN-γ production by T-cells from patients with AD (Chan *et al.*, 1993c).

Functional abnormalities, both biochemical and immunological, have been noted in the infiltrating cells as well as in the circulating leukocytes in AD (Hanifin & Chan, 1995). These aberrations have led to research along different pathways, but centered upon immunological and pharmacological responses in leukocytes. Considerable effort has been expended since the 1980s attempting to distinguish the major effector cells that create the skin damage that results in clinical AD. A very recent report may shed considerable light on this question. This study used a novel and creative approach to investigate the processes that result in the eczematous changes of AD and contact allergy. Using both *in vitro* and *in situ* systems, Trautmann *et al.* (2000) showed that Fas protein is up-regulated on human keratinocytes by IFN-γ and that activated T-cells, in turn, cause apoptotic cell death of the primed keratinocytes, in advance of spongiotic eczematous disease. If confirmed, this process could explain much of what is known to occur in AD: (1) spongiosis, (2) similar histology in AD and ACD (Zachary *et al.*, 1985), (3) increased cytokine expression of IFN-γ in both AD and ACD (Ohmen *et al.*, 1995), and (4) increased IFN-γ production by AD T-cells (Chan *et al.*, 1993c).

Seeking a unifying paradigm

Collectively, the concepts described above provide a basis for unifying the immunological and pharmacophysiological defects that are so ubiquitous in AD leukocytes and in the clinical disease. Deficient cAMP regulation of immune and inflammatory cells can account for the many hyperfunctional cells and mediator pathways that have been demonstrated in AD over the years (Hanifin & Chan, 1995). A key to our understanding of this wide-based regulatory dysfunction was the demonstration that atopic disease, including airways reactivity, eczema and antigen-specific IgE overproduction, could all be transferred by bone marrow transplantation (Agosti *et al.*, 1988). These hematopoietic cells, which infiltrate skin and respiratory mucosa and react inappropriately to cause inflammation and aberrant immunological responses, are likely to reflect the abnormal expression of multiple atopy-associated genes.

A unifying concept depends on resolving two pathophysiological paradigms, one relating to fundamental abnormalities in cyclic nucleotide regulation of the marrow-derived cells, and the other centered on the belief that allergenic overstimulation is the primary event causing the secondary immunological and pharmacophysiological abnormalities.

In the former hypothesis, the core atopic defect results from genetically defined PDE isoforms which cause excessive enzyme hydrolysis, leading to inadequate cellular cAMP, inadequate negative modulation and inflammatory cells that fail to shut off normally. The resulting hyperreactivity can explain many of the features of atopy, including excessive reactivity to irritants (Nassif *et al.*, 1994), excessive release of mast cell histamine (Butler *et al.*, 1983) and increased production of cytokines (IL-4, IFN-γ) and IgE.

This cyclic nucleotide hypothesis is also inclusive of the striking non-immunological characteristics of AD, i.e. skin hyperirritancy and reactive airway disease, even in those 20% of patients lacking allergic IgE reactivity (Barker *et al.*, 1991; Nassif *et al.*, 1994).

In contrast, the allergic hypothesis posits early, possibly *in utero*, antigenic exposures that stimulate, in the genetically susceptible individual, proliferation of Th_2-dominant T-cell clones. After later antigen re-exposure, these preferentially elaborate cytokines such as IL-4, IL-5, IL-6, IL-10 and IL-13 which, in turn, mediate excessive B-cell IgE production and a tendency towards eosinophil-rich inflammation. In this milieu, mast cell-initiated reactions to specific antigens may, if chronically exposed, produce eczematous disease, asthma and allergic rhinitis.

Therapy can sidestep conflicting concepts

The above hypotheses are typical of currently unprovable 'chicken and egg' conflicts and the controversies will remain until atopy is defined at the molecular level. Fortunately, there is no need to wait for conflict resolution to use available information suggesting therapeutically viable approaches. In recent years, the two pathogenic paradigms of cyclic nucleotide dysfunction and allergy have provided some novel therapeutic approaches for AD.

Immune suppressors

Immunosuppressive agents that have been used for treating AD include glucocorticosteroids, azathioprine, methotrexate and the macrolides (Sidbury & Hanifin, 2000). This discussion will focus primarily on the latter group of agents and, particularly, on the newer, more selective drugs for immune intervention. These compounds, known as macrolides or macrolactams, are characterized by large ring structures. All bind to unrelated cytosolic binding proteins, known as immunophilins (Ho *et al.*, 1996; Bieber, 1998), and all function through a common pathway resulting in the formation of complexes that block the phosphatase activity of calcineurin. This, in turn, blocks activation of the nuclear factor of activated T-cells (NF-AT), inhibiting the initiation of cytokine transcription. Immunosuppressive drugs that function through this pathway include cyclosporin A (CsA), FK506 (tacrolimus), rapamycin and the ascomycin derivative SDZ ASM 981 (pimecrolimus).

Oral CsA and FK506 have been available for many years as drugs for the prevention of transplant rejection. While the latter has seen little use in the treatment of AD, oral cyclosporin has been used successfully since the late 1980s as a therapy for severe AD (Sowden *et al.*, 1991). Because of its toxicity as a systemic agent, however, CsA was tested as a topical drug for AD but was found to be ineffective, presumably because of poor transcutaneous penetration (De Rie *et al.*, 1991). In contrast, when FK506, a molecule only slightly smaller than CsA, was tested for topical efficacy, it was found to be highly effective, both in animal models and in clinical trials in AD (Aoyama *et al.*, 1995; Ruzicka *et al.*, 1997). FK506 ointment is absorbed passively through the skin, with relatively little of the drug entering the systemic circulation, and clinical studies suggest that systemic absorption decreases as local eczematous inflammation subsides and conditions improve (Alaiti *et al.*, 1998). This topical drug shows little accumulation in the skin or the systemic circulation, despite prolonged, repeated topical administration. No systemic side-effects or signs of cutaneous immunosuppression have been reported in either short- or long-term clinical trials (Boguniewicz *et al.*, 1998). Only application site burning and itching have been noted, and these symptoms usually cease after healing of the eroded skin.

The other class of drugs being developed for immune intervention comprises the macrolactam inflammatory cytokine inhibitors derived from ascomycins, of which SDZ ASM 981 has been further developed. In preclinical models, SDZ ASM 981 applied topically showed potency comparable to a potent corticosteroid without local side-effects (Meingassner *et al.*, 1997). In contrast to CsA and oral FK506, ASM showed a low potential for systemic immunosuppression (Meingassner *et al.*, 1997). Topical ASM efficacy and safety have been demonstrated in patients with moderate AD (Van Leent *et al.*, 1998). Applications were well tolerated, with localized burning and stinging resembling reactions to topical FK506, but there were no systemic adverse reactions or skin atrophy. Blood levels of the drug showed no accumulation after repeated applications in patients with AD (Meingassner *et al.*, 1997; Van Leent *et al.*, 1998).

This promising preclinical and early clinical profile suggests that the topical macrolactam immunosuppressants may offer the potent activity of a topical corticosteroid without local side-effects such as skin atrophy (Reitamo *et al.*, 1998). Additional clinical investigations are ongoing. Long-term safety evaluations of both FK506 and SDZ ASM 981 will be important in defining the future of these much-needed drugs for treating patients with AD.

Phosphodiesterase inhibitors

PDE inhibitors provide an approach that targets the multiple cell and mediator pathways controlled by cAMP and defective in AD. Aminophylline/theophylline has been used for many years in the treatment of asthma and, given as the intravenous preparation, it can provide dramatic relief from the severe itching of AD (Epstein, 1946). Oral theophylline, however, lacks potency and has little effect in AD (Hanifin *et al.*, 1996). Systemic treatment with more potent PDE inhibitors has not been feasible because they are associated with a high incidence of nausea and vomiting, although newly developed agents appear to hold promise for eliminating the central nervous system toxicity that has previously caused intolerable side-effects (Christensen *et al.*, 1998).

Topical caffeine compounded as a 30% cream showed efficacy in one study, but the compound was weak and cosmetically unacceptable (Kaplan *et al.*, 1978). More potent, type IV PDE inhibitors have been developed over the years and are being studied as topical agents for AD and as oral agents for asthma (Houslay *et al.*, 1998). Topical Ro 20-1724 was studied as a 1% cream and shown to be approximately as effective as hydrocortisone cream, but it was not developed further. A group of related compounds was screened for *in vitro* potency and one, CP 80633, was found to be 100–1000-fold more potent than theophylline (Hanifin *et al.*, 1996). In a randomized, controlled clinical trial, it provided rapid and persistent reduction of inflammatory lesion scores when applied to AD lesions as a 0.5% cream and no adverse reactions. Similar PDE inhibitors are being developed and other even more potent agents can be anticipated in coming years.

Needed: a reliable animal model

Several animal models have been proposed over the years, and these demonstrate that all models need to be thoroughly and critically scrutinized before they are accepted as AD. Hansen (1933) erroneously suggested that rats fed a diet deficient in essential fatty acids developed eczema, whereas in reality it was a scaly, nutritional degenerative condition. At first sight, canine AD would appear to be an ideal model and certainly much has been gleaned from colonies of atopic canines (Schwartzman & Rockey, 1967; Patterson & Kelly, 1974). An AD-like condition was described in asthmatic Basenji–Greyhound dogs, which demonstrated PDE abnormalities identical to those found in human leukocytes (Butler *et al.*, 1983). While canines appear to represent reasonable AD comparators, their size and variability, along with the relative lack of immunological information and reagents compared with mice or other rodent species, has impeded the development of a dog model.

Murine species would appear to provide a more practical area for the development of a model, and considerable progress has been made since the early 1990s. Japanese investigators induced a chronic eczematous condition along with increased serum IgE in mice repeatedly sensitized with DNCB skin applications (Kitagaki *et al.*, 1995). Another Japanese group described an itchy dermatitis and high serum IgE in NC/Nga mice raised in non-germ-free conditions (Matsuda *et al.*, 1996). Recently, two US groups described enhanced IgE responses in mice sensitized to protein antigens through the skin, and in some cases these mice developed eczematous lesions (Spergel *et al.*, 1998; Herrick *et al.*, 2000). One of the most interesting and potentially useful models was reported recently in the form of an IL-4 transgenic mouse (Chan, 2000). This model produces large amounts of IL-4 in the epidermis and develops a severe pruritic eczematous eruption, secondary infections and high serum IgE levels. While all of these models await critical assessment and confirmation, the increasing development of such murine models bodes well for progress in understanding and treating AD.

References

Agosti, J. M., Sprenger, J. D., Lum, L. G., Witherspoon, R. P., Fisher, L. D., Storb, R. *et al.* (1988) Transfer of allergen-specific IgE-mediated hypersensitivity with allogeneic bone marrow transplantation. *New England Journal of Medicine*, **319**, 1623–1628.

Alaiti, S., Kang, S., Fiedler, V. C. *et al.* (1998) Tacrolimus (FK506) ointment for atopic dermatitis: a phase I study in adults and children. *Journal of the American Academy of Dermatology*, **38**, 69–76.

Aoyama, H., Tabata, N., Tanaka, M., Vesugi, Y. & Tagami, H. (1995) Successful treatment of resistant facial lesions of atopic dermatitis with 0.1% FK506 ointment. *British Journal of Dermatology*, **133**, 494–496.

Barker, A. F., Hirshman, C. A., D'Silva, R. & Hanifin, J. M. (1991) Airway responsiveness in atopic dermatitis. *Journal of Allergy and Clinical Immunology*, **87**, 780–783.

Bieber, T. (1998) Topical tacrolimus (FK 506): a new milestone in the management of atopic dermatitis. *Journal of Allergy and Clinical Immunology*, **102**, 555–557.

Bieber, T., Rieger, A., Neuchrist, C., Prinz, J. C., Rieber, E. P., Boltz-Nitulescu, G. *et al.* (1989) Induction of $FceR_2$/CD23 on human epidermal Langerhans' cells by human recombinant interleukin 4 and interferon-γ. *Journal of Experimental Medicine*, **170**, 309–314.

Boguniewicz, M., Fiedler, V. C., Raimer, S., Ellis, C. N., Spurlin, D. V., Fader, D. *et al.* (1998) A randomized vehicle-controlled trial of tacrolimus ointment for treatment of atopic dermatitis in children. *Journal of Allergy and Clinical Immunology*, **102**, 635–642.

Bruijnzeel-Koomen, C. A., Wichen, D. F. van, Toonstra, J., Berrens, L. & Bruijnzeel, P. L. (1986) The presence of IgE molecules on epidermal Langerhans cells in patients with atopic dermatitis. *Archives of Dermatology Research*, **278**, 199–205.

Butler, J. M., Peters, J. E., Hirshman, C. A., White, C. R., Margolin, L. B. & Hanifin, J. M. (1983) Pruritic dermatitis in asthmatic Basenji–Greyhound dogs: a model for human atopic dermatitis. *Journal of the American Academy of Dermatology*, **8**, 33–38.

Chan, L. S. (2000) Expression of interleukin-4 in the epidermis of transgenic mice results in an atopic dermatitis phenotype and severe bacterial infection. *Journal of Investigative Dermatology*, **114**, 779.

Chan, S. C., Reifsnyder, D., Beavo, J. A. & Hanifin, J. M. (1993a) Immunochemical characterization of the distinct monocyte cyclic AMP-phosphodiesterase from patients with atopic dermatitis. *Journal of Allergy and Clinical Immunology*, **91**, 1179–1188.

Chan, S. C., Li, S.-H. & Hanifin, J. M. (1993b) Increased interleukin 4 production by atopic mononuclear leukocytes correlates with increased cyclic AMP-PDE activity and is reversible by PDE inhibition. *Journal of Investigative Dermatology*, **100**, 681–684.

Chan, S. C., Kim, J.-W., Henderson, W. R., Jr & Hanifin, J. M. (1993c) Altered prostaglandin E_2 regulation of cytokine production in atopic dermatitis. *Journal of Immunology*, **151**, 3345–3352.

Christensen, S. B., Guider, A., Forster, C. J., Gleason, J. G., Bender, P. E., Karpinski, J. M. *et al.* (1998) 1,4-Cyclohexanecarboxylates: potent and selective inhibitors of phosphodiesterase 4 for the treatment of asthma. *Journal of Medical Chemistry*, **41**, 821–835.

De Rie, M. A., Meinardi, M. H. M. & Dos, J. (1991) Lack of efficacy of topical cyclosporin A in atopic dermatitis and allergic contact dermatitis. *Acta Dermato-Venereologica*, **71**, 452–454.

Epstein, E. (1946) Theophylline ethylenediamine as an antipruritic agent. *Archives of Dermatology and Syphilology*, **53**, 281–284.

Grewe, M., Walther, S., Gyufko, K., Czech, W., Schopf, E. & Krutmann, J. (1995) Analysis of the cytokine pattern expressed *in situ* in inhalant allergen patch test reactions of atopic dermatitis patients. *Journal of Investigative Dermatology*, **105**, 407–410.

Grewe, S. R., Chan, S. C. & Hanifin, J. M. (1982) Elevated leukocyte cyclic AMP-phosphodiesterase in atopic disease: a possible mechanism for cyclic AMP-agonist hyporesponsiveness. *Journal of Allergy and Clinical Immunology*, **70**, 452–457.

Hanifin, J. M. (1986) Pharmacophysiology of atopic dermatitis. *Clinical Reviews in Allergy*, **4**, 43–65.

Hanifin, J. M. & Chan, S. C. (1995) Monocyte phosphodiesterase abnormalities and dysregulation of lymphocyte function in atopic dermatitis. *Journal of Investigative Dermatology*, **105S**, 84S–88S.

Hanifin, J. M. & Lobitz, W. C. (1977) Newer concepts of atopic dermatitis. *Archives of Dermatology*, **113**, 663–670.

Hanifin, J. M., Chan, S. C., Cheng, J. B., Tofte, S. J., Henderson, W. R., Jr, Kirby, D. S. *et al.* (1996) Type 4 phosphodiesterase inhibitors have clinical and *in vitro* anti-inflammatory effects in atopic dermatitis. *Journal of Investigative Dermatology*, **107**, 51–56.

Hanifin, J. M., Schneider, L. C., Leung, D. Y. M., Ellis, C. N., Jaffe, H. S., Izu, A. E. *et al.* (1993) Recombinant interferon-gamma therapy for atopic dermatitis. *Journal of the American Academy of Dermatology*, **28**, 189–197.

Hansen, A. E. (1933) Study of iodine number of serum fatty acids in infantile eczema. *Proceedings of the Society for Experimental Biology & Medicine*, **30**, 1198–1199.

Herrick, C. A., MacLeod, H., Glusac, E., Tigelaar, R. E. & Bottomly, K. (2000) Th2 responses induced by epicutaneous or inhalational protein exposure are differentially dependent on IL-4. *Journal of Clinical Investigation*, **105**, 765–775.

Ho, S., Clipstone, N., Timmerman, L., Northrop, J., Graef, I., Fiorentino, D. *et al.* (1996) The mechanism of action of cyclosporin A and FK506. *Clinical Immunology and Immunopathology*, **80**, S40–S45.

Houslay, M. D., Sullivan, M. & Bolger, G. B. (1998) The multienzyme PDE_4 cyclic adenosine monophosphate-specific phosphodiesterase family: intracellular targeting, regulation, and selective inhibition by compounds exerting anti-inflammatory and antidepressant actions. *Advances in Pharmacology*, **44**, 225–342.

Jones, H. E., Inouye, J. C., McGerity, J. L. & Lewis, C. W. (1975) Atopic disease and serum immunoglobulin-E. *British Journal of Dermatology*, **92**, 17–25.

Jujo, K. H., Renz, J., Abe, E. W. & Leung, D. Y. M. (1992) Decreased interferon-gamma and increased interleukin 4 production in atopic dermatitis promotes IgE synthesis. *Journal of Allergy and Clinical Immunology*, **90**, 323–331.

Kaplan, R. J., Daman, L., Rosenberg, E. W. & Feigenbaum, S. (1978) Topical use of caffeine with hydrocortisone in the treatment of atopic dermatitis. *Archives of Dermatology*, **114**, 60–62.

Kitagaki, H., Fujisawa, S., Watanabe, K., Hayakawa, K. & Shiohara, T. (1995) Immediate-type hypersensitivity response followed by a late reaction is induced by repeated epicutaneous application of contact sensitizing agents in mice. *Journal of Investigative Dermatology*, **105**, 749–755.

Leiferman, K. M., Ackerman, S. J., Sampson, H. A., Haugen, H. S., Venencie, P. Y. & Gleich, G. J. (1985) Dermal deposition of eosinophil-granule major basic protein in atopic dermatitis. *New England Journal of Medicine*, **313**, 282–285.

Matsuda, H., Watanabe, N., Geba, G. P., Sperl, J., Tsudzuki, M., Hiroi, J. *et al.* (1996) Development of atopic dermatitis-like skin lesion with IgE hyperproduction in NC/Nga mice. *International Immunology*, **9**, 461–466.

Meingassner, J. G., Grassberger, M., Fahrngruber, H., Moore, H. D., Schuurman, H. & Stutz, A. (1997) A novel anti-inflammatory drug, SDZ ASM 981, for the topical and oral treatment of skin diseases: *in vivo* pharmacology. *British Journal of Dermatology*, **137**, 568–576.

Mudde, G. C., Van Reijsen, F. C., Boland, G. J., De Gast, G. C., Bruijnkeel, P. L. & Bruijnkeel-Koomen, C. A. (1990) Allergen presentation by epidermal Langerhans cells from patients with atopic dermatitis is mediated by IgE. *Immunology*, **69**, 335–341.

Nassif, A., Chan, S. C., Storrs, F. J. & Hanifin, J. M. (1994) Abnormal skin irritancy in atopic dermatitis and in atopy without dermatitis. *Archives of Dermatology*, **130**, 1402–1407.

Ohman, S. & Johansson, S. G. (1974) Immunoglobulins in atopic dermatitis. *Acta Dermato-Venereologica*, **54**, 193.

Ohmen, J. D., Hanifin, J. M., Nickoloff, B. J., Rea, T. H., Wyzykowski, R. & Kim, J.-W. (1995) Overexpression of IL-10 in atopic dermatitis: contrasting cytokine patterns with delayed-type hypersensitivity reactions. *Journal of Immunology*, **154**, 1956–1963.

Parker, C. S. & Eisen, A. Z. (1972) Altered cyclic-AMP metabolism in atopic eczema. *Clinical Research*, **20**, 418.

Patterson, R. & Kelly, J. F. (1974) Animal models of the asthmatic state. *Annual Review of Medicine*, **25**, 53–68.

Peterson, R. D., Page, A. R. & Good, R. A. (1966) Wheal and erythema allergy in patients with agammaglobulinemia. *Journal of Allergy*, **33**, 406–411.

Reinhold, U., Wehrmann, W., Kukel, S. & Kreysel, H. W. (1990) Recombinant interferon-γ in severe atopic dermatitis. *Lancet*, **i**, 1282.

Reitamo, S., Rissanen, J., Remitz, A., Granlund, H., Erkko, P., Elg, P. *et al.* (1998) Tacrolimus ointment does not affect collagen synthesis: results of a single-center randomized trial. *Journal of Investigative Dermatology*, **111**, 396–398.

Ruzicka, T., Bieber, T., Schöpf, E., Rubins, A., Dobozy, A., Bos, J. D. *et al.* for the European Tacrolimus Multicenter Atopic Dermatitis Study Group (1997) A short-term trial of tacrolimus ointment for atopic dermatitis. *New England Journal of Medicine*, **337**, 816–821.

Safko, M. J., Chan, S. C., Cooper, K. D. & Hanifin, J. M. (1981) Heterologous desensitization of leukocytes: a possible mechanism of beta adrenergic blockade in atopic dermatitis. *Journal of Allergy and Clinical Immunology*, **68**, 218–225.

Santamaria Babi, L. F., Picker, L. J., Perez Soler, M. T., Drzimalla, K., Flohr, P., Blaser, K. & Hauser, C. (1995) Circulating allergen-reactive T cells from patients with atopic dermatitis and allergic contact dermatitis express the skin-selective homing receptor, the cutaneous lymphocyte-associated antigen. *Journal of Experimental Medicine*, **181**, 1935–1940.

Schwartzman, R. M. & Rockey, J. H. (1967) Atopy in the dog. *Archives of Dermatology*, **96**, 418–422.

Sidbury, R. & Hanifin, J. M. (2000) Atopic dermatitis: old, new and emerging therapies for atopic dermatitis. *Dermatologic Clinics*, **18**, 1–11.

Sowden, J. M., Berth-Jones, J., Ross, J. S., Motley, R. J., Marks, R., Finlay, A. Y. *et al.* (1991) Double-blind, controlled, crossover study of cyclosporin in adults with severe refractory atopic dermatitis. *Lancet*, **338**, 137–140.

Spergel, J. M., Mizoguchi, E., Brewer, J. P., Martin, T. R., Bhan, A. K. & Geha, R. S. (1998) Epicutaneous sensitization with protein

antigen induces localized allergic dermatitis and hyperresponsiveness to methacholine after single exposure to aerosolized antigen in mice. *Journal of Clinical Investigation*, **101**, 1614–1622.
Szentivanyi, A. (1968) The beta-adrenergic theory of the atopic abnormality in bronchial asthma. *Journal of Allergy*, **42**, 203–232.
Taylor, R. S., Baadsgaard, O., Hammerberg, C. & Cooper, K. D. (1991) Hyperstimulatory $CD1a^{+}CD1b^{+}CD36^{+}$ Langerhans cells are responsible for increased autologous T lymphocyte reactivity to lesional epidermal cells of patients with atopic dermatitis. *Journal of Immunology*, **147**, 3794–3802.
Thepen, T., Langeveld-Wildschut, G., Bihari, I. C., Van Wichen, D. F., Van Reijsen, F. C. & Mudde, G. C. (1996) Biphasic response against aeroallergen in atopic dermatitis showing a switch from an initial Th2 response to a Th1 response *in situ*: an immunocytochemical study. *Journal of Allergy and Clinical Immunology*, **97**, 828–837.
Trautmann, A., Akdis, M., Kleemann, D., Altznauer, F., Simon, H.-U., Graeve, T. *et al.* (2000) T cell-mediated Fas-induced keratinocyte apoptosis plays a key pathogenetic role in eczematous dermatitis. *Journal of Clinical Investigation*, **106**, 25–35.
Uno, H. & Hanifin, J. M. (1980) Langerhans cells in acute and chronic epidermal lesions of atopic dermatitis, observed by L-Dopa histofluorescence, glycol methacrylate thin section, and electron microscopy. *Journal of Investigative Dermatology*, **75**, 52–60.
Van Leent, E. J., Graber, M., Thurston, M., Wagenaar, A., Spuls, P. I. & Bos, J. D. (1998) Effectiveness of the ascomycin macrolactam SDZ ASM 981 in the topical treatment of atopic dermatitis. *Archives of Dermatology*, **134**, 805–809.
Zachary, C. B., Allen, M. H. & MacDonald, D. M. (1985) *In situ* quantification of T-lymphocyte subsets and Langerhans cells in the inflammatory infiltrate of atopic eczema. *British Journal of Dermatology*, **112**, 149–156.

4.2

Mast cells: a review of their biology and role in cutaneous inflammation

P.B. Hill BVSc, PhD, DVD, DACVD, MRCVS

The University of Edinburgh, Department of Veterinary Clinical Studies, The Royal (Dick) School of Veterinary Studies, Hospital for Small Animals, Easter Bush Veterinary Centre, Roslin, Midlothian, UK

Summary

Mast cells are normal residents of connective tissue and are found in highest numbers in areas of the body that interface with the environment, such as the skin, lung and gastrointestinal tract. In contrast to blood leucocytes, which differentiate in the bone marrow before being released into the circulation, mast cells do not circulate as mature cells. Morphologically unidentifiable precursors migrate in the blood and invade connective or mucosal tissues, where they proliferate and differentiate into mature mast cells. The differentiation and proliferation of mature mast cells from these progenitor cells is regulated by stem cell factor and interleukins-3,-4,-9 and -10. Under the influence of these cytokine systems, mast cells develop into distinct functional phenotypes with differing biochemical properties, especially with regard to their content of granule proteoglycans and proteases. Once in the peripheral tissues, mast cells play an important role in the defence of the body against parasites and other infectious agents, but they are also involved in more general immune responses and wound healing. Mast cells exert their effects by synthesising and releasing a host of inflammatory mediators such as histamine, proteases and cytokines. This process is usually triggered via the interaction between allergens and allergen-specific immunoglobulin E bound to high-affinity FcεR1 receptors expressed on the mast cell surface. Activation of FcεR1 receptors results in mediator release through a complex series of biochemical reactions involving G-proteins, tyrosine kinases, inositol-trisphosphate, protein kinase C, calcium channel activation and rearrangement of the cytoskeleton. Once released into the intercellular milieu, mast cell mediators participate in an interplay between the microvasculature and other inflammatory cells. However, the precise contribution of these mediators to the pathogenesis of allergic diseases such as canine atopic dermatitis has not been elucidated and awaits further study.

Origin of mast cells

Mast cells have long been recognised as residents of connective tissue, where they are most abundant in parts of the body that interface with the environment, such as the skin, lung and gastrointestinal tract. However, until the recent advent of modern immunological techniques and reagents, the question of how mast cells arrive at these sites has been difficult to resolve.

The initial problem of determining from where mast cells actually originated was solved in 1977 by Kitamura, who performed some elegant experiments using beige mice, a mutant strain analagous to the Chediak–Higashi syndrome in other species (Kitamura *et al.*, 1977). These mice have cellular abnormalities that lead to the formation of giant granules in cells such as neutrophils, melanocytes and mast cells (Chi & Lagunoff, 1975). Kitamura transplanted bone marrow from beige mice into lethally irradiated normal mice and discovered that mast cells with giant granules developed in the recipient (Kitamura *et al.*, 1977). Hence, as with other cells of the haematopoietic series, mast cells were shown to be derived from bone marrow. This can be convincingly demonstrated *in vitro* by culturing rodent bone marrow cells in the presence of appropriate mast cell growth factors (Nabel *et al.*, 1981; Nagao *et al.*, 1981; Razin *et al.*, 1981; Tertian *et al.*, 1981; Haig *et al.*, 1982; Nakahata *et al.*, 1982) (Figure 4.2.1). More recent studies have demonstrated similar findings in the dog (Shull *et al.*, 1992). The specific cell of origin of the mast cell is a multipotential haematopoietic stem cell that is initially capable of differentiating into other leucocytes as well as mast cells (Kitamura *et al.*, 1981; Nakahata & Ogawa, 1982). However, once the lines become committed the cells undergo complete differentiation and cannot change from one type to another.

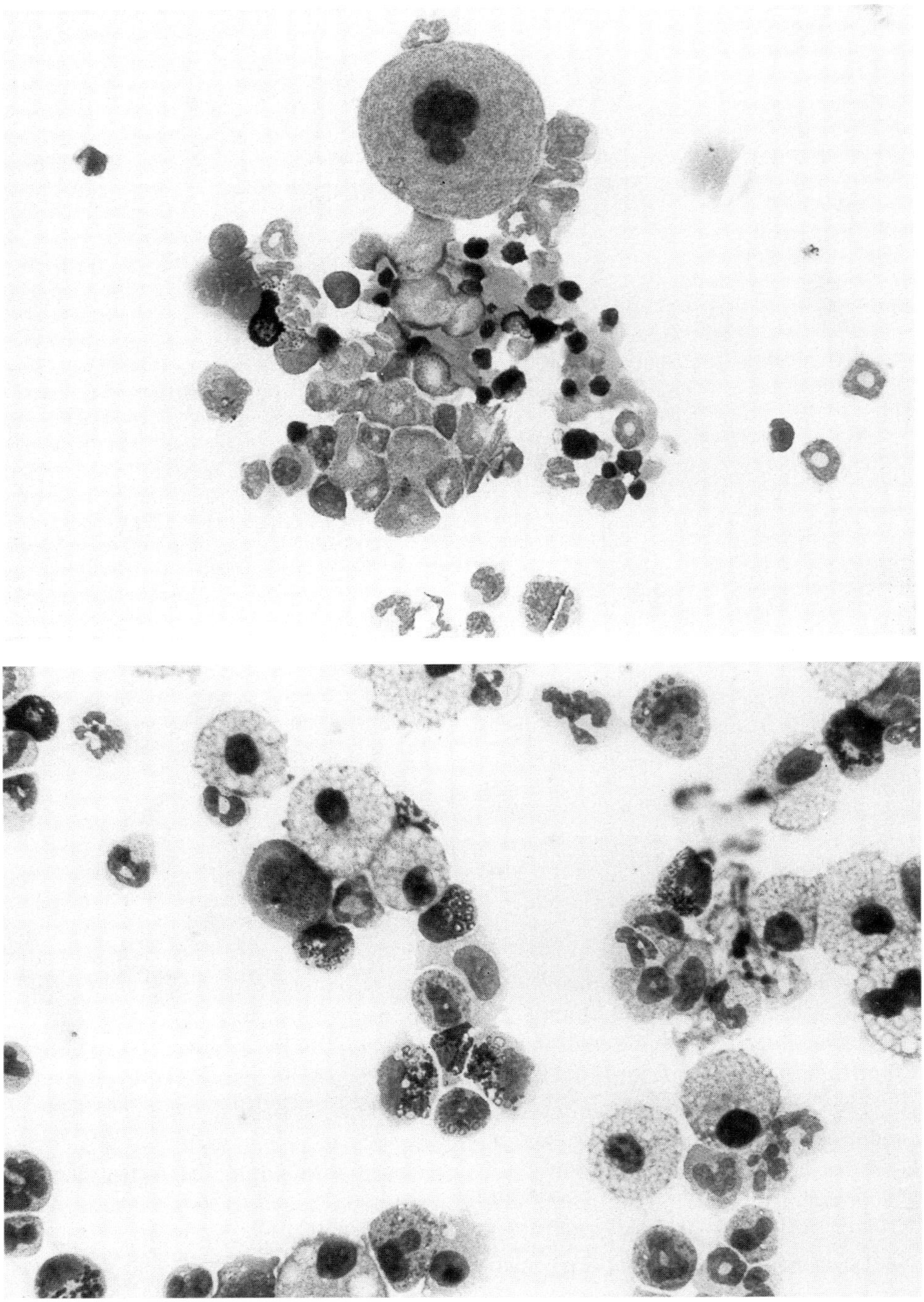

(a)

(b)

Figure 4.2.1. *(Continued on next page.)*

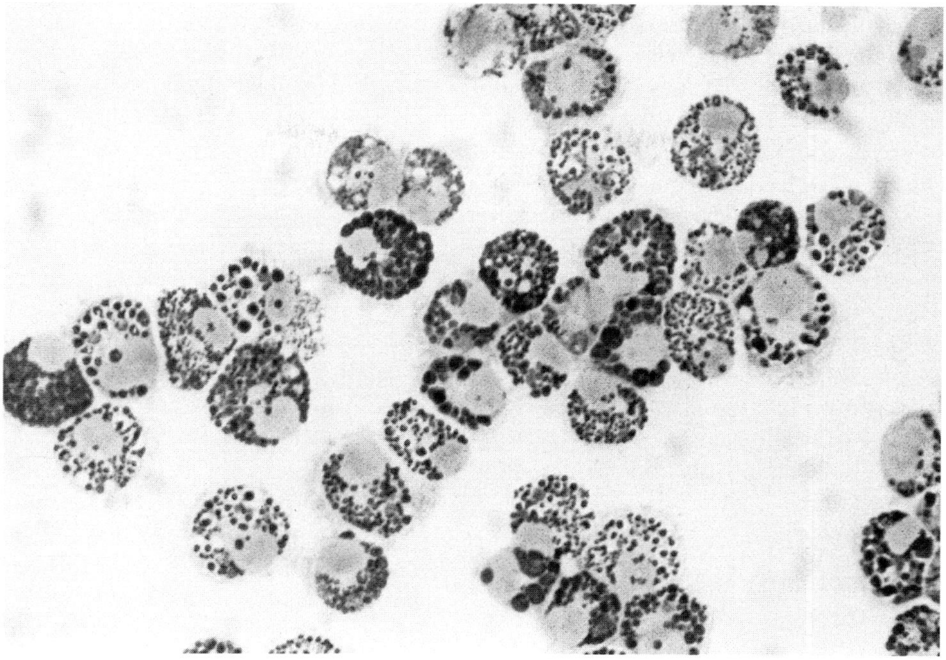

(c)

Figure 4.2.1. (*Continued*) Development of mast cells from bone marrow. (a) Cytospin preparation of bone marrow in tissue culture immediately before addition of mast cell growth factors. (b) Bone marrow culture 5 days after addition of mast cell growth factors (including interleukin-3) showing early development of granulated mast cells. (c) Bone marrow culture after 22 days showing greater than 95% mature mast cells.

Migration of mast cells into the skin

Anyone who routinely evaluates complete blood counts will know that mast cells are not normally found in the circulation. Unlike circulating leucocytes, which fully differentiate in the bone marrow before being released into the bloodstream, mast cells are released as morphologically unidentifiable precursors and not as mature cells (Kitamura *et al.*, 1979; Zucker-Franklin *et al.*, 1981; Sonoda *et al.*, 1982). These circulating cells have recently been characterised using modern immunological reagents and show surface expression of CD34 (a marker for bone marrow pluripotential stem cells), c-kit (the receptor for stem cell factor), RNA coding for mast cell proteases and intracytoplasmic granules (Kirshenbaum *et al.*, 1991; Agis *et al.*, 1993; Rodewald *et al.*, 1996). However, at this stage, the cells do not have the high-affinity immunoglobulin E (IgE) receptor, FcεR1 (Rodewald *et al.*, 1996) (Figure 4.2.2).

Before completing their development, the immature mast cell precursors leave the bloodstream and enter peripheral connective tissues (Kasugai *et al.*, 1995) (Figure 4.2.2). This process is currently incompletely understood but, as with the extravasation of other blood cells, is thought to be regulated by the expression of adhesion molecules and chemotactic factors (Smith & Weis, 1996). Immature mast cells can possess various homing/adhesion molecules such as the $\alpha_4\beta_7$ integrin, the β_2 integrin LFA-1, VLA-5 and L-selectin (Smith & Weis, 1996; Weber *et al.*, 1997). These molecules can interact with molecules on endothelial cells, such as mucosal addressin cell adhesion molecule-1 (MadCAM-1), intercellular adhesion molecule-1 (ICAM-1), P-selectin or extracellular matrix proteins such as laminin and fibronectin (Krugerkrasagakes *et al.*, 1996; Sriramarao *et al.*, 1996; Steegmaier *et al.*, 1997). Adhesion of mast cells to fibronectin is also dramatically enhanced by stem cell factor, a major mast cell growth factor (Dastych & Metcalfe, 1994; Kinashi & Springer, 1994). A recent study has also shown that mast cell precursors can produce matrix metalloproteinase-9, an enzyme that degrades the extracellular matrix to allow transmigration of leucocytes (Tanaka *et al.*, 1999). Furthermore, this mechanism was down-regulated by stem cell factor, suggesting that once mast cells arrive in the connective tissue, the process of migration is inhibited allowing adhesion to the extracellular matrix (Tanaka *et al.*, 1999).

Mast cells are also attracted by various chemotactic factors such as stem cell factor (Meininger *et al.*, 1992), interleukin-3 (Matsuura & Zetter, 1989), interleukin-8 (IL-8) (Lippert *et al.*, 1998; Nilsson *et al.*, 1999), transforming growth factor-β (TGF-β) (Gruber *et al.*, 1994) and complement components C3a and C5a (Hartmann *et al.*, 1997). However, which of these adhesion molecules and chemotactic factors are responsible for the constitutive homing of immature mast cells into normal skin and which are specifically involved in trafficking to sites of inflammation is currently unknown.

Differentiation of mast cell precursors into mature mast cells

The development of mature mast cells from circulating precursors is regulated by two separate cytokine systems. One involves the cytokine stem cell factor (SCF), which is derived from fibroblasts, keratinocytes and stromal cells, whereas the other is dependent on T-cell-derived cytokines such as IL-3, IL-4, IL-9 and IL-10 (Figure 4.2.2).

Stem cell factor is a cytokine that appears to be involved in virtually all aspects of mast cell function (Hill & Martin, 1998). The importance of SCF in mast cell development is graphically illustrated in mutant strains of mice that have abnormalities in the genes for either SCF or its receptor, c-kit (Kitamura *et al.*, 1978; Kitamura & Go, 1979; Galli & Kitamura, 1987). Mice with two mutant alleles at either of these chromosomal sites suffer from macrocytic anaemia, sterility, lack of hair pigmentation and an almost total deficiency of mast cells in all body sites, including the skin (Figure 4.2.3). This combination of abnormalities indicates that SCF is also critically important for the development of other cells, including melanocytes. As would be expected, the mast cell deficiency seen in mice that are unable to produce functional SCF can be reversed by repeatedly injecting soluble SCF (Zsebo *et al.*, 1990). Likewise, if SCF is injected into normal animals, including rodents, monkeys and humans, it induces a striking hyperplasia of the mast cell population in many sites, including the skin (Tsai *et al.*, 1991; Galli *et al.*, 1993; Costa *et al.*, 1996). However, this strategy is not successful if the mice do not have functional c-kit receptors and the lack of mast cells in these mice can only be corrected by transplanting bone marrow cells from normal mice (Kitamura *et al.*, 1978; Galli & Kitamura, 1987).

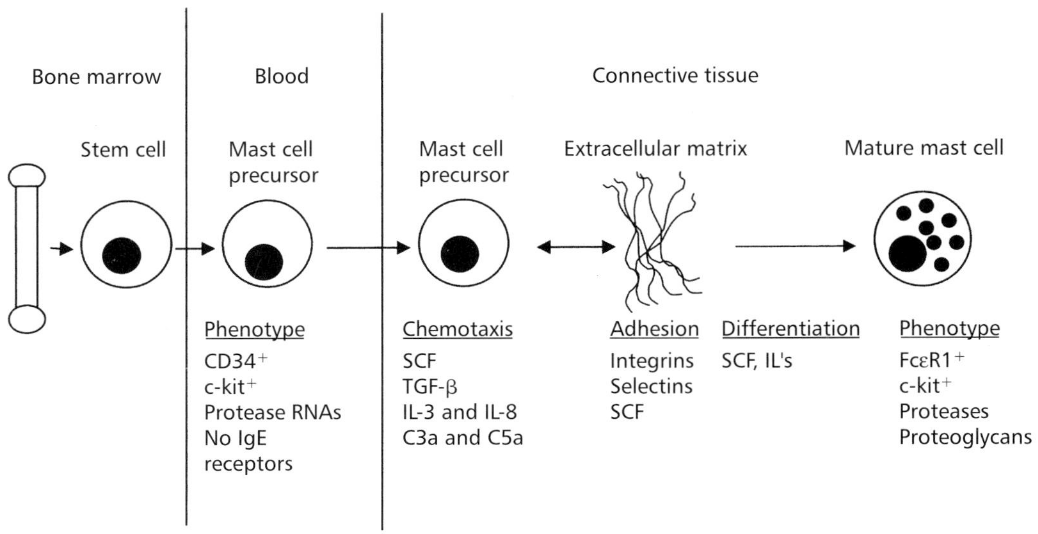

Figure 4.2.2. Development of mast cells. Mast cells originate in the bone marrow and circulate as morphologically unidentifiable precursors. They migrate into connective tissues under the influence of chemotactic factors and bind to the extracellular matrix using adhesion molecules. They then differentiate into mature mast cells in response to various cytokines, especially stem cell factor (SCF). TGF: transforming growth factor; IL: interleukin.

In addition to the mechanisms described above, various T-cell-derived cytokines are able to influence mast cell development. However, these cytokines appear to be more important in regulating the mast cell population in the gut rather than in the skin. In T-cell-deficient rodents, infestation with various intestinal nematodes does not result in the massive proliferation of mucosal mast cells that is seen in normal animals (Ruitenberg & Elgersma, 1976; Mayrhofer & Fisher, 1979; Nawa & Miller, 1979). The key player in this response is IL-3 which, if injected, can restore the host's ability to mount a mast cell response to the parasites (Abe & Nawa, 1988; Abe *et al.*, 1988). IL-3 can also be used as a growth factor in tissue culture to stimulate the growth of mast cells from rodent bone marrow, but the cells that appear are all of the phenotype found in the gut rather than in the skin (Nabel *et al.*, 1981; Nagao *et al.*, 1981; Razin *et al.*, 1981; Schrader *et al.*, 1981; Tertian *et al.*, 1981; Haig *et al.*, 1988; Chiu & Burrall, 1990). This is in contrast to the situation in humans, in which IL-3 leads to the development of basophils in bone marrow cultures and not mast cells (Valent *et al.*, 1989). In fact, human mast cells do not appear to have IL-3 receptors (Valent *et al.*, 1990). Additional T-cell-derived cytokines such as IL-4, IL-9 and IL-10 do not lead to mast cell proliferation when used as sole stimuli, but they all act synergistically with IL-3 to enhance mast cell growth or survival (Schmitt *et al.*, 1987; Moeller *et al.*, 1989; Hultner *et al.*, 1990; Tsuji *et al.*, 1990; Thompson-Snipes *et al.*, 1991).

It is clear from the above data that the constitutive development of mast cells in all parts of the body, including the skin, is critically dependent on a functional interaction between SCF and c-kit. It is also clear that T-cell-derived cytokines are required to initiate the mastocytosis seen in the gut of rodents infested with nematodes. However, the role of interleukins in the development of cutaneous mast cells is less certain. Systemic administration of IL-3 to mast cell-deficient mice can increase the number of mast cells in the skin as well as in other tissues (Ody *et al.*, 1990), but in normal animals it is not clear whether T-cell-derived cytokines play an important role in regulating cutaneous mast cell numbers.

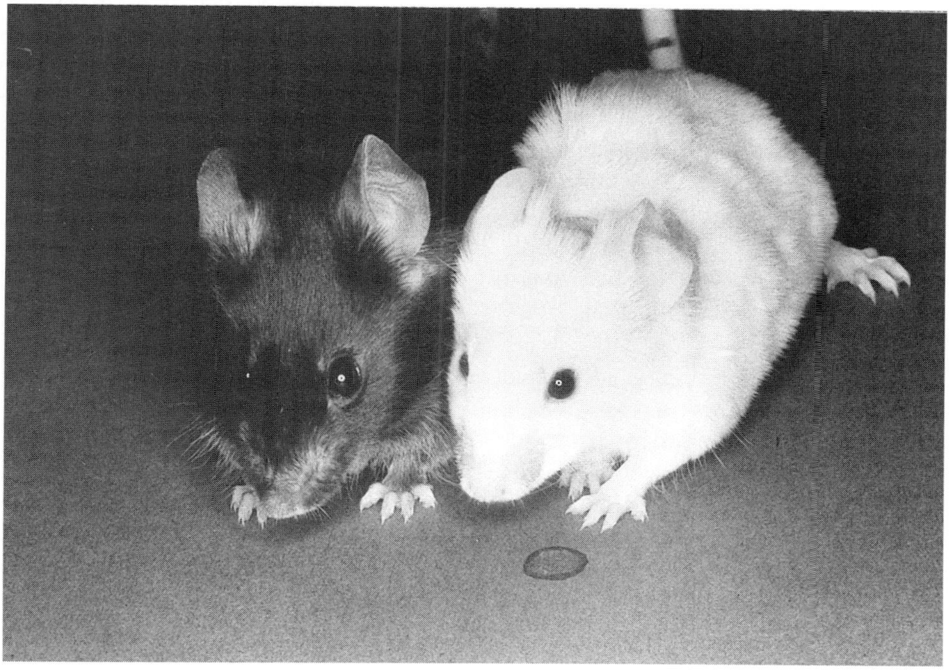

Figure 4.2.3. Appearance of W/Wv mouse compared with normal, congenic mouse. The mouse on the right lacks functional c-kit receptors (the receptor for stem cell factor). These mice are anaemic, lack skin pigmentation and have an almost total deficiency of mast cells. The mouse on the left is normal. (Picture courtesy of Dr S. J. Galli.)

Mast cells in the skin are different from those in the gut and lung

It has become clear from a large body of research that mast cells, like lymphocytes, can be subdivided into two main types. These have been named connective tissue mast cells, which occur predominantly in the skin and peritoneal cavity, and mucosal mast cells, which occur predominantly in the gastrointestinal tract and lung. This mast cell heterogeneity is most obvious in rodents, but it is observed to a lesser degree in humans, sheep and dogs. The difference between these two subpopulations relates to their histochemical properties, the content of their granule mediators and certain functional aspects.

The initial separation of mast cells into two groups was based on their staining properties in histological sections. After sequential staining with alcian blue and safranin, the granules of cutaneous mast cells appear red, whereas intestinal mast cells stain blue (Enerback, 1966a). This staining difference reflects the fact that the two populations of mast cells have different granule proteoglycans: skin mast cells possess heparin and gut mast cells possess chondroitin sulfate (Horner, 1971; Metcalfe *et al.*, 1980; Stevens *et al.*, 1986). There are also distinct differences in the content of granule proteases between the two groups. In rodents, this is characterised by the differential expression of a wide variety of mast cell proteases (reviewed by Hill & Martin, 1998). In humans, the distinction is based on the expression of the proteases chymase and tryptase. Mast cells in the skin contain both tryptase and chymase, whereas those in the intestinal mucosa possess only tryptase (Irani *et al.*, 1986; Schwartz *et al.*, 1987). Mast cell subpopulations also differ in their functional properties. Unlike intestinal mast cells, skin mast cells are known to respond to secretagogues such as compound 48/80 and a variety of neuropeptides (Enerback, 1966b, 1974; Befus *et al.*, 1982; Shanahan *et al.*, 1985).

There is therefore no doubt that mast cells in the skin are different from those in the gastrointestinal tract or lung. However, the concept of mast cell heterogeneity within the skin, as described for the dog, is slightly more controversial. In one study (Becker *et al.*, 1985), the number of mast cells observed in histological sections of dog skin varied depending on whether the tissue had been fixed in formalin or basic lead acetate. Because the counts were lower in the formalin-fixed sections, it was inferred that a subpopulation of 'formalin-resistant' mast cells was present in dog skin, similar to the formalin-resistant mast cells in the rat gastrointesinal tract (Becker *et al.*, 1985). However, no analysis of sequential staining characteristics or granule contents was performed. Despite the limited evidence, Becker extended these observations to mast cell counts in the skin of atopic dogs following antigen challenge (Becker *et al.*, 1986). The number of formalin-resistant, 'atypical' mast cells fell more rapidly in the early phase of the intradermal reaction, whereas the formalin-sensitive, 'typical' mast cells declined gradually over a 24 h period. The authors concluded that the atypical mast cells were primarily involved in the acute response to antigen, whereas the typical mast cells were associated with the late phase reaction (Becker *et al.*, 1986).

More recent studies have focused on the relative amounts of tryptase and chymase in canine mast cells. As in humans, canine cutaneous mast cells possess both tryptase and chymase (Schechter *et al.*, 1988; Kube *et al.*, 1998), whereas those in the gastrointestinal tract are predominantly of the chymase phenotype (Kube *et al.*, 1998). However, the proportion of each cell type seen in various tissues was not as dramatic as that seen in humans and rodents, so that chymase-positive cells could be observed in the skin and chymase/tryptase-positive cells could be observed in the intestinal tract (Kube *et al.*, 1998). As in the previous studies, the relative proportions of each cell type were also dependent on the type of fixative. What is clear from these reports is that mast cell heterogeneity in the dog is not as tissue specific as it is in humans or rodents. However, whether this has any genuine biological significance is currently unknown.

Number and distribution of mast cells in the skin

Once mast cell precursors have migrated from the circulation and differentiated into mature, connective tissue mast cells they take up position in the dermis, predominantly around superficial blood vessels, where they can be visualised in histological sections. It is difficult to provide precise comparative data on the number and distribution of mast cells in the skin because different studies report different methodologies for fixing, staining, counting and recording mast cells. For example, mast cell counts can be reported as per high-power field (HPF), per mm^2, per mm^3, or per unit area (such as a graticule).

Most studies of mast cell density in humans report counts of approximately 7000/mm^3 of dermis (Hellstrom & Holmgren, 1950; Mikhail & Miller-Millinska, 1964). This equates to about 45–50 mast cells/mm^2 in histological sections or approximately 6 per standard HPF (Binazzi & Rampichini, 1959; Eady, 1979; Cowen *et al.*, 1979). However, in one study, the highest mast cell counts were seen in the scrotum, reaching 177/mm^2 (Binazzi & Rampichini, 1959). In mice, mast cell counts of 26/mm^2 are seen in the dermis over the dorsum, but this rises to over 100/mm^2 in the skin of the ears (Galli *et al.*, 1987; Gordon & Galli, 1990).

In dogs, mast cell densities have been reported in standard textbooks as 4–12/HPF (Scott *et al.*, 1995a). Morphometric studies using special stains have yielded similar figures (8.3–10.1/HPF) (Nimmo Wilkie *et al.*, 1990). Other studies have reported approximately 28 (Olivry *et al.*, 1997) to 31 (Welle *et al.*, 1999) mast cells/mm^2 in normal canine skin (equating to about 3.3–3.7/HPF). However, the number of cutaneous mast cells observed in histological sections varies dramatically with body site. Emerson & Cross (1965) reported the highest density of canine mast cells in the ears (16.9/HPF), followed by the vulva (9.7), prepuce and scrotum (9.3), anus (8.3), perineum (8.1), head (7.8), upper eyelid (7.6), dorsal neck (6.8), lower eyelid and lateral thorax (6.5), ventral neck (6.3), lateral thigh (5.7), ventral abdomen (5.5), lip (5.4), dorsum (5.1), medial thigh (5), footpad (3.1) and nasal planum (2.4). In a more recent study, the highest density of canine mast cells was found in the pinnae and ventral interdigital skin (9.2–11.3/HPF) and the lowest density in the nasal planum (2.9) (Auxilia & Hill, 2000). The authors hypothesised that this may be one factor in the frequent occurrence of ear and foot pruritus in canine atopic dermatitis.

In cats, cutaneous mast cell numbers have been reported as 4–20/HPF (Scott *et al.*, 1995a), with most mast cells being present in the superficial dermis (Foster, 1994). Foster found the mean mast cell count in feline skin to be 12.5/HPF (Foster, 1994). However, mast cell counts did not show as much site variation in the cat as they do in the dog. Out of 10 body sites examined, nine had similar counts and a significantly higher number was only observed in the pinna (Foster, 1994).

Hence, although mast cells are present throughout the skin, their numbers vary depending on the body region examined. The mechanisms regulating this site-specific variation and its biological significance are not currently known.

Triggering of mast cell secretion through the IgE receptor

Mast cells exert most of their effects by synthesising and releasing freshly generated or stored inflammatory mediators into the extracellular milieu. This process encompasses degranulation, exocytosis and secretion, and can be triggered by a number of different mechanisms. The most important of these is activation of the high-affinity IgE receptors (FcεR1). There are about 30 000–300 000 of these receptors on the surface of a mast cell, depending on its phenotype (Conrad *et al.*, 1975; Sterk & Ishizaka, 1982; Lee *et al.*, 1985). These receptors are typical G-protein linked receptors that have seven domains that bridge the cell's plasma membrane (Figure 4.2.4). Each receptor is made of four subunits comprising a 45 kDa α-chain, a 33 kDa β-chain and two 9 kDa γ-chains, so that the whole complex is designated $\alpha\beta\gamma_2$ (Alber & Metzger, 1993). The α-chain passes through the membrane only once, with the C-terminal within the cytoplasm and the N-terminal on the outside. The extracellular domain carries the high-affinity binding site for IgE (Kinet, 1990) and can only bind one immunoglobulin molecule at a time (Mendoza & Metzger, 1976). The IgE molecule binds via the Cε3 domain in the Fc region, resulting in a side-on configuration with the antigen-binding sites projected outwards (Baird *et al.*, 1989; Nissim *et al.*, 1991; Nissim & Eshhar, 1992). The specificity of this interaction is almost absolute so IgG cannot bind to this region (Alber & Metzger, 1993).

In an immunofluorescent study, Halliwell (1973) demonstrated that canine dermal mast cells were coated with IgE. This finding has been confirmed in a more recent study that demonstrated high expression of membrane-bound IgE in canine mast cells compared with the low expression seen in epidermal Langerhans' cells (Olivry *et al.*, 1996). Furthermore, the α-chain of the canine high-affinity IgE receptor has recently been cloned and sequenced and is currently used as an IgE-binding reagent in allergy diagnostic immunoassays (C. McCall, personal communication). These studies indicate that similar structures exist in the dog to those that have been described in rodents.

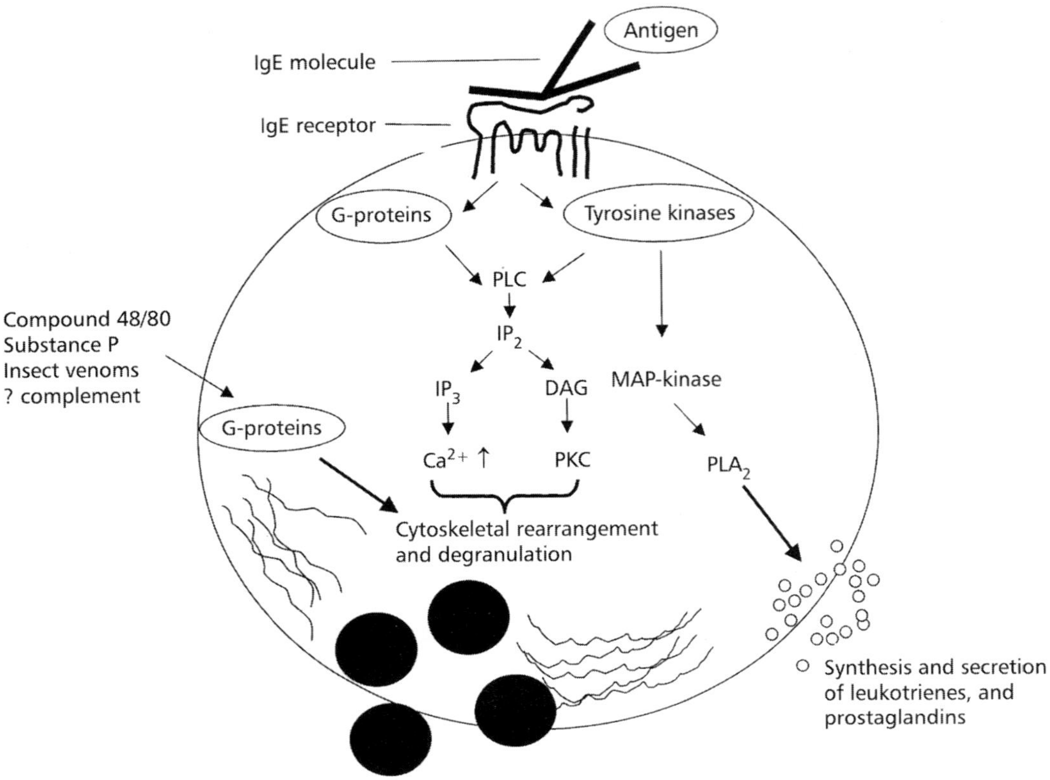

Figure 4.2.4. Summary of the main mechanisms involved in mast cell degranulation. For details, see text. PLC: phospholipase C; IP_2: phosphatidylinositol 4,5-bisphosphate; IP_3: inositol 1,4,5-trisphosphate; DAG: diacylglycerol; PKC: protein kinase C; MAP: mitogen activated protein; PLA: phospholipase A.

The β- and γ-chains of the IgE receptor are not involved in antigen binding, but act as the signalling units between the receptor and cytoplasm (Paolini *et al.*, 1991). The β-unit has four transmembrane domains, whereas each γ-chain has only one (Kinet *et al.*, 1988; Varin-Blank & Metzger, 1990). To activate the signalling mechanisms, two IgE receptors must be brought together and immobilised (Schlessinger *et al.*, 1976; Mao *et al.*, 1991; Tamir *et al.*, 1996). When this happens to multiple receptors they tend to aggregate in patches or at one end of the cell (Stump *et al.*, 1989). Aggregation of IgE receptors is normally brought about by large, specific antigens that are capable of cross-linking two IgE molecules bound to the α-chains. However, the same result occurs if the IgE molecules are cross-linked by anti-IgE antibodies or lectins such as concanavalin A (Roitt *et al.*, 1993). There are several ways in which allergens might gain access to the cutaneous mast cell population to trigger these secretory pathways (Table 4.2.1).

Table 4.2.1. Route by which antigens can gain access to the cutaneous mast cell population

Route of allergen access	Disease or syndrome
Transepidermal penetration	Atopic dermatitis
	Contact dermatitis
	Hypersensitivity to mites
	Hypersensitivity to cutaneous micro-organisms
Cutaneous circulation	Food hypersensitivity
	Drug eruptions
	Urticaria
	Anaphylaxis
Intradermal injection	Flea and fly bites

Aggregation of IgE receptors activates a series of intracellular enzymes

After aggregation of the IgE receptors, a whole series of complex intracellular biochemical reactions commences (Figure 4.2.4). This involves activation of various enzyme systems that transfer phosphate groups from GTP or ATP to amino acids on target proteins. The major components of these pathways are G-proteins and tyrosine kinases. A subfamily of G-proteins known as heterotrimeric G-proteins is involved in signalling through the IgE receptor (Gomperts, 1983). These proteins bind phosphate groups from GTP and are able to activate subsequent enzymes involved in the secretory pathway (Sagi-Eisenberg, 1993). The β-chain of the IgE receptor also activates the Src and Syk group of intracellular tyrosine kinases (Benhamou *et al.*, 1990, 1993; Yu *et al.*, 1991; Connelly *et al.*, 1991; Eiseman & Bolen, 1992; Shiue *et al.*, 1995). These kinases transfer phosphate groups from ATP to tyrosine residues on various target proteins. These target proteins play a critical role in a whole range of mast cell functions, ranging from initiation of secretory pathways to cellular proliferation (Lavens *et al.*, 1992; Jouvin *et al.*, 1994; Hirasawa *et al.*, 1995a).

One of the most critical proteins to be activated by the above mechanisms is phospholipase C-γ-1, a key enzyme in signal transduction (Rhee *et al.*, 1989; Sagi-Eisenberg, 1993; Jouvin *et al.*, 1994). This enzyme catalyses the hydrolysis of phosphatidylinositol 4,5-bisphosphate (an inositol lipid present in the plasma membrane) into inositol 1,4,5-trisphosphate (IP_3) and diacylglycerol (DAG) (Berridge & Irvine, 1984). IP_3 triggers calcium release from the endoplasmic reticulum, leading to a rapid rise in intracellular calcium concentrations (Streb *et al.*, 1983; Spat *et al.*, 1986a, b). This calcium mobilisation is augmented by the release of sphingosine-1-phosphate (a sphingolipid) from the plasma membrane following IgE receptor activation (Choi *et al.*, 1996). The other second messenger generated in this pathway, DAG, is responsible for activating protein kinase C, an enzyme involved in rearrangement of the cytoskeleton (Ludowyke *et al.*, 1989; Barane & Razin, 1991; Ozawa *et al.*, 1993a, b; Dekker & Parker, 1994).

Mast cell degranulation and secretion

Initiation of mast cell degranulation via the IgE receptor occurs owing to a rise in intracellular calcium. This is a self-perpetuating process because the release of calcium from the endoplasmic reticulum activates calcium channels in the plasma membrane, allowing a further influx of calcium ions (Foreman *et al.*, 1973; Ishizaka *et al.*, 1979; White *et al.*, 1984; Hoth & Penner, 1992, 1993; Gericke *et al.*, 1995; Zhang & McCloskey, 1995; Habara & Kanno, 1996). This process can be reproduced *in vitro* by using mast cell secretagogues such as calcium ionophore that create calcium channels in the cell's plasma membrane (Foreman *et al.*, 1973). The intracellular calcium ions are bound by calcium-binding proteins such as calmodulin, which activate additional protein kinases (Chock & Schmauderchock, 1992). These complex enzyme systems, along with protein kinase C, are responsible for altering the conformation of the cytoskeleton, allowing the mast cell granules to move outwards from the interior and fuse with the plasma membrane (Rohlich, 1975; Nielsen *et al.*, 1989; Koffer *et al.*, 1990). The fusion process has not been definitively characterised but it is likely to involve various attachment proteins known as SNAPS and SNARES (Edwardson & Marciniak, 1995). Once the granule has fused, a pore appears that rapidly enlarges, thus allowing release of the granule contents (Monck & Fernandez, 1992).

Ultrastructurally, mast cells can undergo two different types of degranulation known as piecemeal and anaphylactic degranulation (Dvorak, 1993). Piecemeal degranulation involves a slow and partial emptying of mast cell granules and is observed in certain skin disorders such as contact allergy and bullous pemphigoid (Dvorak, 1993). Anaphylactic degranulation is an explosive process in which the mast cell granules are rapidly extruded to the exterior. This pattern of degranulation is typical of that seen in the skin in response to IgE-dependent stimulation and neuropeptides (Dvorak, 1993). However, whether these two patterns of secretion represent distinct mechanisms or a physiological continuum is currently not known.

In addition to granule mediators, mast cells are able to synthesise and secrete various lipid-derived mediators such as leukotrienes and prostaglandins. These are derived from the action of phospholipase A_2 on arachidonic acid in the plasma membrane. As in the pathways described above, phospholipase A_2 is activated by an enzyme cascade commencing with a syk tyrosine kinase, but the mechanisms may then diverge, progressing through a mitogen-activated protein kinase (MAP kinase) rather than phospholipase C (Hirasawa *et al.*, 1995a, b).

Apart from a rise in intracellular calcium, other mechanisms exist for triggering mast cell secretion. Some substances such as the laboratory reagent compound 48/80, neuropeptides such as substance P, and the bee and wasp venoms mellitin and mastoparan are able to activate intracellular G-proteins directly, independent of the IgE receptor (Aridor *et al.*, 1990; Sagi-Eisenberg, 1993; Emadikhiav *et al.*, 1995; Lorenz *et al.*, 1998). These G-proteins can bypass some of the enzyme systems described above and initiate degranulation directly. The complement components C3a and C5a are also known to degranulate mast cells, although it is currently not known whether this is mediated directly by G-proteins or via complement receptors (Foreman, 1993).

Role of mast cells in innate immunity and cutaneous inflammation

Mast cells have long been thought of as effector cells in type 1 hypersensitivity disorders such as asthma, rhinitis, urticaria, anaphylaxis and atopic dermatitis (Brostoff & Hall, 1993). In these settings, mast cells are traditionally viewed as detrimental, causing inflammation that is harmful to the host. This view is now regarded as rather simplistic, because mast cells are involved in a diverse range of inflammatory processes that may or may not involve traditional allergic type reactions. Furthermore, many mast cell functions are protective and represent a component of the innate immune system (Galli *et al.*, 1999).

The most obvious role of mast cells is in the gastrointestinal tract, where they play an important role in the elimination of nematode parasites (Miller, 1993). This is graphically illustrated in rodent and ruminant models, in which a massive infiltration of mast cells occurs following infestation (Miller & Jarrett, 1971; Befus & Bienenstock, 1979). Furthermore, these mast cells are functionally active during expulsion of the parasites, releasing large quantities of granule proteases (Miller, 1971; Miller *et al.*, 1983; Woodbury *et al.*, 1984; Huntley *et al.*, 1987; Tuohy *et al.*, 1990).

In addition to providing protection against intestinal helminths, mast cells form a critical component of the immune response to certain bacterial infections. In experimental models of septic peritonitis or bacterial pneumonia, mast cell-deficient mice are unable to mount a neutrophilic response and rapidly die (Echtenacher *et al.*, 1996; Malaviya *et al.*, 1996). This is due to the lack of mast cell-derived tumour necrosis factor-α (TNF-α), a potent chemoattractant for neutrophils. Furthermore, the innate immunity to bacterial peritonitis can be augmented by treating mice with SCF (Maurer *et al.*, 1998). Hence, it seems plausible that mast cells may also be involved in the defence against cutaneous pyogenic bacteria.

A key role for mast cells has now been recognised in wound healing. Mast cell numbers can increase five-fold in the fibrotic border of a wound and this correlates with the up-regulation of the chemokine monocyte chemoattractant protein-1 (Trautmann *et al.*, 2000). TGF-β, an important wound-healing cytokine, is also a potent chemoattractant for mast cells (Gruber *et al.*, 1994). Mast cell-derived TNF-α and TGF-β can also promote fibroblast proliferation (Kendall *et al.*, 1997), and mast cell extracts can activate fibroblasts, promoting collagen synthesis and the activation of gelatinase A, an enzyme involved in matrix remodelling (Berton *et al.*, 2000). This effect may be partly due to the effect of tryptase, which was shown to stimulate the synthesis of type 1 collagen in human lung (Cairns & Walls, 1997) and dermal fibroblasts (Abe *et al.*, 1998).

From the above studies, it is clear that mast cells are involved in three of the most fundamental defence mechanisms in mammalian species: immunity to parasites, protection against bacteria and wound healing. However, in addition to these functions, mast cells are now known to play a more general role in regulating immune responses. They do this by synthesising and secreting a variety of mediators and cytokines that can influence the function of other inflammatory cells *per se*, or the interaction of these cells with the microvasculature or extracellular matrix (Burd *et al.*, 1989; Plaut *et al.*, 1989; Gordon *et al.*, 1990; Marshall & Bienenstock, 1994; Schwartz, 1994). In addition to the presence of histamine, heparin and proteases, messenger RNA has been detected in mast cells for the cytokines IL-1, -2, -3, -4, -5, -6, -8, -9 and -13, TNF-α, TGF-β γ-interferon (IFN-γ), granulocyte–macrophage colony-stimulating factor (GM-CSF) and the C-C chemokines macrophage inflammatory protein-1α (MIP-1α) and MIP-1β (Galli & Wershil, 1995). However, some caution is warranted in interpreting these data because secretion of active protein has not been demonstrated for all of these cytokines. A consideration of the function of these cytokines would require a separate review for each molecule, but in general terms, these agents are known to regulate IgE synthesis (IL-4 and IFN-γ) and influence a wide range of pathological processes such as cell trafficking, angiogenesis, tissue remodelling and fibrosis (Gordon *et al.*, 1990).

These mechanisms clearly have a dramatic impact on the pathogenesis of cutaneous inflammation. For example, the leucocyte infiltration occurring at sites of IgE-dependent cutaneous inflammation was shown to be totally dependent on the dermal mast cell population in experimental mice (Wershil *et al.*, 1991). Furthermore, 50% of this infiltrate was dependent on mast cell-derived TNF-α (Wershil *et al.*, 1991). Mast cell proteases are also important in regulating the influx of inflammatory cells into the skin. Both chymase and tryptase promote the accumulation of neutrophils and eosinophils following intradermal injection in guinea-pigs (He *et al.*, 1997; He & Walls, 1998). The effect of tryptase may be due to its ability to induce the expression of IL-1 and IL-8 by endothelial cells (Compton *et al.*, 1998). Mast cells can also up-regulate the expression of vascular cell adhesion molecule-1 (VCAM-1) and E-selectin on endothelial cells, again suggesting a modulatory role in inflammatory cell trafficking (van Haaster *et al.*, 1997).

With such a wide range of biological functions, what can be said of the role of mast cells in canine atopic dermatitis, a supposedly typical type 1 hypersensitivity reaction of immense importance to the veterinary dermatologist? It is now clear that the lesions in this disease represent a complex interplay among inflammatory cells, the microvasculature, the extracellular matrix, the epidermis and intercellular signalling mechanisms. However, what is not clear is the precise contribution of mast cells to this overall inflammatory picture.

In contrast to the massive hyperplasia of mast cells that occurs in the intestinal tract following nematode infestation, the numbers of mast cells in the skin of atopic dogs is only marginally increased, if at all. In a subjective evaluation, Scott (1981) reported that mast cell counts in the dermis could be normal, elevated or decreased in canine atopic dermatitis. A more rigorous morphometric study demonstrated that cutaneous mast cell counts could be significantly elevated in canine atopy but not at all sites (Nimmo Wilkie *et al.*, 1990). The authors reported proportional increases of 1.1-fold (lateral neck), 1.5-fold (abdomen) and 1.8-fold (dorsal rump) over the counts in control dogs (Nimmo Wilkie *et al.*, 1990). In other studies, mast cell counts were found to be the same between normal and atopic dogs (Olivry *et al.*, 1997; Welle *et al.*, 1999). Compared with the 100-fold increases that can be seen in parasitised gut, these changes seem relatively trivial. Surprisingly, the number of mononuclear cells infiltrating the lesional skin of dogs with atopic dermatitis is approximately 10 times higher than the mast cell counts (Nimmo Wilkie *et al.*, 1990; Olivry *et al.*, 1997). Hence, in terms of cell numbers alone, it would not be appropriate to say that canine atopic dermatitis is a mast cell-mediated disease.

Although the numbers of mast cells are not dramatically increased in canine atopic dermatitis, their function does appear to be altered. Mast cells isolated from the skin of atopic dogs showed increased 'releasability' compared with those from normal dogs (Demora *et al.*, 1996). The mechanisms underlying this interesting phenomenon are not currently understood, but could represent a predetermined change in the mast cells or the presence of up-regulatory factors. For example, alterations in the c-kit receptor could lead to altered mast cell function (London *et al.*, 1999), as could increased expression of SCF (Columbo *et al.*, 1992; Bischoff & Dahinden, 1992; Bischoff *et al.*, 1996; Hill *et al.*, 1996).

As well as enhanced mast cell function in atopic dermatitis (Bischoff *et al.*, 1996; Hill *et al.*, 1996), there is no doubt that dogs produce allergen-specific IgE (Kleinbeck *et al.*, 1989; Halliwell *et al.*, 1998; Hammerling & De Weck, 1998; Zunic, 1998) and that these antibodies can reside on dermal mast cells (Halliwell, 1973; Olivry *et al.*, 1996). There is also no doubt that canine mast cells degranulate in response to specific antigens in canine atopic dermatitis. A large number of studies involving passive cutaneous anaphylaxis, reverse cutaneous anaphylaxis and the intradermal injection of antigens has confirmed the presence of IgE-dependent mast cell secretory mechanisms in dog skin (Scott *et al.*, 1995b). Despite this, the role of mast cell mediators in canine atopic dermatitis is far from clear. Canine mast cells release histamine following IgE-dependent or independent stimulation (Demora *et al.*, 1993; Brazis *et al.*, 1998), and the cutaneous concentration of histamine is higher in atopic dogs than in normal dogs (Nimmo Wilkie *et al.*, 1990). However, this difference may merely reflect an increased quantity of histamine per cell (Demora *et al.*, 1996) or slightly increased mast cell numbers, or both, because it is not known whether the measured histamine was intracellular or extracellular (Nimmo Wilkie *et al.*, 1990). Furthermore, plasma histamine concentrations are elevated in people with atopic eczema (Ring, 1983), but this was not shown to be the case in dogs (Nimmo Wilkie *et al.*, 1990).

Canine mast cells have been shown to possess both chymase (Schechter *et al.*, 1988) and tryptase (Schechter *et al.*, 1988; Myles *et al.*, 1995). Although the functions of these proteases are becoming increasingly clear, it is not known what contribution they make to the pathogenesis of canine atopic dermatitis. The concentration of tryptase in canine tissues is highest in the duodenum and ileum, indicating the highest mast cell counts in these sites (Myles *et al.*, 1995). The concentration in the skin is similar to or lower than that found in the lung and liver (Myles *et al.*, 1995). However, as stated above, the release of large amounts of chymase and tryptase would be expected to cause the recruitment of neutrophils and eosinophils to the site of inflammation. Intradermal injection of purified canine tryptase was shown to elicit a predominantly neutrophilic response at 16–48 h postinjection (Halliwell *et al.*, 1993). Although these cell types are found in the late phase reaction following intradermal injection of allergens (Becker *et al.*, 1988), they are rare findings in the cutaneous inflammatory infiltrate of spontaneous canine atopic dermatitis (Olivry *et al.*, 1997).

Leukotrienes are known to be produced in the skin of dogs with inflammatory dermatoses (Kietzmann, 1989), but it has not been proven that mast cells are the origin of these mediators. Furthermore, leukotriene concentrations were not higher in atopic skin than in normal skin, suggesting that they did not play a major role in the pathogenesis of the lesions (Marsella & Nicklin, 1999).

To date, the only cytokine shown to be produced by canine mast cells is TNF-α. Although there have been no functional studies reporting the role of this cytokine in canine atopic dermatitis, it seems likely that it would function in the same way as in other species. However, as with chymase and tryptase, the infiltration of neutrophils expected following release of this cytokine is not a feature of atopic dermatitis (Olivry *et al.*, 1997).

Conclusion

Mast cells have evolved to provide a protective and modulatory role at body surfaces. They participate in a wide range of inflammatory reactions that may or may not involve traditional allergic reactions. Although mast cells have been regarded as the predominant effector cell of the inflammation seen in canine atopic dermatitis, the available evidence does not fully support such a view. Hence, further studies are required to delineate accurately the role of mast cells and their mediators in this disease.

References

Abe, M., Kurosawa, M., Ishikawa, O., Miyachi, Y. & Kido, H. (1998) Mast cell tryptase stimulates both human dermal fibroblast proliferation and type I collagen production. *Clinical and Experimental Allergy*, **28**, 1509–1517.

Abe, T. & Nawa, Y. (1988) Worm expulsion and mucosal mast cell response induced by repetitive IL-3 administration in *Strongyloides ratti*-infected nude mice. *Immunology*, **63**, 181–185.

Abe, T., Ochiai, H., Minamishima, Y. & Nawa, Y. (1988) Induction of intestinal mastocytosis in nude mice by repeated injection of interleukin 3. *International Archives of Allergy and Applied Immunology*, **86**, 356–358.

Agis, H., Willheim, M., Sperr, W. R., Wilfing, A., Kromer, E., Kabrna, E. *et al.* (1993) Monocytes do not make mast cells when cultured in the presence of SCF: characterization of the circulating mast cell progenitor as a c-kit$^+$, CD34$^+$, Ly$^-$, CD14$^-$, CD17$^-$, colony-forming cell. *Journal of Immunology*, **151**, 4221–4227.

Alber, G. & Metzger, H. (1993) The high-affinity IgE receptor. In *Immunopharmacology of Mast Cells and Basophils* (Ed. J. C. Freeman), pp. 43–51. Academic Press, London.

Aridor, M., Traub, L. M. & Sagi-Eisenberg, R. (1990) Exocytosis in mast cells by basic secretagogues: evidence for direct activation of GTP-binding proteins. *Journal of Cell Biology*, **111**, 909–917.

Auxilia, S. T. & Hill, P. B. (2000) Mast cell distribution, epidermal thickness and hair follicle density in normal canine skin: possible explanations for the predilection sites of atopic dermatitis? *Veterinary Dermatology*, **11**, 247–254.

Baird, B., Shopes, R. J., Oi, V. T., Erickson, J., Kane, P. & Holowka, D. (1989) Interaction of IgE with its high affinity receptor. *International Archives of Allergy and Applied Immunology*, **88**, 23–28.

Barane, D. & Razin, E. (1991) Protein kinase C regulates proliferation of mast cells and the expression of the mRNA of *fos* and *jun* proto-oncogenes during activation by IgE-Ag or calcium ionophore A23187. *Blood*, **78**, 2534–2364.

Becker, A. B., Chung, K. F., McDonald, D. M., Lazarus, S. C., Frick, O. L. & Gold, W. M. (1985) Mast cell heterogeneity in dog skin. *Anatomical Record*, **213**, 477–480.

Becker, A. B., Chung, K. F., McDonald, D. M., Lazarus, S. C., Frick, O. L. & Gold, W. M. (1986) Cutaneous mast cell heterogeneity: response to antigen in atopic dogs. *Journal of Allergy and Clinical Immunology*, **78**, 937–942.

Becker, A. B., Chung, K. F., McDonald, D. M., Frick, O. L. & Gold, W. M. (1988) Cutaneous allergic response in atopic dogs: relationship of cellular and histamine response. *Journal of Allergy and Clinical Immunology*, **81**, 441–448.

Befus, A. D. & Bienenstock, J. (1979) Immunologically mediated intestinal mastocytosis in *Nippostrongylus brasiliensis* infected rats. *Immunology*, **38**, 95–101.

Befus, A. D., Pearce, F. L., Gauldie, J., Horsewood, P. & Bienenstock, J. (1982) Mucosal mast cells 1. Isolation and functional characteristics of rat intestinal mast cells. *Journal of Immunology*, **128**, 2475–2480.

Benhamou, M., Gutkind, K. C., Robbins, K. C. & Siraganian, R. P. (1990) Tyrosine phosphorylation coupled to IgE receptor-mediated signal transduction and histamine release. *Proceedings of the National Academy of Sciences of the United States of America*, **87**, 5327–5330.

Benhamou, M., Ryba, N. J. P., Kihara, H., Nishikata, H. & Siraganian, R. P. (1993) Protein-tyrosine kinase p72^{syk} in high-affinity IgE receptor signaling: identification as a component of pp72 and association with the receptor gamma-chain after receptor aggregation. *Journal of Biological Chemistry*, **268**, 23318–23324.

Berridge, M. J. & Irvine, R. F. (1984) Inositol trisphosphate, a novel second messenger in cellular signal transduction. *Nature*, **312**, 315–321.

Berton, A., Levischaffer, F., Emonard, H., Garbuzenko, E., Gillery, P. & Maquart, F. X. (2000) Activation of fibroblasts in collagen lattices by mast cell extract: a model of fibrosis. *Clinical and Experimental Allergy*, **30**, 485–492.

Binazzi, M. & Rampichini, L. (1959) Investigations on the regional distributions of mast cells in human skin. *Italian General Review of Dermatology*, **1**, 17–21.

Bischoff, S. C. & Dahinden, C. A. (1992) C-kit ligand: a unique potentiator of mediator release by human lung mast cells. *Journal of Experimental Medicine*, **175**, 237–244.

Bischoff, S. C., Schwengberg, S., Wordelmann, K., Weimann, A., Raab, R. & Manns, M. P. (1996) Effect of *c-kit* ligand, stem cell factor, on mediator release by human intestinal mast cells isolated from patients with inflammatory bowel disease and controls. *Gut*, **38**, 104–114.

Brazis, P., Queralt, M., Demora, F., Ferrer, L. & Puigdemont, A. (1998) Comparative study of histamine release from skin mast cells dispersed from atopic, ascaris-sensitive and healthy dogs. *Veterinary Immunology and Immunopathology*, **66**, 43–51.

Brostoff, J. & Hall, T. (1993) Hypersensitivity – Type I. In: *Immunology*, 3rd edn (Eds I. M. Roitt, J. Brostoff & D. K. Male), pp. 19.1–19.22. Mosby, London.

Burd, P. R., Rogers, H. W., Gordon, J. R., Martin, C. A., Jayaraman, S., Wilson, S. D. *et al.* (1989) Interleukin-3-dependent and -independent mast cells stimulated with IgE and antigen express multiple cytokines. *Journal of Experimental Medicine*, **170**, 245–257.

Cairns, J. A. & Walls, A. F. (1997) Mast cell tryptase stimulates the synthesis of type I collagen in human lung fibroblasts. *Journal of Clinical Investigation*, **99**, 1313–1321.

Chi, E. & Lagunoff, D. (1975) Abnormal mast cell granules in the beige (Chediak–Higashi) mouse. *Journal of Histochemistry and Cytochemistry*, **23**, 117–122.

Chiu, H. F. & Burrall, B. A. (1990) Effect of interleukin-3 on the differentiation and histamine content of cultured bone marrow mast cells. *Agents and Actions*, **31**, 197–203.

Chock, S. P. & Schmauderchock, E. A. (1992) The secretory granule and the mechanism of stimulus–secretion coupling. *Current Topics in Cellular Regulation*, **32**, 183–208.

Choi, O. H., Kim, J.-H. & Kinet, J.-P. (1996) Calcium mobilization via sphingosine kinase in signaling by the FcεR1 antigen receptor. *Nature*, **380**, 634–636.

Columbo, M., Horowitz, E. M., Botana, L. M., MacGlashan, D. W., Bochner, B. S., Gillis, S. *et al.* (1992) The human recombinant c-kit receptor ligand, rhSCF, induces mediator release from human cutaneous mast cells and enhances IgE-dependent mediator release from both skin mast cells and peripheral blood basophils. *Journal of Immunology*, **149**, 599–608.

Compton, S. J., Cairns, J. A., Holgate, S. T. & Walls, A. F. (1998) The role of mast cell tryptase in regulating endothelial cell proliferation, cytokine release, and adhesion molecule expression: tryptase induces expression of mRNA for IL-1β and IL-8 and stimulates the selective release of IL-8 from human umbilical vein endothelial cells. *Journal of Immunology*, **161**, 1939–1946.

Connelly, P. A., Farrell, C. A., Merenda, J. M., Conklyn, M. J. & Showell, H. J. (1991) Tyrosine phosphorylation is an early signalling event common to Fc receptor crosslinking in human neutrophils and rat basophilic leukemia cells (RBL-2H3). *Biochemical and Biophysical Research Communications*, **177**, 192–201.

Conrad, D. H., Bazin, H., Sehon, A. H. & Froese, A. (1975) Binding parameters of the interaction between rat IgE and rat mast cell receptors. *Journal of Immunology*, **114**, 1688–1691.

Costa, J. J., Demetri, G. D., Harrist, T. J., Dvorak, A. M., Hayes, D. F., Merica, E. A. *et al.* (1996) Recombinant human stem cell factor (kit-ligand) promotes human mast cell and melanocyte hyperplasia and functional activation *in vivo*. *Journal of Experimental Medicine*, **183**, 2681–2686.

Cowen, T., Trigg, P. & Eady, R. A. J. (1979) Distribution of mast cells in human dermis: development of a mapping technique. *British Journal of Dermatology*, **100**, 635–640.

Dastych, J. & Metcalfe, D. D. (1994) Stem cell factor induces mast cell adhesion to fibronectin. *Journal of Immunology*, **152**, 213–219.

Dekker, L. V. & Parker, P. J. (1994) Protein kinase C – a question of specificity. *Trends in Biochemical Sciences*, **19**, 73–77.

Demora, F., Garcia, G., Ferrer, L. & Arboix, M. (1993) Canine cutaneous mast cells dispersion and histamine secretory characterization. *Veterinary Immunology and Immunopathology*, **39**, 421–429.

Demora, F., Garcia, G., Puigdemont, A., Arboix, M. & Ferrer, L. (1996) Skin mast cell releasability in dogs with atopic dermatitis. *Inflammation Research*, **45**, 424–427.

Dvorak, A. M. (1993) Ultrastructural analysis of anaphylactic and piecemeal degranulation of human mast cells and basophils. In: *Immunopharmacology of Mast Cells and Basophils* (Ed. J. C. Foreman), pp. 89–113. Academic Press, London.

Eady, R. A. J. (1979) Mast cell population, blood vessel density and histamine content in normal human skin. *British Journal of Dermatology*, **100**, 623–634.

Echtenacher, B., Mannel, D. N. & Hultner, L. (1996) Critical protective role of mast cells in a model of acute septic peritonitis. *Nature*, **381**, 75–77.

Edwardson, J. M. & Marciniak, S. J. (1995) Molecular mechanisms in exocytosis. *Journal of Membrane Biology*, **146**, 113–122.

Eiseman, E. & Bolen, J. B. (1992) Engagement of the high-affinity IgE receptor activates *src* protein-related tyrosine kinases. *Nature*, **355**, 78–80.

Emadikhiav, B., Mousli, M., Bronner, C. & Landry, Y. (1995) Human and rat cutaneous mast cells: involvement of a G-protein in the response to peptidergic stimuli. *European Journal of Pharmacology*, **272**, 97–102.

Emerson, J. L. & Cross, R. F. (1965) The distribution of mast cells in normal canine skin. *American Journal of Veterinary Research*, **26**, 1379–1382.

Enerback, L. (1966a) Mast cells in gastrointestinal mucosa. 2. Dye-binding and metachromatic properties. *Acta Pathologica et Microbiologica Scandinavica*, **66**, 303–312.

Enerback, L. (1966b) Mast cells in gastrointestinal mucosa. 3. Reactivity towards compound 48/80. *Acta Pathologica et Microbiologica Scandinavica*, **66**, 313–322.

Enerback, L. (1974) Ultrastructure of mucosal mast cells in normal and compound 48/80 treated rats. *Cell and Tissue Research*, **150**, 95–101.

Foreman, J. (1993) Non-immunological stimuli of mast cells and basophil leucocytes. In: *Immunopharmacology of Mast Cells and Basophils* (Ed. J. Foreman), pp. 57–69. Academic Press, London.

Foreman, J. C., Mongar, J. L. & Gomperts, B. D. (1973) Calcium ionophores and movement of calcium ions following the physiological stimulus to a secretory process. *Nature*, **245**, 249–251.

Foster, A. P. (1994) A study of the number and distribution of cutaneous mast cells in cats with disease not affecting the skin. *Veterinary Dermatology*, **5**, 17–20.

Galli, S. J. & Kitamura, Y. (1987) Genetically mast cell-deficient W/W^{v} and Sl/Sl^{d} mice: their value for the analysis of the roles of mast cells in biologic responses *in vivo*. *American Journal of Pathology*, **127**, 191–198.

Galli, S. J. & Wershil, B. K. (1995) Mouse mast cell cytokine production: role in cutaneous inflammatory and immunological responses. *Experimental Dermatology*, **4**, 240–249.

Galli, S. J., Arizono, N., Murakami, T., Dvorak, A. M. & Fox, J. G. (1987) Development of large numbers of mast cells at sites of idiopathic chronic dermatitis in genetically mast cell-deficient WBB6F1-W/Wv mice. *Blood*, **69**, 1661–1666.

Galli, S. J., Iemura, A., Garlick, D. S., Gamba-Vitalo, C., Zsebo, K. M. & Andrews, R. G. (1993) Reversible expansion of primate mast cell populations *in vivo* by stem cell factor. *Journal of Clinical Investigation*, **91**, 148–152.

Galli, S. J., Maurer, M. & Lantz, C. S. (1999) Mast cells as sentinels of innate immunity. *Current Opinion in Immunology*, **11**, 53–59.

Gericke, M., Dar, O., Droogmans, G., Pecht, I. & Nilius, B. (1995) Immunological stimulation of single rat basophilic leukemia RBL-2H3 cells co-activates Ca^{2+} entry and K^{+} channels. *Cell Calcium*, **17**, 71–83.

Gomperts, B. D. (1983) Involvement of guanine nucleotide binding protein in the gating of Ca^{2+} by receptors. *Nature*, **306**, 64–66.

Gordon, J. R. & Galli, S. J. (1990) Phorbol 12-myristate 13-acetate induced development of functionally active mast cells in W/Wv but not Sl/Sld genetically mast cell-deficient mice. *Blood*, **75**, 1637–1645.

Gordon, J. R., Burd, P. R. & Galli, S. J. (1990) Mast cells as a source of multifunctional cytokines. *Immunology Today*, **11**, 458–464.

Gruber, B. L., Marchese, M. J. & Kew, R. R. (1994) Transforming growth factor β1 mediates mast cell chemotaxis. *Journal of Immunology*, **152**, 5860–5867.

van Haaster, C. M. C. J., Derhaag, J. G., Engels, W., Lemmens, P. J. M. R., Gijsen, A. P., Hornstra, G. *et al.* (1997) Mast cell mediated induction of ICAM-1, VCAM-1 and E-selectin in endothelial cells *in vitro*: constitutive release of inducing mediators but no effect of degranulation. *Pflugers Archiv, European Journal of Physiology*, **435**, 137–144.

Habara, Y. & Kanno, T. (1996) Perimetric $[Ca^{2+}]_i$ rise and exocytosis detected by ultraviolet laser scanning confocal microscopy in rat peritoneal mast cells. *Experimental Physiology*, **81**, 319–328.

Haig, D. M., Mckee, T. A., Jarrett, E. E. E., Woodbury, R. & Miller, H. R. P. (1982) Generation of mucosal mast cells is stimulated *in vitro* by factors derived from T-cells of helminth-infected rats. *Nature*, **300**, 188–190.

Haig, D. M., McMenamin, C., Redmond, J., Brown, D., Young, I. G., Cohen, S. D. R. & Hapel, A. J. (1988) Rat IL-3 stimulates the growth of rat mucosal mast cells in culture. *Immunology*, **65**, 205–211.

Halliwell, R. E. W. (1973) The localization of IgE in canine skin: an immunofluorescent study. *Journal of Immunology*, **110**, 422–430.

Halliwell, R. E. W., Gilbert, S. M. & Lian, T. M. (1998) Induced and spontaneous IgE antibodies to *Dermatophagoides farinae* in dogs and cats: evidence of functional heterogeneity of IgE. *Veterinary Dermatology*, **9**, 179–184.

Halliwell, R. E. W., Myles, A. D. & Miller, H. R. P. (1993) The inflammatory properties of canine mast cell tryptase and the effects of prednisolone, chlopheniramine and aspirin. In: *Proceedings of the 9th Annual Meeting of the American Academy and American College of Veterinary Dermatology, San Diego*, USA, p. 52.

Hammerling, R. & De Weck, A. L. (1998) Comparison of two diagnostic tests for canine atopy using monoclonal anti-IgE antibodies. *Veterinary Dermatology*, **9**, 191–199.

Hartmann, K., Henz, B. M., Krugerkrasagakes, S., Kohl, J., Burger, R., Guhl, S. *et al.* (1997) C3a and C5a stimulate chemotaxis of human mast cells. *Blood*, **89**, 2863–2870.

He, S. H. & Walls, A. F. (1998) Human mast cell chymase induces the accumulation of neutrophils, eosinophils and other inflammatory cells *in vivo*. *British Journal of Pharmacology*, **125**, 1491–1500.

He, S. H., Peng, Q. & Walls, A. F. (1997) Potent induction of a neutrophil and eosinophil-rich infiltrate *in vivo* by human mast cell tryptase: selective enhancement of eosinophil recruitment by histamine. *Journal of Immunology*, **159**, 6216–6225.

Hellstrom, B. & Holmgren, H. (1950) Numerical distribution of mast cells in the human skin and heart. *Acta Anatomica*, **10**, 81–107.

Hill, P. B. & Martin, R. J. (1998) A review of mast cell biology. *Veterinary Dermatology*, **9**, 145–166.

Hill, P. B., MacDonald, A. J., Thornton, E. M., Newlands, G. F. J., Galli, S. J. & Miller, H. R. P. (1996) Stem cell factor enhances immunoglobulin E-dependent mediator release from cultured rat bone marrow-derived mast cells: activation of previously unresponsive cells demonstrated by a novel ELISPOT assay. *Immunology*, **87**, 326–333.

Hirasawa, N., Scharenberg, A., Yamamura, H., Beaven, M. A. & Kinet, J. P. (1995a) A requirement for Syk in the activation of the microtubule-associated protein kinase/phospholipase-A_2 pathway by FcεR1 is not shared by a G protein-coupled receptor. *Journal of Biological Chemistry*, **270**, 10960–10967.

Hirasawa, N., Santini, F. & Beaven, M. A. (1995b) Activation of the mitogen-activated protein kinase cytosolic phospholipase A_2 pathway in a rat mast cell line: indications of different pathways for release of arachidonic acid and secretory granules. *Journal of Immunology*, **154**, 5391–5402.

Horner, A. A. (1971) Macromolecular heparin from rat skin. *Journal of Biological Chemistry*, **246**, 231–239.

Hoth, M. & Penner, R. (1992) Depletion of intracellular calcium stores activates a calcium current in mast cells. *Nature*, **355**, 353–356.

Hoth, M. & Penner, R. (1993) Calcium release-activated calcium current in rat mast cells. *Journal of Physiology (London)*, **465**, 359–386.

Hultner, L., Druez, C., Moeller, J., Uyttenhouse, C., Schmitt, E., Rude, E. *et al.* (1990) Mast cell growth enhancing activity (MEA) is structurally related and functionally identical to novel T cell growth factor P40/TCGFIII (interleukin 9). *European Journal of Immunology*, **20**, 1413–1416.

Huntley, J. F., Gibson, S., Brown, D., Smith, W. D., Jackson, F. & Miller, H. R. P. (1987) Systemic release of a mast cell proteinase following nematode infections in sheep. *Parasite Immunology*, **9**, 603–614.

Irani, A. A., Schecter, N. M., Craig, S. S., Deblois, G. & Schwartz, L. B. (1986) Two types of human mast cells that have distinct neutral protease compositions. *Proceedings of the National Academy of Sciences of the United States of America*, **83**, 4464–4468.

Ishizaka, T., Foreman, J. C., Sterk, A. R. & Ishizaka, K. (1979) Induction of calcium flux across the rat mast cell membrane by bridging IgE receptors. *Proceedings of the National Academy of Sciences of the United States of America*, **76**, 5858–5862.

Jouvin, M. H. E., Adamczewski, M., Numerof, R., Letourneur, O., Valle, A. & Kinet, J. P. (1994) Differential control of the tyrosine kinases Lyn and Syk by the two signaling chains of the high affinity immunoglobulin E receptor. *Journal of Biological Chemistry*, **269**, 5918–5925.

Kasugai, T., Tei, H., Okada, M., Hirota, S., Morimoto, M., Yamada, M. *et al.* (1995) Infection with *Nippostrongylus brasiliensis* induces invasion of mast cell precursors from peripheral blood to small intestine. *Blood*, **85**, 1334–1340.

Kendall, J. C., Li, X. H., Galli, S. J. & Gordon, J. R. (1997) Promotion of mouse fibroblast proliferation by IgE-dependent activation of mouse mast cells: role for mast cell tumor necrosis factor-α and

transforming growth factor-β1. *Journal of Allergy and Clinical Immunology*, **99**, 113–123.
Kietzmann, M. (1989) Eicosanoid levels in canine inflammatory skin diseases. In: *Advances in Veterinary Dermatology*, Vol. 1 (Eds C. VonTscharner & R. E. W. Halliwell), pp. 211–220. Baillière Tindall, London.
Kinashi, T. & Springer, T. A. (1994) Steel factor and c-kit regulate cell matrix adhesion. *Blood*, **83**, 1033–1038.
Kinet, J.-P. (1990) The high affinity receptor for IgE. *Current Opinion in Immunology*, **2**, 499–505.
Kinet, J.-P., Blank, U., Ra, C., Metzger, H. & Kochan, J. (1988) Isolation and characterization of cDNAs coding for the β subunit of the high-affinity receptor for immunoglobulin E. *Proceedings of the National Academy of Sciences of the United States of America*, **85**, 6483–6487.
Kirshenbaum, A. S., Kessler, S. W., Goff, J. P. & Metcalfe, D. D. (1991) Demonstration of the origin of human mast cells from $CD34^+$ bone marrow progenitor cells. *Journal of Immunology*, **146**, 1410–1415.
Kitamura, Y. & Go, S. (1979) Decreased production of mast cells in Sl/Sl^d anemic mice. *Blood*, **53**, 492–497.
Kitamura, Y., Shimada, M., Hatanaka, K. & Miyano, Y. (1977) Development of mast cells from grafted bone marrow cells in irradiated mice. *Nature*, **268**, 442–443.
Kitamura, Y., Go, S. & Hatanaka, K. (1978) Decrease of mast cells in W/W^v mice and their increase by bone marrow transplantation. *Blood*, **52**, 447–452.
Kitamura, Y., Hatanaka, K., Murakami, M. & Shibata, H. (1979) Presence of mast cell precursors in peripheral blood of mice demonstrated by parabiosis. *Blood*, **53**, 1085–1088.
Kitamura, Y., Yokoyama, M., Matsuda, H., Ohno, T. & Mori, K. J. (1981) Spleen colony-forming cell as common precursor for tissue mast cells and granulocytes. *Nature*, **291**, 159–160.
Kleinbeck, M. L., Hites, M. J., Loker, J. L., Halliwell, R. E. W. & Lee, K. W. (1989) Enzyme linked immunosorbent assay for measurement of allergen-specific IgE antibodies in canine serum. *American Journal of Veterinary Research*, **50**, 1831–1839.
Koffer, A., Tatham, P. E. R. & Gomperts, B. D. (1990) Changes in the state of actin during the exocytotic reaction of permeabilized rat mast cells. *Journal of Cell Biology*, **111**, 919–927.
Krugerkrasagakes, S., Grutzkau, A., Baghramian, R. & Henz, B. M. (1996) Interactions of immature human mast cells with extracellular matrix: expression of specific adhesion receptors and their role in cell binding to matrix proteins. *Journal of Investigative Dermatology*, **106**, 538–543.
Kube, P., Audige, L., Kuther, K. & Welle, M. (1998) Distribution, density and heterogeneity of canine mast cells and influence of fixation techniques. *Histochemistry and Cell Biology*, **110**, 129–135.
Lavens, S. E., Peachell, P. T. & Warner, J. A. (1992) Role of tyrosine kinases in IgE-mediated signal transduction in human lung mast cells and basophils. *American Journal of Respiratory Cell and Molecular Biology*, **7**, 637–644.
Lee, T. D. G., Sterk, A., Ishizaka, T., Bienenstock, J. & Befus, A. D. (1985) Number and affinity of receptors for IgE on enriched populations of isolated rat intestinal mast cells. *Immunology*, **55**, 363–366.
Lippert, U., Artuc, M., Grutzkau, A., Moller, A., KenderessySzabo, A., Schadendorf, D. *et al.* (1998) Expression and functional activity of the IL-8 receptor type CXCR1 and CXCR2 on human mast cells. *Journal of Immunology*, **161**, 2600–2608.
London, C. A., Galli, S. J., Yuuki, T., Hu, Z. Q., Helfand, S. C. & Geissler, E. N. (1999) Spontaneous canine mast cell tumors express tandem duplications in the proto-oncogene c-kit. *Experimental Hematology*, **27**, 689–697.
Lorenz, D., Wiesner, B., Zipper, J., Winkler, A., Krause, E., Beyermann, M. *et al.* (1998) Mechanism of peptide-induced mast cell degranulation: translocation and patch-clamp studies. *Journal of General Physiology*, **112**, 577–591.
Ludowyke, R. I., Peleg, I., Beaven, M. A. & Adelstein, R. S. (1989) Antigen-induced secretion of histamine and the phosphorylation of myosin by protein kinase C in rat basophilic leukemia cells. *Journal of Biological Chemistry*, **264** 12492–12501.
Malaviya, R., Ikeda, T., Ross, E. & Abraham, S. N. (1996) Mast cell modulation of neutrophil influx and bacterial clearance at sites of infection through TNF-alpha. *Nature*, **381**, 77–80.
Mao, S.-Y., Varin-Blank, N., Edidin, M. & Metzger, H. (1991) Immobilization and internalization of mutated IgE receptors in transfected cells. *Journal of Immunology*, **146**, 958–966.
Marsella, R. & Nicklin, C. F. (1999) Investigation on sulfido-leukotriene synthesis from peripheral mononuclear cells and skin of normal and atopic dogs. In: *Proceedings of the 15th Annual Meeting of the American Academy and American College of Veterinary Dermatology*, Maui, Hawaii, USA, pp. 101–102.
Marshall, J. S. & Bienenstock, J. (1994) The role of mast cells in inflammatory reactions of the airways, skin and intestines. *Current Opinion in Immunology*, **6**, 853–859.
Matsuura, N. & Zetter, B. R. (1989) Stimulation of mast-cell chemotaxis by interleukin-3. *Journal of Experimental Medicine*, **170**, 1421–1426.
Maurer, M., Echtenacher, B., Hultner, L., Kollias, G., Mannel, D. N., Langley, K. E. & Galli, S. J. (1998) The c-kit ligand, stem cell factor, can enhance innate immunity through effects on mast cells. *Journal of Experimental Medicine*, **188**, 2343–2348.
Mayrhofer, G. & Fisher, R. (1979) Mast cells in severely T-cell depleted rats and the response to infestation with *Nippostrongylus brasiliensis*. *Immunology*, **37**, 145–155.
Meininger, C. J., Yano, H., Rottapel, R., Bernstein, A., Zsebo, K. M. & Zetter, B. R. (1992) The c-kit receptor ligand functions as a mast cell chemoattractant. *Blood*, **79**, 958–963.
Mendoza, G. R. & Metzger, H. (1976) Distribution and valency of receptor for IgE on rodent mast cells and related tumour cells. *Nature*, **264**, 548–550.
Metcalfe, D. D., Soter, N. A., Wasserman, S. I. & Austen, K. F. (1980) Identification of sulfated mucopolysaccharides including heparin in the lesional skin of a patient with mastocytosis. *Journal of Investigative Dermatology*, **74**, 210–215.
Mikhail, G. R. & Miller-Millinska, A. (1964) Mast cell population in human skin. *Journal of Investigative Dermatology*, **43**, 249–254.
Miller, H. R. P. (1971) Immune reactions in mucous membranes III. The discharge of intestinal mast cells during helminth expulsion in the rat. *Laboratory Investigation*, **24**, 348–354.
Miller, H. R. P. (1993) Mast cells in the gastrointestinal tract. In: *Immunopharmacology of Mast Cells and Basophils* (Ed. J. C. Foreman), pp. 197–215. Academic Press, London.
Miller, H. R. P. & Jarrett, W. F. H. (1971) Immune reactions in mucous membranes. 1. Intestinal mast cell response during helminth expulsion in the rat. *Immunology*, **20**, 277–288.
Miller, H. R. P., Woodbury, R. G., Huntley, J. F. & Newlands, G. (1983) Systemic release of mucosal mast cell protease in primed rats challenged with *Nippostrongylus brasiliensis*. *Immunology*, **49**, 471–479.
Moeller, J., Hultner, L., Schmitt, E. & Dormer, P. (1989) Partial purification of a mast cell growth-enhancing activity and its separation from IL-3 and IL-4. *Journal of Immunology*, **142**, 3447–3451.
Monck, J. R. & Fernandez, J. M. (1992) The exocytotic fusion pore. *Journal of Cell Biology*, **119**, 1395–1404.

Myles, A. D., Halliwell, R. E. W., Ballauf, B. & Miller, H. R. P. (1995) Mast cell tryptase levels in normal canine tissues. *Veterinary Immunology and Immunopathology*, **46**, 223–235.

Nabel, G., Galli, S. J., Dvorak, A. M., Dvorak, H. F. & Cantor, H. (1981) Inducer T lymphocytes synthesize a factor that stimulates proliferation of cloned mast cells. *Nature*, **291**, 332–334.

Nagao, K., Yokoro, K. & Aaronson, S. A. (1981) Continuous lines of basophil-mast cells derived from normal mouse bone marrow. *Science*, **212**, 333–335.

Nakahata, T. & Ogawa, M. (1982) Identification in culture of a class of hemopoietic colony-forming units with extensive capability to self renew and generate multipotential hemopoietic colonies. *Proceedings of the National Academy of Sciences of the United States of America*, **79**, 3843–3847.

Nakahata, T., Spicer, S. S., Cantry, J. R. & Ogawa, M. (1982) Clonal assay of mouse mast cell colonies in methylcellulose culture. *Blood*, **127**, 788–794.

Nawa, Y. & Miller, H. R. P. (1979) Adoptive transfer of the intestinal mast cell response in rats infected with *Nippostrongylus brasiliensis*. *Cellular Immunology*, **42**, 225–239.

Nielsen, E. H., Braun, K. & Johansen, T. (1989) Reorganization of the subplasmalemmal cytoskeleton in association with exocytosis in rat mast cells. *Histology and Histopathology*, **4**, 473–477.

Nilsson, G., Mikovits, J. A., Metcalfe, D. D. & Taub, D. D. (1999) Mast cell migratory response to interleukin-8 is mediated through interaction with chemokine receptor CXCR2/interleukin-8RB. *Blood*, **93**, 2791–2797.

Nimmo Wilkie, J. S., Yager, J. A., Eyre, P. & Parker, W. M. (1990) Morphometric analyses of the skin of dogs with atopic dermatitis and correlations with cutaneous and plasma histamine and total serum IgE. *Veterinary Pathology*, **27**, 179–186.

Nissim, A. & Eshhar, Z. (1992) The human mast cell receptor binding site maps to the third constant domain of immunoglobulin E. *Molecular Immunology*, **29**, 1065–1072.

Nissim, A., Jouvin, M.-H. & Eshhar, Z. (1991) Mapping of the high affinity Fcε receptor binding-site to the third constant domain of IgE. *EMBO Journal*, **10**, 101–107.

Ody, C., Kindler, V. & Vassali, P. (1990) Interleukin 3 perfusion in W/W^v mice allows the development of macroscopic spleen colonies and restores cutaneous mast cell number. *Journal of Experimental Medicine*, **172**, 403–406.

Olivry, T., Moore, P. F., Affolter, V. K. & Naydan, D. K. (1996) Langerhans cell hyperplasia and IgE expression in canine atopic dermatitis. *Archives of Dermatological Research*, **288**, 579–585.

Olivry, T., Naydan, D. K. & Moore, P. F. (1997) Characterization of the cutaneous inflammatory infiltrate in canine atopic dermatitis. *American Journal of Dermatopathology*, **19**, 477–486.

Ozawa, K., Szallasi, Z., Kazanietz, M. G., Blumberg, P. M., Mischak, H., Mushinski, J. F. & Beaven, M. A. (1993a) Ca^{2+}-dependent and Ca^{2+}-independent isozymes of protein kinase C mediate exocytosis in antigen stimulated rat basophilic RBL-2H3 cells – reconstitution of secretory responses with Ca^{2+} and purified isozymes in washed permeabilized cells. *Journal of Biological Chemistry*, **268**, 1749–1756.

Ozawa, K., Yamada, K., Kazanietz, M. G., Blumberg, P. M. & Beaven, M. A. (1993b) Different isozymes of protein kinase C mediate feedback inhibition of phospholipase C and stimulatory signals for exocytosis in rat RBL-2H3 cells. *Journal of Biological Chemistry*, **268**, 2280–2283.

Paolini, R., Jouvin, M. H. & Kinet, J. P. (1991) Phosphorylation and dephosphorylation of the high-affinity receptor for immunoglobulin E immediately after receptor engagement and disengagement. *Nature*, **353**, 855–858.

Plaut, M., Pierce, J. H., Watson, C. J., Hanleyhyde, J., Nordan, R. P. & Paul, W. E. (1989) Mast cell lines produce lymphokines in response to cross-linkage of FcεR1 or to calcium ionophores. *Nature*, **339**, 64–67.

Razin, E., Cordon-Cardo, C. & Good, R. A. (1981) Growth of a pure population of mouse mast cells *in vitro* with conditioned medium derived from concanavalin A-stimulated splenocytes. *Proceedings of the National Academy of Sciences of the United States of America*, **78**, 2559–2561.

Rhee, S. G., Shu, P. G., Ryu, S. H. & Lee, S. Y. (1989) Studies of inositol phospholipid-specific phospholipase C. *Science*, **244**, 546–550.

Ring, J. (1983) Plasma histamine concentrations in atopic eczema. *Clinical Allergy*, **13**, 545–552.

Rodewald, H. R., Dessing, M., Dvorak, A. M. & Galli, S. J. (1996) Identification of a committed precursor for the mast cell lineage. *Science*, **271**, 818–822.

Rohlich, P. (1975) Membrane-associated actin filaments in the cortical cytoplasm of the rat mast cell. *Experimental Cell Research*, **93**, 293–298.

Roitt, I., Brostoff, J. & Male, D. (1993) *Immunology*, pp.1.1–25.16. Mosby, London.

Ruitenberg, E. J. & Elgersma, A. (1976) Absence of intestinal mast cell response in congenitally athymic mice during *Trichinella spiralis* infection. *Nature*, **264**, 258–260.

Sagi-Eisenberg, R. (1993) Signal-transmission pathways in mast cell exocytosis. In: *Immunopharmacology of Mast Cells and Basophils* (Ed. J. C. Foreman), pp. 71–88. Academic Press, London.

Schechter, N. M., Slavin, D., Fetter, R. D., Lazarus, G. S. & Fraki, J. E. (1988) Purification and identification of two serine class proteinases from dog mast cells biochemically and immunologically similar to human proteinases tryptase and chymase. *Archives of Biochemistry and Biophysics*, **262**, 232–244.

Schlessinger, J., Webb, W. W., Elson, E. L. & Metzger, H. (1976) Lateral motion and valence of Fc receptors on rat peritoneal mast cells. *Nature*, **264**, 550–552.

Schmitt, E., Fassbender, B., Beyreuther, K., Spaeth, E., Schwarzkopf, R. & Rude, E. (1987) Characterization of a T cell-derived lymphokine that acts synergistically with IL-3 on the growth of murine mast cells and is identical with IL-4. *Immunobiology*, **174**, 406–419.

Schrader, J. W., Lewis, S. J., Clark-Lewis, I. & Culvenor, J. G. (1981) The persistent (P) cell: histamine content, regulation by a T cell-derived factor, origin from a bone marrow precursor and relationship to mast cells. *Proceedings of the National Academy of Sciences of the United States of America*, **78**, 323–327.

Schwartz, L. B. (1994) Mast cells: function and contents. *Current Opinion in Immunology*, **6**, 91–97.

Schwartz, L. B., Irani, A. A., Roller, K., Castells, M. C. & Schecter, N. M. (1987) Quantitation of histamine, tryptase and chymase in dispersed human T and TC mast cells. *Journal of Immunology*, **138**, 2611–2615.

Scott, D. W. (1981) Observations on canine atopy. *Journal of the American Animal Hospital Association*, **17**, 91–100.

Scott, D. W., Miller, W. H. & Griffin, C. E. (1995a) *Small Animal Dermatology*, p. 32. W. B. Saunders, Philadelphia, PA.

Scott, D. W., Miller, W. H. & Griffin, C. E. (1995b) Immunological skin diseases. In: *Small Animal Dermatology*, 5th edn. (Eds D. W. Scott, W. H. Miller & C. E. Griffin), pp. 484–626. W. B. Saunders, Philadelphia, PA.

Shanahan, F., Denburg, J. A., Fox, J., Bienenstock, J. & Befus, D. (1985) Mast cell heterogeneity: effects of neuroenteric peptides on histamine release. *Journal of Immunology*, **135**, 1331–1337.

Shiue, L., Zoller, M. J. & Brugge, J. S. (1995) Syk is activated by phosphotyrosine-containing peptides representing the tyrosine-based activation motifs of the high-affinity receptor for IgE. *Journal of Biological Chemistry*, **270**, 10498–10502.

Shull, R. M., Suggs, S. V., Langley, K. E., Okino, K. H., Jacobsen, F. W. & Martin, F. H. (1992) Canine stem cell factor (c-kit ligand) supports the survival of hematopoietic progenitors in long term canine marrow culture. *Experimental Hematology*, **20**, 1118–1124.

Smith, T. J. & Weis, J. H. (1996) Mucosal T-cells and mast cells share common adhesion receptors. *Immunology Today*, **17**, 60–63.

Sonoda, T., Ohno, T. & Kitamura, Y. (1982) Concentration of mast cell precursors in bone marrow, spleen and blood of mice determined by limiting dilution analysis. *Journal of Cellular Physiology*, **112**, 136–140.

Spat, A., Fabiato, A. & Rubin, R. P. (1986a) Binding of inositol trisphosphate by a liver microsomal fraction. *Biochemical Journal*, **233**, 929–932.

Spat, A., Bradford, P. G., McKinney, J. S., Rubin, R. P. & Putney, J. W. (1986b) A saturable receptor for ^{32}P-inositol-1,4,5-trisphosphate in hepatocytes and neutrophils. *Nature*, **319**, 514–516.

Sriramarao, P., Anderson, W., Wolitzky, B. A. & Broide, D. H. (1996) Mouse bone marrow-derived mast cells roll on P-selectin under conditions of flow *in vivo*. *Laboratory Investigation*, **74**, 634–643.

Steegmaier, M., Blanks, J. E., Borges, E. & Vestweber, D. (1997) P-selectin glycoprotein ligand-1 mediates rolling of mouse bone marrow-derived mast cells on P-selectin but not efficiently on E-selectin. *European Journal of Immunology*, **27**, 1339–1345.

Sterk, A. R. & Ishizaka, T. (1982) Binding properties of IgE receptors on normal mouse mast cells. *Journal of Immunology*, **128**, 838–843.

Stevens, R. L., Lee, T. D. G., Seldin, D. C., Austen, K. F., Befus, A. D. & Bienenstock, J. (1986) Intestinal mucosal mast cells from rats infected with *Nippostrongylus brasiliensis* contain protease-resistant chondroitin sulfate di-B proteoglycans. *Journal of Immunology*, **137**, 291–295.

Streb, H., Irvine, R. F., Berridge, M. J. & Schulz, I. (1983) Release of Ca^{2+} from a non-mitochondrial intracellular store in pancreatic acinar cells by inositol 1,4,5-trisphosphate. *Nature*, **306**, 67–69.

Stump, R. F., Pfeiffer, J. R., Schneebeck, M. C., Seagrave, J. C. & Oliver, J. M. (1989) Mapping gold-labelled receptors on cell surfaces by back scattered electron imaging and digital image analysis: studies of the IgE receptor on mast cells. *American Journal of Anatomy*, **185**, 128–141.

Tamir, I., Schweitzerstenner, R. & Pecht, I. (1996) Immobilization of the type-1 receptor for IgE initiates signal transduction in mast cells. *Biochemistry*, **35**, 6872–6883.

Tanaka, A., Arai, K., Kitamura, Y. & Matsuda, H. (1999) Matrix metalloproteinase-9 production, a newly identified function of mast cell progenitors, is downregulated by c-kit receptor activation. *Blood*, **94**, 2390–2395.

Tertian, G., Yung, Y. P., Guy-Grand, D. & Moore, M. A. S. (1981) Long term *in vitro* culture of murine mast cells. 1. Description of a growth factor-dependent culture technique. *Journal of Immunology*, **127**, 788–794.

Thompson-Snipes, L. A., Dhar, V., Bond, M. W., Mosmann, T. R., Moore, K. W. & Rennick, D. M. (1991) Interleukin-10: a novel stimulatory factor for mast cells and their progenitors. *Journal of Experimental Medicine*, **173**, 507–510.

Trautmann, A., Toksoy, A., Engelhard, E., Brocker, E. B. & Gillitzer, R. (2000) Mast cell involvement in normal human skin wound healing: expression of monocyte chemoattractant protein-I is correlated with recruitment of mast cells which synthesize interleukin-4 *in vivo*. *Journal of Pathology*, **190**, 100–106.

Tsai, M., Shih, L. S., Newlands, G. F. J., Takeishi, T., Langley, K. E., Zsebo, K. M. *et al.* (1991) The rat c-kit ligand, stem cell factor, induces the development of connective tissue type and mucosal mast cells *in vivo*: analysis by anatomical distribution, histochemistry, and protease phenotype. *Journal of Experimental Medicine*, **174**, 125–131.

Tsuji, K., Nakahata, T., Takagi, M., Kobayashi, T., Ishiguro, A., Kikuchi, T. *et al.* (1990) Effects of interleukin-3 and interleukin-4 on the development of connective tissue-type mast cells: interleukin-3 supports their survival and interleukin-4 triggers and supports their proliferation synergistically with interleukin-3. *Blood*, **75**, 421–427.

Tuohy, M., Lammas, D. A., Wakelin, D., Huntley, J. F., Newlands, G. F. J. & Miller, H. R. P. (1990) Functional correlations between mucosal mast cell activity and immunity to *Trichinella spiralis* in high and low responder mice. *Parasite Immunology*, **12**, 675–685.

Valent, P., Schmidt, G., Besmer, J., Mayer, P., Zenke, G., Liel, E. *et al.* (1989) Interleukin-3 is a differentiation factor for human basophils. *Blood*, **73**, 1763–1769.

Valent, P., Besemer, J., Sillaber, C., Butterfield, J. H., Eher, R., Majdic, O. *et al.* (1990) Failure to detect IL-3-binding sites on human mast cells. *Journal of Immunology*, **145**, 3432–3437.

Varin-Blank, N. & Metzger, H. (1990) Surface expression of mutated subunits of the high affinity mast cell receptor for IgE. *Journal of Biological Chemistry*, **265**, 15685–15694.

Weber, S., Babina, M., Feller, G. & Henz, B. M. (1997) Human leukaemic (HMC-1) and normal skin mast cells express β2-integrins: characterization of β2-integrins and ICAM-1 on HMC-1 cells. *Scandinavian Journal of Immunology*, **45**, 471–481.

Welle, M. M., Olivry, T., Grimm, S. & Suter, M. (1999) Mast cell density and subtypes in the skin of dogs with atopic dermatitis. *Journal of Comparative Pathology*, **120**, 187–197.

Wershil, B. K., Zhen-Sheng, W., Gordon, J. R. & Galli, S. J. (1991) Recruitment of neutrophils during IgE-dependent cutaneous late phase reactions in the mouse is mast cell dependent. Partial inhibition of the reaction with antiserum against tumor necrosis factor-alpha. *Journal of Clinical Investigation*, **87**, 446–453.

White, J. R., Ishizaka, T., Ishizaka, K. & Shaafi, R. I. (1984) Direct demonstration of increased intracellular concentration of free calcium as measured by quin-2 in stimulated rat peritoneal mast cells. *Proceedings of the National Academy of Sciences of the United States of America: Biological Sciences*, **81**, 3978–3982.

Woodbury, R. G., Miller, H. R. P., Huntley, J. F., Newlands, G. F. J., Palliser, A. C. & Wakelin, D. (1984) Mucosal mast cells are functionally active during spontaneous expulsion of intestinal nematode infections in rat. *Nature*, **312**, 450–452.

Yu, K. T., Lyall, R., Jariwala, N., Zilberstein, A. & Haimovich, J. (1991) Antigen- and ionophore-induced signal transduction in rat basophilic leukemia cells involves protein tyrosine phosphorylation. *Journal of Biological Chemistry*, **266**, 22564–22568.

Zhang, L. & McCloskey, M. A. (1995) Immunoglobulin E receptor-activated calcium conductance in rat mast cells. *Journal of Physiology*, **483**, 59–66.

Zsebo, K. M., Williams, D. A., Geissler, E. N., Broudy, V. C., Martin, F. H., Atkins, H. L. *et al.* (1990) Stem cell factor is encoded at the Sl-locus of the mouse and is the ligand for the c-kit tyrosine kinase receptor. *Cell*, **63**, 213–224.

Zucker-Franklin, D., Grusky, G., Hirayama, N. & Schnipper, E. (1981) The presence of mast cell precursors in rat peripheral blood. *Blood*, **58**, 544–551.

Zunic, M. (1998) Comparison between IMMUNODOT tests and the intradermal skin test in atopic dogs. *Veterinary Dermatology*, **9**, 201–205.

4.3

Feline atopic dermatitis: a review

P.J. Roosje DVM,[1] T. Thepen PhD,[2] V.P.M.G. Rutten PhD[3] and T. Willemse DVM, PhD[4]

[1] Interdisciplinary Dermatology Unit, Faculty of Veterinary Medicine, University of Bern, Bern, Switzerland
[2] Laboratory of Immunotherapy, Department of Immunology, University Medical Center, Utrecht, The Netherlands
[3] Institute of Infectious Diseases and Immunology, Department of Immunology, The Netherlands
[4] Department of Clinical Sciences of Companion Animals, Faculty of Veterinary Medicine, Utrecht University, Utrecht, The Netherlands

Summary

In humans, research on atopy in general and atopic dermatitis specifically has revealed a wealth of information about the possible underlying pathogenesis. Although the exact pathogenesis is still unknown the acquired understanding has led to many new therapies trying to modulate specific steps in the disease process. Knowledge about feline allergic skin disease is far behind the knowledge gathered in the human field. Recently, new information on the immunopathogenesis of feline atopic dermatitis has become available, comparing findings in cats with the observations in human atopic dermatitis. Although species differences will exist, the information on human atopic dermatitis can be of great benefit in our understanding of feline atopic dermatitis. Knowledge of the pathogenesis of feline atopic dermatitis can lead to better therapies.

Introduction

The first reports published on selected feline allergic skin diseases appeared in the early 1980s (Reedy, 1982; McDougal, 1986). In these publications the use and effects of allergy testing and hyposensitisation were described, indicating that a pathogenesis comparable to atopic dermatitis (AD) in humans was hypothesised. Feline AD is now a commonly diagnosed disease and various studies estimate that it accounts for approximately 12–15% of the cases of feline allergic dermatitis (Scott, 1986; O'Dair *et al.*, 1996).

Atopy in humans is defined as the tendency to develop immunoglobulin E (IgE) antibodies to commonly encountered environmental allergens and the subsequent development of disease (Ring, 1991). Allergic rhinitis, asthma and atopic dermatitis are clinical manifestations of atopy. Atopic dermatitis in humans is a common chronic, eczematous skin disease characterised by remissions and exacerbations. The diagnosis of AD is based on clinical observations, consisting of the patient's history, family history, and a distinct clinical morphology and distribution of skin lesions (Hanifin & Rajka, 1980). There is no objective laboratory test for the diagnosis of AD. The diagnosis is generally based on the criteria proposed by Hanifin & Rajka (1980) and consists of major and minor criteria.

Pathogenesis

The aetiology of AD in humans is multifactorial. Genetic factors, bacterial infections, aeroallergens, irritants, food allergens and psychological factors may play a role (Bos *et al.*, 1994).

A multitude of evidence indicates the importance of genetic factors in humans. Twin studies showed a 85% concordance for AD among monozygotic twins (Schultz Larsen, 1993). It is likely that several genes are involved in the development of allergic disease (Leung, 1999). The increasing prevalence of AD in humans, however, is difficult to explain on the basis of genetics alone (Williams, 1992).

In cats a genetic background is suspected because a personal or family diagnosis of atopy has been described (Scott, 1986; Cieslicki & Cieslicki, 1989; Moriello, 2001). Unfortunately, it is often difficult to gather information about a familial history in cats because of the consistency of the cat population. Asthma, one of the other symptoms of the atopy complex, is well known and feline allergic airway responsiveness has been used as an animal model (Barch & Talbott, 1976; Padrid *et al.*, 1995). Concurrent signs of asthma and atopic dermatitis, however, seem to be rare in cats.

Aeroallergens

The role of aeroallergens in the pathogenesis of AD in humans has been a subject of debate and investigations. The fact that more than 80% of the AD patients have elevated serum IgE, with specificity to a variety of the aeroallergens (Juhlin *et al.*, 1969), to which they also demonstrate immediate-type skin reactions (Mackie *et al.*, 1979), indicates a role for aeroallergens in sensitisation. The current concept is that aeroallergens may enter the body via inhalation or skin contact. A limited number of allergen inhalation studies has been performed in AD patients. Tupker *et al.* (1996) showed that skin lesions could be induced or exacerbated by bronchial challenge with aeroallergens in a great number of AD patients. In support of the hypothesis of local allergen transmission, allergen binding was elegantly demonstrated by Tanaka *et al.* (1990), who found house dust mite allergens localised on the membrane of Langerhans' cells after epicutaneous allergen application. In addition, patients with AD often have dry skin (xerosis) and it was shown that a disturbed epidermal barrier function, facilitating allergen penetration, exists in these patients (Imokawa *et al.*, 1991; Fartasch & Diepgen, 1992).

In cats the hypothesis of involvement of aeroallergens is based on the occurrence of positive intradermal skin test reactions to common aeroallergens (Reedy, 1982; McDougal, 1986; Bevier, 1990). In addition, the occurrence of allergen-specific antibodies in serum has been described (Halliwell, 1997). How relevant this is for disease pathogenesis is unknown because allergen-specific IgE levels in normal household cats were not significantly different to those in AD cats (Gilbert & Halliwell, 1998a). Results of hyposensitisation of AD cats, after intradermal skin testing or serology, have been described in open studies only, with a variable success rate depending on the publication (Reedy, 1982; McDougal, 1986; Prost, 1992; Halliwell, 1997). Patient follow-up was often not elaborately described.

The fact is that similarly to humans, the living environment of cats has changed recently and many cats have a different role as pets. Compared with the recent past, more cats live a life that is primarily indoors and therefore are exposed more to indoor aeroallergens. Reactions to house dust mites are frequent among positive intradermal skin reactions. These observations may be skewed because investigators mainly use allergens that commonly cause AD in humans (or in dogs). Cats, however, may be sensitive to other aeroallergens as well.

Food allergens play a pathogenic role, especially in infants and children with AD (Sicherer & Sampson, 1999). The role of food allergens is obscure in AD cats; however, food hypersensitivity is recognised in cats. Cats are generally fed commercial diets, which is different from years ago when the diet consisted more of, for example, mice, birds, and rabbits. The influence of this dietary change is unknown.

Discussion exists about the route of allergen exposure, but evidence supports the concept of both percutaneous allergen penetration (Tanaka *et al.*, 1990) and allergen transmission via the respiratory mucosa in humans (Tupker *et al.*, 1996). The skin of cats is covered by a dense coat, in contrast to humans, suggesting an additional barrier for allergen skin penetration. However, sparsely haired areas do exist (i.e. head, pinnae and abdomen). To the authors' knowledge, percutaneous allergen penetration in feline haired skin has not been studied. Evidence for the respiratory route exists in sensitised cats with bronchial hyperreactivity (Padrid *et al.*, 1995). In addition, the occurrence of a disturbance of the epidermal barrier function facilitating allergen penetration, as in humans with AD, is unknown in cats with AD. This disturbance may occur during the disease process in cats through licking and inflammation but its role in cats is unknown.

Antigen presentation

The Langerhans' cells are part of the skin immunosurveillance system and are important antigen-presenting cells (APC). They are present in increased numbers in the epidermis of human patients with chronic AD (Leung, 1995). It was demonstrated in humans that IgE bound on epidermal Langerhans' cells induced allergen-specific T-cell activation more efficiently. Moreover, eczematous reactions to aeroallergens could be better induced via skin regions harbouring IgE-bearing dendritic cells (Mudde *et al.*, 1990). Langerhans' cells with surface-bound IgE could only be found in AD patients with high serum IgE levels (Bieber & Bruijnzeel, 1990). The discovery of the expression of the high-affinity receptor for IgE (FcεR1) by Langerhans' cells (Bieber *et al.*, 1992; Wang *et al.*, 1992; Osterhoff *et al.*, 1994) supported earlier findings of the presence of IgE^+ dendritic cells in the epidermis and dermis of AD patients (Bruijnzeel-Koomen *et al.*, 1986; Leung *et al.*, 1987). In the skin of healthy control patients no evidence for such cells was found. One of the more specific markers for the Langerhans' cell is the CD1a molecule, which is considered to be part of a third family (CD1) of antigen-presenting molecules, next to major histocompatibility complex class I (MHC I) and MHC II molecules (Beckman & Brenner, 1995). The most reliable morphological way to identify Langerhans' cells is by detection of their Birbeck granules, rod-shaped organelles with unknown function. This can be done by means of electron microscopy or with an antibody that specifically stains for the Lag-antigen, which is part of the membranes of Birbeck granules and related structures (Kashihara *et al.*, 1986). After leaving the epidermis, Langerhans' cells undergo developmental and functional maturation and form part of the dermal dendritic cell population. They change from antigen-capturing and -processing cells into antigen-presenting cells. During the migratory phase the dendritic cells adapt to antigen presentation to T-cells in the dermis or in the draining lymph nodes. Up-regulation of MHC II, adhesion molecules and costimulatory markers entails these phenotypic changes (Neiß *et al.*, 1995).

In the dermis, a number of dendritic cell populations exist which express different markers. One group consists of migrating $CD1a^+$ cells, which are former Langerhans' cells that have lost their Birbeck granules after migration out of the epidermis. The $CD1a^+$ dermal dendritic cells proved to be more important APC than $CD1a^-$ macrophage-like cells in a stimulation assay of peripheral blood mononuclear cells (PBMC) (Sepulveda-Merrill *et al.*, 1994). Osterhoff *et al.* (1994) demonstrated that $FcεR1^+$ cells in the dermis belonged to the Langerhans' cells ($CD1a^+$)/dendritic cell ($RFD1^+$) cell lineage or to mast cells, and not to dermal macrophages ($FXIIIa^+$), suggesting that these $FcεR1^+/RFD1^+$ cells are more important APC.

In AD cats lesional skin contained significantly increased numbers of $CD1a^+$ and MHC II^+ dendritic-like cells in the epidermis and dermis compared with the skin of healthy control animals (Roosje *et al.*, 1997). A variable increase in factor $XIIIa^+$ cells was described in cats with miliary dermatitis and eosinophilic plaques (Anttila *et al.*, 1994). Further differentiation of the dermal dendritic cell population in cats has not been performed.

T-cells

An imbalance has been demonstrated in the generation of Th_1 and Th_2 cytokines in AD in humans, which seems to be related to disease symptoms (Wierenga *et al.*, 1990; van der Heijden *et al.*, 1991). In lesional skin of AD patients a high CD4/CD8 T-cell ratio was found (Sillevis Smitt *et al.*, 1986). van der Heijden *et al.* (1991) and van Reijsen *et al.* (1992) demonstrated that a considerable part of this T-cell population consists of allergen-specific Th_2-cells, implying an important role for these cells in the cutaneous inflammatory reaction of AD. By *in situ* hybridisation it was demonstrated that acute AD lesions are associated with an increased expression of interleukin-4 (IL-4) and IL-13 mRNA compared with chronic lesional skin. In chronic lesions IL-4-producing cells are still found but an increased number of cells expressing IL-5 and IL-12 is present (Hamid *et al.*, 1994, 1996). Moreover, recent studies have demonstrated the overexpression of IL-16 in acute lesions and granulocyte–macrophage colony-stimulating factor (GM-CSF) overexpression in chronic AD lesions (Bratton *et al.*, 1995; Laberge *et al.*, 1998). In addition, uninvolved skin of AD patients contained a significantly greater number of cells that were positive for IL-4 and IL-13 but not IL-5 or γ-interferon (IFN-γ) mRNA (Hamid *et al.*, 1994). This means that at least initially Th_2-cells are predominate over Th_1- and Th_0-cells. The increase in IL-12 and IFN-γ in chronic lesional skin underlines the biphasic expression pattern because these cytokines play a role in Th_1-cell development and modulate the switch from a Th_2- to a Th_1-cell pattern (Hamid *et al.*, 1996; Thepen *et al.*, 1996).

In contrast to the skin, in the peripheral blood an increased number of $CD4^+$ T-cells compared with $CD8^+$ T-cells is not always present. Data exist on increased ratios (Sowden *et al.*, 1992), but decreased ratios have also been found (Blok *et al.*, 1991).

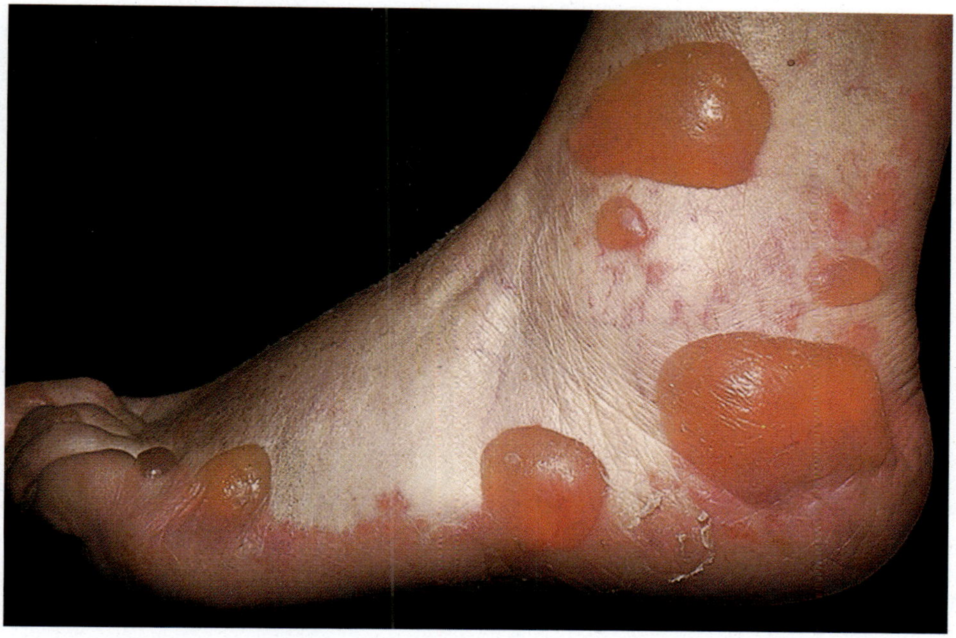

Plate 1. Bullous pemphigoid in a human. Erythematous turgid vesicles, bullae and epidermal collarettes are present on the foot.

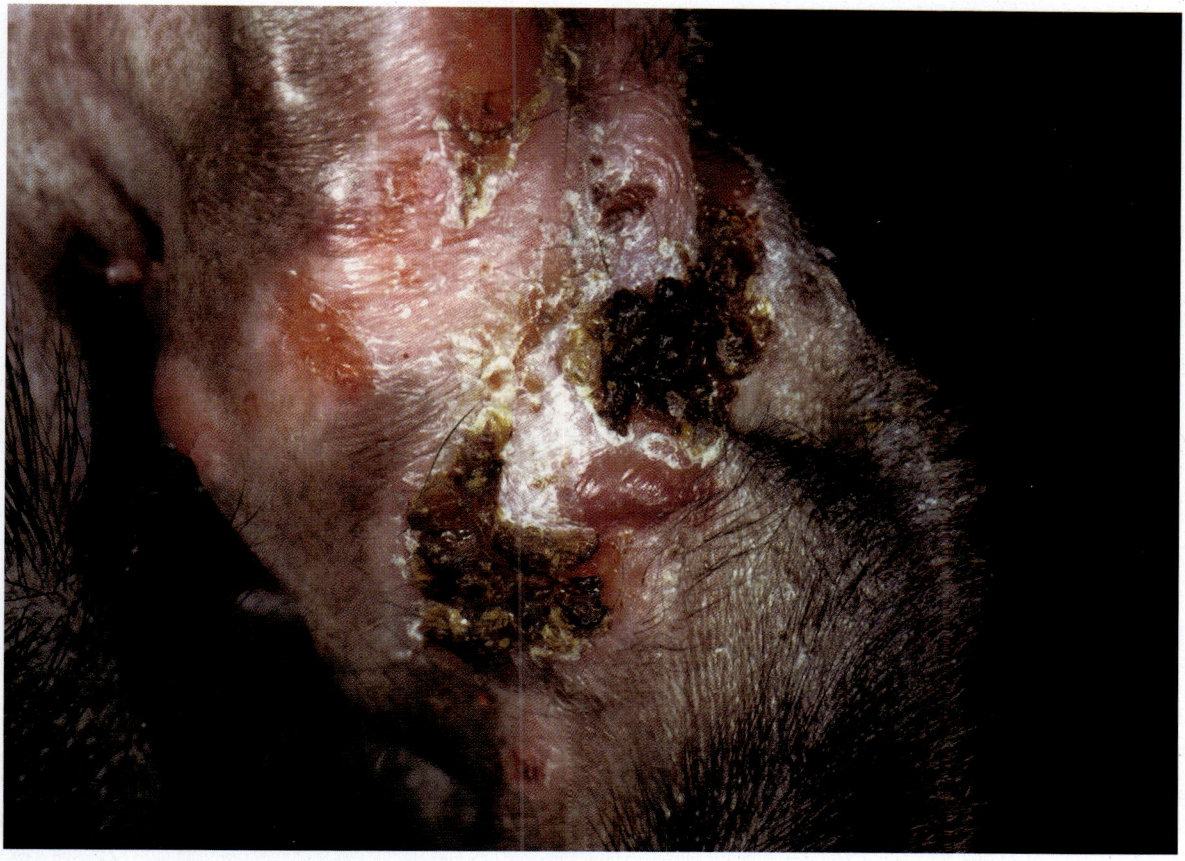

Plate 2. Bullous pemphigoid in a dog. Erythema, hemorrhagic turgid vesicles, erosions and crusts on the concave p nna.

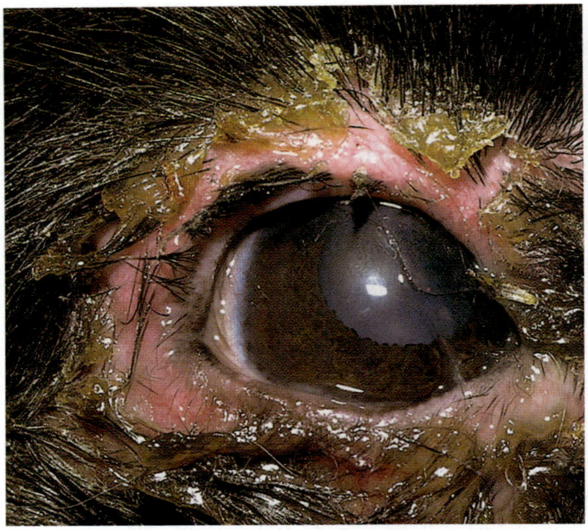

Plate 3. Mucous membrane pemphigoid in a dog. Erosive conjunctivitis and blepharitis occasionally are observed (Courtesy of Dr B. Gilger, NC State University, USA.)

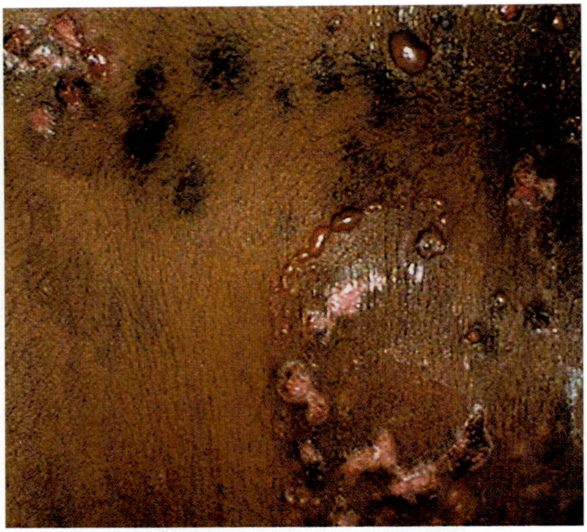

Plate 4. Linear IgA disease in humans. Vesicles, erosions and hypopigmented scars exhibit a polycyclic arrangement.

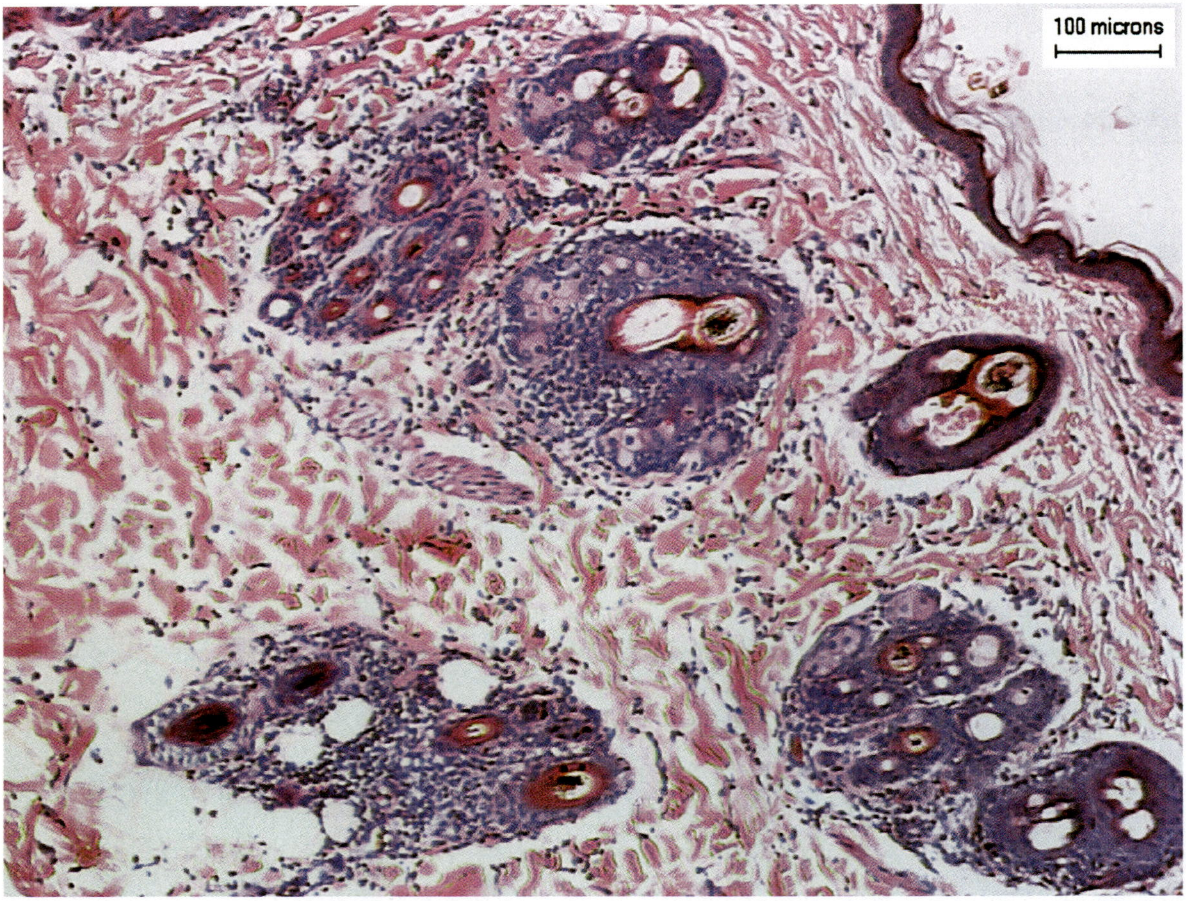

Plate 5. Section of a skin biopsy specimen taken from the site of intradermal injection with soluble *Microsporum canis* antigen, 72 h after injection. There is a perifollicular and follicular infiltrate of predominantly lymphocytes and macrophages. (H&E.)

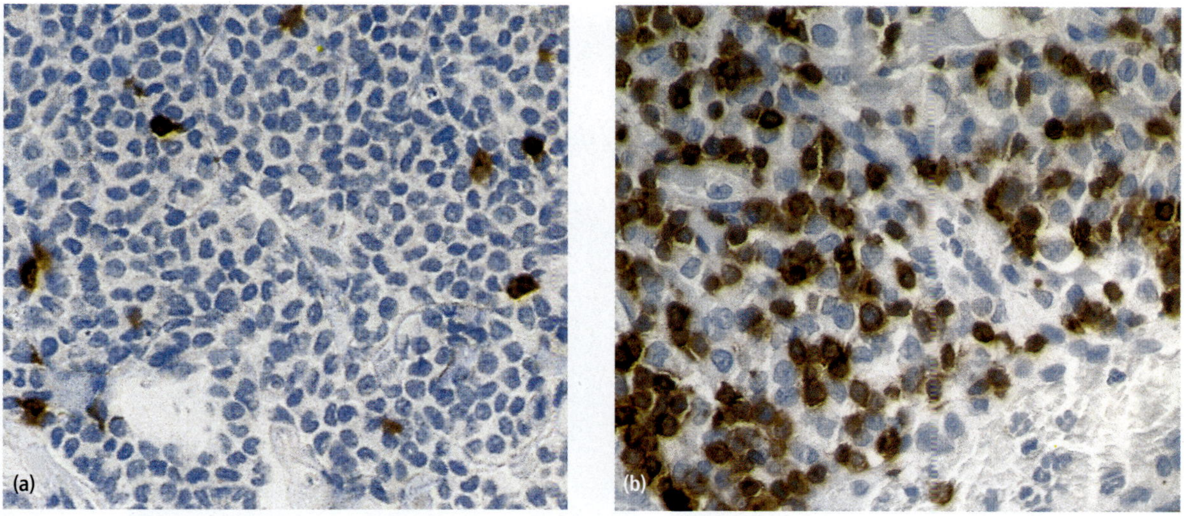

Plate 6. Histological sections of a canine cutaneous histiocytoma labelled with an antibody specific for CD3. (a) A tumour in the early proliferative phase showing a uniform population of large histiocytic cells and scant CD3$^+$ T-cells. (B) A late lesion showing a widespread infiltrate of CD3$^+$ T-cells. (DAB chromogen and Mayer's haematoxylin, × 100.)

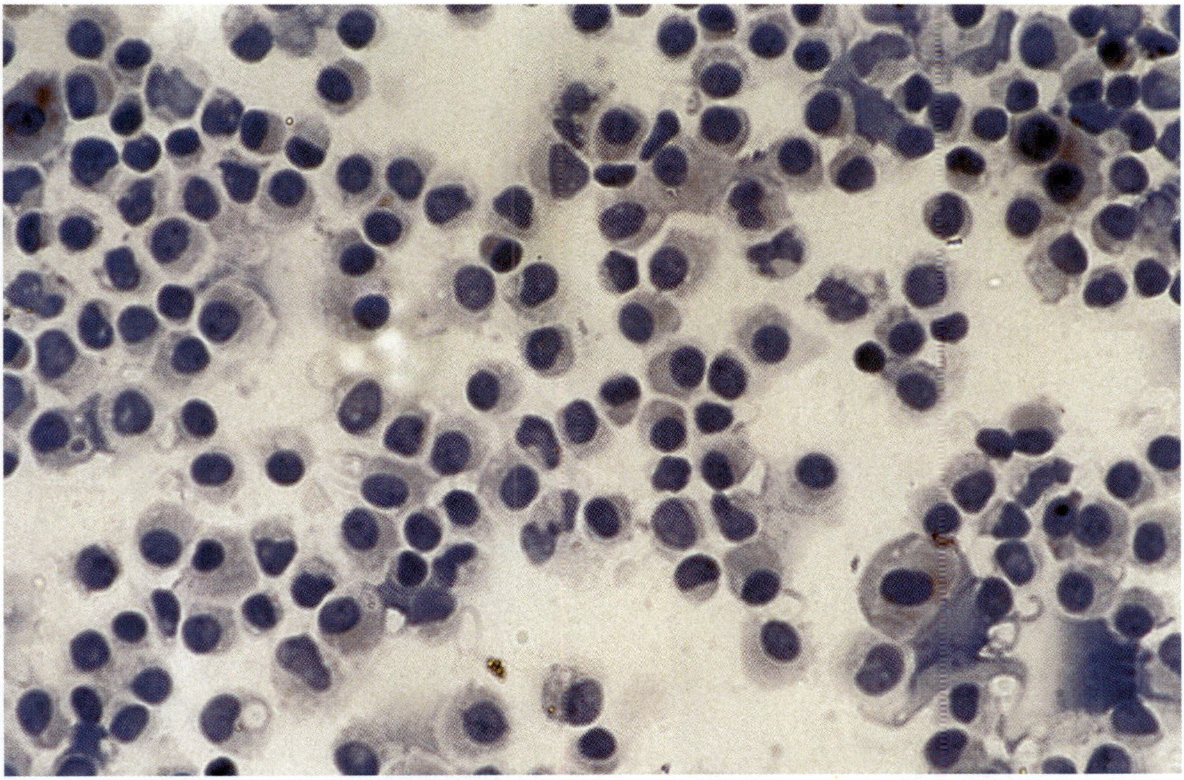

Plate 7. Cytospin preparation of cells isolated from a cutaneous histiocytoma. Large cells with histiocytic morphology, typified by voluminous cytoplasm and a large, round or indented nucleus, are present. (Giemsa, × 400.)

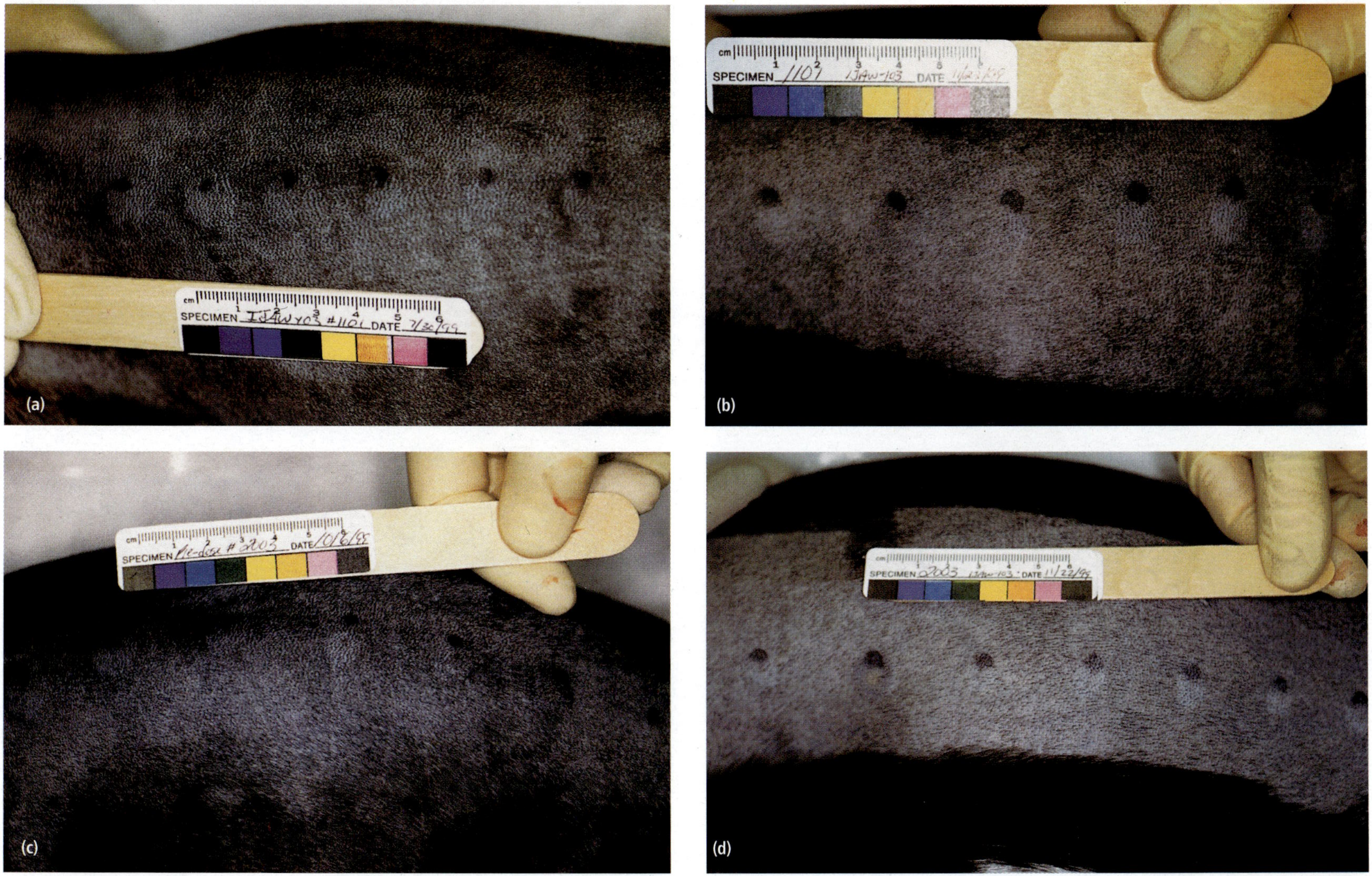

Plate 8. (a) Control dog before the study; (b) control dog after the feasiblity experiment; (c) test dog before the study; (d) test dog after the feasibility experiment. Skin testing was performed as described in Figure 4.4.5. (There was no difference in skin-test sensitivity to ragweed allergen in the control dog before and after the experiment. (c) The pre-experimental skin test for one of the treated animals is shown. A positive skin test is evident at the first three dilutions of allergen, characterized by swelling and infusion of Evans blue dye. (d) After c15A2 treatment there was no swelling or infusion of dye at any allergen concentration. From left to right: 1000 protein nitrogen units (PNU)/ml, 100 PNU/ml, 10 PNU/ml, 1 PNU/ml, 0.1 PNU/ml, histamine, saline.

In lesional skin of AD cats a significant total increase in T-cell numbers was found with a CD4/CD8 T-cell ratio of 3.9 ± 2.0 (mean ± SD) (Roosje *et al.*, 1998). In the skin of healthy control cats one or two $CD4^+$ cells and no $CD8^+$ cells were found. In addition, in non-lesional skin there was a significant increase in $CD4^+$ T-cells. In another study, significantly more $IL\text{-}4^+$ positive cells were found in lesional and in non-lesional skin of AD cats than in healthy control cats (Roosje *et al.*, 1995). Double staining with antibodies against feline CD4 or feline pan-T and human IL-4 revealed that all $IL\text{-}4^+$ cells were T-cells. Further investigations into the presence of feline T-cell subsets were not possible because the tested antibodies against IFN-γ were not reactive with feline IFN-γ. The ratio of CD4/CD8 cells in the peripheral blood of AD cats was not significantly different from that of healthy control animals.

IgE

By definition, allergen-specific IgE is often associated with the development of AD. There are several mechanisms by which IgE molecules can contribute to the inflammatory cell infiltrate in human AD: mast cell release, IgE-dependent late phase skin reaction, facilitated allergen presentation by Langerhans' cells and IgE autoreactivity to human proteins (Leung, 1999). In contrast, a group of human patients with the typical clinical appearance of AD exists who have the 'intrinsic' variant. In these patients no specific IgE can be detected (Werfel & Kapp, 1999).

Evidence exists for the existence of feline IgE. Passive transfer of reaginic antibodies in cats is possible and this reaction is heat sensitive (Powell *et al.*, 1980; Bevier, 1990). These data were confirmed in later studies (Baldwin *et al.*, 1993; Foster *et al.*, 1995). Cross-reactivity of antibodies against feline IgA and IgM hampered further antibody development (DeBoer *et al.*, 1994). More recently, the isolation and development of a polyclonal antibody reactive with feline IgE was described (Gilbert & Halliwell, 1998b). Unfortunately, to the authors' knowledge, research has not resulted in a widely available, well-defined, specific, monoclonal or polyclonal antibody against feline IgE. The recently developed *in vitro* test using a recombinant truncated version of the human high-affinity IgE receptor α-chain (rHuFcεR1α) as an IgE detection reagent (McCall *et al.*, 1997) may help to shed further light on the presence and role of feline IgE in disease pathogenesis.

In addition, cloning and expression of complementary DNA (cDNA) encoding the feline IgE heavy chain may result in development of feline IgE-specific reagents (Griot-Wenk *et al.*, 2000; Weber *et al.*, 2000).

In human AD patients not only allergen-specific IgE but also allergen-specifc IgG_4 (Kemeny *et al.*, 1989) can be found and Foster *et al.* (1997) used this to develop an enzyme-linked immunosorbent assay (ELISA). They described that cats with confirmed allergic skin disease have significantly more IgG directed against some pollen, dust and flea allergens than healthy cats, cats with non-dermatological illness and cats with undiagnosed pruritus. In addition, heat-stable cytophilic antibodies were described in cats with miliary dermatitis and eosinophilic plaques (Roosje & Willemse, 1995).

Mast cells

The exact role of connective tissue mast cells in human AD is unknown. In humans, in acute lesional AD skin, mast cells numbers are not increased but degranulation of mast cells is observed (Soter, 1989). Mast cell numbers, however, are increased in more chronic lesional AD skin (Soter, 1989). Mast cells and basophils were the first recognised cells expressing the high-affinity IgE receptor (FcεR1), which triggers these cells to release their contents upon bridging of these receptors by the antigen–IgE complex. Evidence for this mechanism is provided by the finding of degranulated mast cells in acute lesional AD skin (Soter, 1989) and the staining of mast cells binding IgE through the FcεR1 *in situ* (Klubal *et al.*, 1997). Different subtypes of mast cells exist. Mast cells can release prestored substances such as histamine, proteoglycans and proteases, and secrete synthesised leukotrienes, chemokines and prostaglandins. Different subtypes of mast cell exist and in normal human skin most are of the MC_{TC} type that contain the proteases chymase, tryptase, carboxypeptidase and a cathepsin G-like proteinase (Järvikallio *et al.*, 1997). The produced collection of cytokines includes IL-1, -3, -4, -5, -6, -8, -10, -13 and -16, GM-CSF, tumour necrosis factor-α (TNF-α) and IL-12 (Mécheri & David, 1997; Rumsaeng *et al.*, 1997). In accordance with this, it has been shown that the leucocyte infiltration at sites of IgE-dependent cutaneous reactions in mice was entirely mast cell dependent and was in part dependent on TNF-α (Galli & Costa, 1995). IL-5 produced by mast cells acts as a potent growth activator and chemoattractant for eosinophils (Wang *et al.*,

1989). The perivascular localisation of mast cells is in concordance with these findings. Most of the knowledge on mast cells has been gathered from mucosal mast cells and mast cell lines. Because mast cells are very heterogeneous cells that are strongly influenced by their microenvironment, findings relating to mast cells from mast cell lines or mucosal mast cells may not always be applicable to connective tissue mast cells.

Thepen *et al.* (1996) described only T-cell staining with an antibody against human IL-4 and could not find concurrent staining of mast cell tryptase with an antibody against human tryptase. Horsmanheimo *et al.* (1994) demonstrated IL-4 immunoreactivity of mast cells after enzyme histochemical staining for tryptase and a different (polyclonal) antibody reactive with human IL-4.

Mast cells are predominant cells in the perivascular infiltrate in lesional skin of allergic cats. They are present in increased numbers compared with the skin of non-allergic cats and are primarily located in the upper dermis (Koeman *et al.*, 1998). In the skin of normal cats, mast cell density in various body locations was not significantly different, except for the skin of the pinnae which has a significantly higher mast cell number than other body locations (Foster, 1994).

Nearly all skin mast cells of healthy cats contain chymase and tryptase (Beadleston *et al.*, 1997). McCusker (1965) demonstrated that the skin of feline eczema cats contained four-fold higher levels of mast cells and histamine, indicating a role for mast cells in the disease process. Two years later, a study was published describing mast cell degranulation after direct skin testing in cats (McCusker & Aitken, 1967). Many studies on the identification of feline IgE have used the passive cutaneous anaphylaxis (PCA), reverse cutaneous anaphylaxis (RCA) or Prausnitz–Küstner (PK) tests, which all are based on the principle of erythema and weal formation upon mast cell degranulation as sequelae to binding of antigen to antigen-specific IgE bound to the FcεR1 (Baldwin *et al.*, 1993; Foster *et al.*, 1995; Roosje *et al.*, 1995; Gilbert & Halliwell, 1998b). A disadvantage of this technique can be the variation in sensitivity between recipient cats (Foster *et al.*, 1995).

Further studies on feline mast cells are limited to electron microscopy describing the mast cell granules of feline mast cell tumours (Ward & Hurvitz, 1972). Recently, Bevier & Dunston (1998) described the ultrastructural changes of mast cell degranulation in positive intradermal skin-test reactions. Feline dermal mast cells exhibited primarily one type of granule structure. In humans, however, four different types of granules have been described, with variable occurrence of mast cells depending on tissue type.

Eosinophils

Although intact eosinophils are not often prominent in lesional human AD skin, eosinophil-derived proteins such as major basic protein (MBP) and eosinophilic cationic protein (ECP) are found in abundance, indicating eosinophil degranulation at the site of inflammation causing tissue damage (Leiferman *et al.*, 1985). In the peripheral blood of AD patients ECP can be measured and can even function as a parameter for severity of the disease (Czech *et al.*, 1992).

Eosinophils influence the inflammatory reaction not only by the release of the toxic protein granule content but also by the cytokines and chemokines that they produce. Eosinophils can produce many cytokines, such as IL-1α, -3, -5, -6 and -8, GM-CSF, TGF-α, TGF-β, TNF-α and IL-10 (Weller, 1994). Moreover, eosinophils produce and secrete bioactive IL-12 upon stimulation with IL-4 (Grewe *et al.*, 1998). Beside this effect, eosinophils can also function as APC by means of their FcεR1 and FcεR2. Up-regulation of FcεR1 on eosinophils was seen in AD lesions and atopy patch test lesions in connection with mite antigen-bearing eosinophils (Tanaka *et al.*, 1995). In addition, IL-4 induced chemotaxis of eosinophils from AD patients but not from healthy individuals (Dubois *et al.*, 1994).

Eosinophils are an important indicator for feline allergic dermatitis (Koeman *et al.*, 1998). Blood eosinophilia often occurs but its value in cats is limited as it can be caused by many diseases or endoparasitic and ectoparasitic infestations (Center *et al.*, 1990). Although the exact content of feline eosinophil granules is not known, comparable substances to human eosinophils are to be expected as collagenolysis due to massive eosinophil degranulation is observed in lesions of the eosinophilic granuloma complex (Yager & Wilcock, 1994). Recently, however, it was debated whether these collagen changes are true collagenolysis (Fernandez *et al.*, 2000).

Clinical signs and history of AD cats

The onset of symptoms in AD cats occurs early in life (6 months to 2 years), although a wide range is described (6 months to 14 years) (Scott, 1986).

Both seasonal and non-seasonal patterns occur and a breed or sex predilection does not occur. The most consistent clinical feature of feline AD is pruritus (Scott & Miller, 1993; Chalmers & Medleau, 1994). In addition, the disease should be recurrent. A few studies report a familial involvement in feline atopy, suggesting a genetic component (Scott, 1986; Cieslicki & Cieslicki, 1989; Moriello, 2001). A distinct common clinical atopic dermatitis phenotype has not been described. The most commonly reported cutaneous reaction patterns are miliary dermatitis, self-induced alopecia, eosinophilic granuloma complex lesions and an initially non-lesional pruritus of the face, neck and pinnae (Scott *et al.*, 2001). Combinations of these patterns are seen. Lesions belonging to the eosinophilic granuloma complex, however, can have different aetiologies as well. This was shown by Power *et al.* (1990) in a closed, inbred colony of cats. Concurrent signs of feline asthma are rare. Combinations of atopic dermatitis and food hypersensitivity or flea-bite hypersensitivity occur. In some cases, the relevance of a diagnosis of atopic dermatitis based on positive intradermal skin-test results is debatable if cats respond to a rigorous flea-control programme.

Miliary dermatitis consists of papules and small crusts which can be present virtually all over the body with an emphasis on the head, neck and trunk. Eosinophilic plaques can vary in size and may have an eroded surface or secondary crusts. These plaques are often observed on the neck and the abdominal skin and can occur in combination with miliary dermatitis (Yager & Wilcock, 1994; Scott *et al.*, 2001).

The histopathological reaction patterns of miliary dermatitis, eosinophilic plaques and pruritic facial and neck dermatitis share the dermal infiltration with mast cells, eosinophils, macrophages and lymphocytes. Flea-bite hypersensitivity, food hypersensitivity and 'feline atopic dermatitis' cannot be distinguished on this archetypal reaction pattern (Gross *et al.*, 1986, 1992; Yager & Wilcock, 1994).

Diagnosis

With the different clinical presentations the differential diagnosis of feline atopic dermatitis can vary.

Other causes of miliary dermatitis and pruritic dermatitis of the face and neck include infestations with fleas, *Notoedres cati*, *Otodectes cynotis*, *Cheyletiella* spp., *Demodex* spp. or *Sarcoptes* spp., or lice, flea-bite, mosquito or other insect bite hypersensitivity, dietary hypersensitivity, dermatophytosis, mastocytosis and epitheliotropic cutaneous lymphosarcoma. When self-induced alopecia is the primary clinical sign the differential diagnosis includes, in addition, psychogenic alopecia and hyperthyroidism. Lesions of the eosinophilic granuloma complex can be related to flea-bite, mosquito or other insect bite hypersensitivity, dietary hypersensitivity, neoplasia, bacterial infections (e.g. [atypical] mycobacterial infection, fighting abscesses, nocardiosis, actinobacillosis), genetic background and idiopathy. Because of the multitude of other causes a presumptive diagnosis of atopic dermatitis should only be made after a thorough work-up involving exclusion of these diseases and often in combination with a dermatohistopathology compatible with an allergic dermatitis. This work-up should include an elimination diet (preferably home-cooked) for at least 8 weeks, followed by provocation with the previous food, and a rigorous flea-control programme for at least 6–8 weeks in geographical areas where fleas occur. Flea-bite hypersensitivity is still the most common cause of allergic dermatitis. Further evidence could theoretically be obtained from *in vivo* and *in vitro* allergy tests. Intradermal allergy testing is used to confirm a tentative diagnosis of feline atopy. Unfortunately, this test is often difficult to interpret because of softer, non-erythematous weals and weal formation that often occurs and disappears more quickly than the reactions seen in dogs. The use of intravenous dyes (fluorescent or Evans blue dye, for example) can improve visualisation of positive reactions (Ovary, 1958). Only a limited number of publications exists on the validity of the intradermal allergy test as it is used in cats (Moriello & McMurdy, 1989; Bevier, 1990; Codner, 1996).

Many of the available *in vitro* tests for diagnosis of feline atopic disease have proved to be unreliable and therefore *in vitro* testing was not considered to be a useful diagnostic method (Anderson, 1993). In addition, no significant difference was found in a study comparing *Dermatophagoides farinae* specific-IgE levels of atopic cats and normal household cats (Gilbert & Halliwell, 1998a). Newer tests, such as the FcεR1α-based ELISA, have been developed since and are promising. Examination of sera submitted to a diagnostic laboratory revealed that 75% of the cats had IgE to both *D. farinae* and *D. pteronyssinus*. An IgE response directed towards Der f 2 was found in 42% of the cats, whereas the rate of anti-Der f I positivity was 32%. In addition, the *D. farinae* chitinase (98 kDa protein) is a major allergen for cats, with a frequency of 68% positives. House dust mite-positive cats show a complex pattern of reactivity to house dust mite allergens which clearly differentiates cats from dogs (McCall, 2000). So far, results of hyposensitisation following intradermal allergy testing in cats have only been described in open studies (Reedy, 1982; McDougal, 1986; Prost, 1992; Foster & O'Dair, 1993; O'Dair *et al.*, 1996; Bettenay, 1998), with reported success rates of 50–75%.

Conclusion

With the current knowledge and available techniques it might be more prudent to talk about feline atopic dermatitis-like skin disease until further information has been gathered. For the individual patient, a diagnosis of atopic dermatitis can only be made after a thorough work-up and exclusion of the previously mentioned diseases. Negative results from *in vitro* or *in vivo* tests cannot exclude the diagnosis of feline AD, whereas positive results have to fit the clinical history and may include false-positive results. The clinical signs of atopic dermatitis can wax and wane in severity over time and influence the interpretation of the efficacy of the hyposensitisation. Therefore, to estimate the true efficacy rate of hyposensitisation, further investigations in controlled trials are needed.

References

Anderson, R. K. (1993) *In vitro* testing for feline atopic disease. In: *Proceedings of the 10th ESVD Annual Congress*, Aalborg, Denmark, p. 72.

Anttila, M., Smith, C. & Suter, M. (1994) Dermal dendrocytes and T cells in inflammatory dermatoses in dogs and cats. In: *Proceedings of the 10th Annual Members' Meeting AAVD & ACVD*, Charleston, USA, p. 43.

Baldwin, C. I., Medeiros, F. de & Denham, D. A. (1993) IgE responses in cats infected with *Brugia pahangi*. *Parasite Immunology*, **15**, 291–296.

Barch, G. K. & Talbott, M. W. (1976) Allergic bronchoconstriction and its drug-induced reversal in anesthetized ovalbumin-sensitized cats. *Research Communications in Chemical Pathology and Pharmacology*, **13**, 623–633.

Beadleston, D. L., Roosje, P. J. & Goldschmidt, M. H. (1997) Chymase and tryptase staining of normal feline skin and of feline cutaneous mast cell tumors. *Veterinary Allergy and Clinical Immunology*, **5**, 54–58.

Beckman, E. M. & Brenner, M. B. (1995) MHC class I-like, class II-like and CD1 molecules: distinct roles in immunity. *Immunology Today*, **16**, 349–352.

Bettenay, S. (1998) Response to hyposensitization in 29 atopic cats. In: *Advances in Veterinary Dermatology* (Eds K. W. Kwochka, T. Willemse & C. von Tscharner), Vol. 1, pp. 517–518. Butterworth Heinemann, Oxford.

Bevier, D. E. (1990) The reaction of feline skin to the intradermal injection of allergenic extracts and passive cutaneous anaphylaxis using serum from skin test positive cats. In: *Advances in Veterinary Dermatology* (Eds C. von Tscharner & R. E. W. Halliwell), Vol. 1, pp. 126–136. Bailliere Tindall, London.

Bevier, D. E. & Dunston, S. (1998) Ultrastructural changes in feline dermal mast cells during antigen-induced degranulation *in vivo*. In: *Advances in Veterinary Dermatology* (Eds K. W. Kwochka, T. Willemse & C. von Tscharner), Vol. 3, pp. 213–222. Butterworth Heinemann, Oxford.

Bieber, T. & Bruijnzeel-Koomen, C. (1990) Langerhans cells in the physiopathology of atopic dermatitis. *Annales de Dermatologie et de Vénéréologie*, **117**, 185–193.

Bieber, T., Salle, H. de la, Wollenberg, A., Hakimi, J., Chizzonite, R., Ring, J. *et al.* (1992) Human epidermal Langerhans cells express the high affinity receptor for immunoglobulin E (Fc epsilon RI). *Journal of Experimental Medicine*, **175**, 1285–1290.

Blok, B., Taylor, R. S., Gonzales, A., Simon, M., Solomon, W., Ellis, C. *et al.* (1991) Peripheral blood leukocyte subsets in atopic dermatitis: effect of Gamma Interferon. *Journal of Investigative Dermatology*, **96**, 604.

Bos, J. D., Kapsenberg, M. L. & Smitt, J. H. (1994) Pathogenesis of atopic eczema. *Lancet*, **343**, 1338–1341.

Bratton, D. L., Hamid, Q., Boguniewicz, M., Doherty, D. E., Kailey, J. M. & Leung, D. Y. (1995) Granulocyte macrophage colony-stimulating factor contributes to enhanced monocyte survival in chronic atopic dermatitis. *Journal of Clinical Investigation*, **95**, 211–218.

Bruijnzeel-Koomen, C., Wichen, D. F. van, Toonstra, J., Berrens, L. & Bruijnzeel, P. L. (1986) The presence of IgE molecules on epidermal Langerhans cells in patients with atopic dermatitis. *Archives of Dermatological Research*, **278**, 199–205.

Center, S. A., Randolph, J. F., Erb, H. N. & Reiter, S. (1990) Eosinophilia in the cat: a retrospective study of 312 cases (1975 to 1986). *Journal of the American Animal Hospital Association*, **26**, 349–358.

Chalmers, S. A. & Medleau, L. (1994) Feline atopic dermatitis: its diagnosis and treatment. *Veterinary Medicine*, **89**, 342–352.

Cieslicki, M. & Cieslicki, P. (1989) Auftreten von endogenem Ekzem und Kardiomyopathie in einer Abessinier-Katzenzucht. *Kleintierpraxis*, **34**, 395–402.

Codner, E. C. (1996) Reactivity to intradermal injections of extracts of house dust mite and flea antigen in normal cats and cats suspected of being allergic. In: *Proceedings of the 12th Annual Members' Meeting AAVD & ACVD*, Las Vegas, USA, pp. 26–27.

Czech, W., Krutmann, J., Schopf, E. & Kapp, A. (1992) Serum eosinophil cationic protein (ECP) is a sensitive measure for disease activity in atopic dermatitis. *British Journal of Dermatology*, **126**, 351–355.

DeBoer, D. J., Yue, X. & Donner, R. (1994) Monoclonal antibodies against feline immunoglobulin E. In: *Proceedings of the 10th Annual Members Meeting AAVD & ACVD*, Charleston, USA, p. 11.

Dubois, G. R., Bruijnzeel Koomen, C. A. & Bruijnzeel, P. L. (1994) IL-4 induces chemotaxis of blood eosinophils from atopic dermatitis patients, but not from normal individuals. *Journal of Investigative Dermatology*, **102**, 843–846.

Fartasch, M. & Diepgen, T. L. (1992) The barrier function in atopic dry skin. Disturbance of membrane-coating granule exocytosis and formation of epidermal lipids? *Acta Dermato-Venereologica* **176** (Suppl.), 26–31.

Fernandez, C. J., Scott, D. W. & Erb, H. E. (2000) Staining abnormalities of dermal collagen in eosinophil- or neutrophil-rich inflammatory dermatoses of horses and cats as demonstrated with Masson's trichrome stain. *Veterinary Dermatology*, **11**, 43–48.

Foster, A. P. (1994) A study of the number and distribution of cutaneous mast cells in cats with disease not affecting the skin. *Veterinary Dermatology*, **5**, 17–20.

Foster, A. P. & O'Dair, H. A. (1993) Allergy skin testing for skin disease in the cat *in vivo* vs *in vitro* tests. *Veterinary Dermatology*, **4**, 111–115.

Foster, A. P., Duffus, W. P. H., Shaw, S. E. & Gruffydd-Jones, T. J. (1995) Studies on the isolation and characterization of a cat reaginic antibody. *Research in Veterinary Science*, **58**, 70–74.

Foster, A. P., O'Dair, H. A. & DeBoer, D. J. (1997) Allergen-specific IgG antibodies in cats with allergic skin disease. *Research in Veterinary Science*, **63**, 239–243.

Galli, S. J. & Costa, J. J. (1995) Mast-cell–leukocyte cytokine cascades in allergic inflammation. *Allergy*, **50**, 851–862.

Gilbert, S. & Halliwell, R. E. (1998a) Feline immunoglobulin E: induction of antigen-specific antibody in normal cats and levels in spontaneously allergic cats. *Veterinary Immunology and Immunopathology*, **63**, 235–252.

Gilbert, S. & Halliwell, R. E. (1998b) Production and characterisation of polyclonal antisera against feline IgE. *Veterinary Immunology and Immunopathology*, **63**, 223–233.

Grewe, M., Czech, W., Morita, A., Werfel, T., Klammer, M., Kapp, A. *et al.* (1998) Human eosinophils produce biologically active IL-12: implications for control of T cell responses. *Journal of Immunology*, **161**, 415–420.

Griot-Wenk, M. E., Obexer-Ruff, G. & Marti, E. (2000) Partial sequences of feline and caprine immunoglobulin epsilon heavy chain cDNA and comparative binding studies of recombinant IgE fragment-specific antibodies across different species. *Veterinary Immunology and Immunopathology*, **75**, 59–69.

Gross, T. L., Kwochka, K. W. & Kunkle, G. A. (1986) Correlation of histologic and immunologic findings in cats with miliary dermatitis. *Journal of the American Veterinary Medical Association*, **189**, 1322–1325.

Gross, T. L., Ihrke, P. J. & Walder, E. J. (1992) *Veterinary Dermatopathology*, pp. 122–123. Mosby Yearbook, St Louis, MO.

Halliwell, R. E. W. (1997) Efficacy of hyposensitization in feline allergic diseases based upon results of *in vitro* testing for allergen-specific immunoglobulin E. *Journal of the American Animal Hospital Association*, **33**, 282–288.

Hamid, Q., Boguniewicz, M. & Leung, D. Y. (1994) Differential *in situ* cytokine gene expression in acute versus chronic atopic dermatitis. *Journal of Clinical Investigation*, **94**, 870–876.

Hamid, Q., Naseer, T., Minshall, E. M., Song, Y. L., Boguniewicz, M. & Leung, D. Y. (1996) *In vivo* expression of IL-12 and IL-13 in atopic dermatitis. *Journal of Allergy and Clinical Immunology*, **98**, 225–231.

Hanifin, J. M. & Rajka, G. (1980) Diagnostic features of atopic dermatitis. *Acta Dermato-Venereologica (Stockholm)*, **92**, 44–47.

Heijden, F. L. van der, Wierenga, E. A., Bos, J. D. & Kapsenberg, M. L. (1991) High frequency of IL-4-producing $CD4^+$ allergen-specific T lymphocytes in atopic dermatitis lesional skin. *Journal of Investigative Dermatology*, **97**, 389–394.

Horsmanheimo, L., Harvima, I. T., Jarvikallio, A., Harvima, R. J., Naukkarinen, A. & Horsmanheimo, M. (1994) Mast cells are one major source of interleukin-4 in atopic dermatitis. *British Journal of Dermatology*, **131**, 348–353.

Imokawa, G., Abe, A., Jin, K., Higaki, Y., Kawashima, M. & Hidano, A. (1991) Decreased level of ceramides in stratum corneum of atopic dermatitis: an etiologic factor in atopic dry skin? *Journal of Investigative Dermatology*, **96**, 523–526.

Järvikallio, A., Naukkarinen, A., Harvima, I. T., Aalto, M. L. & Horsmanheimo, M. (1997) Quantitative analysis of tryptase- and chymase-containing mast cells in atopic dermatitis and nummular eczema. *British Journal of Dermatology*, **136**, 871–877.

Juhlin, L., Johansson, S., Bennich, H., Hogman, C. & Thyresson, N. (1969) IgE in dermatoses. *Archives of Dermatology*, **100**, 12–16.

Kashihara, M., Ueda, M., Horiguchi, Y., Furukawa, F., Hanaoka, M. & Imamura, S. (1986) A monoclonal antibody specifically reactive to human Langerhans cells. *Journal of Investigative Dermatology*, **87**, 602–607.

Kemeny, D. M., Urbanek, R., Ewan, P., McHugh, S., Richards, D., Patel, S. & Lessof, M. H. (1989) The subclass of IgG antibody in allergic disease: II. The IgG subclass of antibodies produced following natural exposure to dust mite and grass pollen in atopic and non-atopic individuals. *Clinical and Experimental Allergy*, **19**, 545–549.

Klubal, R., Osterhoff, B., Wang, B., Kinet, J. P., Maurer, D. & Stingl, G. (1997) The high-affinity receptor for IgE is the predominant IgE-binding structure in lesional skin of atopic dermatitis patients. *Journal of Investigative Dermatology*, **108**, 336–342.

Koeman, J. P., Roosje, P. J. & Willemse, T. (1998) Quantity and distribution of mast cells and eosinophils in feline allergic miliary dermatitis. In: *Advances in Veterinary Dermatology* (Eds K. W. Kwochka, T. Willemse & C. von Tscharner), pp. 480–481. Butterworth Heinemann, Oxford.

Laberge, S., Ghaffar, O., Boguniewicz, M., Center, D. M., Leung, D. Y. & Hamid, Q. (1998) Association of increased $CD4^+$ T-cell infiltration with increased IL-16 gene expression in atopic dermatitis. *Journal of Allergy and Clinical Immunology*, **102**, 645–650.

Leiferman, K. M., Ackerman, S. J., Sampson, H. A., Haugen, H. S., Venencie, P. Y. & Gleich, G. J. (1985) Dermal deposition of eosinophil-granule major basic protein in atopic dermatitis. Comparison with onchocerciasis. *New England Journal of Medicine*, **313**, 282–285.

Leung, D. Y. (1995) Atopic dermatitis: the skin as a window into the pathogenesis of chronic allergic diseases. *Journal of Allergy and Clinical Immunology*, **96**, 302–318.

Leung, D. Y. (1999) Pathogenesis of atopic dermatitis. *Journal of Allergy and Clinical Immunology*, **104**, S99–S108.

Leung, D. Y., Schneeberger, E. E., Siraganian, R. P., Geha, R. S. & Bhan, A. K. (1987) The presence of IgE on macrophages and dendritic cells infiltrating into the skin lesion of atopic dermatitis. *Clinical Immunology and Immunopathology*, **42**, 328–337.

McCall, C. (2000) Allergy to flea and house dust mites in the cat – recent developments in allergen identification. In: *Proceedings of the British Veterinary Dermatology Study Group*, Birmingham, UK, pp. 23–26.

McCall, C., Stedman, K.E., Bevier, D. E., Kunkle, G. A., Foil, F. S. & Foil, L. D. (1997) Correlation of feline IgE, determined by FcεRIα-based ELISA technology, and IDST to *Ctenocephalides felis* salivary antigens in a feline model of flea bite allergic dermatitis. *Supplement to Compendium on Continuing Education for the Practicing Veterinarian*, **19**, 29–32.

McCusker, H. B. (1965) Histamine and mast cells in the normal skin and eczematous skin in the cat. In: *Comparative Physiology and Pathology of the Skin* (Eds A. J. Rook & G. S. Walton), pp. 427–434. F.A. Davis, Philadelphia, PA.

McCusker, H. B. & Aitken, I. D. (1967) Immunological studies in the cat. II–Experimental induction of skin reactivity to foreign proteins. *Research in Veterinary Sciences*, **8**, 265–271.

McDougal, B. J. (1986) Allergy testing and hyposensitization for 3 common feline dermatoses. *Modern Veterinary Practice*, **67**, 629–633.

Mackie, R. M., Cobb, S. J., Cochran, R. E. I. & Thompson, J. (1979) Total and specific IgE levels in patients with atopic dermatitis. *Clinical and Experimental Dermatology*, **4**, 187–195.

Mécheri, S. & David, B. (1997) Unravelling the mast cell dilemma: culprit or victim of its generosity? *Immunology Today*, **18**, 212–215.

Moriello, K. A. (2001) Feline atopy in three littermates. *Veterinary Dermatology*, **12**, 177–181.

Moriello, K. A. & McMurdy, M. A. (1989) The prevalence of positive intradermal skin test reactions to flea extract in clinically normal cats. *Companion Animal Practice*, **19**, 298–302.

Mudde, G. C., Van Reijsen, F. C., Boland, G. J., Gast, G. C. de, Bruijnzeel, P. L. & Bruijnzeel Koomen, C. A. (1990) Allergen presentation by epidermal Langerhans' cells from patients with atopic dermatitis is mediated by IgE. *Immunology*, **69**, 335–341.

Neiß, U., Deimleitner, K., Marx, A., Mehlig, M., Scheicher, C. & Reske, K. (1995) Antigen presentation by Langerhans/dendritic cells. In: *The Immune Functions of Epidermal Langerhans Cells* (Ed. H. Moll), pp. 87–101. R. G. Landes, Austin, TX.

O'Dair, H. A., Markwell, P. J. & Maskell, I. E. (1996) An open prospective investigation into aetiology in a group of cats with suspected allergic skin disease. *Veterinary Dermatology*, **7**, 193–202.

Osterhoff, B., Rappersberger, K., Wang, B., Koszik, F., Ochiai, K., Kinet, J. P. & Stingl, G. (1994) Immunomorphologic characterization of Fc epsilon RI-bearing cells within the human dermis. *Journal of Investigative Dermatology*, **102**, 315–320.

Ovary, Z. (1958) Passive cutaneous anaphylaxis in the mouse. *Journal of Immunology*, **81**, 355–357.

Padrid, P., Snook, S., Finucane, T., Shiue, P., Cozzi, P., Solway, J. & Leff, A. R. (1995) Persistent airway hyperresponsiveness and histologic alterations after chronic antigen challenge in cats. *American Journal of Respiratory and Critical Care Medicine*, **151**, 184–193.

Powell, M. B., Weisbroth, S. H., Roth, L. & Wilhelmsen, C. (1980) Reaginic hypersensitivity in *Otodectes cynotis* infestation of cats and mode of mite feeding. *American Journal of Veterinary Research*, **41**, 877–882.

Power, H. T. (1990) Eosinophilic granuloma in a family of specific pathogen-free cats. *Proceedings of the 6th Annual Members' Meeting AAVD & ACVD*, San Francisco, USA, p. 45.

Prost, C. (1992) Atopy in the cat: 28 cases. In: *Proceedings of the 2nd world Congress of Veterinary Dermatology*, Montreal, Canada, p. 87.

Prost, C. (1998) Diagnosis of feline allergic diseases: a study of 90 cats. In: *Advances in Veterinary Dermatology* (Eds K. W. Kwochka, T. Willemse & C. von Tscharner), pp. 516–517. Butterworth Heinemann, Edinburgh.

Reedy, L. M. (1982) Results of allergy testing and hyposensitization in selected feline skin diseases. *Journal of the American Animal Hospital Association*, **18**, 618–623.

Reijsen, F. C. van, Bruijnzeel Koomen, C. A., Kalthoff, F. S., Maggi, E., Romagnani, S., Westland, J. K. & Mudde, G. C. (1992) Skin-derived aeroallergen-specific T-cell clones of Th2 phenotype in patients with atopic dermatitis. *Journal of Allergy and Clinical Immunology*, **90**, 184–193.

Ring, J. (1991) Atopy: condition, disease or syndrome? In: *Handbook of Atopic Eczema* (Eds J. Ring, T. Ruzicka & B. Przybilla), pp. 3–8. Springer, Berlin.

Roosje, P. J. & Willemse, T. (1995) Cytophilic antibodies in cats with miliary dermatitis and eosinophilic plaques: passive transfer of immediate-type hypersensitivity. *Veterinary Quarterly*, **17**, 66–69.

Roosje, P. J., Kooten, P. J. van, Thepen, T., Rutten, V. P. M. G. & Willemse, T. (1995) A role for Th2 cells in the pathogenesis of allergic dermatitis in cats? Abstracts, Joint Congress of the British and Netherlands Societies for Immunology, Brighton, UK. *Immunology*, **86** (Suppl. 1), 98 W93.93.

Roosje, P. J., Whitaker-Menezes, D., Goldschmidt, M. H., Moore, P. F., Willemse, T. & Murphy, G. F. (1997) Feline atopic dermatitis. A model for Langerhans cell participation in disease pathogenesis. *American Journal of Pathology*, **151**, 927–932.

Roosje, P. J., Kooten, P. J. van, Thepen, T., Bihari, I. C., Rutten, V. P., Koeman, J. P. & Willemse, T. (1998) Increased numbers of $CD4^+$ and $CD8^+$ T cells in lesional skin of cats with allergic dermatitis. *Veterinary Pathology*, **35**, 268–273.

Rumsaeng, V., Cruikshank, W. W., Foster, B., Prussin, C., Kirshenbaum, A. S., Davis, T. A. *et al.* (1997) Human mast cells produce the $CD4^+$ T lymphocyte chemoattractant factor, IL-16. *Journal of Immunology*, **159**, 2904–2910.

Schultz Larsen, F. (1993) Atopic dermatitis: a genetic–epidemiologic study in a population-based twin sample. *Journal of the American Academy of Dermatology*, **28**, 719–723.

Scott, D. W. (1986) Feline dermatology 1983–1985: 'the secret sits'. *Journal of the American Hospital Association*, **23**, 255–274.

Scott, D. W. & Miller, W. H., Jr (1993) Medical management of allergic pruritus in the cat, with emphasis on feline atopy. *Journal of the South African Veterinary Association*, **64**, 103–108.

Scott, D. W., Miller, W. H. & Griffin, C. E. (2001) Skin immune system and allergic skin diseases. In: *Muller & Kirk's Small Animal Dermatology*, pp. 543–666. W. B. Saunders, Philadelphia, PA.

Sepulveda Merrill, C., Mayall, S., Hamblin, A. S. & Breathnach, S. M. (1994) Antigen-presenting capacity in normal human dermis is mainly subserved by $CD1a^+$ cells. *British Journal of Dermatology*, **131**, 15–22.

Sicherer, S. H. & Sampson, H. A. (1999) Food hypersensitivity and atopic dermatitis: pathophysiology, epidemiology, diagnosis, and management. *Journal of Allergy and Clinical Immunology*, **104**, S114–S122.

Sillevis Smitt, J. H., Bos, J. D., Hulsebosch, H. J. & Krieg, S. R. (1986) *In situ* immunophenotyping of antigen presenting cells and T cell subsets in atopic dermatitis. *Clinical and Experimental Dermatology*, **11**, 159–168.

Soter, N. A. (1989) Morphology of atopic eczema. *Allergy*, **44** (Suppl. 9), 16–19.

Sowden, J. M., Powell, R. J. & Allen, B. R. (1992) Selective activation of circulating $CD4^+$ lymphocytes in severe adult atopic dermatitis. *British Journal of Dermatology*, **127**, 228–232.

Tanaka, Y., Anan, S. & Yoshida, H. (1990) Immunohistochemical studies in mite antigen-induced patch test sites in atopic dermatitis. *Journal of Dermatological Science*, **1**, 361–368.

Tanaka, Y., Takenaka, M., Matsunaga, Y., Okada, S., Anan, S., Yoshida, H. & Ra, C. (1995) High affinity IgE receptor (Fc epsilon RI) expression on eosinophils infiltrating the lesions and mite patch tested sites in atopic dermatitis. *Archives of Dermatological Research*, **287**, 712–717.

Thepen, T., Langeveld-Wildschut, E. G., Bihari, I. C., Wichen, D. F. van, Reijsen, F. C. van, Mudde, G. C. & Bruijnzeel-Koomen, C. A. F. M. (1996) Biphasic response against aeroallergen in atopic dermatitis showing a switch from an initial TH2 response to a TH1 response *in situ*: an immunocytochemical study. *Journal of Allergy and Clinical Immunology*, **97**, 828–837.

Tupker, R. A., De Monchy, J. G., Coenraads, P. J., Homan, A. & Meer, J. B. van der (1996) Induction of atopic dermatitis by inhalation of house dust mite. *Journal of Allergy and Clinical Immunology*, **97**, 1064–1070.

Wang, B., Rieger, A., Kilgus, O., Ochiai, K., Maurer, D., Fodinger, D. *et al.* (1992) Epidermal Langerhans cells from normal human skin bind monomeric IgE via Fc epsilon RI. *Journal of Experimental Medicine*, **175**, 1353–1365.

Wang, J. M., Rambaldi, A., Biondi, A., Chen, Z. G., Sanderson, C. J. & Mantovani, A. (1989) Recombinant interleukin 5 is a selective eosinophil chemoattractant. *European Journal of Immunology*, **19**, 701–705.

Ward, J. M. & Hurvitz, A. I. (1972) Ultrastructure of normal and neoplastic mast cells of the cat. *Veterinary Pathology*, **9**, 202–211.

Weber, E. R., Helps, C. R., Foster, A. P., Perry, A. C. F., Gruffyd-Jones, T. J., Hall, L. *et al.* (2000) Molecular cloning and phylogenetic analysis of a cDNA encoding the cat (*Felis domesticus*) Ig epsilon constant region. *Veterinary Immunology and Immunopathology*, **76**, 299–308.

Weller, P. F. (1994) Eosinophils: structure and functions. *Current Opinion in Immunology*, **6**, 85–90.

Werfel, T. & Kapp, A. (1999) What do we know about the etiopathology of the intrinsic type of atopic dermatitis? In: *The Atopy Syndrome in the Third Millennium* (Ed. B. Wüthrich), pp. 29–33. Karger, Basel.

Wierenga, E. A., Snoek, M., Bos, J. D., Jansen, H. M. & Kapsenberg, M. L. (1990) Comparison of diversity and function of house dust mite-specific T lymphocyte clones from atopic and non-atopic donors. *European Journal of Immunology*, **20**, 1519–1526.

Williams, H. C. (1992) Is the prevalence of atopic dermatitis increasing? *Clinical and Experimental Dermatology*, **17**, 385–391.

Yager, J. A. & Wilcock, B. P. (1994) *Color Atlas and Text of Surgical Pathology of the Dog and Cat; Dermatopathology and Skin Tumors*, pp. 148–149. Wolfe, London.

4.4

Recombinant chimeric canine anti-immunoglobulin E monoclonal antibody therapy removes free and total serum immunoglobulin E and eliminates skin-test reactivity in ragweed-sensitized dogs

A. Aiyappa PhD, H. Guo PhD, S. Faust BS, R. Regan BS, R. Krah PhD, A. Siefring MS, S. Brewer BS, B. Bartol MS, G. Francoeur MS and T. Lawton MD, PhD

Department of Molecular and Cellular Biology, IDEXX Laboratories Inc., Westbrook, Maine, USA

Summary

A chimeric anti-canine immunoglobulin E (IgE) monoclonal antibody was constructed by fusing the variable region of an anti-canine IgE mouse monoclonal antibody with the constant region of canine IgG. The resulting chimeric antibody, designated c15A2, was generated in a baculovirus expression system and tested in ragweed-sensitized dogs for its ability to bind serum IgE and prevent the inter-action of IgE with the high-affinity IgE receptor (FcεR1) on mast cells. Levels of measurable, free serum IgE were undetectable in experimental dogs 1 h after infusion of the chimeric antibody. Total IgE levels dropped to undetectable levels by day 20. Flow-cytometric analysis showed that basophil high-affinity IgE receptor density was reduced after c15A2 infusion, suggesting that elimination of free serum IgE resulted in a negative feedback loop on receptor expression. Furthermore, the animals were evaluated for their ability to produce a skin-test response to ragweed allergen before and after treatment with the chimeric antibody. In two post-treatment skin tests there was no response to ragweed challenge in the treated dogs, while the response to ragweed was unchanged in the control dogs. It is possible that in dogs suffering from allergen-induced atopic dermatitis, a reduction in free serum IgE and concomitant reduction in IgE receptor expression may lower the threshold for mast cell triggering. These experiments demonstrate the feasibility of using anti-IgE monoclonal antibody therapy for the treatment of canine atopic dermatitis.

Introduction

Immunoglobulin E (IgE) is the antibody type that is understood to be an important mediator of allergic responses, including type I immediate hypersensitivity. IgE molecules bind to high-affinity receptor molecules designated FcεR1 on mediator cells such as mast cells and basophils. When IgE bound to FcεR1 on mediator cells then binds to an allergen, the allergen cross-links multiple IgE molecules on the cell surface. IgE cross-linking induces the release of histamine and other soluble mediators of inflammation that produce the symptoms and clinical signs associated with allergy. In humans the concentration of IgE in serum is correlated with the presence of allergic disease. In dogs, serum IgE is present at much higher levels than in humans but is not diagnostic of an allergic condition (Hill & DeBoer, 1994). Although the levels of serum IgE may not correlate with allergic disease in dogs, it may be desirable to decrease serum IgE levels as a mechanism for alleviating allergic symptoms. Recent developments in human therapy for allergy suggest that reducing the concentration of IgE in serum may result in the reduction of allergic symptoms (Corne *et al.*, 1997; Holgate *et al.*, 1998b; Chang, 2000).

To address this question, a mouse–dog chimeric anti-IgE antibody, designated c15A2, was constructed and tested in ragweed-sensitized dogs for its capacity to bind and neutralize free IgE in serum. Furthermore, the antibody was evaluated for its ability to prevent the interaction of IgE with its high-affinity receptor on mast cells and to effect a subcutaneous skin response to allergen.

Materials and methods

Five dogs were used in the feasibility experiment. Three dogs were infused with the chimeric anti-canine IgE antibody c15A2. Two control dogs received sterile saline. Free and total IgE enzyme-linked immunosorbent assays (ELISA) were used to monitor pretreatment and post-treatment IgE levels. 'Free' IgE refers to IgE that was unbound in serum and was available to bind to the high-affinity IgE receptor. Total IgE included free IgE plus IgE associated with the chimeric antibody as a complex and was thus incapable of binding to the high-affinity receptor. Free and total IgE could be differentiated using monoclonal antibodies raised against distinct epitopes on the canine IgE molecule. IgE levels were undetectable by ELISA below 1 ng/ml in serum.

Chimeric anti-canine antibody was administered to dogs at approximately 5 day intervals for eight consecutive treatments. The amount of c15A2 administered in the first treatment was equivalent to 10 times the concentration of measurable free serum IgE 3 days before the start of the feasibility experiment. The concentration of c15A2 in the second dose was also 10 times the initial free serum IgE level. All subsequent dosages were established at half of the initial dose. The chimeric antibody was diluted into sterile phosphate-buffered saline (PBS) at the appropriate potency and infused intravenously (i.v.) over a 30 min period.

Results

Free and total IgE levels in experimental dogs after administration of chimeric anti-canine IgE c15A2 antibody

Figure 4.4.1 illustrates the concentration of free and total serum IgE in representative test and control dogs

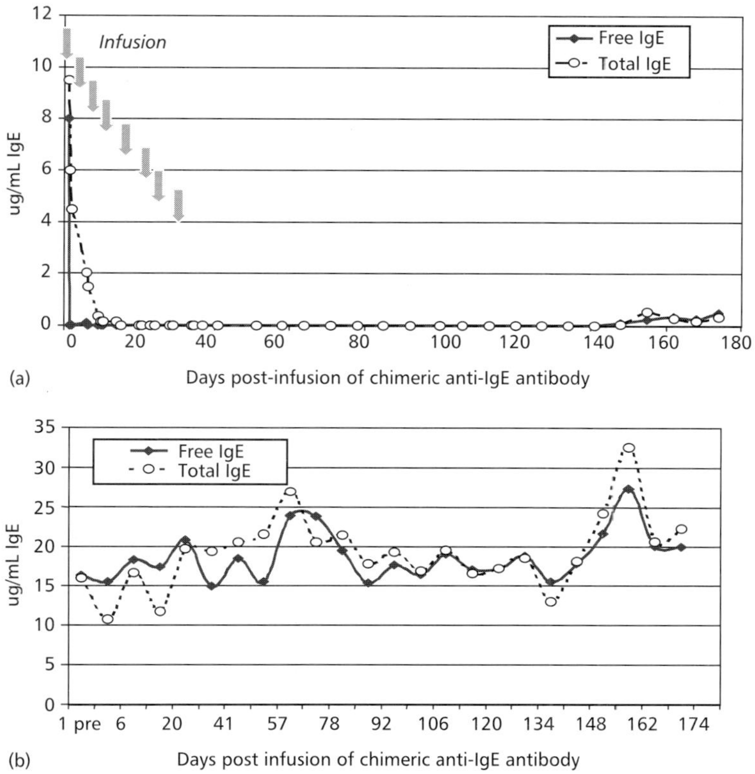

Figure 4.4.1. Free and total immunoglobulin E (IgE) in typical (a) chimeric c15A2 antibody-treated and (b) control dog. Sandwich enzyme-linked immunosorbent assays (ELISA) were used to detect free and total IgE in experimental dogs. Free IgE was defined as IgE in serum that was able to bind to high-affinity IgE receptors, FcεR1, on mast cells or basophils. A monoclonal antibody specific for domain 3 of canine IgE was used as the capture antibody. Bound IgE was then detected using a canine IgE domain 4 specific monoclonal antibody that had been labeled with horseradish peroxidase (HRP). Total IgE which included IgE in association with the chimeric anti-IgE antibody was measured by domain 4 specific antibody capture followed by detection with an HRP labeled monoclonal antibody that was specific for an epitope of canine IgE which was distinct from the chimeric anti-IgE molecule. Free and total IgE in serum remained unchanged in dogs receiving only saline. In normal dogs serum IgE fluctuates slightly over time. In dogs treated with the chimeric anti-IgE c15A2, free IgE was undetectable in serum 1 h after infusion. There was a temporal drop in total IgE in dogs receiving anti-IgE therapy and total IgE was undetectable by day

versus time. Free IgE in the experimental dogs dropped to undetectable levels within 60 min (Figure 4.4.1a). Total IgE concentration in serum dropped over a period of 2 weeks and became undetectable at approximately day 15. Free and total IgE levels remained at undetectable levels for approximately 5 months. The temporal reduction in total IgE suggested the formation of chimeric antibody–IgE immune complexes and reflected the clearance of these complexes over a 2 week period. When c15A2–IgE immune complexes were measured directly by ELISA (Figure 4.4.2), the decline in immune complexes reflected the result seen in the total IgE ELISA. In this assay, immune complexes were captured using an anti-IgE antibody solid phase (domain 4 specific monoclonal antibody (mAb) capture) and then detecting the complex using a polyclonal anti-dog immunoglobulin Fc specific antibody conjugated to horseradish peroxidase (HRP). By day 28 no immune complexes were detected in dogs receiving c15A2. This result suggests that the complexes were cleared from the circulating pool of serum immunoglobulin and that synthesis of new IgE in this time frame was reduced or eliminated. Free and total serum IgE in control dogs receiving only saline did not change significantly during this period (Figure 4.4.1b).

The presence of free chimeric 15A2 in the serum of dogs was determined by ELISA using a chimeric antibody specific peptide mimetope as a capture molecule. Detection of the free chimeric was accomplished using HRP-conjugated polyclonal rabbit anti-canine IgG antibody. Figure 4.4.3 shows that the levels of c15A2 in serum increased and decreased consistently with the beginning and end of each 5 day administration period. Free c15A2 was still detectable in the serum of experimental dogs 24 days after infusion. No changes were observed in control dogs. There was no detectable chimeric antibody in the serum of the experimental dogs after 60 days.

These results are surprising given that serum IgE is understood to have a short half-life, of about 2 days, and that recombinant or chimeric molecules may likewise exhibit relatively short half-lives *in vivo* (Capon *et al.*, 1989). An early pharmacokinetic experiment before the initiation of the feasibility experiment demonstrated that the half-life of the chimeric anti-IgE molecule in serum was approximately 5–7 days (data not shown). Circulating serum IgE is believed to be entirely replenished every 4–5 days, but following administration of a canine anti-IgE mAb, serum IgE levels remained suppressed below the level of detection for 5 months. These results suggest that IgE synthesis did not replenish serum IgE in treated dogs, because IgE was undetectable long after there was no free chimeric anti-IgE antibody present in the serum of these animals. The results further imply that IgE-producing B-cells may have been eliminated or induced into a

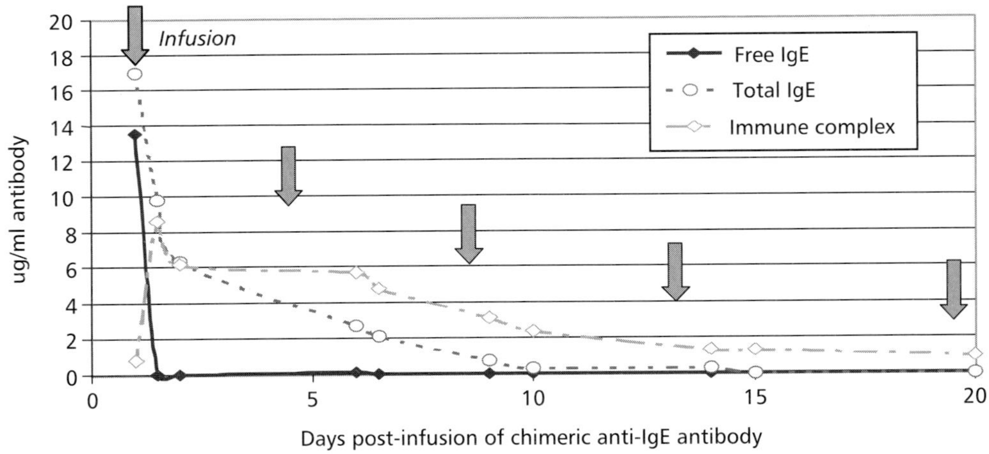

Figure 4.4.2. Immune complex clearance in c15A2-treated dogs. Chimeric anti-immunoglobulin E (IgE) c15A2–IgE immune complexes were detected using an anti-canine IgE domain 4 specific monoclonal antibody to capture the complexed molecules. The complex was then detected using a horseradish peroxidase-labeled polyclonal anti-dog immunoglobulin Fc specific antibody. Chimeric 15A2 antibody–IgE immune complexes could be detected immediately after infusion of the molecule into dogs. The complexed molecules were then cleared from the system over a 3 week period, reflecting the drop in total IgE. No immune complexes were detected 28 days post-treatment.

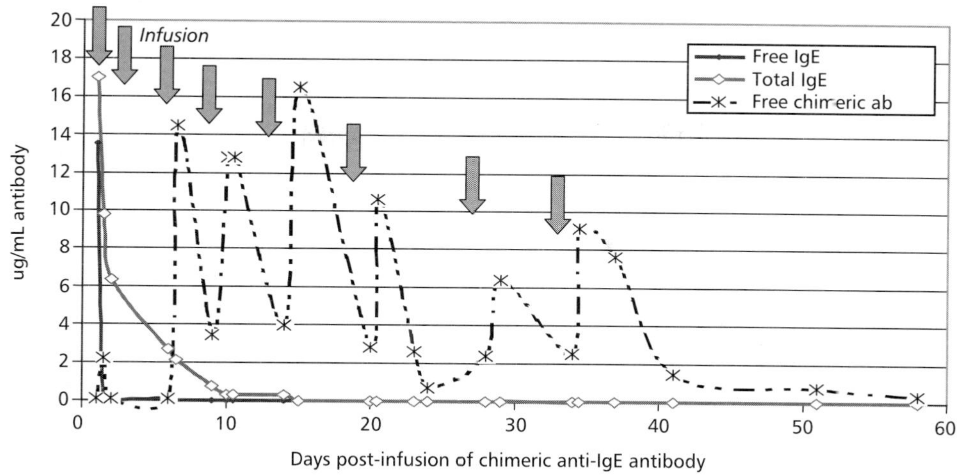

Figure 4.4.3. Detection of free chimeric anti-canine immunoglobulin E (IgE) antibody c15A2 in treated dogs. Free chimeric antibody was detected by a sandwich enzyme-linked immunosorbent assay (ELISA) in which a chimeric antibody peptide mimetope served as the solid phase. The chimeric molecule was detected using a horseradish peroxidase-labeled polyclonal rabbit anti-dog antibody. Serum c15A2 levels consistently rose and fell with each 5 day administration period. Free chimeric antibody was still detectable 24 days after infusion.

state of anergy after treatment with the chimeric antibody. Low levels of both free and total IgE (approximately 200 ng/ml) were measured during the 5th month after the start of the experiment. Serum IgE levels remained low and did not return to pre-experimental levels. The increase in IgE may reflect the generation of a new population of IgE-secreting B-cells in the treated dogs. This result is supported by *in vitro* IgE synthesis experiments. When peripheral blood lymphocytes (PBL) were collected on day 40 and cultured with mitogen there was no detectable IgE synthesis in experimental dogs, while secreted IgE was detected in day 180 PBL (data not shown). Control dogs demonstrated *in vitro* IgE synthesis from PBL taken on both day 40 and day 180 (data not shown).

Effect on level of expression of the high-affinity IgE receptor on basophils upon administration of canine anti-IgE mAb c15A2

At 6 and 16 days following the administration of c15A2, flow-cytometric analyses were performed to investigate the level of high-affinity IgE receptor expression on circulating basophils. The data for a single chimeric antibody-treated dog are depicted in Figure 4.4.4 and are representative results. The number of double-staining cells in quadrant 4 decreased after the administration of c15A2. The data show that the level of expression of high-affinity IgE receptors in basophils was reduced by over 80% after the administration of c15A2 to the experimental dog during this time. In humans, elimination of serum IgE over time leads to a reduction in expression of receptors for IgE on basophils and may reflect a similar response in skin mast cells (MacGlashan *et al.*, 1997, 1998; Saini *et al.*, 1999). An analogous correlation of receptor level expression and serum IgE concentration may exist in dogs. It follows that reduced mast cell expression of high-affinity IgE receptors could lead to a reduction in or elimination of skin-test reactivity to allergen.

Effect on ragweed skin-test reactivity of administration of canine anti-IgE mAb c15A2

Three experimental and two control dogs were challenged with ragweed allergen, as described in Figure 4.4.5, before administration of c15A2, and then at 3 days and 7 days after the last administration (days 36 and 41, respectively). Figure 4.4.5 and the photographs of representative skin tests (Plate 8) show that in control dogs the skin response to ragweed allergen was similar throughout the study. For the control dog depicted, the ragweed skin response actually increased over time. In experimental dogs 2 and 3 the ragweed sensitivity after administration of c15A2 was completely absent for at least 7 days after completion of the dosing regimen. Only dog 1 showed any ragweed sensitivity at the highest ragweed concentration on day 36

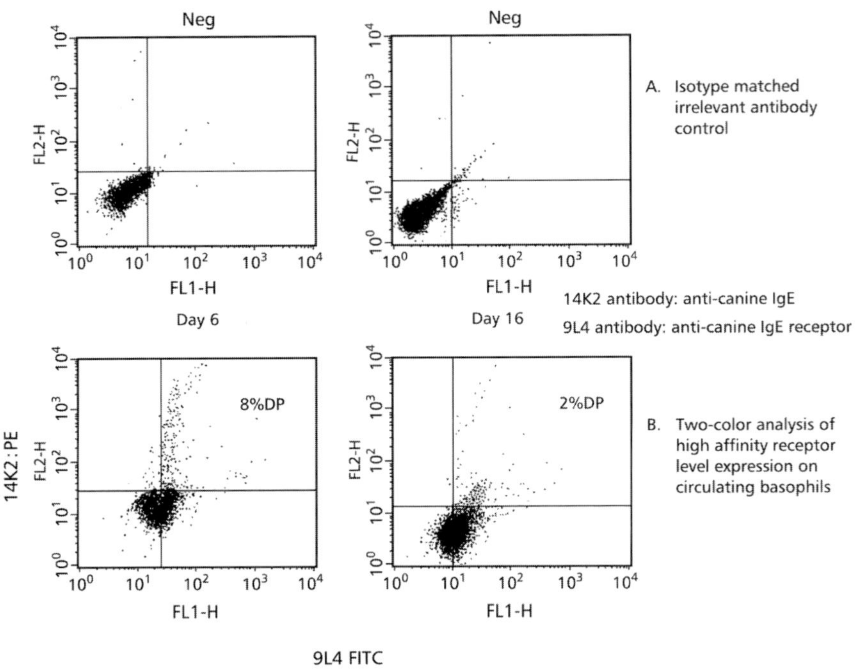

Figure 4.4.4. Down-regulation of high-affinity immunoglobulin E (IgE) receptor expression on circulating basophils. At 6 days and 16 days following the administration of c15A2 10 ml of whole blood was removed. Semipurified populations of peripheral blood leukocytes were prepared by density gradient centrifugation and stained with reagents for two-dimensional flow-cytometric analyses. The reagents used in these experiments were fluoroscein isothiocyanate (FITC)-conjugated, anti-canine high-affinity IgE receptor FcεR1 antibody and phycoerythrin (PE)-conjugated anti-IgE antibody. The cells double staining (double positive, DP cells) for these antibodies were basophils and are observed in quadrant 4.

and that response was given a rating of 1 because of the spread of dye. It did not have the characteristic swelling seen in the rating of 1 observed and recorded for the control dogs. At day 41 or 7 days after the final infusion a response rating of 1 was given to this animal for allergen injections of 1000 protein nitrogen units (PNU)/ml, 100 PNU/ml and 10 PNU/ml. Again, there was only color diffusion and no swelling. Given the fact that this dog had no detectable free or total IgE during this skin-testing period, it seems likely that the skin reactions observed may not have been due to cross-linking of IgE on the mast cell high-affinity IgE receptors. The skin response observed could have been the result of some other skin reaction associated with the testing procedure. Alternatively, receptor-bound IgE may not have been completely removed from the skin mast cells in this animal, even though serum IgE was undetectable. The efficacy of the chimeric molecule may have been reduced in this animal or the dosing regimen may not have been optimized for this particular dog.

Discussion

This study reports the potential utility of a recombinant mouse–dog chimeric anti-canine IgE antibody. Monoclonal anti-IgE antibody will bind serum IgE and affect the ability of skin mast cells to undergo degranulation upon allergen challenge. Characterization of the chimeric antibody, designated c15A2, before the feasibility experiments suggested that it possessed attributes for efficacy as a therapeutic molecule. It had a high affinity for soluble, native canine IgE. The interaction of c15A2 and canine IgE *in vitro* prevented IgE from binding to a recombinant high-affinity IgE receptor. Furthermore, c15A2 had no affinity for canine IgE prebound to immobilized recombinant canine high-affinity IgE receptor in *in vitro* ELISA experiments (data not shown). The *in vitro* data suggested that the chimeric molecule recognized an overlapping or a proximate epitope on canine IgE that interacted with the high-affinity receptor. Alternatively, it was possible that c15A2–canine IgE complexes were unable to bind to the high-affinity IgE receptor FcεR1 as the result of a conformational change induced in IgE by c15A2 binding. Furthermore, an *in vivo* receptor cross-linking experiment in which c15A2 was injected intradermally in dogs produced no weal and flare, thus demonstrating that the antibody would not cross-link receptor-bound IgE and induce a potentially fatal anaphylactic response (data not shown).

To evaluate the ability of c15A2 to effect immunological changes *in vivo*, dogs that had been sensitized

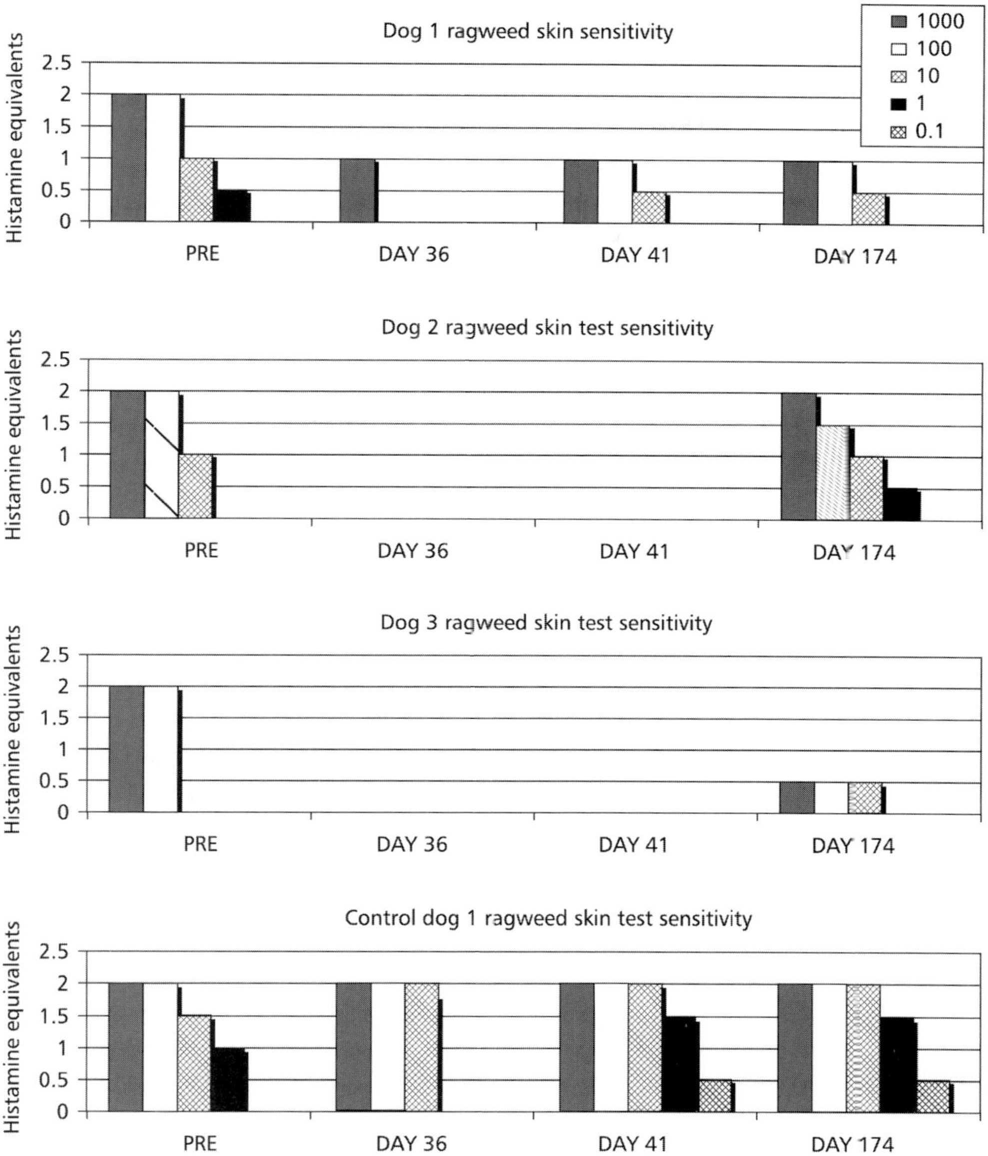

Figure 4.4.5. Skin-test reactivity of chimeric anti-immunoglobulin E (IgE)-treated dogs. Ragweed-sensitized and control dogs were infused with a 0.5% solution in phosphate-buffered saline (PBS) of Evans blue dye at 0.2 ml/kg and then challenged with allergen 10 min later. Five 10-fold serial dilutions of ragweed allergen in PBS starting at 1000 protein nitrogen units (PNU)/ml were prepared and 100 μl was injected intradermally in a shaved section of the torso. Saline (PBS) served as a negative control and histamine (100 μl of a 0.275 μg/ml dilution of histamine in PBS) served as a positive control. Reactivity was measured 10 min later as the swelling and blue-dye diffusion in the skin compared with the histamine control. A rating of 2 was given to an allergen dilution in which the reaction was equivalent in size and color to the histamine reaction. A rating of 1 was given for a reaction that was half of the histamine control and a rating of 0 was equivalent to the saline negative control.

from birth to ragweed allergen were treated with the chimeric antibody by i.v. infusion. It was presumed that, based on *in vitro* data, c15A2 would bind serum IgE and prevent further interaction with the IgE receptor on basophils and mast cells. IgE bound by c15A2 was predicted either to circulate as immune complexes or to be cleared from the circulation. An unknown component to this scenario was the fate of the IgE that existed in interstitial spaces or was bound to high-affinity IgE receptors at the time of infusion.

This non-serum IgE component is referred to as the IgE reservoir. Previous pharmacokinetic experiments had shown that it was possible to remove free IgE rapidly from the serum of dogs (data not shown). Once IgE was removed from serum, the equilibrium between serum IgE and reservoir IgE would become disrupted. The model predicted that IgE should then diffuse from the reservoir, as dictated by the law of mass action, until a new equilibrium was established. As long as free chimeric anti-IgE antibody was present, this IgE would be continually mopped up. The condition described should result in changes in basophil and mast cell-bound IgE. IgE removed, whether by changes in serum IgE concentration or by normal turnover on the cell surface, would eventually disarm the mast cell. The length of time required to induce these effects was unknown. It was assumed, however, that disarming the mast cells would be critical to effect a change in the skin response to ragweed.

In humans it has been shown that, as IgE levels decrease in serum, the density of the high-affinity IgE receptor on basophils and mast cells is down-regulated (MacGlashan *et al.*, 1998; Saini *et al.*, 1999). In an effort to determine whether or not c15A2 infusion would result in similar responses in canine cells, IgE receptor expression on circulating basophils was evaluated by flow cytometry. Comparisons of receptor expression between 6 and 16 days after the initiation of the study revealed an 80% reduction in receptor expression. These data suggest that a regulatory mechanism similar to that observed in humans functions in dogs, whereby there is an inverse correlation between circulating IgE levels and IgE receptor expression on basophils.

Down-regulation of receptor expression further implied that the sensitivity of these animals to allergen challenge had been reduced. To address this possibility, intradermal skin testing was performed. On days 36 and 41 after infusion of c15A2, there was no detectable sensitivity to ragweed allergen in two of the experimental animals. In the third treated animal, although a slight skin reaction was observed at the highest allergen dilution, the skin-test response remained far below pretreatment levels. In a final skin test performed 6 months after the start of the study, the response remained below pretreatment levels in two of the dogs but returned to preinfusion levels in the third animal. This effect was due, presumably, to re-arming of the mast cells by newly synthesized IgE. Free and total IgE in the serum of the treated animals were again detectable in the 5th month of the study, but the levels remained depressed compared with the pre-experimental serum IgE concentration.

It was surprising that free and total IgE in serum remained at undetectable levels long after any free chimeric antibody was measured in the serum of the experimental dogs. This observation strongly suggests that the IgE-secreting B-cell population had been eliminated or induced into a state of anergy. Mechanisms to account for this effect include apoptosis induced by chimeric antibody binding to IgE^+ B-cells or complement-mediated lysis of B-cells following the binding of c15A2. The chimeric antibody was able to lyse canine IgE-coated sheep red blood cells (data not shown), suggesting that complement lysis was a possible mechanism for the elimination of IgE^+ B-cells. At least four isotypes of canine IgG have been shown to exist (Mazza *et al.*, 1993). It is not known which isotype is represented by the heavy-chain structure of c15A2, but the molecule is able to fix complement and that may have been important in the sustained reduction in IgE synthesis observed. By engineering the mouse IgE binding region with other canine heavy chains it may be possible to increase serum half-life and improve the efficacy of its therapeutic effect.

In the studies reported here, only a very low-titer, anti-chimeric response was measured in one dog. This response was not directed against the mouse variable region of the chimeric molecule. It was possible that the response generated was the result of unique baculoviral-derived epitopes created by non-mammalian glycosylation of the chimeric antibody. Mammalian expression should eliminate this problem. In addition, a mammalian expressed protein should have a longer serum half-life. Future experiments are underway to address these issues. The data indicate that anti-IgE antibody therapy in dogs with allergen-induced atopic dermatitis should be investigated and that anti-IgE antibody therapy may prove efficacious for the treatment of canine atopic dermatitis.

References

Capon, D. J., Chamow, S. M., Mordenti, J., Marsters, S. A., Gregory, T., Mitsuya, H. *et al.* (1989) Designing CD4 immunoadhesins for AIDS therapy. *Nature*, **337**, 525–531.

Chang, T. (2000) The pharmacological basis of anti-IgE therapy. *Nature Biotechnology*, **18**, 57–162.

Corne, J., Djukanovic, R., Warner, J., Botta, L., Grandordy, B., Gygax, D. *et al.* (1997) The effect of intravenous administration of a chimeric anti-IgE antibody on serum IgE levels in atopic subjects: efficacy, safety, and pharmacokinetics. *Journal of Clinical Investigation*, **99**, 879–887.

Hill, P. B. & DeBoer, D. J. (1994) Quantification of serum total IgE concentration in dogs by use of an enzyme-linked immunosorbent assay containing monoclonal murine anti-canine IgE. *American Journal of Veterinary Research*, **55**, 944–948.

Holgate, S. T., Corne, J., Jardieu, P., Fick, R. B. & Heusser, C. H. (1998) Treatment of allergic airway disease with anti-IgE. *Allergy*, **53**, 83–88.

MacGlashan, D. W., Bochner, B., Adelman, D., Jardieu, P., Togias, A., White, J. *et al.* (1997) Down-regulation of FcεRI expression on human basophils during *in vivo* treatment of atopic patients with anti-IgE antibody. *Journal of Immunology*, **158**, 1438–1445.

MacGlashan, D. W., Lavens-Phillips, S. & Miura, K. (1998) IgE mediated desensitization in human basophils and mast cells. *Frontiers in Bioscience*, **3**, 746–756.

Mazza, G., Duffus, W. P. H., Elson, C. J., Stokes, C. R., Wison, D. A. & Whiting, A. H. (1993) The separation and identification by monoclonal antibodies of dog IgG fractions. *Journal of Immunological Methods*, **161**, 193–203.

Saini, S. S., MacGlashan, D. W., Sterbinsky, S. A., Togias, A., Adelman, D. C., Lichtenstein, L. M. & Bochner, B. S. (1999) Down-regulation of human basophil IgE and FcεRIα surface densities and mediator release by anti-IgE infusions is reversible *in vitro* and *in vivo*. *Journal of Immunology*, **162**, 5624–5630.

4.5

Effects of phosphodiesterase-4 inhibitors in a model of allergic dermatitis

M. Kietzmann Dr med vet, A.M. Ehinger Dr med vet, G. Gorr Dr rer nat, J. Hoppmann Dr rer nat and E. Telser Dr med vet

Institute of Pharmacology, Toxicology and Pharmacy, School of Veterinary Medicine Hannover, Hannover, Germany

Summary

This study was performed to investigate effects of phosphodiesterase-4 (PDE_4) inhibitors (SB 207499, RPR 73401) on an allergic skin reaction. To simulate an immunological inflammation, mice were sensitised to dinitrochlorobenzene (DNCB) or toluenediisocyanate (TDI). In sensitised mice, DNCB or TDI was given topically as a challenge during repeated local and systemic treatment with the test compounds. Vehicle-treated controls showed a significant increase in ear thickness after challenge with DNCB and TDI, whereas the PDE_4 inhibitors administered topically or systemically reduced this reaction significantly. In conclusion, allergic contact dermatitis or even other immunological skin diseases such as atopic dermatitis may be an indication for PDE_4 inhibitors.

Introduction

In atopic dermatitis (AD), various mediators released from keratinocytes and inflammatory cells initiate and promote the progress of this allergic skin disease (Hanifin, 1991; Kaiserlian & Etchart, 1999). In the regulation of the mediator release, cyclic AMP (cAMP) and cyclic GMP (cGMP) play a pivotal role. The second messenger cAMP suppresses the inflammatory reaction by activation of protein kinases, especially in lymphocytes (Palfreyman & Souness, 1996). Cell-specifically distributed phosphodiesterase (PDE) isoenzymes catalyse the breakdown of the cyclic nucleotides (Nicholson *et al.*, 1991).

In leucocytes of patients with AD, very high PDE_4 activities were found (Grewe *et al.*, 1982; Cooper *et al.*, 1985). It is hypothesised that an excessive stimulation of antigen-presenting cells (APC) in the skin (Langerhans' cells) occurs, leading to the activation of Th_2-cells (Hanifin & Chan, 1996). Interleukin-1 (IL-1) from APC and also from keratinocytes increases the interleukin secretion by activated T-lymphocytes. IL-4 from Th_2-cells, for example, induces the release of immunoglobulin E (IgE) from B-cells (Hanifin & Chan, 1996). The Th_1-cell expansion is inhibited by IL-10 from Th_2-cells and APC. Owing to the characteristic existence of PDE_4 in immune and inflammatory cells (Torphy, 1998), PDE_4 inhibitors seem to be especially suited for the treatment of AD (Chan & Hanifin, 1993; Crocker & Townley, 1999; Ferrer *et al.*, 1999; Marsella & Nicklin, 2000).

Whereas methylxanthines (e.g. theophylline or isobutylmethylxanthine) inhibit the PDE isoenzymes weakly and unspecifically (Rabe *et al.*, 1995; Palfreyman & Souness, 1996), the development of novel PDE_4 inhibitors is of major interest (Dent & Rabe, 1996). Since the use of the first specific PDE_4 inhibitor, rolipram, is limited by its emetic side-effects (Palfreyman, 1995; Duplantier & Biggers, 1996), PDE_4 inhibitors that show a low affinity to the rolipram binding site were synthesised (Polymeropoulos & Höfgen, 1997). For example, substances such as RPR 73401 (Piclamilast), SB 207499 (Ariflo) and BY 217 (Roflumilast) are newer PDE_4

inhibitors with lower affinity to the rolipram binding site (Torphy *et al.*, 1997; Poppe & Szelenyi, 1999; Aoki *et al.*, 2000; Bundschuh *et al.*, 2001).

The experiments described here were performed to investigate the effects of PDE_4 inhibitors on an allergic inflammatory skin reaction. The test compounds, SB 207499 and RPR 73401, were administered systemically and topically. To simulate an immunological inflammation, an ear swelling test (Gad *et al.*, 1986) with mice sensitised to dinitrochlorobenzene (DNCB) or toluenediisocyanate (TDI) was used, representing a model for type IV hypersensitivity with delayed allergic reaction (Tominaga *et al.*, 1985).

Materials and methods

Animals

Female BALB/c-mice were housed in groups of four to six mice per cage at 22°C with a 12 h light/dark cycle. Water and a standard diet (Altromin; Lage/Lippe, Germany) were available *ad libitum*.

Animal model

After shaving and depilating of the abdominal skin, Freund's adjuvant was injected intradermally. Then, the horny layers of the abdominal skin were stripped off 10 times with adhesive tape. For active sensitisation, dinitrochlorobenzene (DNCB) (100 μl of a 0.5% solution in acetone/dimethylsulfoxide) or toluenediisocyanate (TDI) (100 μl of a 5% solution in acetone) was administered on the abdominal skin for 4 consecutive days. After 10 days, the allergic reaction was challenged by administration of DNCB (10 μl of a 1% solution in acetone/DMSO) or TDI (10 μl of a 0.5% solution in acetone) each onto the inner and outer surface of the left ear skin. The right ears remained untreated and were used as individual controls. The development of oedema was controlled by measurement of the ear thickness with a cutimeter (Mitutoyo, Tokyo, Japan) before challenge as well as 24 and 48 h afterwards. Mice with a mean swelling of more than 20% after challenge were used as sensitised animals for the experiments.

Experiments with PDE_4 inhibitors (SB 207499 and RPR 73401)

As positive controls, TDI-sensitive mice ($n = 6$ per group) were treated with 30 mg/kg cyclosporin A intraperitoneally (i.p.) or 1 mg/kg dexamethasone phosphate subcutaneously (s.c.) twice in 24 h, or with 0.05% diflorasone diacetate topically once. Other TDI-sensitive mice were treated with either 10 mg/kg SB 207499 i.p. three times in 24 h, 5 mg/kg RPR 73401 i.p. four times every 3 h, 3% SB 207499 topically once or 3% RPR 73401 topically four times every 3 h as test compounds. DNCB-sensitive mice were treated with 10 mg/kg SB 207499 i.p. five times every 3 h or 1 mg/kg RPR 73401 i.p. twice in 24 h. Negative controls were treated with the vehicle alone. The animals were challenged topically with TDI and DNCB 2 h after the first (RPR 73401 in the TDI model, SB 207499, diflorasone diacetate) or second (RPR 73401 in the DNCB model, dexamethasone phosphate, cyclosporin A) treatment. The ear thickness was measured 24 and 48 h after allergen exposure.

TDI-sensitive mice were killed 8 h after rechallenge. Their blood was sampled and heparinised (20 IU/ml). Plasma was obtained by centrifugation (2000 *g*, 10 min, 4°C) and frozen at −80°C. Then tumour necrosis factor-α (TNF-α) was measured by bioassay with a modified methyltetrazolium assay (Mosmann, 1983), owing to its cytotoxic activity on the tumour cell line L929 (Earle *et al.*, 1943). Ear tissue was sampled immediately: one half was fixed in 4% formaldehyde for histological sectioning, stained with haematoxylin and eosin to score granulocyte accumulation, and the other half was shock-frozen in liquid nitrogen and stored at −80°C. After homogenisation of the tissue under liquid nitrogen, the homogenates were taken in RPMI 1640 medium (Biochrom, Berlin, Germany), 1 mmol Pefabloc® (Boehringer Mannheim, Germany) was added and the probes were mixed intensively. After centrifugation (10 000 *g*, 10 min, 4°C), the supernatant was collected and IL-4 was determined by enzyme-linked immunosorbent assay (ELISA) according to the manufacturer's instructions (monoclonal anti-mouse IL-4 and horseradish peroxidase (HRP)-conjugated anti-mouse IL-4; R&D Systems, Wiesbaden, Germany). For quantification of the homogenised tissue, the amount of protein in the supernatant was measured according to the method of Lowry *et al.* (1951) (Biorad®, München, Germany).

Statistical evaluation

Differences between the treatment groups were evaluated using the non-parametric Mann–Whitney *U*-test. A *p*-value of < 0.01 was considered to be significant.

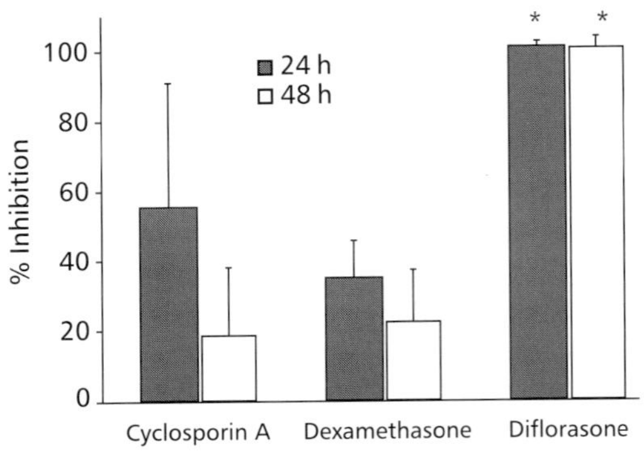

Figure 4.5.1. Inhibition of ear swelling 24 and 48 h from local toluenediisocyanate (TDI) challenge after treatment with 30 mg/kg cyclosporin A intraperitoneally, 1 mg/kg dexamethasone phosphate subcutaneously twice in 24 h or 0.05% diflorasone diacetate topically once. Animals were challenged with TDI 2 h after the first (diflorasone diacetate) or second (cyclosporin A and dexamethasone phosphate) treatment. Data are given as the mean (% inhibition of ear swelling compared with vehicle controls after TDI challenge) and standard deviation of six mice per group. *Significant difference from vehicle controls ($p < 0.01$, *U*-test).

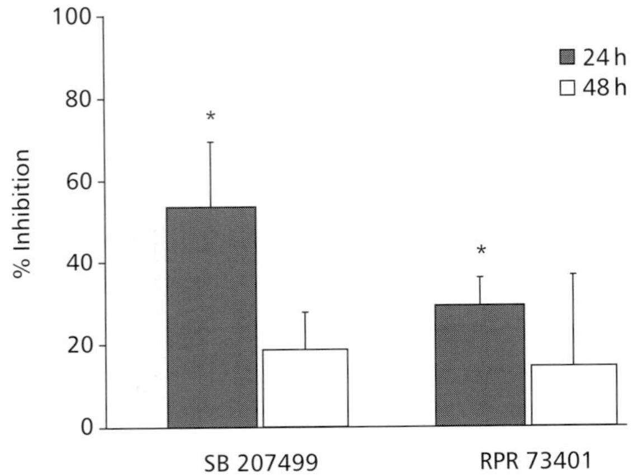

Figure 4.5.2. Inhibition of ear swelling 24 and 48 h from local dinitrochlorobenzene (DNCB) challenge after intraperitoneal treatment with SB 207499 (10 mg/kg, five times every 3 h) or RPR 73401 (1 mg/kg, twice in 24 h). Animals were challenged with DNCB 2 h after the first (SB 207499) or second (RPR 73401) treatment. Data are given as the mean (% inhibition of ear swelling compared with vehicle controls after DNCB challenge) and standard deviation of six mice per group. *Significant difference from vehicle controls ($p < 0.01$, *U*-test).

Results

In both DNCB- and TDI-sensitive mice, the vehicle control with systemic treatment showed a significant ($p < 0.01$) increase in ear thickness 24 and 48 h after challenge, respectively (data not shown). After TDI challenge, the ear swelling was nearly prevented by topically administered diflorasone diacetate and to a lesser extent by cyclosporin A as well as dexamethasone phosphate (Figure 4.5.1). In experiments with DNCB-sensitive mice, the effect of diflorasone diacetate was comparable.

After repeated intraperitoneal administration of SB 207499 and RPR 73401, the ear swelling was reduced in TDI- and DNCB-sensitive mice. Significant ($p < 0.01$) inhibitory effects were obvious only after 24 h in DNCB-sensitive mice (Figure 4.5.2). In contrast to SB 207499, RPR 73401 showed no significant effects at this time point in TDI-sensitised mice (Figure 4.5.3).

After topical treatment with both test compounds, a nearly complete inhibition of ear swelling was obvious in TDI-sensitised mice after 24 h as well as after 48 h (Figure 4.5.4). In the additional experiment with TDI-sensitised mice treated topically with the test compounds, an increased granulocyte infiltration was observed in the vehicle controls after 8 h. Topical treatment with the PDE_4 inhibitors diminished this cellular infiltration. In the challenged ear skin of vehicle-treated mice, an IL-4 concentration of 480 pg/mg protein was measured. In SB 207499 and RPR 73401-treated mice, the concentrations were 270 and 290 pg/mg protein, respectively. The concentration

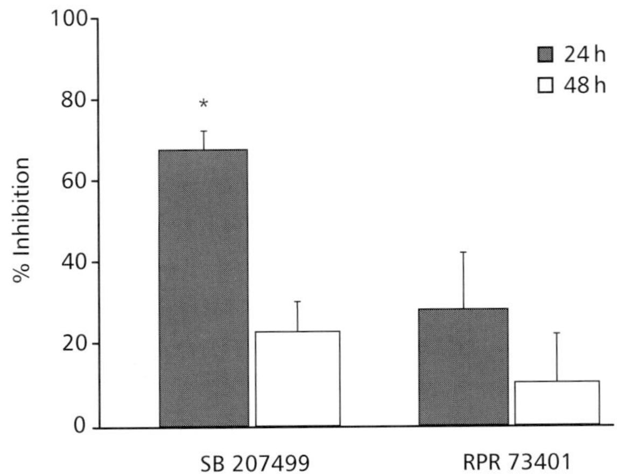

Figure 4.5.3. Inhibition of ear swelling 24 and 48 h from local toluenediisocyanate (TDI) challenge after intraperitoneal treatment with SB 207499 (10 mg/kg, three times in 24 h) or RPR 73401 (5 mg/kg, four times every 3 h). Animals were challenged with TDI 2 h after the first treatment. Data are given as the mean (% inhibition of ear swelling compared with vehicle controls after TDI challenge) and standard deviation of six mice per group. *Significant difference from vehicle controls ($p < 0.01$, *U*-test).

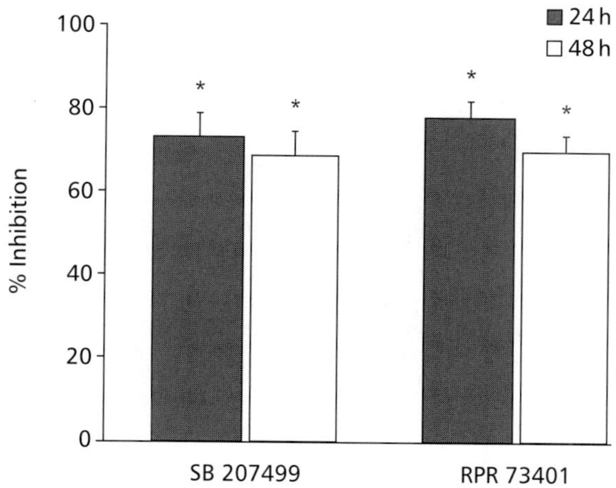

Figure 4.5.4. Inhibition of ear swelling 24 and 48 h from local toluenediisocyanate (TDI) challenge after topical treatment with SB 207499 (3%, once) or treatment with RPR 73401 (3%, four times every 3 h). The animals were challenged with TDI 2 h after the first treatment. Data are given as the mean (% inhibition of ear swelling compared with vehicle controls after TDI challenge) and standard deviation of six mice per group. *Significant difference from vehicle controls ($p < 0.01$, *U*-test).

of active TNF-α in plasma was 0.7 pg/ml in the sensitized controls. In animals treated with the PDE_4 inhibitors, the TNF-α concentration was below the detection limit of the bioassay.

Discussion

In sensitised mice, the challenge with DNCB and TDI was followed by an inflammatory reaction which was demonstrated by a significant swelling of the treated ears. In addition, cyclosporin A, dexamethasone phosphate and diflorasone diacetate prevented the increase in ear swelling significantly. Glucocortiocids are frequently used in the treatment of allergic skin diseases. In severe cases, immunosuppressive drugs are also administered (Hanifin & Chan, 1996). The use of these drugs is limited by their side-effects. From the literature it is known that PDE_4 inhibitors are anti-inflammatory drugs (Torphy, 1998). Beneficial effects were shown in human and veterinary patients with asthma or AD (Chan & Hanifin, 1993; Crocker & Townley, 1999; Ferrer *et al.*, 1999; Marsella & Nicklin, 2000). Currently, the mammalian PDE isoenzymes are divided into 11 gene families that are pharmacologically differentiated by their special substrate (cAMP, cGMP) and selective inhibitors (Torphy & Page, 2000). The gene families include isogene subtypes and within these isoform splice variants (Dousa, 1999). Table 4.5.1 summarises data concerning the gene families 3, 4 and 7, as well as their distribution in inflammatory cells.

Table 4.5.1. Phosphodiesterase (PDE) families 3, 4 and 7, their characteristics and existence in immune and inflammatory cells, according to Torphy (1998)

Family	Isoenzyme	K_m (μmol/l)		Subtypes
		cAMP	cGMP	
3	cGMP-inhibited	0.2	0.3	2
4	cAMP-specific	4.0	>3000	4
7	cAMP-specific, highly	0.2	>1000	1

Cells	PDE family
Basophils	3, 4
B-lymphocytes	?
Eosinophils	4
Macrophages	3, 4
Mast cells	3, 4
Monocytes	3
Neutrophils	3
T-lymphocytes	3, 4, 7

The experiments described herein were performed to demonstrate the anti-inflammatory effects of PDE_4 inhibitors in a model of allergic contact dermatitis. TDI and DNCB were used as allergens. Whereas DNCB increases the production and secretion of IL-2 in Th_1-cells, TDI increases Th_2-cell-specific cytokines such as IL-4 (Dearman *et al.*, 1996). According to Gad *et al.* (1986), the expression of the secondary response to TDI application started more quickly and faded rapidly within 48 h. The difference between DNCB and TDI may be caused by the varying ability of these compounds to penetrate the epidermal barrier, apart from the different types of allergic reaction onset.

The inflammatory reaction (ear swelling) was diminished by systemically and topically administered PDE_4 inhibitors. By the topical route, both test compounds had a more pronounced and longer lasting effect. This may be caused pharmacokinetically owing to prolonged influx of the test compounds after local administration and a poor penetration from the vasculature into the cutaneous compartment after systemic treatment (Griswold *et al.*, 1998). The results described are confirmed by the measured concentrations of IL-4 and TNF-α as well as by an observed diminished leucocyte infiltration.

Conclusion

The mouse ear swelling test (Gad *et al.*, 1986) was successfully established as an *in vivo* model for immunological skin inflammation, as nearly every animal was sensitive to DNCB or TDI after induction and the positive controls showed the expected effect. Independently of the route of administration, the PDE_4 inhibitors SB 207499 and RPR 73401 reduced the increase in ear thickness. The drugs showed a longer lasting effect after topical treatment than after systemic administration. These and other results indicate a use for PDE_4 inhibitors in allergic contact dermatitis or even other immunological skin diseases such as AD, especially with direct application to the epidermis, which may diminish systemic side-effects (Palfreyman & Souness, 1996). Following the development of suitable formulations for systemic and topical use in animals, clinical studies are necessary to confirm the experimental results of this new class of drugs in the treatment of allergic skin diseases.

References

Aoki, M., Kobayashi, M., Ishikawa, J., Saita, Y., Terai, Y., Takayama, K. *et al.* (2000) A novel phosphodiesterase type 4 inhibitor, YM976 (4-(3-chlorophenyl)-1,7-diethylpyrido[2,3-*d*]pyrimidin-2(1*H*)-one), with little emetogenic activity. *Journal of Pharmacology and Experimental Therapeutics*, **295**, 255–260.

Bundschuh, D. S., Eltze, M., Barsig, J., Wollin, L., Hatzelmann, A. & Beume, R. (2001) *In vivo* efficacy in airway disease models of roflumilast, a novel orally active PDE_4 inhibitor. *Journal of Pharmacology and Experimental Therapeutics*, **297**, 280–290.

Chan, S. C. & Hanifin, J. M. (1993) Differential inhibitor effects on cyclic AMP phosphodiesterase isoforms in atopic and normal leukocytes. *Journal of Laboratory and Clinical Medicine*, **121**, 44–51.

Cooper, K. D., Kang, K. F., Chan, S. C. & Hanifin, J. M. (1985) Phosphodiesterase inhibition by Ro 20-1724 reduces hyper-IgE synthesis by atopic dermatitis cells *in vitro*. *Journal of Investigative Dermatology*, **84**, 477–482.

Crocker, I. C. & Townley, R. G. (1999) Therapeutic potential of phosphodiesterase 4 inhibitors in allergic diseases. *Drugs of Today*, **35**, 519–535.

Dearman, R. J., Basketter, D. A. & Kimber, I. (1996) Characterization of chemical allergens as a function of divergent cytokine secretion profiles induced in mice. *Toxicology and Applied Pharmacology*, **138**, 308–316.

Dent, G. & Rabe, K. F. (1996) Effect of theophylline and non-selective xanthine derivatives on PDE isoenzymes and cellular function. In: *Phosphodiesterase inhibitors* (Eds C. Schudt, G. Dent & K. F. Rabe), pp. 41–64. Academic Press, New York.

Dousa, T. P. (1999) Cyclic-3′,5′-nucleotide phosphodiesterase isoenzymes in cell biology and pathophysiology of the kidney. *Kidney International*, **55**, 29–62.

Duplantier, A. J. & Biggers, M. S. (1996) Biarylcarboxylic acids and -amides: inhibition of phosphodiesterase type IV versus [^{3}H]rolipram binding activity and their relationship to emetic behavior in the ferret. *Journal of Medical Chemistry*, **39**, 120–125.

Earle, W. R., Schilling, E. L., Stark, T. H., Straus, N. P., Brown, M. F. & Shelton, E. (1943) The mouse fibroblast cultures and changes in the living cells. *Journal of the National Cancer Insitute*, **4**, 165–212.

Ferrer, L., Alberola, J., Queralt, M., Brazis, P., Rabanal, R., Llenas, J. & Puigdemont, A. (1999) Clinical anti-inflammatory efficacy of arofylline, a new selective phosphodiesterase 4 inhibitor, in dogs with atopic dermatitis. *Veterinary Record*, **145**, 191–194.

Gad, S. C., Dunn, B. J., Dobbs, D. W., Reilly, C. & Walsh, R. D. (1986) Development and validation of an alternative dermal sensitization test: the mouse ear swelling test (MEST). *Toxicology and Applied Pharmacology*, **84**, 93–114.

Grewe, S. R., Chan, S. C. & Hanifin, J. M. (1982) Elevated leukocyte cyclic AMP-phosphodiesterase in atopic disease: a possible mechanism for cyclic AMP-agonist hyporesponsiveness. *Journal of Allergy and Clinical Immunology*, **70**, 452–457.

Griswold, D. E., Webb, E. F., Badger, A. M., Gorkycki, P. D., Levandoski, P. A., Barnette, M. A. *et al.* (1998) SB-207499 (Ariflo), a second generation phosphodiesterase 4 inhibitor, reduces tumor necrosis factor α and interleukin-4 production *in vivo*. *Journal of Pharmacology and Experimental Therapeutics*, **287**, 705–711.

Hanifin, J. M. (1991) Atopic dermatitis: new therapeutic considerations. *Journal of the American Academy of Dermatology*, **24**(6, Suppl. II), 1097–1101.

Hanifin, J. M. & Chan, S. C. (1996) Diagnosis and treatment of atopic dermatitis. *Dermatologic Therapy*, **1**, 9–18.

Kaiserlian, D. & Etchart, N. (1999) Epicutaneous and transcutaneous immunization using DNA of proteins. *European Journal of Dermatology*, **9**, 169–176.

Lowry, O. H., Rosebrough, N. J., Farr, A. L. & Randall, R. J. (1951) Protein measurement with the Folin reagent. *Journal of Biological Chemistry*, **193**, 265–275.

Marsella, R. & Nicklin, C. F. (2000) Double-blinded cross-over study on the efficacy of pentoxifylline for canine atopy. *Veterinary Dermatology*, **11**, 255–260.

Mosmann, T. (1983) Rapid colorimetric assay for cellular growth and survival: application to proliferation and cytotoxicity assays. *Journal of Immunological Methods*, **65**, 55–63.

Nicholson, C. D., Challiss, R. A. J. & Shahid, M. (1991) Differential modulation of tissue function and therapeutic potential of selective inhibitors of cyclic nucleotide phosphodiesterase isoenzymes. *Trends in Pharmacological Sciences*, **12**, 19–27.

Palfreyman, M. N. (1995) Phosphodiesterase type IV inhibitors as antiinflammatory agents. *Drugs of the Future*, **20**, 793–804.

Palfreyman, M. N. & Souness, J. E. (1996) Phosphodiesterase type IV inhibitors. *Progress in Medical Chemistry*, **33**, 1–52.

Polymeropoulos, E. E. & Höfgen, N. (1997) A pharmacophore model for PDE IV inhibitors. *Quantitative Structure–Activity Relationship*, **16**, 231–234.

Poppe, H. & Szelenyi, I. (1999) Effect of the new selective PDE_4-inhibitor AWD 12-281 and RPR 73401 on LPS-induced neutrophilia in ferret lung and emetogenic effects in concious ferrets. *Naunyn-Schmiedeberg's Archives of Pharmacology*, **359** (Suppl. 3), 443.

Rabe, K. F., Magnussen, H. & Dent, G. (1995) Theophylline and selective PDE inhibitors as bronchodilators and smooth muscle relaxants. *European Respiratory Journal*, **8**, 637–642.

Tominaga, M., Kohno, S., Tanaka, K. & Ohata, K. (1985) Studies on toluene diisocyanate (TDI)-induced delayed type hypersensitivity. *Japanese Journal of Pharmacology*, **39**, 163–171.

Torphy, T. J. (1998) Phosphodiesterase isoenzymes. *American Journal of Respiratory and Critical Care Medicine*, **157**, 351–370.

Torphy, T. J. & Page, C. (2000) Phosphodiesterases: the journey towards therapeutics. *Trends in Pharmacological Sciences*, **21**, 157–159.

Torphy, T. J., Christensen, S. B., Barnette, M. S., Burman M., Cieslinsk, L. B. & Dewolf, W. E. (1997) Molecular basis for an improved therapeutic index of SB 207499, a second generation phosphodiesterase 4 inhibitor. *European Respiratory Journal*, **10**, 313s.

4.6

Immunoglobulin G responses to *Malassezia pachydermatis* antigens in atopic and normal dogs

T.A. Chen BVM, R.E.W. Halliwell MA, VetMB, PhD, DACVD, DECVD, MRCVS and P.B. Hill BVSc, PhD, DVD, DACVD, MRCVS

Department of Veterinary Clinical Studies, The Royal (Dick) School of Veterinary Studies, The University of Edinburgh, UK

Summary

Overgrowth of *Malassezia pachydermatis* is a common occurrence on the skin of dogs with atopic dermatitis, but the interaction between the organism and the host's immune system has not been extensively investigated. The aim of this study was to characterise one arm of the humoral immune response to *M. pachydermatis* by comparing immunoglobulin G (IgG) responses to antigens separated by sodium dodecyl sulfate–polyacrylamide gel electrophoresis in 18 atopic dogs with *Malassezia* dermatitis, 20 atopic dogs without *Malassezia* dermatitis and 18 clinically normal dogs using Western immunoblotting. Numerous IgG-binding proteins were detected with sera from atopic dogs with *Malassezia* dermatitis. Strong bands with molecular weights of 25, 29, 42, 45–51, 61, 82 and 90 kDa were seen in more than 50% of the dogs. However, antigens of 28–30, 42, 45–51, 61, 82 and 90 kDa were also recognised by most atopic dogs without *Malassezia* dermatitis. Approximately half of the normal dogs showed faint IgG binding to multiple indistinct bands between 42 and 68 kDa, but clearer bands could be seen at 42, 45 and 82 kDa. These results indicate that the majority of atopic dogs with *Malassezia* dermatitis have a greater IgG response than normal dogs, and show responses to an additional protein of 25 kDa. This antigen may therefore be clinically important in cases of *Malassezia* dermatitis associated with canine atopy.

Introduction

Malassezia pachydermatis is a lipophilic, unipolar-budding yeast that can be isolated from the skin and ear canals of healthy dogs (Baxter, 1976; Gedek *et al.*, 1979; Bond *et al.*, 1994, 1995; Bond & Anthony, 1995; Kennis *et al.*, 1996). However, since the early 1980s, a dermatitis has been reported that is associated with elevated cutaneous populations of *M. pachydermatis* and shows a beneficial response to antifungal therapy (Dufait, 1983; Larsson *et al.*, 1988; Mason & Evans, 1991). The factors that have been suggested to cause overgrowth of the organism are alterations in skin-surface microclimate, such as increased temperature, moisture and sebum production as well as defective host immunity (Mason, 1992). Such changes may be associated with various underlying skin diseases, including hypersensitivity disorders, bacterial skin infections, keratinisation defects and endocrine diseases (Scott & Miller, 1989; Mason & Evans, 1991; Mason, 1992; Morris, 1999).

Atopic dermatitis is one of the most common diseases associated with *Malassezia* overgrowth in dogs. It has been demonstrated that some atopic dogs carry higher numbers of *M. pachydermatis* on the skin than normal dogs (Bond & Sant, 1993; Bond *et al.*, 1994; White *et al.*, 1996), and cytological evidence of *Malassezia* overgrowth is a common finding in atopic dogs in the authors' clinic (personal observations).

The interaction between *M. pachydermatis* and the host's immune system has not been widely studied either in normal or atopic dogs. Morris *et al.* (1998)

showed that atopic dogs may mount an immunoglobulin E (IgE) response to *M. pachydermatis*, and Nuttall showed that atopic dogs had elevated levels of *Malassezia*-specific IgG (Nuttall, 1997) and IgE (Nuttall, 1998) in their serum.

The aim of this study was to characterise further one arm of the humoral immune response to *M. pachydermatis* by comparing IgG responses to individual antigens of the yeast in atopic dogs with and without *Malassezia* dermatitis and normal dogs, using sodium dodecyl sulfate–polyacrylamide gel electrophoresis (SDS–PAGE) and Western immunoblotting.

Materials and methods

Serum samples

Serum samples were collected from 18 atopic dogs with *Malassezia* dermatitis and 20 atopic dogs without *Malassezia* dermatitis presenting to the dermatology clinic at the Royal (Dick) School of Veterinary Studies in Edinburgh. Sera of clinically normal dogs were collected from 18 dogs presenting for euthanasia at a rescue centre.

The diagnosis of atopic dermatitis was based on a combination of consistent history and clinical signs, exclusion of other causes of pruritic skin disease and the presence of at least one positive intradermal skin-test reaction. Coat brushings, skin scrapings and trial therapy were used to eliminate ectoparasites. A 6 week, home-cooked diet trial was conducted to eliminate food intolerance. No anti-inflammatory medication was given for at least 3 weeks before examination. The intradermal skin tests were performed with 57 allergens using 0.05 ml of each allergen extract on the lateral flank after the dogs were sedated with 0.15 mg/kg xylazine intramuscularly (i.m.) and clipped. Histamine (1/100 000 w/v) and saline diluent were also injected as positive and negative controls. Test sites were assessed after 20 min and scored from 0 (negative control) to 4 (positive control) compared with the controls. Reactions ≥ 2 were considered positive (Scott *et al.*, 2001).

Malassezia dermatitis was diagnosed by microscopic observation of Diff-Quik® (Dade AG, Switzerland) stained tape strips (Mason, 1992; Bond & Sant, 1993; Charach, 1997). Samples were obtained from the groin, axilla and interdigital web, and *Malassezia* overgrowth was characterised as an average of five or more *Malassezia* organisms per 400 × field. *Malassezia* otitis was diagnosed by sampling the external ear canal with a cotton swab and transferring the material to a glass slide prior to heat fixing and staining. The criteria for demonstrating overgrowth were as described for the tape strips.

Normal dogs had no history or clinical signs of skin disease and had no lesions on dermatological examination.

Culture of M. pachydermatis

An isolate of *M. pachydermatis* was obtained from the ear canal of a dog with *Malassezia* otitis. This was deemed appropriate because previous studies have shown that *M. pachydermatis* was the only *Malassezia* species isolated from the skin and external ear canal of dogs with either otitis externa or skin infections, and all isolates of *M. pachydermatis* had similar electrophoretic karyotypes (Senczek *et al.*, 1999). The sample was cultured on Sabouraud Dextrose agar (Oxoid, Basingstoke, UK) containing 20 mg/ml chloramphenicol (Intramycetin®; Parke-Davis Veterinary, Eastleigh, UK) for 48 h at 37°C, and the colonies were identified as *M. pachydermatis* by microscopic examination. The colonies were then subcultured onto large numbers of plates to obtain enough organisms for subsequent studies.

Extraction of M. pachydermatis proteins

Malassezia colonies were carefully harvested and suspended in phosphate-buffered saline (PBS, pH 7.4) for a washing procedure that consisted of three cycles of centrifugation at 500 *g* for 5 min followed by removal of the supernatant and resuspension in PBS. After the last washing cycle, the cells were resuspended in extraction buffer (pH 7.4) containing 125 mM NH_4HCO_3 (Sigma, Poole, UK) and protease inhibitors (20 mM ϵ-aminocaproic acid, Sigma, UK; 5 mM ethylenediaminetetraacetic acid, Sigma, UK; and 1 mM phenylmethylsulfonyl fluoride, BDH, UK) (Jensen-Jarolim *et al.*, 1992; Morris *et al.*, 1998).

Preliminary experiments were performed using three different methods to determine the optimum method for protein extraction. First, the *Malassezia* colonies in the extraction buffer were mixed vigorously with an equal volume of glass beads (0.4 mm, 40 mesh, BDH, UK) on a vortex mixer for 10 min to disrupt the cell membranes mechanically. A second suspension of *Malassezia* organisms was subjected to three cycles of freezing and thawing by alternately immersing the container in a dry ice–methanol mixture and warm tap water. This was intended to fracture the cell membranes and allow release of cytoplasmic contents. Thirdly, a *Malassezia* suspension was placed in an ultrasonic water bath for 5 min to fragment the organisms physically. Ten agar plates were prepared for each method, and equal weights of colonies (3.07 g) were added to 5 ml of extraction buffer. After extraction, the cell suspensions were stored at 4°C overnight, then centrifuged at 6000 *g* for 5 min, and the supernatants were collected. The amount of protein obtained from each method was measured with BCA Protein Assay Reagent (Pierce Chemical Company, Rockford, IL, USA) and the extracts were analysed by SDS–PAGE. The protein concentrations of the extracts obtained from the three methods (glass beads, freeze–thaw cycles and ultrasonification) were 16.35, 0.58, and 0.22 mg/ml, respectively. Figure 4.6.1 shows the Coomassie blue-stained protein profiles of the three different extracts on an SDS–PAGE gel. Much stronger protein bands were seen in the extract obtained by glass bead disruption. This method was therefore used in subsequent studies.

SDS–PAGE and immunoblotting

The gel electrophoresis was performed according to the method of Laemmli (1970) using 12% separating polyacrylamide gel and 4% stacking gel in a discontinuous buffer system containing 0.025 M Tris (Sigma, UK), 0.2 M glycine (Fisher Scientific, Loughborough, UK) and 0.1% SDS (Fisher Scientific, UK), pH 8.3. The extracts and molecular weight standards were diluted 1:1 with reducing sample buffer (containing 5% β-mercaptoethanol; Sigma, UK) and heated at 95°C for 5 min. They were then added to the wells of the gel and the electrophoresis was run at 200 V for 60 min.

The separated proteins and molecular weight standards were transferred from the gel to a polyvinylidene difluoride microporous membrane (Millipore Immobilon™-P Transfer Membrane; Millipore Corporation, Bedford, MA, USA) in a BioRad Trans-Blot® SD Semi-Dry Electrophoretic Transfer Cell according to

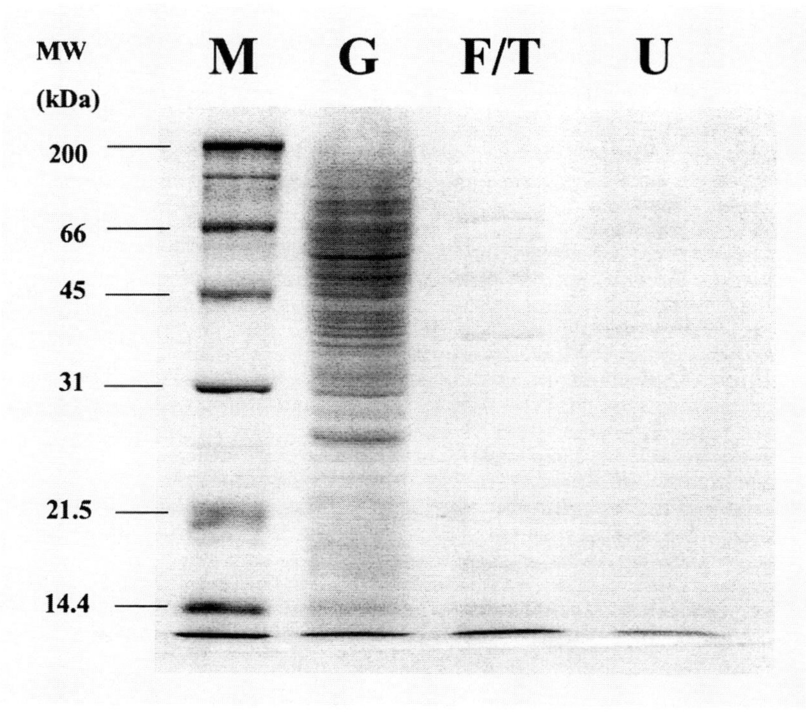

Figure 4.6.1. Extracts of *Malassezia pachydermatis* obtained using three different methods in a Coomassie blue-stained sodium dodecyl sulfate–polyacrylamide gel electrophoresis gel. M: broad-range molecular weight standard; G: glass beads; F/T: three freeze–thaw cycles; U: ultrasonification. Molecular weights are shown in kilodaltons. The extract produced using glass bead disruption was selected for the immunoglobulin G study.

the manufacturer's instructions. The transfer buffer contained 10 mM (cyclohexylamino)-1-propane sulfonic acid (CAPS, Sigma, Poole, UK) and 10% methanol (Fisher Scientific, UK) (LeGendre *et al.*, 1993). The transfer was run at 80 mA per minigel for 1 h. The quality of transfer was checked by staining gels and molecular weight standards blotted onto the membrane with Coomassie brilliant blue R-250 (BDH, Poole, UK).

For detection of IgG binding proteins, one broad well of *Malassezia* extract (123 μg, 150 μl of 1/20 dilution) running across the top of the gel was used. This allowed the membrane to be cut into narrow strips so that they could be probed with individual sera. They were then blocked for 1 h with 1% skimmed milk in Tris-buffered saline (TBS) containing 0.02 M Tris and 0.5 M NaCl (Sigma, UK), pH 7.5. After washing with TBS containing 0.05% Tween 20 (Fisher Scientific, UK) (TTBS) for 15 min (3 × 5 min rinses), each strip was incubated with 10 μl of dog serum diluted to 1 ml in dilution buffer (1% skimmed milk in TTBS) for 30 min. The strips were then washed again in TTBS for a further 15 min. Bound IgG was detected by incubating the strips for 1 h with horseradish peroxidase-conjugated goat anti-dog IgG heavy and light chain (Bethyl Laboratories, Montgomery, TX, USA) diluted 1:10 000 in dilution buffer. After further washing with TTBS for 15 min, the strips were developed with 3,3′-diaminobenzidine (DAB) peroxidase substrate (Vector Laboratories, Burlingame, CA, USA) for about 1 min. The molecular weights of IgG binding proteins were determined using standard curves generated by analysing the position of molecular weight markers on Coomassie blue-stained membranes.

Results

The IgG immunoblots of individual dog sera from the three different groups are shown in Figure 4.6.2a–c. The amount of staining seen in the normal dogs (Figure 4.6.2a) was much weaker than that seen in the atopic dogs with cytological evidence of *Malassezia* overgrowth (Figure 4.6.2b). The binding pattern seen in atopic dogs without *Malassezia* dermatitis was between that of the other two groups (Figure 4.6.2c).

More than half of the normal dogs showed multiple indistinct bands between 42 and 68 kDa, but clearer bands could be seen at 42 (in 83% of dogs), 45 (61%) and 82 kDa (67%) (Figure 4.6.3a). Two dogs showed relatively strong binding patterns (nos 9 and 18) and one dog had a prominent band at 27 kDa (no. 15).

In the atopic dogs with *Malassezia* dermatitis, there was more intense staining of indistinct bands between 45 and 51 kDa. However, distinct IgG binding proteins with molecular weights of 25 (78%), 29 (67%), 42 (94%), 61 (67%), 82 (89%) and 90 kDa (61%) were recognised by more than 50% of the atopic dogs with *Malassezia* dermatitis (Figure 4.6.3b). Some atopic dogs also showed binding to various low molecular weight proteins between 14 and 42 kDa. Antigens of 28–30 (55%), 42 (95%), 45–51 (80%), 61 (50%), 82 (65%) and 90 (55%) kDa were also recognised by more than 50% of the atopic dogs without *Malassezia* dermatitis (Figure 4.6.3c).

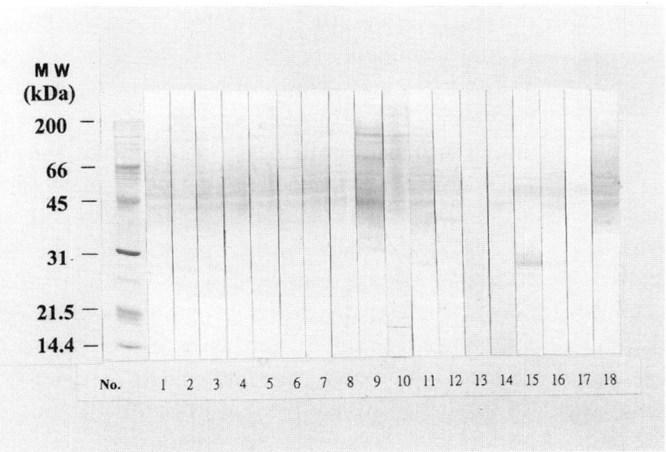

(a)

Figure 4.6.2. Immunoglobulin G-binding components in extracts of *Malassezia pachydermatis* detected by immunoblotting with dog sera from three different groups: (a) normal dogs, (b) atopic dogs with *Malassezia* dermatitis, and (c) atopic dogs without *Malassezia* dermatitis. The numbers along the bottom signify the strips probed with individual dog sera. The molecular weight standards on the left are 200, 66, 45, 31, 21.5 and 14.4 kDa.

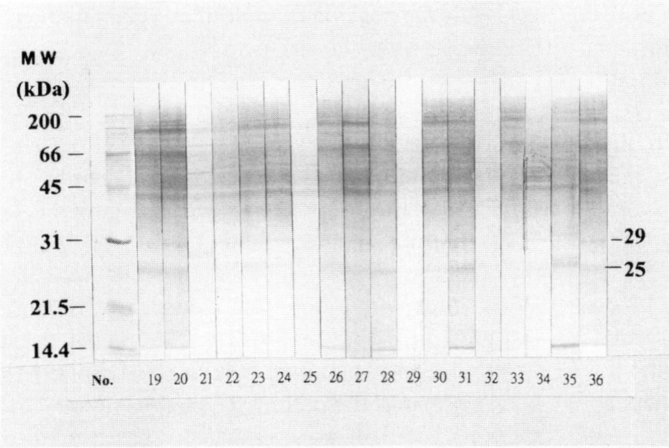

(b)

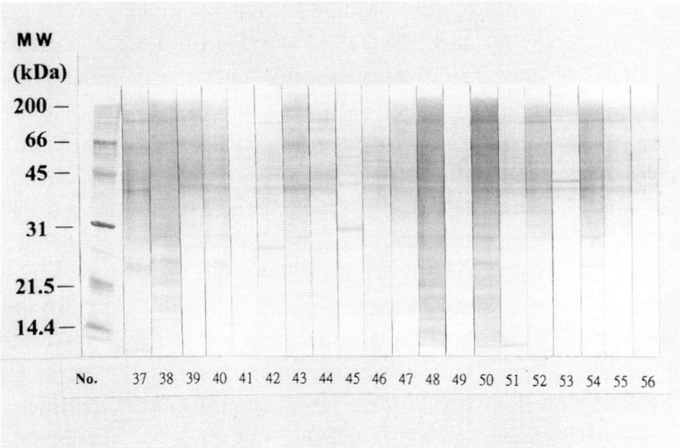

(c)

Figure 4.6.2. *(Continued)*

The blots of the three groups demonstrated that most dogs showed IgG binding to multiple *Malassezia* antigens. However, atopic dogs with *Malassezia* dermatitis had a much greater IgG response than the normal dogs, and the majority showed binding to a protein of 25 kDa which was not seen in most dogs of the other two groups.

Discussion

The results of the immunoblotting with individual dog sera indicate that most dogs have an IgG response to multiple antigens of *M. pachydermatis*. Approximately half of the normal dogs showed faint IgG binding to multiple indistinct bands between 42 and 68 kDa, but clearer bands could be seen at 42, 45 and 82 kDa. These difficulties in distinguishing bands could be overcome using two-dimensional SDS–PAGE and immunoblotting (Onishi *et al.*, 1999). Nevertheless, the results suggest that the commensal population of *M. pachydermatis* is recognised by the dog's immune system, leading to an antibody response. Whether or not this IgG response is protective in any way remains to be determined.

The degree and intensity of staining on the blots from the atopic dogs with *Malassezia* dermatitis was much greater than that seen in the normal dogs, indicating that the majority of atopic dogs with *Malassezia* dermatitis had a greater IgG response to *M. pachydermatis*. This result is in accordance with a recent finding that dogs with skin disease associated with *M. pachydermatis* develop high serum titres of *M. pachydermatis*-specific IgG (Bond *et al.*, 1998). Furthermore, more numerous IgG binding proteins were observed on the blots from the atopic dogs with *Malassezia* dermatitis than from the normal dogs. Some of these proteins were the same in

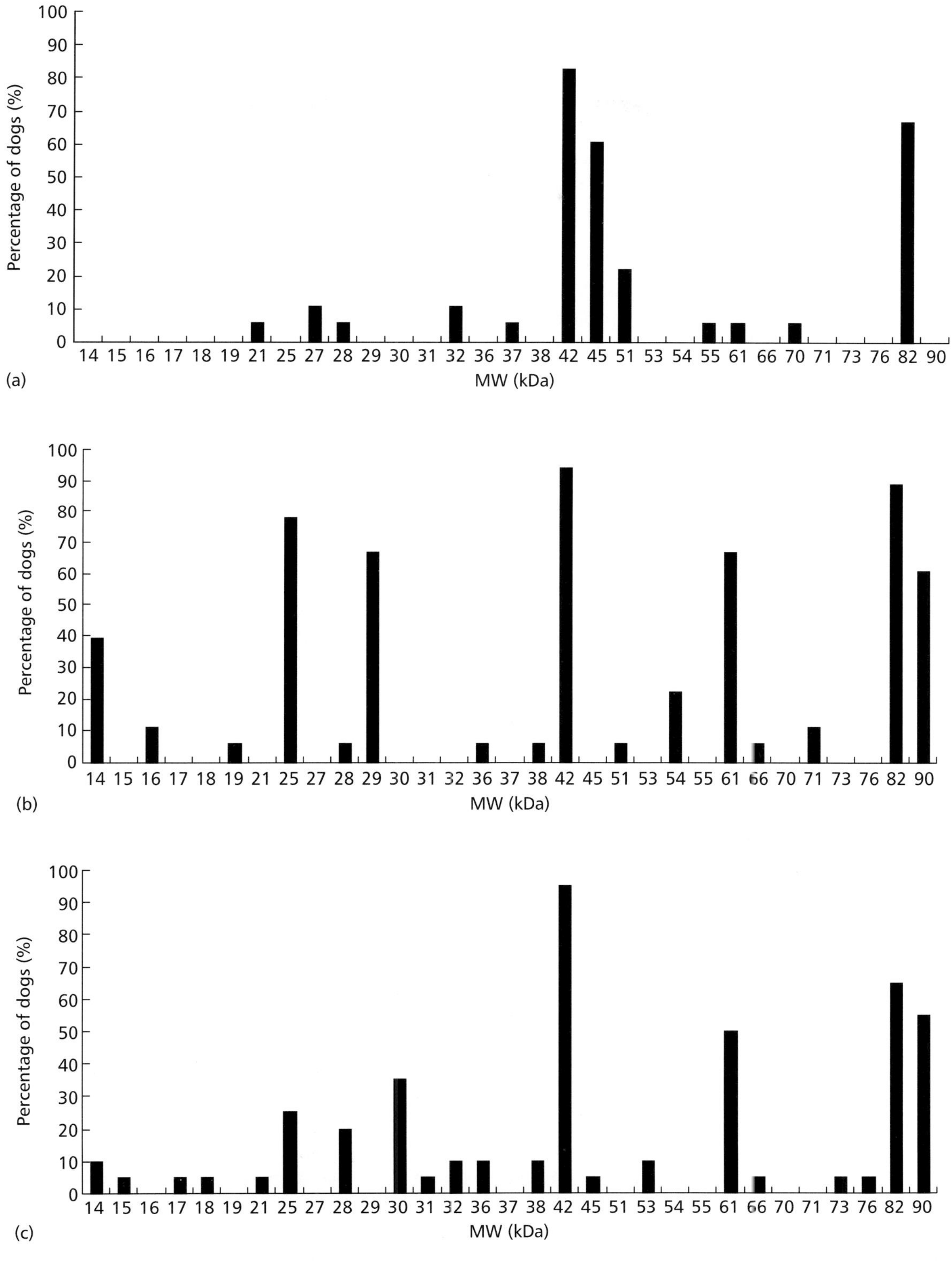

Figure 4.6.3. Percentage of dogs from three different groups showing immunoglobulin G binding to individual antigenic components in extracts of *Malassezia pachydermatis*: (a) normal dogs, (b) atopic dogs with *Malassezia* dermatitis, and (c) atopic dogs without *Malassezia* dermatitis. *x*-Axis: molecular weights of the bands detected on the strips; *y*-Axis: percentage of dogs reacting to these bands.

both groups (molecular weights of 42, 45–51 and 82 kDa). However, an antigen of 25 kDa was recognised by the majority of atopic dogs with *Malassezia* dermatitis but was not recognised by most dogs in the other two groups. At this stage, the identity and function of this protein are unknown, as is the significance of the IgG response to this antigen in the atopic dogs. The IgG may act as an opsonin to facilitate phagocytosis of *Malassezia* antigens. This could have a protective function but it could also activate the complement system and exacerbate the underlying inflammation. It has been shown that *Malassezia furfur* is capable of activating both the classical and alternative complement pathways (Belew *et al.*, 1980; Sohnle & Collins-Lech, 1983). It has also been suggested that zymogen in the cell wall of *M. pachydermatis* might activate complement, leading to epidermal damage and inflammation (Mason, 1993). Despite the uncertainty surrounding the role of this antigen, the IgG response seen in the atopic dogs with *Malassezia* overgrowth but not in the normal dogs suggests that it may have some clinical relevance in the disease.

IgG binding components in extracts of *M. pachydermatis* have also been investigated with sera of healthy dogs and non-atopic dogs with *Malassezia* dermatitis (Bond & Lloyd, 1999). Proteins of 132, 66 and 50–54 kDa were recognised by most sera, but affected dogs showed immunoreactivity mainly to proteins of 219, 110, 71 and 42 kDa (Bond & Lloyd, 1999). Comparing the relative positions of bands and molecular weight standards, it may be inferred that some of these results are likely to represent the same bands as those seen in the present study. However, the 25 kDa antigen was not recognised in the non-atopic dogs with *Malassezia* dermatitis, again suggesting a degree of specificity for this response in dogs with atopic dermatitis.

The pattern of IgG binding seen in the atopic dogs without *Malassezia* dermatitis was between that of the normal dogs and atopic dogs with *Malassezia* dermatitis. Most of these dogs also recognised antigens of 28–30, 42, 45–51, 61, 82 and 90 kDa. Owing to the difficulty in precisely resolving the molecular weight of proteins on SDS–PAGE gels, it is possible that the bands detected at 28 and 30 kDa are the same as the 29 kDa antigen seen in the group with *Malassezia* overgrowth. There are some possible explanations for this intermediate pattern. White *et al.* (1996) compared the carriage of *M. pachydermatis* on clinically normal skin of the intradermal skin-test area in atopic dogs and trunkal glabrous skin in healthy dogs. They found that atopic dogs had significantly higher yeast culture scores than healthy dogs. Hence, the atopic dogs without *Malassezia* dermatitis could still have had elevated populations of the yeast without having cytological evidence of an overgrowth. In addition, some of the atopic dogs in the present study may have had *Malassezia* dermatitis in the past, leading to a residual IgG response. Finally, the immune system of atopic dogs may be sensitized to the normal population of the commensal through their frequent scratching behaviour. It has been suggested that disruption of stratum corneum barrier function by scratching may enhance exposure of the skin immune system to yeast allergens (Morris *et al.*, 1998). However, the 25 kDa antigen was only seen in less than 25% of the atopic dogs without *Malassezia* overgrowth, suggesting that an IgG response to this protein is clinically relevant in the disease.

In human beings, *M. furfur* is believed to be significant in the pathogenesis of atopic dermatitis, and numerous IgE binding proteins have been identified in crude extracts using immunoblotting techniques (Johansson & Karlstrom, 1991; Jensen-Jarolim *et al.*, 1992; Zargari *et al.*, 1994; Lintu *et al.*, 1997). Furthermore, type I hypersensitivity responses towards intradermally injected extracts of *M. pachydermatis* have been reported in atopic dogs with *Malassezia* dermatitis (Morris *et al.*, 1998). Hence, to complement the IgG data presented in this paper, and to elucidate further the role of *M. pachydermatis* in atopic dermatitis, studies are currently underway to define the IgE response to *Malassezia* antigens in atopic dogs.

Acknowledgements

The authors would like to thank Miss L. Hume for technical assistance with the *Malassezia* cultures, Mr T. Nuttall for providing the dog serum samples and the laboratory of Professor H. R. P. Miller for technical assistance.

References

Baxter, M. (1976) The association of *Pityrosporum pachydermatis* with the normal external ear canal of dogs and cats. *Journal of Small Animal Practice*, **17**, 231–234.

Belew, P. W., Rosenberg, E. W. & Jennings, B. R. (1980) Activation of the alternative pathway of complement by *Malassezia ovalis* (*Pityrosporum ovale*). *Mycopathologia*, **70**, 187–191.

Bond, R. & Anthony, R. M. (1995) Characterization of markedly lipid-dependent *Malassezia pachydermatis* isolates from healthy dogs. *Journal of Applied Bacteriology*, **78**, 537–542.

Bond, R. & Lloyd, D. H. (1999) Investigation of the humoral immune response to *Malassezia pachydermatis* in healthy dogs and dogs with *Malassezia* dermatitis using western immunoblotting (Abstract). In: *Proceedings of the BSAVA Annual Congress*, Birmingham, UK, p. 241.

Bond, R. & Sant, R. E. (1993) The recovery of *Malassezia pachydermatis* from canine skin. *Veterinary Dermatology Newsletter*, **15**, 25–27.

Bond, R., Collin, N. S. & Lloyd, D. H. (1994) Use of contact plates for the quantitative culture of *Malassezia pachydermatis* from canine skin. *Journal of Small Animal Practice*, **35**, 68–72.

Bond, R., Saijonmaa-Koulumies, L. E. & Lloyd, D. H. (1995) Population sizes and frequency of *Malassezia pachydermatis* at skin and mucosal sites on healthy dogs. *Journal of Small Animal Practice*, **36**, 147–150.

Bond, R., Elwood, C. M., Littler, R. M., Pinter, L. & Lloyd, D. H. (1998) Humoral and cell-mediated responses to *Malassezia pachydermatis* in healthy dogs and dogs with *Malassezia* dermatitis. *Veterinary Record*, **143**, 381–384.

Charach, M. (1997) *Malassezia* dermatitis. *Canadian Veterinary Journal*, **38**, 311–314.

Dufait, R. (1983) *Pityrosporum canis* as a cause of canine chronic dermatitis. *Veterinary Medicine/Small Animal Clinician*, **78**, 1055–1057.

Gedek, B., Brutzel, K., Netzer, F., Rocken, H., Unger, H. & Symoens, J. (1979) The role of *Pityrosporum pachydermatis* in otitis externa of dogs: evaluation of a treatment with miconazole. *Veterinary Record*, **104**, 138–140.

Jensen-Jarolim, E., Poulsen, L. K., With, H., Kieffer, M., Ottevanger, V. & Stahl, S. P. (1992) Atopic dermatitis of the face, scalp, and neck: type I reaction to the yeast *Pityrosporum ovale*? *Journal of Allergy and Clinical Immunology*, **89**, 44–51.

Johansson, S. & Karlstrom, K. (1991) IgE-binding components in *Pityrosporum orbiculare* identified by an immunoblotting technique. *Acta Dermato-Venereologica*, **71**, 11–16.

Kennis, R. A., Rosser, E. J. J., Olivier, N. B. & Walker, R. W. (1996) Quantity and distribution of *Malassezia* organisms on the skin of clinically normal dogs. *Journal of the American Veterinary Medical Association*, **208**, 1048–1051.

Laemmli, U. K. (1970) Cleavage of structural proteins during the assembly of the head of bacteriophage T_4. *Nature*, **227**, 680–685.

Larsson, C. E., Larsson, M. H. M. A., Amaral, R. C., Gandra, C. R. P. & Hagiwara, M. K. (1988) Dermatitis in dogs caused by *Malassezia (Pityrosporum) pachydermatis*. *Ars Veterinaria*, **4**, 63–68.

LeGendre, N., Mansfield, M., Weiss, A. & Matsudaira, P. (1993) Purification of proteins and peptides by SDS–PAGE. In: *A Practical Guide to Protein and Peptide Purification for Microsequencing*, 2nd edn (Ed. P. Matsudaira), pp. 71–85. Academic Press, San Diego, CA.

Lintu, P., Savolainen, J. & Kalimo, K. (1997) IgE antibodies to protein and mannan antigens of *Pityrosporum ovale* in atopic dermatitis patients. *Clinical and Experimental Allergy*, **27**, 87–95.

Mason, K. V. (1992) *Malassezia* dermatitis and otitis. In: *Current Veterinary Therapy: Small Animal Practice* (Eds R. W. Kirk & J. D. Bonagura), pp. 544–546. W. B. Saunders, Philadelphia, PA.

Mason, K. V. (1993) Cutaneous *Malassezia*. In: *Current Veterinary Dermatology* (Eds C. E. Griffin, K. W. Kwochka, & J. M. MacDonald), pp. 44–48. Mosby Year Book, St Louis, MO.

Mason, K. V. & Evans, E. G. (1991) Dermatitis associated with *Malassezia pachydermatis* in eleven dogs. *Journal of the American Animal Hospital Association*, **27**, 13–20.

Morris, D. O. (1999) *Malassezia* dermatitis and otitis. *Veterinary Clinics of North America: Small Animal Practice*, **29**, 1303–1310.

Morris, D. O., Olivier, N. B. & Rosser, E. J. (1998) Type-1 hypersensitivity reactions to *Malassezia pachydermatis* extracts in atopic dogs. *American Journal of Veterinary Research*, **59**, 836–841.

Nuttall, T. J. (1997) Serum specific IgG levels to cutaneous *Malassezia* in normal and atopic dogs (Abstract). In: *Proceedings of 14th Annual Congress of the ESVD-ECVD*, Pisa, Italy, p. 166.

Nuttall, T. J. (1998) *Malassezia* specific IgE levels in normal and atopic dogs (Abstract). In: *Proceedings of 15th Annual Congress of the ESVD-ECVD*, Maastricht, The Netherlands, p. 155.

Onishi, Y., Kuroda, M., Yasueda, H., Saito, A., Sono-Koyama, E., Tunasawa, S. *et al.* (1999) Two-dimensional electrophoresis of *Malassezia* allergens for atopic dermatitis and isolation of Mal f 4 homologs with mitochondrial malate dehydrogenase. *European Journal of Biochemistry*, **261**, 148–154.

Scott, D. W. & Miller, W. H. (1989) Epidermal dysplasia and *Malassezia pachydermatis* infection in West Highland white terriers. *Veterinary Dermatology*, **1**, 25–35.

Scott, D. W., Miller, W. H. & Griffin, C. E. (2001) Canine atopic disease. In: *Muller & Kirk's Small Animal Dermatology*, 6th edn, pp. 574–601. W. B. Saunders, Philadelphia, PA.

Senczek, D., Siesenop, U. & Bohm, K. H. (1999) Characterization of *Malassezia* species by means of phenotypic characteristics and detection of electrophoretic karyotypes by pulsed-field gel electrophoresis (PFGE). *Mycoses*, **42**, 409–414.

Sohnle, P. G. & Collins-Lech, C. (1983) Activation of complement by *Pityrosporum orbiculare*. *Journal of Investigative Dermatology*, **80**, 93–97.

White, S. D., Bourdeau, P., Blumstein, P., Ibish, C., Scott, K. V., Salman, M. D. & Chapman, P. L. (1996) Comparison via cytology and culture of carriage of *Malassezia pachydermatis* in atopic and healthy dogs. In: *Advances in Veterinary Dermatology*, Vol. 3 (Eds K. W. Kwochka, T. Willemse & C. V. Tscharner), pp. 291–298. Butterworth Heinemann, Oxford.

Zargari, A., Harfast, B., Johansson, S., Johansson, S. G. & Scheynius, A. (1994) Identification of allergen components of the opportunistic yeast *Pityrosporum orbiculare* by monoclonal antibodies. *Allergy*, **49**, 50–56.

Part 5

Workshop reports

5.1

Antibiotic use in chronic otitis externa

Lynette K. Cole[1] (Chairperson) and Marcia Schwassmann[2] (Secretary)

[1] The Ohio State University, Columbus, Ohio, USA
[2] Veterinary Dermatology Center, Winter Park, Florida, USA

Lynette Cole *USA* I would like to thank everyone for attending this workshop and particularly those colleagues I have invited to make specific contributions: Drs Carlotti, Foster, Noxon and Nuttall. I would also like to thank Pfizer for sponsoring this workshop.

I want to give you an overview of the topics we want to cover. Questions we will address include: what is the definition of chronic otitis, what is our work-up protocol for these cases, how do we treat infected ears and what specific treatments do we use for *Pseudomonas aeruginosa*? We will also discuss otitis media, fluoroquinolone usage in the treatment of otitis, any adjunctive therapies people are using, and if time permits, treatment of concurrent yeast infections. I thought I would start by asking the panel how they define chronic otitis externa.

Tim Nuttall *UK* It sounds easy to define chronic otitis externa, but in my experience it actually is not. There is certainly a gray area with respect to what is chronic otitis externa and what is recurrent, acute otitis externa. From a clinical point of view, anything that has chronic pathological changes I automatically define as chronic otitis externa, despite the fact that those changes can arise fairly rapidly. Beyond that, any dog that has had recurrent bouts of otitis externa for more than 3–4 months I would define as chronic. Any dog that has had 3 weeks of treatment but has not resolved, I also consider chronic.

Lynette Cole I would agree with those points. Does anyone else on the panel have anything to add?

Jim Noxon *USA* Along with the time frame mentioned, I would add extension of the disease beyond one season. I live in a temperate climate and we have very distinct seasons.

Steve Melman *USA* Can you differentiate between chronic and recurrent?

Lynette Cole I consider chronic and recurrent cases in the same category, different from the acute case.

Steve Melman So a chronic otitis case could be one that did not necessarily extend from one season to the next, but recurred the following year in the same season?

Lynette Cole Definitely. The next question I want to ask is, what is included in the work-up of these dogs? What are our basic initial diagnostic procedures for otitis?

Aiden Foster *UK* Most of my cases with otitis will undergo routine otoscopy. We use the MedRx® video endoscope system with the dog conscious. We normally do some cytology. In some cases where there is no exudate, the returns are low. If cytology is positive for rods, we definitely culture. If cytology reveals cocci, then we might do culture and sensitivity. Those samples will be collected with the dog conscious, under sedation, or under general anesthesia depending upon animal and owner compliance. The baseline would be at least cytology, and possibly culture and sensitivity.

Lynette Cole I think that a thorough otic examination is very important. If you have a dog with a chronic ear infection, this may require sedation. Or you may have to send the dog home with topical or systemic medication to decrease the inflammation and ulceration, and then look in the ear later. In my opinion, cytology is one of the most underused diagnostic techniques that we have available. You or your technician can take and read the slides in less than 10 min. I see many people who do a culture before they do cytology or even look in the ear.

Jim Noxon I think cytology should be done on every ear every time a case comes in, not just at the first visit. It is part of the database. Also remember to do both ears.

Lynette Cole How many people in the audience routinely do cytology? [Most audience members indicated that they do cytology.] You might see yeasts on cytology that your laboratory may not even culture for.

Marcy Murphy *USA* I do an ear clinic at North Carolina State University 1–2 days a week. The other thing I would like to emphasize about cytology is that it can differentiate an ongoing problem from a recurring problem. I see many cases where we are not sure if the problem ever resolved because repeat cytology was not done. The ears will usually look better after treatment because most ear medications contain a steroid, but without cytology you do not know if the infection has resolved. That is why it is important to repeat cytology even if the ear appears to be normal. I will also see dogs being treated with antibiotics whose infections are not clearing because they actually have a yeast infection.

Kevin Shanley *USA* This is a follow-up to what Marcy was saying. It is amazing how good an ear can look on otoscopic examination and there can still be large numbers of *Malassezia* present, even without any wax, erythema or hypertrophy.

Didier Carlotti *France* I think it is important to have a standard procedure for each case. In my clinic, we always follow the same procedure. If we have an erythematous otitis externa, i.e. an otitis externa which may be pruritic with thick ceruminous exudate, we will first do a parasitological examination to look for mites. Then we will do the cytology. In such a case we will probably not do culture and sensitivity testing. Then we will do the flushing. In contrast, if we have a suppurative otitis externa the first thing we will do is sample for culture and sensitivity testing. Then we will do the cytology. If the slide shows many rods, then the sample for culturing will be used. In contrast, if the cytology shows cocci and *Malassezia*, we may not use the sample for culture. Then we will do the flushing.

Lynette Cole That is a good point. If you have standard procedures, you are less likely to miss something.

John Angus *USA* I was wondering if the panel could comment on the presence or absence of leukocytes on cytology?

Didier Carlotti I think that when you have pus, it is extremely likely your cytology will show many degenerate neutrophils. In contrast, when I have cocci and *Malassezia* and thick cerumen, neutrophils are rare.

Jim Noxon I personally think it is a very important thing to look at. I base a lot of therapy on whether there are leukocytes present or just free bacteria and yeast. If there are leukocytes present, then I believe systemic antimicrobial therapy is indicated. I base that decision on some biopsy results from ears that showed folliculitis in many cases. We don't treat folliculitis in skin elsewhere on the body with only topical therapy and I feel we should treat ears in the same way.

Tim Nuttall It is also important to be able to differentiate a mature, degenerate neutrophil from a mature, non-degenerate neutrophil. The degenerate neutrophils are very commonly associated with a severe infection, and in that case I would treat with systemic antibiotics. I would possibly also culture, depending on the results of cytology. The most common cause I find for non-degenerate neutrophils is not infection but, rather, overly aggressive flushing and cleaning. Possibly the second most common reason for non-degenerate neutrophils is a drug reaction to one of the components of a topical cleaner or medication.

Steve Melman How do you recommend we do cytology?

Lynette Cole That is a good question. Do you [panel members] use a Gram's stain, Diff-Quik®, or something different?

Didier Carlotti I mainly use Diff-Quik.

Jim Noxon I also use Diff-Quik.

Lynette Cole I heat-fix slides and I use Diff-Quik. I don't use Gram's stain because it is too messy and I always forget how to do it. Do you (members of the panel) heat-fix slides for cytology?

Jim Noxon I heat-fix anything that is greasy. If it's not greasy, I don't heat-fix it.

Steve Melman I think if you don't heat-fix when you are looking for bacteria you are going to lose a lot of yeast. Also, if you are looking for polymorphonuclear leukocytes, are you also looking for epidermal cells?

Lynette Cole When I stain a slide, I look for cellular debris, epidermal cells and inflammatory cells.

Helen Power *USA* We did two sets of slides in parallel for 2 months and heat-fixing did not seem to make any difference.

Marcy Murphy The microbiologist at North Carolina State University strongly recommends heat-fixing. My impression is I see more yeast when I heat-fix my slides.

Lynette Cole I think the important take-home message is both Diff-Quik and Gram's stain are equally as effective. It is important to look for specific organisms, leukocytes and epithelial cells. The question of heat-fixing remains undecided.

Ally Blesham *USA* Do you include the fee for cytology in your examination or do you charge separately?

[**Tim Nuttall, Aiden Foster** and **Jim Noxon** all said they charged separately.]

Didier Carlotti It is included in my examination fee.

Lynette Cole I think that is at your discretion. I charge separately.

The next topic is one that I think is very important, and that is diagnostics for the primary problem. We often forget that there is a primary triggering problem and these infections are only perpetuating factors. However, since this workshop deals with antibiotic treatment, we will save this topic for later. If time allows we will discuss with the panel what they do for evaluating primary problems.

Before we begin discussing flushing techniques I would like to ask the panel whether they are doing specific diagnostics for otitis media.

Didier Carlotti Sometimes I am concerned about otitis media and in that case I would recommend a computed tomography (CT) scan or magnetic resonance imaging (MRI). I do not have these facilities in our dermatology clinic so I refer these cases.

Jim Noxon I will frequently radiograph dogs when they are under anesthesia for flushing. We do not have CT or MRI facilities in-house and it takes about one and a half months to get them scheduled. I feel they are very useful if the client can afford them.

Lynette Cole If an animal is going to have an ear flush, is it something you will try to encourage?

Jim Noxon As you showed earlier today, the sensitivity of radiography is not very good. I like to get radiographs if possible, but if finances were limited, I would rather put that money towards therapy.

Aiden Foster If I think a case is going to have an ear flush and is going to be anesthetized, I will try to get radiographs. I feel that radiography provides potentially useful diagnostic information. Our surgeons frequently get cases of ear disease referred to them and they will often ask for consultations from us. Their standard work-up includes radiography. It gives them more information when they are planning for surgery. I think if you are going to anesthetize an animal, for the cost of a radiograph, it is worth doing.

Lynette Cole Do you do one view or multiple views?

Aiden Foster We routinely do ventrodorsal and intraoral views.

Tim Nuttall Virtually all our chronic ear cases will be anesthetized for an ear flush, and while they are under anesthesia we will radiograph them. I agree that the sensitivity of radiography is poor, but it can often be helpful when making a decision about whether to treat an animal medically or send it directly for surgery. An owner is not going to thank you for running through several hundred dollars of medical therapy that does not work, when that dog may have been better off going straight for surgery, and then coming back to you to work up its primary problem.

Lynette Cole We have CT now in addition to radiographs and I cannot tell you yet if I think the sensitivity is better. If I suspect otitis media I treat for it, even if I don't find radiographic evidence. If I see lysis or sclerosis of the tympanic bulla on radiography, I will tell the client we will try medical management, but the bulla looks bad and we may be looking at surgery. Radiographs do add to the bill, but I think if you explain these things to the owner ahead of time, they will understand the reasons for doing them. These radiographs are not that hard to position.

Marcy Murphy About 4 or 5 years ago we did a study at North Carolina State University comparing CT to radiography. There were 20 dogs in the study, and 19 out of 20 were cocker spaniels. These were dogs that were scheduled for surgery so these were very chronic ears. Fifteen out of 20 ears were positive for otitis media on radiographs, but 19 out of 20 ears were positive for otitis media on CT scan. The conclusion was that CT was more sensitive than radiography for detecting otitis media.

Lynette Cole The difference was not statistically significant in that study.

Marcy Murphy No it was not, but my impression is that CT is more sensitive. We charge $100 for radiographs and $125 for CT so we always do CT. We can often do a good evaluation of the external ear canal on CT scan and see if there are chronic changes such as mineralization that would indicate the case is going to be very difficult to manage.

Lynette Cole Let's move on to ear flushing. When you do ear flushing, do you use sedation or general anesthesia, or does it depend on what you anticipate finding?

Tim Nuttall I always anesthetize. I have found that even under heavy sedation, dogs will still shake their heads once you start flushing. If you use deeper sedation, it is actually safer to anesthetize them. The other reason to anesthetize them is you have control of the airway. If the eardrum is ruptured, you can push fluid straight through the eustachian tube and it can be aspirated quite easily.

Lynette Cole I also use general anesthesia for ear flushing. I think it is important for me to do a very good job of cleaning and evaluating the tympanic membrane and middle ear. Do you [the audience] use general anesthesia or sedation for ear flushing? [Most members of the audience indicated that they do ear flushing and most use general anesthesia. A few use sedation only.]

Didier Carlotti So far we have been talking about flushing for chronic suppurative otitis externa. I do some flushing regularly for mild otitis externa in dogs with atopy, for example. This would be part of my on-site treatment and would be done with or without sedation.

Aiden Foster Certainly, if you have atopic dogs you are sedating for intradermal skin testing and they have otitis externa, you can clean the ear while they are under sedation.

Lynette Cole Yes, although I still worry about them moving, and if the tympanic membrane is not intact, flushing something down the airway. So exactly how do you flush ears? Do you use any special cleaners?

Tim Nuttall We use a urinary catheter or a feeding tube and attach that to a three-way valve. We use a 10–20 ml syringe for suction, depending on the type of dog. We then attach another syringe filled with sterile saline to the valve. The three-way valve allows you to flush, aspirate and take the syringe off to discard the aspirated material without having to keep removing and replacing the catheter. This minimizes trauma to the ear canal.

Aiden Foster We use a surgical suction technique. We place the otoscope in the ear canal and use long catheters to flush a saline and povidone iodine solution. We do the initial cleaning with a proprietary ear cleaner to get down to the eardrum. When we go further, that is when we use the saline and povidone iodine mixture. I think Tim's comment about connecting and disconnecting is good, because it is incredibly time consuming to effectively do an ear flush.

Lynette Cole How much time do you spend on an ear?

Aiden Foster If the otitis is bilateral, you can sometimes spend nearly an hour. It is a very arduous process and the owner needs to be aware it is going to take quite some time. Surgical suction does make it a fairly rapid process because we can pump considerable quantities of fluid into the ear canal.

Lynette Cole Do you have a video endoscope? Are you doing any flushing through that?

Aiden Foster We tend not to flush through the video endoscope but we do use it to show students and owners what we are doing, and to record images. When the dog comes back for a recheck, we have pictures to compare to.

Didier Carlotti I do something quite similar. I use bulbs from time to time. I think that the pressure of the bulb is appropriate, particularly in large dogs. But I use diluted ear cleanser (Epi-Otic®) and I mix it with lukewarm water.

John Angus Dr Cole, you mentioned in your talk earlier today that you soak the canal in a ceruminolytic prior to flushing. Could you elaborate on that, and do you have any concerns if you do not know if the tympanum is intact?

Lynette Cole That is a good question, because if you read labels, most ceruminolytics are ototoxic. When I first started my residency I would not put anything potentially ototoxic in an ear, and I could not get ears clean. Sterile saline is safe, but not very effective for removing thick, ceruminous exudate or pus. I use

Pan-Otic®. It contains dioctyl sodium succinate (DSS) that is potentially ototoxic, but once I get the ear clean, if the tympanic membrane is not intact, I flush until all the cleanser is rinsed out. Clinically I have never had a problem; however, I don't routinely do bone evoked auditory responses. My concern is if I only partially clean the ear and leave it filled with debris, I really have not done that patient a service.

John Angus How long do you leave the ceruminolytic in before you flush it out?

Lynette Cole For a ceruminous exudate, I leave it for 10 min. For a purulent exudate 5 min is usually enough. I massage the ear canal while it is soaking. I use a flushing technique very similar to that of the panel members. I use a bulb syringe first, and then I use a polypropylene urinary catheter. These are more rigid than the feeding tubes. I feel I can get the urinary catheters down the ear better. I feed the tube through the otoscope so I can visualize what I am doing. This prevents me from inadvertently doing a myringotomy too early.

Tom Manning *USA* I would like to remind everyone to protect dogs' eyes when doing ear flushing (especially brachycephalic breeds). Some *Pseudomonas* organisms can rupture a cornea in 24 h.

Lynette Cole That is a good point.

Jim Noxon now has a presentation on some other flushing techniques.

Jim Noxon What I would like to comment on today are some techniques for ear cleaning that have simplified and speeded up the process for me. We are using human pediatric gastric sump tubes. These are essentially a tube within a tube. The larger tube is hooked up to suction and a 60 ml syringe is attached to the other tube for flushing with saline. I use DSS with it after I see if the tympanic membrane is intact. We hook the suction to the larger tube so the larger chunks of debris can pass through the tube. I would prefer the flushing tube to be about half the size it is to get a stronger fluid stream. When we pass this tube we are doing pulsatile flushing with the syringe, at the same time that the suction is running. You need to hold the connection between the syringe and the tube otherwise it can come apart. We have made our own version of this type of tube by gluing together two red rubber feeding tubes and it sort of works. However, they do tend to come apart. There is an advantage to this figure-of-eight configuration in that it prevents you from inadvertently forming a seal. With a circular tube, if you use a large tube attached to constant suction, you can create a sealed chamber and inadvertently aspirate an eardrum. With the figure-of-eight configuration, there is always a channel along the side for air to pass through. Actually, both times I have damaged an eardrum were when I tried to do this through a video endoscope. The pediatric gastric tubes can be hard to find, but they work nicely. The tubes do come in different diameters; however, they are too large for most cats with chronic ear problems. For cats, we make our own tubes with the smaller diameter red rubber feeding tubes.

Aiden Foster Do you sterilize them and reuse them?

Jim Noxon Yes, we gas-sterilize them a few times, then discard them.

Aiden Foster Are they expensive?

Jim Noxon Yes, but the cost is not too high if you sterilize them and reuse them.

Lynette Cole I would like next to talk about treatment of otitis externa. If time allows we will talk about specific treatment for otitis media. Tim, how do you initially start treating once you have cleaned the ear?

Tim Nuttall Treatment is based on cytology and culture in the sense that I try to read those together. The cytology will sometimes tell me which is the more important organism, particularly if I wind up with a mixed culture. If cytology shows coccoid bacteria and they look like *Staphylococci*, it is usually easy to guess what the sensitivity pattern will be. In that case I don't need to do culture and sensitivity and will choose an antibiotic empirically. The topical products I tend to prefer are the fucidin-containing products. I don't think you have these in the USA. Fucidin is a very good anti-staphylococcal antibiotic and is very safe. Gentamycin is the other topical I tend to use.

I use systemic antibiotics if there is any chronic thickening of the ear canal. That is no longer a surface infection, that is a pyoderma. Pyoderma anywhere else on the body you would treat with systemic antibiotics and the ear is no different. I usually use a cephalosporin or clavulanic acid-potentiated amoxycillin. A trimethoprim–sulfonamide combination would be acceptable as a first-line antibiotic, but I do not tend to use it if the ear has received antibiotic therapy beforehand. For *Malassezia*, I tend to use miconazole (present in Surolan®) or nystatin (present in the fucidin preparation). If it is a chronic infection and there is thickening of the ear canal, it is doubtful if you are going to be able to distribute a topical product adequately throughout the length of the ear canal. Certainly, if there is middle ear involvement, it is doubtful that an owner applying topical medication will get it into the bulla, so I tend to use systemic therapy for that. I use ketoconazole as my routine. I have used itraconazole in a few cases, but that drug is quite a bit more expensive.

Aiden Foster I think the prospect of using topical therapy raises the issue of whether you can get the topical medication down the ear canal, especially if any hyperplastic change is present. Systemic glucocorticoid therapy may be needed to reduce the hyperplasia, and reduction of hyperplasia will significantly influence the success of medical therapy. The ability to reduce hyperplastic changes may also affect the decision to go to surgery. The short-term use of glucocorticoids in the face of infection may seem strange, but it can be a valuable aid in turning some of these cases around.

Lynette Cole This is a good time to talk about glucocorticoid use in otitis. Most topical products available in the USA contain glucocorticoids. We make extralabel preparations, and sometimes we put steroids in these also. Many ears with serious infection will need glucocorticoid therapy in addition to antibiotics to open up the ear canals. This brings up another point. I do not attempt to flush an ear canal that is rolled up like a carpet. I open that ear canal first, and that may require aggressive topical and possibly systemic glucocorticoid therapy.

Aiden Foster will now give a presentation on sensitivity testing for *Pseudomonas* comparing Kirby–Bauer (KB) disk diffusion versus minimum inhibitory concentration (MIC). From here on we will discuss primarily treatments for *Pseudomonas*. Most of us do a fairly good job treating infections with cocci. The *Pseudomonas* infections seem to be the more difficult ones to deal with.

Aiden Foster In preparation for this workshop I looked at some of the data we had with respect to *Pseudomonas* infections. These data do not give any clear-cut answers, but hopefully will spark some good discussion. In our laboratory we have access to KB disk diffusion sensitivity testing. We set up a system whereby we could look at MIC data using another laboratory. Two populations of dogs were used for the collection of swabs for bacterial culture and sensitivity testing. Group 1 consisted of samples collected from the deep horizontal ear canal from cases referred for investigation of severe otitis externa and/or media. The second group consisted of samples mailed in from veterinarians in practice from dogs with presumed ear disease. Sensitivity testing was carried out using agar gel disk diffusion and any *Pseudomonas* isolates were then submitted to a second laboratory for MIC estimation. Antibacterial sensitivity testing of *Pseudomonas* isolates was carried out using a wide variety of antibacterial agents including amoxycillin, amoxycillin with clavulanic acid, cephalexin, chloramphenicol, enrofloxacin, framycetin, gentamycin, neomycin, nitrofurantoin, oxytetracycline, polymyxin B, streptomycin, sulfamethoxazole and trimethoprim-sulfonamide combination. Many of these antibiotics are totally irrelevant for *Pseudomonas* because they simply don't work. The two groups of antibiotics that are particularly important are the fluoroquinolones and the aminoglycosides. They form the mainstay of therapy for *Pseudomonas* spp. whether given topically or systemically.

There was no resistance of *Pseudomonas* isolates in either group of dogs to polymyxin B. The rates of resistance to aminoglycosides and enrofloxacin in both groups of dogs were similar to what has been previously reported in the literature. The rate of enrofloxacin resistance is particularly disturbing and the likelihood is that these isolates will be equally resistant to ciprofloxacin or marbofloxacin.

Dawn Boothe *USA* We have done similar studies looking at a number of tissues, not just ears, and we have found the same proportion of resistance in *Pseudomonas*. My question to you is, are you using the newer breakpoint MIC of 4 μg/ml or the old one of 2 μg/ml?

Aiden Foster I believe we used the 2 μg/ml.

Dawn Boothe You might want to look at your data with the new number and see if it changes. It's still scary.

Aiden Foster Table 5.1.1 shows the KB versus MIC data for our *Pseudomonas* isolates ($n = 18$). For enrofloxacin, paired disk diffusion and broth microdilution MIC patterns of *Pseudomonas aeruginosa* were compared. Six of 18 (33.3%) *P. aeruginosa* isolates

Table 5.1.1. Minimum inhibitory concentration (MIC)/Kirby–Bauer (KB) sensitivity patterns of *Pseudomonas* isolates from 18 dogs with severe otitis

Antibiotic	% Sensitive MIC/KB	% Intermediate MIC/KB	% Resistant MIC/KB
Gentamycin	55/94	22/0	22/5
Neomycin	39/78	27/0	33/22
Enrofloxacin	11/61	33/11	55/27

were identical on disk diffusion and broth microdilution susceptibility testing. Of the 11 *P. aeruginosa* isolates susceptible on disk diffusion susceptibility testing, five (45.5%) were intermediate and four (36.4%) were resistant on broth microdilution susceptibility testing. Of the two *P. aeruginosa* isolates intermediate on disk diffusion susceptibility testing, all were resistant on broth microdilution susceptibility testing. My concern is the considerable discrepancy between the values for the two methods. The MIC data showed much more resistance than the KB data. I don't think I have seen *Pseudomonas* resistant to polymyxin B.

Marcy Murphy I have seen it.

Aiden Foster Table 5.1.2 shows the KB sensitivity results for *Pseudomonas* isolates from dogs with severe otitis submitted from outside clinics.

In most of the cases in group 1, the dogs made a good response to aggressive medical therapy for their ear infection including cleaning with Epi-Otic®, medicating the ear canal topically with an ear preparation containing polymyxin B, enrofloxacin 10–20 mg/kg once daily per os (p.o.), and if necessary, 1–2 mg/kg prednisolone to reduce ear canal hyperplasia. The decision to use high-dose enrofloxacin was based on the results of agar disk diffusion testing rather than MIC testing. Since the MIC is proported to be the more appropriate test, the question arises from the above results as to whether the MIC test should be the standard test employed before committing to fluoroquinolone use. Would the results of either method of sensitivity testing for *Pseudomonas* be important if one used topical fluoroquinolone solutions rather than parenteral therapy? When we use enrofloxacin topically we are reaching concentrations in the ear canal that are much higher than what is used in both KB and MIC testing.

In most of the cases, the infections responded to aggressive medical therapy, but it is not known whether the response was due to the high dosages of

Table 5.1.2. Kirby–Bauer sensitivity results for *Pseudomonas* isolates from dogs with severe otitis submitted from outside clinics

Antibiotic	% Sensitive	% Intermediate	% Resistant
Gentamycin	83	5	11
Neomycin	72	5	22
Enrofloxacin	61	11	28

enrofloxacin (10–20 mg/kg p.o. once daily), or the topical polymyxin B, or a combination. Therefore, future studies are needed to evaluate oral enrofloxacin as the sole therapy for treatment based on the results of both agar broth microdilution and MIC for *Pseudomonas* isolates from the ear canal to determine the clinical significance of the discrepancies between susceptibility testing for enrofloxacin. The bottom line is that we don't understand ear disease very well.

Marcia Schwassmann *USA* You mentioned that if a *Pseudomonas* isolate was sensitive to enrofloxacin you felt it would be sensitive to marbofloxacin or orbifloxacin.

Aiden Foster As far as I understand it, sensitivity testing to enrofloxacin can be used as a guide to sensitivity to marbofloxacin and the other fluoroquinolones.

Marcia Schwassmann On the panel of antibiotics I get, we get sensitivity to ciprofloxacin, enrofloxacin and orbifloxacin. The results are usually the same for all these, but sometimes the results are different, and I don't know what to make of that.

Jim Noxon We get the same sort of panel. It seems to me that once the bacteria develop resistance to one of the fluoroquinolones, the others follow quickly. If the panel says sensitive to one of the fluoroquinolones and we switch antibiotics, it seems clinically it doesn't work as well as we would like.

Dawn Boothe In the study we are doing, we looked at 300 different organisms and compared the fluoroquinolones marbofloxacin, difloxacin, orbifloxacin, enrofloxacin and ciprofloxacin. Usually if an organism was sensitive on MIC testing to one, it was sensitive to all of them. A very small percentage of organisms were sensitive to one fluoroquinolone, but resistant to others. Usually if an organism was sensitive to enrofloxacin, it was sensitive to marbofloxacin. Difloxacin and orbifloxacin were a little different. The other point I will make about orbifloxacin is that their KB data are not NCCLS tested, so be a little careful with that. This was true 4 months ago but I am not sure if it has changed.

Lynette Cole There is no KB disk for marbofloxacin in the USA yet. David Lloyd did a study in which he compared the MIC data for enrofloxacin versus marbofloxacin. At the time he did the study, enrofloxacin had been available for 10 years, I think, and marbofloxacin had been available for 3 years. The MIC 100 for skin and ears for enrofloxacin was 8 μg/ml, and it was much lower for marbofloxacin (0.63 μg/ml for skin and 1.25 μg/ml for ears). The suggestion was the difference was due to the length of time enrofloxacin had been available compared to marbofloxacin.

I try to save the fluoroquinolones for my horrible ears and not use them for simple staphylococcal infections. I feel if we use these drugs for everything, they will not be effective when we need them for severe infections, because of the resistance that has developed. How and when does the panel use fluoroquinolones?

Jim Noxon I tend to use fluoroquinolones mostly for difficult ear cases, when *Pseudomonas* is involved, or occasionally when there is a mixed population of bacteria. I sometimes use fluoroquinolones for deep pyodermas.

Didier Carlotti I use fluoroquinolones when there is no other option.

Aiden Foster I use fluoroquinolones mainly for ear disease. I also use them for the deep pyoderma case where I feel the penetration properties of the fluoroquinolones would be useful.

Tim Nuttall I do the same. I use fluoroquinolones when I have to, and not otherwise. I don't think that the convenience of once-a-day dosing is sufficient reason for using them. Unfortunately, I see practitioners using fluoroquinolones to treat cat-bite abscesses simply because they feel they get better owner compliance with once-a-day dosing. I use them once a day, but I frequently increase the dose above the manufacturer's recommended dose.

John Angus Can you elaborate on once-a-day dosing versus twice-a-day? Is the situation the same for all the fluoroquinolones?

Dawn Boothe There are a number of studies that support once-a-day dosing for the fluoroquinolones. They are concentration-dependent drugs. I would like to remind everyone that neither KB nor MIC testing is the answer. It may be that in the end KB versus MIC doesn't ultimately make a difference. I tend to use MICs more as a guideline for dosage. I don't care if you use the fluoroquinolones once a day or twice a day, but when you use them, make sure you use the higher dose.

Lynette Cole I agree. Because these drugs are concentration dependent, you need to get the high initial dose. It is not important that the concentration of the drug remains above the MIC for the whole 24 h period. It is important to get the drug concentration as high above the MIC as you can. You definitely don't want to use anything lower than the recommended dose. If I have a *Pseudomonas* that shows intermediate susceptibility to enrofloxacin, I will still use the drug, but I will use the higher dose of 20 mg/kg. With marbofloxacin, we do not have the KB disks yet but I have had good success using that drug at the high end of the recommended dose range (5.5 mg/kg). Both of these drugs are very expensive.

Didier will now present some data using marbofloxacin to treat *Pseudomonas* otitis.

Didier Carlotti This is a study I have already presented in Europe. It was done in cooperation with Vetoquinol, the European laboratory that sells marbofloxacin. We did two studies. The first study was done by our colleagues at Vetoquinol (V. Guiral and E. Thomas) and I and three other dermatological specialist practitioners (E. Guaguère, H.-J. Koch and J. Fontaine) did a second study. The *in vitro* study used two *Pseudomonas* isolates from canine otitis. They were both susceptible to marbofloxacin. We had two strains. One was more susceptible to marbofloxacin with an MIC of 0.25 μg/ml, and one was less susceptible with an MIC of 1 μg/ml. They tested six marbofloxacin concentrations, 0.5, 1, 2, 4, 8 and 16 times the MIC, and they counted colonies at 1, 2, 4, 6 and 24 h after exposure. The results showed concentration-dependent bactericidal activity. They obtained complete bacterial eradication at eight times the MIC at 4 h postexposure for the first strain (MIC 0.25 μg/ml), and at four times the MIC at 2 h postexposure for the other strain (MIC 1 μg/ml). They therefore concluded that a 5 mg/kg per day dose was appropriate for *Pseudomonas aeruginosa* infections. This might apply to pyodermas as well as to otitis externa in the dog.

We did a field trial in order to answer the question 'is systemic antibiotic therapy useful in chronic, suppurative otitis externa?' We enrolled 58 dogs from 11 practices in France, Belgium and Germany. The inclusion criteria were simple: suppurative otitis externa and pain. The exclusion criteria were non-suppurative otitis externa, parasitic otitis externa, otitis externa due to autoimmune skin diseases and the presence of foreign bodies or tumors. Treatment with any medication during the past 7 days, treatment with short-acting glucocorticoids during the past 14 days, and treatment with long-acting glucocorticoids during the previous 60 days were prohibited. We did parasitological examination of ear exudate, cytological examination and culture and sensitivity testing. We treated these animals with marbofloxacin at 5 mg/kg per day. Dogs were treated for 21 days and if the animal was not cured at day 21, treatment was extended to 42 days. We cleaned the external ear canal with saline and nothing else. No topical antibiotic therapy was allowed during the study. This is perhaps why we could not recruit more cases. We monitored the quantity of pus, the amount of pain and the degree of ulceration at days 0, 7, 21 and 35 if we had a cure at day 21. We monitored the animal at days 0, 7, 21, 42 and 56 if the dog was not cured at day 21.

Pseudomonas aeruginosa was cultured from slightly less than half of the cases. Sometimes no bacteria were cultured and sometimes Gram-positive cocci or Enterobacteriaceae were cultured. This may be due to the fact that all samples were sent to a central laboratory and perhaps the duration of transport affected bacterial viability. We had a total cure in 28% of the animals, a clear improvement in about 6% of the animals and a partial improvement in 37% of the animals. We had failure in 30% of the cases. The quantity of pus in the external ear canals decreased in most animals. Pain and ulceration also decreased in most cases. Some dogs had no ulceration at the start of the study since this was not obligatory for inclusion. We concluded that marbofloxacin could be used at a dose of 5 mg/kg once a day for *P. aeruginosa* otitis externa.

With no topical antibacterial treatment, we had 28% cure and 43% clear to partial improvement. It remains to be seen whether we can improve results if we combine this systemic antibacterial therapy with topical treatment.

Lynette Cole Now we go to the flip side of the coin. Tim Nuttall will present some results from a study using very aggressive topical and parenteral therapy.

Tim Nuttall This is some work I first presented several years ago now, but it is a protocol we have been using since then. As we have been discussing, *Pseudomonas* is possibly the most important complication of chronic otitis externa that we see. Aminoglycosides and fluoroquinolones are normally our treatments of choice but it is not uncommon to see resistant strains of *Pseudomonas*. We then must use alternative antibiotic therapy. These antibiotics are often human drugs that are being used off-label. Ticarcillin is one that we have tried. This is a human anti-*Pseudomonas* penicillin. The dosage is 15–40 mg/kg intramuscularly or intravenously three times daily. The dosage was adjusted some years ago and we now tend to use 15–25 mg/kg three times daily. Side-effects are uncommon and are related to the usual penicillin hypersensitivity reactions. It is reasonably expensive. The preparation we use is Timentin®, made by SmithKline Beecham. It comes in a crystalline form for reconstitution. We chose Timentin because it is clavulanate potentiated and we see a lot of *Pseudomonas* with β-lactamase production.

When I first presented these data we had eight cases, and since then we have treated many more. This study was not controlled since the control would have been surgery or euthanasia. Prior therapies included various topical ear preparations, ear cleaners, steroids and systemic enrofloxacin. In my experience, virtually all of the *Pseudomonas* that is referred to me will have had a lot of systemic and topical fluoroquinolone treatment. The key thing is that most of these animals have not had adequate ear flushes. I find if you put a lot of fluoroquinolones into an animal, but leave all that pus sitting in the ear canal to protect the bacteria, you don't get a cure, but you do get resistance. In none of these cases was a primary cause identified. Many of these cases were severe, proliferative otitis externa with some thickening of the ear canals. Tympanic membranes were ruptured in half the cases, so otitis media was present, although none of the cases had bony abnormalities on radiography. Cytology showed numerous neutrophils and rod bacteria. *Pseudomonas* was grown in pure culture and KB sensitivity testing suggested resistance to aminoglycosides and fluoroquinolones and sensitivity to ticarcillin.

Treatment was very aggressive in these animals as we were aiming for a 100% cure rate rather than looking at how well the antibiotic worked alone. Most of these cases were already receiving high doses of marbofloxacin or enrofloxacin (topically and systemically) and were not responding. The catheter method we have previously discussed was used to flush the ears. Ear flushing was done under general anesthesia every other day except on weekends, until no purulent discharge or bacteria were seen. These dogs also had an otoscopic examination and otic cytology every day. Prednisolone was used fairly aggressively until the ear canals opened. Epi-Otic was used as the ear cleaner prior to flushing and on days when flushing was not done. I prefer Epi-Otic because it has very good cleansing and drying action and some degree of antimicrobial effect. The ticarcillin comes in a 1.6 g vial and is made up with sterile water for injection. For mild to moderate cases of otitis externa, we put in three or four drops topically three times a day after cleaning the ear first with Epi-Otic. Severe otitis externa and cases in which otitis media was also present would receive systemic therapy in addition to topical treatment. Ticarcillin can be given intramuscularly, but it is extremely painful, so we administered it intravenously. Most of the dogs were being anesthetized every other day so they already had intravenous catheters in place. Duration of therapy was anywhere between 2 weeks and 1 month.

All our cases thus far have been clinically cured. A cure is defined as the presence of a healed tympanic membrane, resolution of secondary chronic changes, resolution of pain, absence of pus in the ear canal, and no bacteria or leukocytes present on cytology. If you culture ears, you will still pick up occasional bacteria, but generally not *Pseudomonas*. I don't think you can sterilize an ear canal. We saw no adverse effects in the original group of dogs, but since then we have had one dog that developed sensitivity to ticarcillin. This patient had an exfoliative skin eruption and a head tilt. Those signs resolved upon discontinuation of the ticarcillin. We had an 80–100% cure rate with these dogs. We wanted these clients to go home with cured animals and I think we have to use a combination approach to achieve that.

Cleaning is of primary importance. If we don't clean the ear and remove the pus and debris, we seem to get nowhere with treatment. Reversing secondary pathological changes is also important. Leaving the ear canal closed reduces the chances you will be able to clean properly, and the debris and chronic thickening provide a nice home for bacteria. Make a big effort to identify otitis media by CT scan or radiography, or visualization. If you are in any doubt at all, treat as if it is present. Specific antibiotic therapy is very important. We have tried the combination approach using empirical antibiotic therapy for *Pseudomonas* and we don't get the same results. We do think we need to do sensitivity testing and use it. We are quite happy with our results with ticarcillin. Remember to look for the primary factors as well. The ear is always attached to a dog, and that dog invariably has some sort of generalized disease that is causing this problem. The ticarcillin therapy is safe and effective, but is very expensive and ticarcillin can only be administered by injection.

Steve Melman Is it my understanding that these dogs were put under anesthesia every other day for 36 days?

Tim Nuttall That was the outlier dog. Most dogs were in the 14–21 day group. We now have treated some dogs within 7 days as well.

Steve Melman Has there been any follow-up of these cases to see if there has been recurrence?

Tim Nuttall Yes, we followed up these dogs for 11–19 months and I think three out of 12 dogs relapsed, but only one of those was with *Pseudomonas* infection. That was a dog that had been taken swimming despite our instructions not to allow this. The sensitivity data were different so we think it was a different strain of *Pseudomonas*.

Lynette Cole I would like to wrap up the discussion of *Pseudomonas* otitis with some of my comments, then I will ask the panel how they treat *Pseudomonas* otitis. I do cytology and culture on my chronic ears because I want to know the susceptibility pattern of the organism. Unfortunately, we have also seen polymyxin B-resistant *Pseudomonas* infections, and that is really scary. Polymyxin B is only available as a topical preparation, but it has saved many ears for me. I flush my ears, and evaluate for otitis media. If I have a systemic antibiotic that I can use, I treat with that. I also do aggressive topical therapy because if you use topical therapy, you are going to get concentrations in the ear 100–1000 times higher than any MIC level that you would get on your susceptibility testing. Most of my topical therapy for *Pseudomonas* is extralabel. I will mix one part Baytril® injectable with four parts of a vehicle such as saline or 1% hydrocortisone. We have mixed up ticarcillin. I also use tobramycin. It comes as an ophthalmic preparation, Tobradex®, and it is incredibly expensive. I also use silver sulfadiazine. Jim Noxon did a nice study demonstrating that one part silver sulfadiazine in nine parts of water is very effective against *Pseudomonas*. We have many topical ear preparations in the USA that are a combination of neomycin, polymyxin B and hydrocortisone. These are relatively inexpensive. Sometimes I have clients putting three different topical preparations in the ear. I don't know if there is interaction between these various drugs.

Steve Melman I have seen that you use edetate trisodium (Tris–EDTA).

Lynette Cole I do use Tris–EDTA, but I do not mix other antibiotics with it. Some people mix gentamicin in with it. Steve has his own product, Triz-EDTA®, that he sells under DermaPet. There are pharmacists that can compound Tris–EDTA for you. It is very difficult to make in your practice because it should be pH balanced. I will use that prior to the antibiotic. It breaks down the cell wall and allows the antibiotic to penetrate. Here is a list of my topical favorites for *Pseudomonas* infections:

- Tris–EDTA: 1.2 g EDTA, 6.05 g Tris buffer, 1 l distilled water, pH 8, autoclave for 15 min (compounded by a pharmacist), or use Triz–EDTA (DermaPet). Fill the ear 15 min prior to topical application of an antibacterial agent of your choice twice daily.
- To prepare topical enrofloxacin use one part injectable enrofloxacin (22.7 mg/ml) and four parts of vehicle (saline, Synotic® or hydrocortisone). This gives you a 4.5 mg/ml solution. Five to 10 drops should be instilled into the ear twice daily.
- Silver sulfadiazine 1% cream: mix one part silver sulfadiazine with nine parts of water (weigh on gram scale or a rough estimate would be 0.33 of a 20 g tube with 54 ml water for a 60 ml solution). Use five to10 drops per ear twice daily.
- Topical ticarcillin: add 30 ml sterile water to a 3 g bottle of injectable ticarcillin. Take 1.8 ml of the mixture and add 88.2 ml of propylene glycol to get a 2 mg/ml solution. Refrigerate and shake well before using. The preparation is stable for 2 weeks. Use five to10 drops per ear twice daily.
- Neomycin, polymyxin B and hydrocortisone otic solutions (many generics available).
- Tobramycin ophthalmic solutions with dexamethasone (Tobradex®, Alcon) or without dexamethasone (Tobrex®, Alcon and generic).

Does the panel have any other comments?

Didier Carlotti It is surprising how beautifully you can cure some apparently severe otitis externa cases if you are very aggressive topically. In some instances, systemic antibiotic therapy is indispensable, but in some cases it is not.

Jim Noxon I would first like to commend Tim on his work with Timentin®, because it inspired me. I was struggling with many bad cases at the time I first read his paper. We were not able to use the intravenous route three times a day because of the expense and difficulty of maintaining an intravenous catheter. But we did formulate our own topical form of ticarcillin. You dilute a vial of ticarcillin to a 3% solution and freeze it. It maintains potency for about a month. We put the solution into 1 ml syringes, and the client thaws those out and treats two or three times a day, using 1 ml per ear. I have two other comments about topical therapy. One is, what volume of medication do you have to put in an ear for it to reach the deep horizontal canal? I am concerned with both volume and viscosity. I tend to use aqueous material because I don't know how well lipid-based materials get down ears. I can tell you that most of the popular commercial ear preparations don't get anywhere near the horizontal canal, especially when an owner is instructed to use two to three drops. I had my students do a project whereby we determined with dyes of different viscosity that it took at least 10 drops (close to 1 ml) to touch the tympanic membrane. I don't know how much diffusion over time contributes to medication spreading.

Lynette Cole I think if you have a really bad ear and you put an ointment in, you end up with concretions in the ear. I don't use ointment-based ear medications very often. I think it is important to use adequate amounts of ear medication, certainly more than two to three drops.

We will have to finish this now. Some key points are: we need to do cytology, and culture if indicated, based on cytology. Whether you do KB or MIC testing is still controversial. Base your antibiotic therapy on sensitivity testing results, remembering that topical therapies can get much higher concentrations. Remember to use adequate amounts of topical medication at each application.

I hope you have enjoyed this discussion and thank you for attending.

5.2

Food allergy and nutritionally related skin disease

Terese DeManuelle[1] (Chairperson) and Emily Rothstein[2] (Secretary)

[1] Northwest Veterinary Specialists, Clackamas, Oregon, USA, and Washington State University, Pullman, Washington, USA
[2] Animal Allergy and Dermatology Service of Connecticut, Southington, Connecticut, USA

Terese DeManuelle *USA* I would like to thank the sponsor of this workshop, Hill's Pet Nutrition, and there are handouts at the back on adverse food reactions that you are welcome to take. This workshop will be fun and we have some interesting presentations at this workshop. First, I would like to introduce the panel: Dr Randy Thomas, Dr Emily Rothstein, Dr Helen Globus, Dr Kim Boyanowski, Dr Andrea Cannon and Dr Pat White.

Kim Boyanowski *USA* I am going to talk about two cases of feline food allergy that have some degree of mural folliculitis in their skin biopsies. Hopefully, this will stimulate discussion on what role mural folliculitis has or does not have in food hypersensitivity.

Mural folliculitis was defined in a wonderful paper by Drs Gross and Stannard. There are five patterns: interface (with the hallmark being apoptosis of follicular basal cells, e.g. erthyema multiforme, graft-versus-host disease, vasculopathy), infiltrative (inflammatory cells into the follicular outer root sheath in the middle third of the follicle), necrotizing (necrosis at or below the isthmus, typically eosinophilic, e.g. eosinophilic folliculitis and furunculosis, mosquito-bite hypersensitivity in the feline, *Culicoides* hypersensitivity in the equine), pustular (pustules in the superficial hair follicle generally above the isthmus, e.g. pemphigus foliaceus and erythematosus), and bulbitis and luminal [targeting the bulb or intraluminal area, e.g. alopecia areata (bulbitis), bacterial folliculitis/furunculosis, dermatophytosis, demodicosis (luminal)]. I am going to concentrate on the infiltrative form in feline patients. There are new classifications in our feline patients starting to evolve: four to six categories and they are clinically diverse. These categories are feline dermatophytosis, feline sebaceous adenitis-like disease, pseudopalade-like disease, degenerative mucinotic (cats are often ill, but food allergy may fall into this class in a few reports), T-cell-type lymphoma and idiopathic (case report of food allergy).

The first case presented as a moderately pruritic cat. It was 14 years old, with some alopecia, had *Malassezia* dermatitis and a greasy coat. Preliminary work-up by the referring veterinarian showed no evident abnormalities. Skin biopsy was performed and showed infiltrative mural folliculitis and perifollicular and perivascular disease suggestive of an allergic disorder. It also showed superficial pyoderma. Treatment included topical and systemic therapy for both *Malassezia* dermatitis and superficial pyoderma with absolutely no change in clinical signs. A duck and potato commercial food trial was started and the pruritus improved in about 3 weeks. In several more weeks the cat responded totally. It then developed pancreatitis and a lower fat diet was tried and the cat got pruritic and greasy. This was tolerated until the cat's pancreatitis was resolved, then a different low-fat and limited antigen diet was started and its clinical signs again improved. Unfortunately, we did not re-biopsy the cat when its clinical signs were again seen with this diet change.

John Gordon *USA* Does infiltrative mural folliculitis suggest that there is more than pyoderma occurring?

Kim Boyanowski There are two points: the pyoderma seen was histologically in just the superficial epidermis and was not noted clinically. There was no luminal disease. The mural folliculitis was not related to the superficial pyoderma.

Ed Rosser *USA* What low-fat diet did you use?

Kim Boyanowski It went on to Hill's I/D® for pancreatitis when it relapsed, then we put in on Hill's D/D® and it did fine.

The second case was more typically a food allergic cat: typical head and neck pruritus in an 11-year-old cat. This cat was biopsied at the owner's request. We found no problems in the minimum database but the biopsy showed changes typical of allergic dermatitis. However, the infiltrate also went into the hair follicle as infiltrative mural folliculitis. A commercial venison and potato diet was used and the cat responded quickly (3–4 weeks). If the cat ate the dog food, it would relapse.

So the take-home message is that is mural folliculitis related to food allergy in the cat? What should we do and what should we think when we get a biopsy with mural folliculitis in the cat? A thorough minimum database would be helpful to collect the most information so we can to try to understand this pattern in the cat. Also, if you biopsy a cat with a dermatosis that is suspicious of food allergy, ask your pathologist to be sure to check for mural folliculitis, even if subtle. It may only be a perifollicular/perivascular extension of allergic disease, or that we are just more aware. Also, it may mean we need to include food allergy in our differential diagnosis when mural folliculitis is seen. And a biopsy with mural folliculitis may come from a cat that does not look like your typical food-allergic case.

Some observations of food allergy in the cat: these two cases responded quickly to dietary modification, they relapsed quickly and they were mature cats. And they did not have eosinophils in their biopsy, as many people think they might. Also, I should like to give you my particular thoughts on food hypersensitivity in the cat. Trials are difficult due to the fact that many cats find diets unpalatable, more cats seem to have food allergy than do dogs, there is a quicker response to the dietary change than in dogs, there are fewer secondary complications (infection) in our food-allergic cat patients, some develop new food hypersensitivities after several years and we may see mural folliculitis on biopsy.

Ed Rosser There were several cases of mural folliculitis in cats presented 6–7 years ago that responded to steroids and eventually came off steroids. I recognized some cats years ago that had mural folliculitis that did not respond to steroids and then worked them up for food allergy. But I do not see a lot of food-allergic cats in my practice.

Terese DeManuelle Kim, do you have an idea that all food-allergic cats have a similar histopathological presentation with mural folliculitis?

Kim Boyanowski Mine were lymphocytic and plasmacytic. Dr Declercq wrote up a case in *Veterinary Dermatology* a few months ago of a cat with lymphocytic, plasmacytic mural folliculitis.

Terese DeManuelle Were any antipruritic drugs used on these cats?

Kim Boyanowski Nothing on either of the cats. We really went stepwise on the first cat; the second cat had historical Depo-Medrol® injections, but since the biopsy came back quickly and we started the food trial and it started to respond, we really did not need to use anything. I see a lot more cats in private practice than as a resident, so maybe I am appreciating this more.

Bruce Hammerberg *USA* I am an immunologist and we are developing monoclonal antibody against cat IgE and we are quantitating total IgE. Some of the samples I am using are samples collected by Thierry Olivry and they are from cases of mural folliculitis in the cat. These cats show some of the highest levels of total IgE in serum.

Kim Boyanowski Do you know which classification of mural folliculitis they were in?

Bruce Hammerberg No, unfortunately not. So if anyone has cases of mural folliculitis in which they would like me to check serum total IgE, please contact me.

Emily Rothstein *USA* This is a short presentation about a 4-year-old husky with zinc-responsive dermatosis that may stimulate a discussion on therapy for difficult cases. This dog presented with severe crusting and pruritus of the ears, periocular area, muzzle and legs for years and the primary veterinarian suggested euthanasia. A minimum database showed only *Malassezia* and bacterial dermatitis. Sarcoptic mange was also suspected based on clinical signs, yet mites were not found on skin scrapings. These were all treated and the dog showed some response. A biopsy was then performed and suggested zinc-responsive dermatosis and/or *Malassezia* dermatitis, so the therapy for *Malassezia* was continued and zinc sulfate started at 1 mg/kg elemental zinc daily. Although the pruritus responded, there was minimal response of the crusting in 1 month, and the dose was doubled. The dog still showed little improvement and glucocorticoids (prednisone 0.5 mg/kg per day) and DermCaps® were added. For a while she did better, then the crusts and pruritus returned. Infections were treated when needed over the next year, but the crusts typical of zinc-responsive disease responded poorly. At their financial and personal tolerance limits, no further work-up was done. The dog continued to take 0.25 mg/kg prednisone on alternate days with the zinc supplement until its acute death. Unfortunately, necropsy was not permitted.

Ed Rosser I see many of what Dr Dunstan (when he was still at Michigan) and I would call 'non-zinc-responsive zinc-responsive' dermatosis as an entity. I am starting to entertain that this may be an interesting and unique cutaneous reaction pattern of certain breeds with a multifactorial underlying etiology. Zinc works for some of them. I would like to share with you a classic parakeratotic zinc-responsive dermatosis case in an atopic individual, which was being treated with zinc and immunotherapy. The owners questioned if the dog needed zinc and immunotherapy and unilaterally stopped the zinc. They called me 6 months later and said there were no plaque-like parakeratotic lesions just on the allergy therapy. We should also consider food trials in cases like this with 'non-zinc responsive zinc-responsive' dermatosis.

Terese DeManuelle Dr Sousa in California taught me that the diet you feed the dog along with the zinc might affect the absorption of oral zinc. It was thought a beef-based diet might help with the absorption of oral zinc. Unfortunately I do not have a reference from her; it was something she remembered from many years ago. Does anyone have any thoughts on that?

Dottie LeFlamme *USA* That thought is likely to be an extrapolation that we all know: fiber, phytates and some vegetable proteins interfere with the absorption of zinc, so the beef-based diet just moves you away from the high-fiber foods. Certainly, if an animal is on a fiber-based diet and they are zinc responsive, that will interfere with zinc absorption.

Karin Beale *USA* I have had extremely frustrating cases like this. The ZinPro® product is a chewable zinc methionine supplement. I have had better response with that than zinc sulfate. Most of the dogs that I have had problems with have had other problems like allergy as well.

Kim Boyanowski I had a zinc-responsive dog that took the prescription form of zinc sulfate. The dog did well. When that ran out, the owner purchased the over-the-counter product of the same strength (220 mg). After 1 month, the owner reported that the dog was much worse on the over-the-counter product. When she used the prescription form again, the dog did better. I found that interesting.

John Gordon I have a lot of dogs that do better with the chewable canine variety of zinc methionine with beef.

Ed Rosser Yes, zinc methionine is still available (it was unavailable for a short time in the transitional buy-out) in the chewable beef product called NutroVet/ZinPro® available through Butler (in the USA).

Terese DeManuelle So are most people using zinc methionine or sulfate?

[**Many people** responded that they use zinc sulfate and they were happy to hear that ZinPro is available again.]

Phil Rodebush *USA* There is research looking at zinc bioavailability in many zinc preparations at Hill's. We looked at bone zinc levels in normal dogs. Bone zinc levels are probably the best depot sites for zinc determination. We did not biopsy skin. We looked at bone and gonad zinc levels, manipulating calcium and phytates, and there is no better deposition in those organs using different types of zinc (methionine, sulfate) without high levels of phytates and calcium. The base diet may have something to do with absorption. I do not know if skin behaves in the same way but I would assume so. So it is the diet and the supplement together that seems to make a difference more than whether zinc is proteinated or sulfated.

Åke Hedhammar *Sweden* Shouldn't we be working harder on finding the underlying defects rather than just trying different products? It is important to know the physiology of the defect. I am not doing research on this but I think it is important.

Pat White *USA* While we wait for the primary cause to be identified, it is important when we are supplementing with vitamins, minerals or other things, that we know the source and bioavailability of what we are giving. Kim's cases dramatically pointed that out. How do we treat with nutrients that are not pharmaceutical products and are not scrutinized except by the company itself?

Terese DeManuelle Kim, did you look at the grade and quality of the two zinc products used by your client?

Kim Boyanowski Yes, and they had adequate labeling. All I can assume is that the over-the-counter product had less bioavailability of zinc. The brand the owner bought over the counter was not a well-known supplement brand. Or, possibly, something changed in this dog at the same time the supplement changes took place, but I doubt that.

Pat White I am going to present two cases of diet-responsive eosinophilic granuloma/dermatitis in cats. I would like to generate discussion on eosinophilic disease and how it is treated. Dr Helen Powers showed that eosinophilic dermatoses are associated with a variety of conditions. Clinicians must identify the problems that cause these clinical signs. Eosinophilic disease is typically glucocorticoid responsive, so owners must be educated that it is important to find the underlying cause so the cat does not only receive long-term glucocorticoid therapy. If it is not steroid responsive, it is very important to go back to the history.

The first case is a 12-year-old cat with a history of 3–4 years of pruritus and an indolent ulcer. The cat was intermittently steroid responsive and the owner was happy with that over the years. The main concern to the owner at the time of presentation was not really the pruritus or the lip lesion but a large swelling in the throat. The cat was somehow able to eat and swallow and not only its food but also the food of all the other species of animals in the house. In preparation for biopsy and because of the history of the ulcer and that possibly the cat's lip improved with certain foods, the cat was started on a food trial. The throat swelling improved but the lip ulcer worsened. I felt at that time, the mass in the throat was a dietary-responsive process. The throat biopsy showed ulcerated eosinophilic granuloma with collagen degeneration and with no evidence of neoplasia. Because the lip was not improving, intradermal testing was performed and immunotherapy started and the lip improved with that and antihistamine therapy.

Terese DeManuelle How did you get the owner to do the food trial with so many animals in the house?

Pat White I basically told the owner they had to isolate the cat for the trial to work. The owner isolated the cat for 2 weeks and the throat improved. If the cat ate the dog's food, it worsened.

Terese DeManuelle I would like to ask the group a question. When we have cases that are 'intermittently' responsive to glucocorticoids, what does that mean in relation to food allergy?

Karin Beale I think that if they do not respond, then think food allergy, but some food-allergic cats are responsive. I had a similar case of eosinophilic granuloma in the tonsils of a cat that had plaques on its ventral abdomen and indolent ulcer. I think of lip ulcers in cats as a sign of food allergy until proven otherwise. I also think cats with lip ulcers on the sides/commissures respond better to food trials than do those with the ulcer in the middle of their lip.

Andrea Cannon *USA* I am not sure which older paper gave many people the impression that food-allergic animals do not respond to glucocorticoids, but if you read them carefully, they just say that food-allergic animals may not respond. If they are truly type IV hypersensitivities, they should respond. If they do not, we should consider the non-responsive animals to have another immunological response.

Ed Rosser What about the concept of different response to different steroids? Dr Ed Robinson was an advocate that chronic obstructive pulmonary disease (COPD) was not prednisone responsive since horses do not absorb prednisone, nor can you measure it in their blood. Tony Stannard taught me to use prednisolone in the horse. I brought it to Dr Robinson's attention that horses are prednisolone responsive. I think cats are like small horses.

Pat White I tend to use prednisolone in cats as against prednisone because I feel they do not respond well to prednisone. I also think they respond to triamcinolone better than to Depo-Medrol.

The second case is an 11-year-old cat with a 2 year history of a granulomatous, pruritic dermatosis with alopecia in the axilla. Historically, it worsened with glucocorticoid therapy, improved with clavulanic acid–amoxycillin therapy, but progressively deteriorated. The initial work-up showed only hyperglobulinemia. The biopsy showed severe, ulcerative eosinophilic plaque. Bacterial culture and sensitivity grew many bacteria with sensitivity to Clavamox®. A food trial was started as well as oral antibiotics, an Elizabethan collar, T-shirt and instructions to clean the lesion. After 3 weeks, there was a dramatic improvement. I am sure the antibiotics and barriers helped. After 10 weeks, the area was healed. The owner refused a food challenge and I did not question this, as the cat had been uncomfortable with the lesions for 2 years. I cannot be sure, then, that this was food-responsive disease. However, since the cat had taken antibiotics and used barriers before without resolution of the disease and the only new therapy was dietary change, I have to strongly suspect the diet.

Randy Thomas *USA* I wonder if anyone has seen cases of what ultimately turned out to be food-allergic dermatitis in the cat but there was a poor response to dietary change until glucocorticoid was used concurrently. I have had a few cats that do not initially improve on glucocorticoids, do not initially respond to an 8–10 week dietary trial, but when glucocorticoids are then given concurrently, the cats respond. They continue to do well after withdrawal of the drug, eating only the food on the trial. I think that the reaction of eosinophilic degranulation and inflammation is self-perpetuating and removing the allergen may not be the only thing that stops the itch. So by using glucocorticoids with the food, then stopping them, they do well.

Terese DeManuelle I use low-dose dexamethasone in cats at the beginning of the food trial for 2–3 weeks and then taper the dexamethasone. Pat, are there any problems with palatability?

Pat White There are some problems. I use canned food nearly exclusively since most cats enjoy canned food. I limit my choices to commercial rabbit and potato and venison and potato.

Andrea Cannon I will be discussing a group of cases of sebaceous adenitis from the University of California at Davis, and the use of vitamin A. The use of vitamin A in these cases was influenced by Dr Candace Sousa. Sebaceous adenitis is characterized by follicular casting, adherent scale, alopecia, broken hairs, easy epilation of hair and, in short-coated breeds, a nodular or granulomatous form. Because of the histopathological changes in sebaceous adenitis including follicular keratosis, I wondered if vitamin A would work.

Breeds commonly affected by sebaceous adenitis are the akita, standard poodle, vizsla and samoyed, but other breeds are affected as well. Although the exact pathogenesis is unknown, we do know through breeding studies that it is an autosomal recessive trait in the standard poodle. There was a study from the Czech Republic that CD4 and CD8 T-cells predominate in the lesions. But there have been many cells shown to be CD4 and CD8 negative. Therefore, the pathogenesis may be immunological. Also, there is the keratinization defect theory and that is supported by the response to retinoids. Dr Stewart, in 1991, reported two vizslas that responded to isotretinoin and, in 1995, Dr White reported a reasonably good response to retinoids in many dogs. Retinoids improve keratinization.

There are side-effects of vitamin A therapy. In humans, 300 000–500 000 IU causes worse adverse effects than synthetic retinoids. Chelitis, facial dermatitis, dry mucous membranes, conjunctivitis, arthropathy and paronychia can be seen. Elevations in triglycerides (TG) and cholesterol may also occur. In humans, 1250–25 000 IU of vitamin A per day over 5 years did not result in changes in TG or liver enzymes. We did not want to harm these dogs, so we used lower doses.

The Association of American Feed Control Officials permits up to 50 000 IU/kg per day in their guidelines for dog food, which seems quite high. The dosage we tried on our cases was extrapolated: 10 000 IU twice a day per dog. We evaluated Schirmer tear tests (STT), liver enzymes and TG prior to and during therapy. Other treatments were used as needed, such as antibiotics for secondary bacterial infections and topical therapy. I always used 75% propylene glycol as a daily mist, as well as antiseborrhoeic baths followed by emollients in all cases.

We found very good response to vitamin A in vizslas, akitas, dobermans and mixed breeds. I actually discontinued the topicals in these dogs (and future cases taking vitamin A) to less than once weekly. Eventually, I discontinued recommending propylene glycol as well. Seven of 11 in this group showed an 80% response to vitamin A at 10 000 IU orally twice a day. At 20 000 IU we had 90% response.

[**Terese DeManuelle** and **Kim Boyanowski** both still use propylene glycol at the beginning of therapy, even with vitamin A.]

Andrea Cannon Kim Boyanowski suggested that in cases that did not respond to 10 000 IU of vitamin A twice a day, the dosage could be increased to 20 000–30 000 IU twice daily. These cases did better.

The few cases that did not do well with vitamin A were given retinoids and improved. However, when retinoids became too expensive, the dogs were changed back to 30 000 IU vitamin A and, although they got a little scalier, the owners were content.

These dogs have been taking high doses for at least 2 years with no side-effects. Using 10 000 IU, 80% of dogs respond in approximately 3 months. At that time, you can probably decrease the topical therapy. After preliminary monitoring, blood parameters are checked once yearly. I think the first change will be dry eye, so I always check an STT before starting treatment. The only real problem I have heard of is a case I consulted on which was a dog already taking retinoids (the veterinarian did not tell me) and when vitamin A was added the dog became icteric. On stopping both medications and with the use of intravenous fluids, the dog recovered. It is recommended that vitamin A and retinoids not be used in combination.

In conclusion, vitamin A is a less expensive alternative to retinoids for sebaceous adenitis and is safe and convenient. I do recommend baseline STT, liver enzymes and TG levels. Does anyone else use vitamin A for this disease? I am trying it with other scaling diseases as well.

Emily Rothstein I have used it in at least a half-dozen dogs with very good success and no side-effects. I start with 10 000 IU twice a day in smallish dogs and 20 000 IU twice daily in large dogs. I am also using it in ichthyosis in two golden retrievers.

Ed Rosser Are you using vitamin A by itself? I know many breeders that are getting what sounds like similar results with topicals only (propylene glycol) every 2–3 weeks.

Andrea Cannon I agree that topical therapy can play a large role but many owners of large dogs that are not breeders find it difficult. Again, I do not recommend aggressive topical therapy any more.

Ins Reichler *Switzerland* I have worked with akitas and find that bathing/rinsing helps a lot. I also use fish oil. I start with bathing once a week and then reduce to once a month. I have one case on fish oil only without topical agents.

Andrea Cannon I have a few cases that, when vitamin A was stopped and bathing only used, they relapsed. I also think the referral cases I see may be more severe than the milder cases never referred. I think there is probably a spectrum to this disease.

Randy Thomas I am going to discuss a fairly simple but interesting case of recurrent pyoderma that was food responsive. It is not anything new but interesting in that the only complaint was pyoderma. The dog was a 5-year-old, aggressive neutered male Shetland sheepdog with a 1.5 year history of non-seasonal, non-pruritic pyoderma. It was antibiotic responsive but would relapse with antibiotic withdrawal within 2–4 weeks. A typical clinical picture of pyoderma was seen with multifocal crusts on the trunk and mostly ventral collarettes, with mild erythema in the ears. A full diagnostic work-up showed only a pyoderma. Treatment was cephalexin, benzoyl peroxide shampoo and a commercial venison and potato food trial. The dog did very well for several months. With beef exposure it would relapse. We then tried a commercial lamb and rice diet and the dog did fine as well. So I think of food allergy as a differential diagnosis in dogs with recurrent pyoderma.

Terese DeManuelle Would you describe this as a typical 'superficial spreading pyoderma'?

Randy Thomas Yes, although that was mainly the description given by the referring veterinarian. When I saw this dog, the lesions were not so dramatic because it had recently been taking antibiotics. Unfortunately, there was not a lot of personal follow-up as the dog was aggressive. We also discussed that if the dietary restriction did not help, we would try Staphage Lysate®.

Ed Rosser In 1980, Dr Halliwell described collies, Shetland sheepdogs and other breeds that had non-pruritic recurrent pyoderma. He said underlying allergy should be considered in these dogs. Food trials and skin tests were done and many were allergic. I found this true in my practice with some dogs being skin-test positive.

Randy Thomas I didn't think of skin testing dogs that were not pruritic before, but I have had a few cases of pyoderma that were skin-test positive as well.

Helen Globus *USA* This is a case of my own, a 15-year-old, male-neutered domestic short-haired cat. When he was young, I diagnosed flea allergy dermatitis and it responded to treatment. We then moved and it developed head and neck pruritus over the next several months. The cat would have erythematous pinnae with some papules and crusts all over, but mainly on the head and neck. It would excoriate areas of the face and neck. After the initial work-up, a food trial was done and the pruritus decreased within 3 weeks eating Hill's D/D®, but plateaued at only 90% improvement. The facial lesions remained, but to a milder degree. Because the problem waxed and waned without changing his food, I did an intradermal skin test that was negative. I then tried a commercial dry venison and potato diet with subsequent severe worsening in clinical signs. The dry lamb and potato did the same thing. I decided to live with this 90% improvement.

The cat then developed chronic renal failure. I was afraid to change to a commercial renal diet (Hill's K/D®) because of the results of previous challenges. Then Craig Griffin's study was published. He suggested that mites existing in dry food could lead to allergic reactions in animals. I wondered whether that was why my cat worsened with the dry foods. I tried dry Hill's K/D and he did fine. I then tried his original dry food and he was still no longer pruritic! Did the adverse food reaction resolve? I have treated some pruritic cats that go through a thorough work-up, improve on their food trial and finally during the food challenge they seem normal.

Pat White I have seen that. I think they were diet sensitive or food allergic, because they are challenged to confirm their food trial response. Then, for whatever reason, another food is introduced and the animal is fine.

Åke Hedhammar Do you think they changed the recipe of the cat's original diet?

Helen Globus That was considered. The major ingredients were the same, but perhaps something in the formulation changed. Some cats do not react to the ingredients per se, but the processing.

Pat White I had a case of a dog that was exquisitely food allergic. The owner found a food without meat and meat byproducts and the dog did very well. He bought a new bag of the same food and the dog had an adverse reaction again. They had changed the ingredients in the food.

Terese DeManuelle Thanks to all the presenters and participants.

5.3

House dust mites and allergy

Chiara Noli[1] (Chairperson) and Andrew Hillier[2] (Secretary)

[1]Via Sismondi 62, 20133 Milano, Italy
[2]College of Veterinary Medicine, The Ohio State University, Columbus, Ohio, USA

Chiara Noli *Italy* House dust mites (HDM) play the major role as allergens for dogs and cats, with 30–80% of atopic animals having positive intradermal reactions, and yet there is remarkably little known about this topic. *Dermatophagoides farinae* and *D. pteronyssinus* are pyroglyphid mites and belong to the same sub-order (Acaridides) as *Psoroptes, Otodectes, Sarcoptes* and storage mites, which may be the cause of some cross-reactivity in intradermal tests (IDT) and serum tests (ST). HDM live best at high relative humidity (>60–70%) and temperatures of 21–25°C. High mite concentration and humidity are considered risk factors for development of allergy in humans. The main source of allergens is the mite faeces. More than 10 groups of allergens have been recognized to cause HDM allergy in humans. Most of these are enzymes with molecular weights of 14–60 kDa. The low molecular weight allergens Der p I and II, Der f I and II (14–25 kDa) are not considered to be major allergens in dogs, whereas a *D. farinae* high molecular weight molecule of >90 kDa has been suggested to be the most important. Purified allergens could help to standardize and improve allergy testing and hyposensitization. Recombinant allergens have been produced in human allergology.

Cathy McCall *USA* There are 14 official *Dermatophagoides* allergens recognized by the International Union of Immunologic Societies subcommittee for Allergen Nomenclature and these do not appear to be major allergens for dogs. On Western blots, most dog serum reacts with a 98 kDa band and a 109 kDa band: these two molecules appear to be the same protein based on their N-terminal amino acid sequences. The protein portion of the 98 kDa molecule is about 60 kDa molecular weight. This protein is heavily O-glycosylated, shows high homology to chitinases and has been shown with immunohistochemical localization to be a digestive chitinase found intracellularly in the mite intestine. The canine 98 kDa allergen has been difficult to express as a recombinant because of the extensive glycosolation. Much of the immunoglobulin E (IgE) to this molecule is directed at the carbohydrate and the clinical relevance of this carbohydrate-specific IgE has yet to be determined. This molecule is also allergenic to dust mite-allergic humans, but is not a major allergen. Humans have been shown to be IgE reactive with another 98 kDa *Dermatophagoides* allergen, but this allergen is a paramyosin and is not related to the 98 kDa allergen of dogs. The *D. pteronyssinus* homologue of the *D. farinae* 98 kDa allergen is very similar, but does not appear to be as heavily glycosylated.

Another dominant band on Western blot has been seen to be a 60 kDa molecule, which appears to be important in dogs and even more important in cats. This molecule has also been cloned and is also a chitinase. By Western blot, it appears that the 98 kDa molecule is not as important in cats as it is in dogs, and cats have more reactivity to lower molecular weight allergens, including Der f I and II allergens. In *in vitro* studies with 88 cat sera, more cats were reactive to both *D. farinae* and *D. pteronyssinus* compared to dogs, where there is less reactivity to *D. pteronyssinus* compared to *D. farinae*. Of these 88 cat sera, 32% reacted to Der f I, 42% to Der f II, 70% to the 98 kDa molecule and, in a second panel of putatively atopic cat sera, 31 of 36 (86%) to the 60 kDa molecule.

In summary, dogs have hypersensitivity to *D. farinae* predominantly, show low reactivity to the low molecular weight allergens and react mostly with 98 kDa and 60 kDa chitinase molecules of the dust mites. By contrast, >50% of cats react to both *D. farinae* and *D. pteronyssinus* and show strong reactivity to low molecular weight allergens as well as the 60 and 98 kDa chitinases.

Doug DeBoer *USA* Is there much reactivity (skin or *in vitro*) to the recombinant allergens of the 98 kDa allergens produced by Heska?

Cathy McCall About 20% of sera that were positive to the native allergen were positive to the recombinant. The *Escherichia coli* expression system does not produce carbohydrate and the other two systems (Baculovirus and the yeast *Pichio pastoris*) express the wrong carbohydrate. Studies with sera from Heska high IgE-responder beagles artificially sensitized to *D. farinae* showed the presence of IgE to the protein portion of the 98 kDa molecule, but the reactivity appears to be highly variable from dog to dog. The carbohydrate determinants are not likely to be important for immunotherapy so long as the correct protein portion of the molecules is present. The lack of carbohydrates poses a problem for the use of recombinant allergens in a diagnostic test in animals whose IgE recognizes glycan epitopes.

Doug DeBoer Is there cross-reactivity between the carbohydrate on the dust mite 98 kDa allergen with carbohydrates on other insect (flea, mites, ticks) allergens?

Cathy McCall The best characterized carbohydrates (glycans) of plants and insects that appear to elicit anti-carbohydrate IgE are N-glycosylated. The 98 kDa allergen, in contrast, is heavily O-glycosylated along an extensive portion of the molecule. Flea-hypersensitive dogs do not show cross-reactivity with this allergen. There is much debate and speculation regarding the clinical relevance of IgE directed at carbohydrate moieties. In humans, IgE to the glycans on plant and insect allergens are thought to be irrelevant as they cannot cross-link IgE, but nobody knows if the glycoprotein in its entirety (i.e. peptide plus carbohydrate epitopes) may be able to cross-link adjacent IgE molecules. Some of the discrepancy between skin and serum test results is due to the cross-reactivity to the glycans of taxonomically unrelated plants. IgE to these glycans is readily detected *in vitro*, but because of the apparent inability of these IgEs to be cross-linked at the mast cell surface, they do not give rise to a positive skin test.

Bob Esch *USA* The HDM extracts are very stable and resistant to denaturation. We have observed in some cases (e.g. after trypsin treatment of extracts) that there may be increased reactivity, which may suggest the existence of 'buried' allergenic epitopes which are exposed after such treatment. Is there a relationship between the 98 kDa and 60 kDa allergens?

Cathy McCall Although we believe that both of these allergens are chitinases, they have different sequences and are therefore antigenically different.

Andrew Hillier *USA* You have reported a high percentage of reactivity to the 98 kDa and 60 kDa allergens in animals that were positive to crude *D. farinae* and/or *D. pteronyssinus* extracts. Have you looked at animals with atopic dermatitis that were negative to the crude extracts and seen reactivity to these two high molecular weight allergens?

Cathy McCall Only very occasional cases have been seen where animals were negative to the crude whole mite extracts and yet positive to either of the two specific allergens.

Bob Esch We have examined the relationship between IDT reactivity and IgE levels on enzyme-linked immunosorbent assay (ELISA) for all allergens, and have found that there is only correlation between IDT and ST with HDM allergens. When animals have been skin tested with doubling dilutions of HDM extract, we find the best correlation with ELISA is seen with the 1:10 000 w/v crude HDM extract on the IDT. For lot-to-lot reproducibility and potency testing, we use the ELISA inhibition assay, using canine control serum and an HDM extract formulated for use in veterinary medicine. Using human control serum or the human HDM extract, we do not see the correlation with IDT in dogs that we see with canine sera and the canine crude HDM extracts.

Most dog sera submitted to our laboratory have IgE to *D. farinae* or to both *D. farinae* and *D. pteronyssinus*. We rarely see reactivity to *D. pteronyssinus* alone. To examine the possibility of cross-reactivity between *D. farinae* and *D. pteronyssinus*, we have used reciprocal ELISA inhibition (EI) assays. We have found that the correlation coefficient between IgE and IgG to *D. farinae* is between 0.4 and 0.5 and the situation is similar for *D. pteronyssinus*. However, the correlation coefficient between IgE to *D. farinae* and IgE to *D. pteronyssinus* is only between 0.1 and 0.2, indicating a lack of significant cross-reactivity. This is further demonstrated by the fact that *D. pteronyssinus* has little inhibitory potency on *D. farinae* binding in the EI. However, *D. farinae* can be a potent inhibitor of *D. pteronyssinus* binding in the EI with some sera, which leads us to believe that there are two major profiles in dogs: (1) independent sensitization to each species of HDM in some dogs, and (2) many cases where sensitization to *D. pteronyssinus* is induced by *D. farinae*.

Andrew Hillier In our recent study of intradermal reactivity to HDM extracts in 90 dogs with atopic dermatitis, 53% of dogs with reactivity to *D. farinae* and/or *D. pteronyssinus* had positive reactions to both mite species. Have you done any studies to determine if these dogs may have cross-reactivity and, if so, with which specific allergens is there cross-reactivity?

Bob Esch We have performed immunoblot inhibition studies to determine if cross-reactivity is across a few allergens or many allergens. There is little cross-reactivity with the 98 kDa allergen and we think there may be cross-reactivity over many minor allergens.

Kenichi Masuda *Japan* We examined cross-reactivity between crude *D. farinae* and *D. pteronyssinus*, Der f I and Der p I, and Der f II and Der p II in three dogs with atopic dermatitis using EI. We found poor inhibition with the crude HDM extracts. For the group I and II allergens, we found that some dogs have high IgE to these allergens but there was no consistency between the dogs. In one dog, Der f I completely inhibited the binding of IgE to Der p I, but Der p I did not inhibit the IgE binding to Der f I. In other dogs, there was no inhibition. We have demonstrated that dogs have IgE to the crude dust mite extracts and to group I and group II allergens and there is variable cross-reactivity, and we think that some dogs may recognize different conformational epitopes of these allergens from other dogs. It appears that dogs are different to humans and are thus not a good model of HDM allergy in humans.

Bob Esch What is the prevalence of hypersensitivity to the two species of HDM in Japan?

Kenichi Masuda About 80% of dogs have hypersensitivity to HDM and almost all have reactivity to both species of mites.

Chiara Noli That is very similar to my experience in Italy, where I very rarely see reactivity to *D. pteronyssinus* alone, occasionally see reactivity to *D. farinae* alone, and very often see reactivity to both species of HDM in dogs with HDM hypersensitivity.

Ross Bond *UK* It may also depend on which allergens one uses for IDT. When I used Greer allergens, I routinely saw positive reactions to both dust mite species. However, when I started to use ARTU allergens, I routinely saw positive reactions to *D. farinae* and negative reactions to *D. pteronyssinus*.

Fleming Kristensen *Denmark* I think that we must also consider the narrow gene pools that we are each looking at in our various regions. The gene pool in a certain breed of dog in one country is not the same as that in another country, and this may also affect the prevalence of HDM hypersensitivity and possible cross-reactivity.

Doug DeBoer It seems that these presentations confirm that some dogs do have reactivity to the human *Dermatophagoides* group I and II allergens, even if they are not major allergens. This has not previously been clear in the literature.

Bob Esch The subject of major allergens is controversial. Although a majority of dogs may not have IgE to the group I or II allergens, for some dogs these may be the major allergens. In our laboratory, we see dog sera with IgE to the group I and II allergens, but it is usually only about 10% of the IgE that is directed towards the crude extract, whereas about 80% is directed towards the 98 kDa allergen.

Cathy McCall Humans with hypersensitivity to HDM do react to the 98 kDa chitinase, but in the human serum samples that we have looked at from The Netherlands, less than 50% of humans have IgE to the 98 kDa allergen, and this allergen does not appear to be able to degranulate basophils *in vitro*.

Bob Esch The Greer extract of HDM used for IDT in dogs is a different preparation to that used in humans and is qualitatively different. We believe that the optimal concentration for the IDT in dogs is 1:5000 to 1:10 000, depending on the area of the country.

Kim Stedman *USA* The storage mites (SM), including the genera *Lepidoglyphus*, *Tyrophagus*, *Acarus* and *Glycyphagus* are found throughout the world, in ranges dependent upon temperature and humidity. These mites are related to the more widely studied HDM, being fungivorous species commonly found in stored grain products, hay and sometimes house dust. HDM group II allergen homologues have been characterized in both *L. destructor* and *T. putrescentiae*, and the anti-SM IgE observed in many patients may result from direct exposure, cross-reactivity with HDM allergens or both. The role, if any, played by storage mites in canine and feline atopic dermatitis is not known. For the last 3 years, Heska AG has included extracts of *L. destructor* and *T. putrescentiae* in the indoor panel of all ALLERCEPT® tests run on European serum samples. A high rate of positive tests to *L. destructor* and *T. putrescentiae* has been observed. For example, in a series of 69 putatively atopic dogs submitted for testing, 18 (26%) were negative to all mites tested, 43 (62%) were positive to *D. farinae*, 36 (52%) were positive to *T. putrescentiae* and 25 (36%) were positive to *L. destructor*. There were very few sera that had IgE to *D. farinae* only and four of 69 (6%) had IgE to *Tyrophagus* or *Lepidoglyphus* only.

We have recently examined a larger series of 547 sera from American dogs submitted for ALLERCEPT testing: 51% were positive to *D. farinae*, 66% were positive to *T. putrescentiae* and 37% were positive to *L. destructor*. Of these, 3% were positive to only *D. farinae*, 18% only to *Tyrophagus* and about 10% of those with IgE to *Lepidoglyphus* did not have IgE to *D. farinae*, although most of these had anti-*Tyrophagus* IgE. Thus, *Lepidoglyphus* appears to be secondary to *Tyrophagus*.

Forty-eight cat sera submitted to Heska Corporation for IgE screening were tested in an FcεR1α-based research ELISA. *Tyrophagus putrescentiae* was the most significant mite allergen for these cats (94% positive), followed by *D. pteronyssinus* (77% positive), *D. farinae* (75% positive) and *L. destructor* (63% positive). IgE to *Tyrophagus* was seen independently in 21% of the cats but none had IgE to *Lepidoglyphus* exclusively.

Thus, in all sample populations, certain sera contained anti-SM IgE in the absence of IgE directed against the HDM extracts, suggesting that the observed prevalence of anti-storage mite IgE cannot be explained purely on the basis of antibody cross-reactivity. Storage mites may, therefore, be an important, but underappreciated, cause of perennial atopic dermatitis in dogs and cats.

5.4

Non-inflammatory, non-thyroidal, non-Cushing's: puzzling alopecias

Lynn P. Schmeitzel[1] (Chairperson) and Patricia F. Ashley[2] (Secretary)

[1] College of Veterinary Medicine, University of Tennessee, Knoxville, Tennessee, USA
[2] Oregon Veterinary Referral Associates, Springfield, Oregon, USA

Lynn Schmeitzel *USA* This workshop will review alopecias that lack specific diagnoses and overlap in their clinical presentation (i.e. alopecia X/pseudo-Cushing's disease, canine recurrent flank alopecia, pattern baldness and sex hormone dermatoses) and how melatonin relates to the treatment of these disorders. There will be mini-talks by myself on alopecia X, Dr Linda Frank on sex hormones in Cushing's syndrome patients, Dr Trish Ashley on the effects of melatonin administration on sex hormone concentrations, Dr Manon Paradis on melatonin and pattern baldness, Dr Wayne Rosenkrantz on alopecia X in the Arctic fox and mitotane and its effects on various disorders, and Dr Alan Mundell on cyclic canine flank alopecia.

Lynn Schmeitzel Alopecia X was initially called pseudo-Cushing's disease, a term coined by Dr Edward Segal in 1977. He noted that the disorder occurred most often in poodles. They had alopecia and hyperpigmentation typical of hyperadrenocorticism but had normal adrenal function tests and routine blood work. He gave several dogs growth hormone (GH), based on experience with pituitary dwarfism and hair regrowth when GH was given to affected people. The dogs responded and Segal suggested this could be a disorder of hyposomatotropism. The disease has undergone a number of name changes (such as castration-responsive alopecia and black skin disease of Pomeranians), often due to responses to different therapeutic interventions.

Alopecia X affects Nordic breeds (breeds with plush coats developed in northern climates) most commonly. There are 30 breeds in this group, including the Chinese shar pei. It is seen in young adult dogs, either neutered or intact. The ventrum is affected early and the alopecia then extends to the perineum, caudal thighs, tail and tail base and around the neck. The trunk is affected later in the disease. Marked hyperpigmentation is common. The head and distal extremities are often spared. Some dogs present only after clipping. We suspect that these dogs are in telogen when they are clipped. In Pomeranians and poodles, the skin can be thin and hypotonic. Secondary seborrhea and mild, superficial pyoderma are also common. The hyperpigmented skin may lose pigment from the resultant inflammation. Commonly, dogs will regrow hair where the skin is biopsied. I suspect this results from the local release of cytokines.

The cause of this disorder is unknown, but I will present the pros and cons for theories of hyposomatotropism and adrenal sex hormone imbalance. Dr Clint Lothrop and I evaluated xylazine-stimulated GH release in chow chows and samoyeds. We found that two-thirds of clinically affected dogs had suppressed release of GH but one-third had a normal response. Somatomedin C levels were normal in those with low GH, indicating that the GH may be low, secondary to one or more other problems. Additionally, not all dogs responded to GH therapy.

We suspected the GH deficiency was secondary to a sex hormone imbalance and when the sex hormone balance was altered, hair was stimulated to grow. When sex hormone concentrations were evaluated in Pomeranians and other dogs, we saw a variety of high sex hormone concentrations, even in neutered animals. These changes might alter hair growth by either binding to receptors on hair follicles or affecting sex hormone receptor levels. Dr Lothrop and I proposed there was a partial deficiency of the 21-hydroxylase or 11-hydroxylase enzyme in the pathway of steroid (cortisol and aldosterone) production in the adrenal glands causing the high 17-hydroxyprogesterone (17-OHP), androstendione, progesterone and testosterone. This alteration would stimulate the pituitary gland to produce more adrenocorticotropic hormone (ACTH), thus driving the steroid pathway toward sex hormone production. This is similar to congenital adrenal hyperplasia in people.

I suspect because normal Pomeranians have abnormal adrenal sex hormone profiles, that these Nordic breeds are genetically primed to produce such a hair coat in response to the excess hormones. The dogs that become alopecic are unique in the lack of response by their hair follicles to the 'abnormal' sex hormone concentrations. I also proposed that it could be a combined effect of sex hormone and GH abnormalities. Yet some dogs fail to respond to either GH or sex hormone alterations. This points towards a primary hair cycle or hair growth disorder. I propose that there may be a local defect at the hair follicle level, a hormone metabolism abnormality or a receptor problem. Thus, a change in sex hormones such as neutering will kick-start hair growth but eventually the dog will become alopecic again. Another indication of this being a primary hair follicle disorder is that some dogs fail to respond to any medical treatments.

The diagnosis of this disorder is made by ruling out other causes of non-pruritic symmetrical alopecia such as hypothyroidism, hyperadrenocorticism, Sertoli's cell tumors and other gonadal abnormalities, cyclic flank alopecia, follicular dysplasia, postclipping alopecia (if that is indeed a separate entity) and anagen and telogen defluxion. The latter two disorders tend to affect the head and distal extremities, unlike alopecia X.

Presentation of alopecia in certain breeds such as the Pomeranian leads to a high index of suspicion. Cutaneous histopathology will show some degree of flame follicles and miniaturization of hair follicles. Measuring GH is difficult because there are no assays available to my knowledge. Somatomedin C concentrations can be measured. However, Pomeranians have little to no measurable somatomedin C. Also, it may be low secondary to other endocrine imbalances. So this test is of limited value. The adrenal sex hormone panel is available through the University of Tennessee. The panel is expensive, so I recommend doing it if neutering and medical therapy have failed. The test is an ACTH response test with a baseline serum sample, administration of 0.5 IU/kg of cosyntropin (Cortrosyn®) intravenously and a 1 h postcosyntropin serum sample.

Bill Miller *USA* Have the normal ranges for the adrenal sex hormone profile changed?

Lynn Schmeitzel Yes, they have, particularly because the assay was changed.

Regarding treatment, the first step is to neuter an intact animal. The next suggestion is a trial with melatonin. The dose is very empirical. I recommend 3 or 6 mg orally twice a day for small dogs and large dogs, respectively. Side-effects are minimal but include lethargy. I recommend giving melatonin for 2–3 months to effect hair growth. Another treatment is methyltestosterone, but it has potential deleterious side-effects such as hepatotoxicity. I recommend a maximum dose of 30 mg every other day and then decrease it to a maintenance dose once hair growth occurs. Overall, when dogs with alopecia X are treated, hair growth may be stimulated but the coat does not return to its original quality.

[**Lynn Schmeitzel** asked how many people in the audience were using neutering as a treatment and had seen 50% or more of cases respond. Ten people said that they had. When she asked how many of the group were seeing good long-term results, only two people said that they were.]

Wayne Rosenkrantz *USA* I seem to see more dramatic responses from castration than spaying. [Other people noticed no difference.]

Lynn Schmeitzel and Wayne Rosenkrantz In the USA, most female dogs are neutered by 6 months of age, so we have a biased population.

[**Lynn Schmeitzel** asked how many of the group were using melatonin to treat this problem. Approximately 15 people said they were.]

Manon Paradis *Canada* Approximately 40% of the cases I see respond. [Other people said they saw a 20–25% response rate.]

[**Lynn Schmeitzel** asked whether any of the group had seen responses to methyltestosterone. Two or three people had seen very poor responses.]

Wayne Rosenkrantz I see a more dramatic response in dogs with high progesterone and 17-OHP concentrations. I also see a better response with injectable methyltestosterone than when it is given orally. I get the preparation from a local distributor and give it monthly at 1 mg/kg (maximum dose 30 mg) intramuscularly. We have treated approximately 15 dogs this way and have an overall response rate of approximately 20%. I have not seen hepatotoxicity.

Lynn Schmeitzel Mitotane therapy will be discussed later by Dr Rosenkrantz. I feel mitotane is more effective in neutered animals. I use 15–25 mg/kg daily orally for approximately 5–7 days and then do an ACTH response test. Then I start giving a maintenance dose every 4–10 days. Perhaps mitotane only needs to be used to initiate hair growth and should then be discontinued.

Other miscellaneous treatments include prednisone to suppress ACTH and sex hormone production and ketoconazole to alter adrenal steroid production. L-Deprenyl has not been effective in suppressing ACTH production. Gonadotropin agonists suppress gonadotropin release. If the adrenal tissue is sensitive to gonadotropins, then this therapy may be effective. A chow chow I treated with lupronide initially responded but subsequently became refractory to treatment.

Jean Greek *USA* The H_2 antagonist cimetidine has been used successfully on occasions for this disorder. What is its proposed method of action?

Wayne Rosenkrantz I believe it has antiandrogenic effects and I have used it when there has been no response from other treatments and the androgen concentrations were high.

Linda Frank *USA* These are preliminary data on a study evaluating adrenal sex hormone concentrations with alopecia X in different canine breeds. In this study we hope to find more insight into the pathomechanism of the alopecia and if certain abnormalities are seen consistently in certain breeds, it may change our treatment recommendations. Data were taken from adrenal panels submitted to the University of Tennessee. Patients with Cushing's disease, hypothyroidism or sexually intact animals were excluded from this study. Breeds evaluated included the chow chow, cocker spaniel, keeshond, Alaskan malamute, Pomeranian, poodle and samoyed. With the exception of the Pomeranian, poodle and Alaskan malamute, 50% or fewer animals had values outside the normal range. Alaskan malamutes had no abnormal concentrations. Keeshonds had slightly higher estrogen concentrations compared with other breeds. The Pomeranian had higher progesterone and 17-OHP concentrations compared with other breeds. These differences may signify differences in the mechanism of disease in the individual breeds. Also of interest was that not all of the dogs with the characteristic hair loss have adrenal sex hormone abnormalities, which makes me speculate that the alopecia may stem from a dysfunction of the hair follicle, its receptors or the receptor interactions with hormones.

A second study evaluated the response of adrenal sex hormones to ACTH stimulation in neutered Cushing's syndrome patients. The study found that nine of 10 dogs had high concentrations of one or more hormones in the pre- or post-ACTH samples. Testosterone was not increased in any sample. Dihydroepiandrostenedione (DHEAS) was high in two dogs, androstendione was high in five and 17-OHP was high in four. The hormone altered most frequently was progesterone. I speculate that the hair coat changes seen in Cushing's disease may be influenced by which sex hormone(s) is (are) abnormal. I encouraged veterinarians submitting adrenal sex hormone panels to the laboratory from patients with endocrine alopecia to rule out Cushing's disease first. Interestingly, people with Cushing's disease do not have increases in sex hormones.

Trish Ashley *USA* Drs Frank and Schmeitzel and I did a study evaluating the effect of oral melatonin on sex hormone concentrations in dogs. Ten adult, intact dogs (five males, five females) were given 25 mg of melatonin (approximately 1 mg/kg) twice daily for 28 days. Adrenal sex hormone concentrations were measured prior to and on days 7, 14 and 28 of the study. A control group of dogs received a placebo twice daily and adrenal sex hormone concentrations were evaluated on the same days. The hormone concentrations in the treatment and control groups were analysed for significant differences over time. Serum melatonin concentrations were measured in four of the melatonin-treated dogs.

Female dogs treated with melatonin had significant decreases in serum estradiol, testosterone and DHEAS between days 0 and 28. Male dogs treated with melatonin had significant decreases in serum estradiol and 17-OHP between days 0 and 28. Serum melatonin concentrations increased significantly in the dogs tested. I propose that melatonin may affect sex hormone concentrations by enhancing or inhibiting the negative feedback of sex hormones on gonadotropin-releasing hormone (GnRH) from the hypothalamus. Whether melatonin's effect is enhancing or inhibiting may depend upon how the individual species is affected by light. In species that reproduce during long, light days, melatonin inhibits GnRH release. The opposite is true for short-day breeders. A second possible theory is that melatonin affects sex hormone production at the level of adrenal or gonadal tissue. Lastly, it is possible that melatonin influences hair growth by altering hormone concentrations at the level of the hair follicle.

I caution the interpretation of these findings. They should be taken in light of the small number of dogs in the study and the great variation in concentration of sex hormones from individual to individual, especially in intact animals. It would be interesting to do a similar follow-up study using only sexually neutered animals.

Melatonin concentration in the dogs in which it was measured revealed significant increases after oral administration, but the half-life of melatonin is rather short (approximately 8 h). If we need to maintain high serum concentrations of melatonin, administration every 8 h is necessary. However, we do not know if we need to maintain high blood levels of melatonin in order to influence hair growth. No side-effects were noted from the high dose of melatonin.

Unknown participant What was the source of melatonin?

Trish Ashley I used a purified, chemical-grade source, not implants or over-the-counter sources, for purity and consistency. This source is too expensive for practical use.

Unknown participant Were you able to clarify whether some of the changes in steroid hormone concentrations were a direct effect of melatonin on steroid hormone protein binding?

Trish Ashley There was no information on the effect of melatonin on protein binding in my literature searches.

Wayne Rosenkrantz I agree that we tend to include several different alopecias, such as sex hormone imbalances, under the category of alopecia X. I believe that dogs that have postclipping alopecia are in follicular arrest that is not uncovered until they are clipped. I believe these alopecias are due to an interaction of hormones, extrinsic factors and the hair follicle and its receptors. It is the hair follicle and its receptors and their interactions with hormones that need to be studied in normal and abnormally coated dogs before we can understand what is happening in these patients. Some work has been done. I believe Dr Eigenmann was the first to describe the estrogen receptor sites in female dogs with ovarian imbalances and flank alopecia. A limiting factor to this work is the expense; its cost even limits work in the human field of alopecia.

Why do we see the pattern of alopecia that we do? Why is the head unaffected? This, to me, indicates there is more than just hormone imbalance going on. There has to be something happening locally at the hair follicle. A frustrating problem is not being able to measure hormones at the level of the hair follicle. To compound this, it becomes even more confusing because the peripheral hormones are converted to other hormones at the site of the hair follicle. For example, testosterone may be converted peripherally to 17-β-estradiol.

Regarding the pattern of the alopecia, I see many chow chows with alopecia X. They show alopecia especially in areas of friction, for example, under the collar. They tend to have varying degrees of alopecia, hyperpigmentation and a dull coat. It has been mentioned that traumatizing the skin, such as by skin biopsy, stimulates hair growth. However, if we look at the hair regrowth at the biopsy site, it is not normal. There are soluble hair growth factors in fibroblasts that can be found at the level of the dermal papillae of the follicle, so trauma may influence follicle–receptor interaction and stimulate hair to grow, but is not correcting the basic problem.

I have seen alopecia in a neutered male Arctic fox. It looked very much like alopecia X. The head and extremities were fairly normal but, on the body, the coat was dull with loss of primary hairs. Thyroid function was borderline low based on canine values and the fox was receiving thyroid supplementation. ACTH stimulation testing was normal. Adrenal panels have not been done. We put the fox on melatonin 4–6 weeks prior to this meeting and there was minor regrowth of hair. As a side note, I have not seen the superficial pyoderma associated with alopecia X that Dr Schmeitzel mentioned previously.

Regarding treatment of alopecia X, many different drugs may be effective. Most of us first spay or neuter an intact animal. I believe that the dogs that respond to neutering tend to grow a nicer hair coat than the dogs that we treat medically. I have used GH with some success. It is difficult to acquire and can create diabetes mellitus. There is a source of GH in the Los Angeles area. I have not used it for several years. I have used ketoconazole with no success. I have treated a few cases with prednisone and it has helped some dogs. What is the mechanism? Perhaps, as mentioned previously, there is a central effect of prednisone on the hypothalamus or pituitary gland and their products. I use melatonin at approximately the same dose as others who use it. Approximately 25% or fewer of my cases respond to it. Responses to methyltestosterone are 20% or less. I use it when I have done the adrenal panel and find high progesterone or 17-OHP, because progesterone has reported antiandrogen effects. I use the injectable form of methyltestosterone. Occasionally I will try estrogen (diethylstilbestrol) and I use the urinary incontinence protocol.

The drug I use most often is Lysodren® (mitotane). Over time I have become more conservative with dosing with this drug, not because of side-effects but because it works at a lower dosage. Initially, I used 25 mg/kg per day for 5–7 days. Now I use a dose of 15 mg/kg per day for 2–3 days and then do an ACTH stimulation test on day 4 or 5. I aim for 138–276 nmol/l (5–10 μg/dl) of cortisol post-ACTH. I also agree with Dr Schmeitzel that some dogs just need to be kick-started and can come off the mitotane once hair has started to grow, while in others the hair-coat deteriorates when the drug is stopped. I keep a number of dogs on a pulse dose of mitotane (10–15 mg/kg) every 14 days. I divide my maintenance dose and give it two to three times a week for both alopecia X and Cushing's patients. I find my Cushing's patients have much better control and fewer side-effects when maintained this way. Most patients take 2–3 months to respond to mitotane, although some respond more quickly. Certainly, we have a significant number of failures and that is when we try other medications. I recall a spayed female Pomeranian that we treated with all medications already mentioned and the dog spontaneously regrew hair years later. Again, most of the patients that regrow hair are more cosmetically acceptable to the owners but do not develop a normal coat.

Manon Paradis I am going to talk about melatonin and pattern alopecia. The textbooks describe three possible syndromes of pattern alopecia. The first is a pinnal alopecia of the dachshund and Chihuahua. I have seen three or four of these in the past 20 years. It occurs in young dogs. The pinnae become progressively alopecic and hyperpigmented. I have not treated any of these with melatonin. I have seen one case spontaneously regrow hair. I see this syndrome more in Siamese cats.

Wayne Rosenkrantz Melatonin has worked in a few cases I have treated and not worked in many others.

Manon Paradis The second syndrome is an alopecia of the American water spaniel and Portuguese water dog. Alopecia is restricted to the ventral neck, medial thighs and tail and starts at a young age. In the Irish water spaniel, hypotrichosis of the tail and ventral neck is a breed standard. I think it is likely that all these breeds are closely related and I suspect they are genetically programmed to have pattern alopecia. I have no experience using melatonin in this syndrome.

The third syndrome is seen more commonly and occurs in female dogs that develop alopecia of the postauricular area, ventral neck, thorax and medial thighs. It also starts at young age in short-coated breeds (e.g. the dachshund, Boston terrier and boxer). The differential diagnoses are follicular dysplasia and colour dilution alopecia. However, I wonder whether this is the same condition as estrogen-responsive dermatosis (ovarian imbalance type 2). They look the same in textbook pictures, except estrogen-responsive dermatosis is seen in older females spayed earlier in life. I have never diagnosed type 2 ovarian imbalance. Do members of the group believe type 2 ovarian imbalance and syndrome 3 of pattern alopecia are the same or different diseases? [There was no consensus among the participants.]

Bill Miller A pattern alopecia should not respond to estrogen and most cases of this type of alopecia are a pattern alopecia rather than ovarian imbalance type 2. The two diseases do exist but most of the animals we see are pattern alopecias and not estrogen-responsive conditions.

Manon Paradis So, perhaps we can agree that, after careful questioning of the owner, most of the dachshunds we see with this problem developed it at a young age and there may be a few cases in which the alopecia resolves or fluctuates in intensity over time.

To diagnose this problem I do not feel a biopsy is very useful. The biopsy often leaves a scar where hair will not grow back. I prefer to use my clinical impression for diagnosis. In the textbooks, the histopathology of pattern alopecia is a miniaturization of the hair follicle, whereas in estrogen-responsive alopecia there is an altered appearance of the hair follicle. I question that these descriptions may be different degrees of the same disease.

I used melatonin in this disorder rather by accident. I was treating two boxers for cyclic flank alopecia with melatonin and their concurrent pattern baldness (on the chest) responded. So I did a pilot study using melatonin implants in dogs with pattern baldness. Several responded, including boxers, Chihuahuas and a greyhound. Some skin hyperpigmentation reduced as well. One dog improved maximally after 6 months of treatment. Some lost hair again after stopping the melatonin; others did not, especially two boxers. Whether, and for how long, melatonin will work in these cases is unpredictable. I estimate that 70–75% of dogs with this form of pattern alopecia respond well. The drug seems to be very safe.

Karen Helton-Rhodes *USA* Some 50–60% of greyhounds with 'bald thigh syndrome' will spontaneously regrow hair several months after being adopted from the track. I believe that greyhound skin disease has not been studied well enough to categorize their alopecia as a pattern alopecia.

Alan Mundell *USA* I see many greyhounds recently removed from the track that have received much exogenous androgenic stimulation that may be contributing to their alopecia.

Karen Helton-Rhodes If you look at literature given to adoptive greyhound owners, there is a long list of drugs and supplements the new owners are told to give to these dogs. There are many things that could affect hair growth.

Linda Frank In ancient history, when men were castrated, it was noted that any male pattern baldness present at the time of castration did not reverse after castration. So, stopping androgen treatment may not be what is permitting hair regrowth.

Alan Mundell I am going to talk about cyclic flank alopecia. I see much cyclic flank alopecia in the Seattle, Washington, area and I believe we see more in the northern latitudes. I see it in a number of different breeds (boxers, bulldogs, Labrador retrievers and pugs) and it is not always seasonal. Some dogs may become alopecic at different times of the year and some may not develop the condition every year. It can be a diffuse or partial, symmetrical or asymmetrical alopecia. The site of the alopecia may vary during the cycle: what I call a 'lava lamp effect'.

Many bulldogs and boxers lose hair starting in late spring and regrow it in the late summer. Others, especially Labrador retrievers, begin losing hair in late autumn and winter and regrow it in the spring. Melatonin seems to work on both groups. The summer-cycling dogs regrow hair on melatonin faster than we would expect them to. Melatonin has been effective in approximately 70% of my cases. I use up to 0.5 mg/kg twice daily, but I usually start with a lower dose. If the history of alopecia is a seasonal one, I will start treating 2 months ahead of the predicted time of development of the alopecia. I keep some dogs on melatonin all year and that has controlled the alopecia as well.

Tony Yu *USA* I use injectable melatonin at 10 mg/ml subcutaneously in an alcohol base with dimethylsulfoxide (DMSO). I give an injection every 2 weeks, for three injections. Is there a standard way of measuring melatonin?

Trish Ashley In our study, I used a research-only kit for measuring melatonin that was both expensive and difficult to obtain at that time. More recent work in validating a melatonin assay was done by Dr Juli Gunter when she was at Auburn. They used a different kit and I believe the endocrinology laboratory there validated the assay.

Karen Helton-Rhodes Has anybody used melatonin in horses with partial facial and head alopecia? This alopecia is a fairly common problem. [None of the participants had used melatonin for this problem.]

Kerstin Bergvall *Sweden* In Sweden, I have two horses that develop recurrent hypotrichosis (thin, miniaturized hairs, not complete alopecia) of the face and thighs every autumn that resolves in the spring.

Alan Mundell Tony Yu and I consulted with a nutritionist at the San Diego zoo, where there was a bear that developed recurrent, seasonal flank alopecia in November. Melatonin was considered cautiously because it is not to be used during pregnancy and interferes with reproduction.

5.5
Treatment options for hyperadrenocorticism

Ralf S. Mueller[1] (Chairperson) and Michael A. Shipstone[2] (Secretary)

[1] Colorado State University, Fort Collins, Colorado, USA
[2] Dermatology for Animals, Brisbane, Queensland, Australia

Ralf Mueller *USA* We will start this workshop on treatment options for hyperadrenocorticism with three short presentations. The first will be a brief overview on o,p′-DDD (mitotane or Lysodren®) by Dominique Heripret.

Dominique Heripret *France* I will present my own opinions on treating these cases.

There are many different protocols and many very large-scale studies reporting the use of o,p′-DDD. In my hands it is very rare to have side-effects if it is used carefully. Furthermore, I do not use concurrent glucocorticoid supplementation, making control and the interpretation of monitoring tests easier. The problems associated with this drug are cost and relapses, and these will be covered later.

o,p′-DDD is fat soluble and therefore must be given with food and fat as there is minimal absorption of the drug if given on an empty stomach. Fat absorption decreases as the disease is controlled. Thus, early in treatment with the disease uncontrolled, the drug is more easily absorbed. As it is brought under control, fat absorption and therefore drug absorption is decreased. Thus, with time, the maintenance dosage may need to be adjusted and increased.

Discussion with owners is very important and should cover a number of things. The disease is chronic and there is no urgency to treat it. Thus, if the owner observes any problem, the treatment should be stopped while assessment is carried out. If the abnormality is not associated with o,p′-DDD, treatment can begin again. If induction is going smoothly, always monitor progress with an adrenocorticotropic hormone (ACTH) stimulation test after the first 10 days. o,p′-DDD accumulates in body fat with time and thus there is a lag effect once the drug is stopped, i.e. it continues to work for a period after it is withdrawn. Owners should monitor water input and urine output during induction. Costs of treatment and monitoring must be explained. An ACTH stimulation test should be carried out 10 days after beginning induction, then 1 month after beginning induction and every 3–4 months thereafter.

It is important to remember that one is treating a particular dog, not a population with the same disease. Each animal will have its own unique presentation and problems. A thorough examination of the dog and its problems will determine the dosage that should be used for induction. For example, a dog that is very ill from the disease should be treated with a lower induction dose (e.g. 15 mg/kg every 12 h). If this lower induction dose is used, it must be continued for longer, e.g. 3–4 weeks. This dose has the advantage of giving a smoother induction, with less risk of side-effects, and should be easier for the owner to monitor with less risk of overdosage. A lower induction dose may also be recommended to owners who find the treatment protocol difficult to understand. However, I do not find this lower dose to work as well as my normal induction dose of 25 mg/kg every 12 h.

Other treatment options include radiotherapy, ketoconazole and L-Deprenyl. Radiotherapy is satisfactory for microadenomas where dogs have neurological signs. I feel more confident using radiotherapy than pituitary surgery, as radiotherapy can be done at the same cost but with less morbidity. I have only treated two dogs with hyperadrenocorticism using radiotherapy and both have no signs 12 months later.

I use ketoconazole at 30 mg/kg per day, but increase the dose slowly over 2–3 weeks for cases with adrenal tumours, either to prepare for adrenal surgery, in cases where the owners do not want surgery, or if there is metastasis. I find approximately 50% of cases with adrenal tumours do not respond to ketoconazole.

I have been very disappointed with L-Deprenyl in treating Cushing's disease, but have been happy with its effect on behavioural changes and general attitude of the dogs. In the cat it may be interesting as the drug is only acting on the posterior pituitary gland, but there are no published studies and the number of cats with spontaneous hyperadrenocorticism is low.

I find that o,p′-DDD is not well tolerated in approximately 10% of cases, so trilostane, which will be discussed later, may be an interesting alternative.

Greg Burton *Australia* I will present a study involving six dogs diagnosed with pituitary-dependent hyperadrenocorticism (PDH). The aim of the study was to determine whether what we use as a clinical endpoint in o,p′-DDD induction correlates with a laboratory endpoint as measured by ACTH stimulation testing.

Six dogs were hospitalised for 5 days prior to induction. During this time, they were fed twice daily and their food and water intake was assessed. The clinical criteria for induction treatment with o,p′-DDD were reduced appetite, increased time taken to eat and reduction in water intake to less than 60 ml/kg per day. However, we noted that some of the dogs that were polydipsic at home were not so in the hospital setting. Thus, water intake was found to be a poor clinical criterion and reliance on behaviour and enthusiasm to eat was used.

The treatment protocol was the administration of o,p′-DDD at approximately 35 mg/kg per day (range 33–44 mg/kg per day) divided into two equal doses every 12 h. An ACTH stimulation test was performed each day. Blood was separated and the samples were batched. Thus, clinical parameters were the sole means of assessing the endpoint, with the ACTH stimulation test results available only after the trial had been completed.

The aims of the trial were: to determine whether the plasma cortisol level dropped in a linear fashion and whether this could enable paired ACTH stimulation tests done early in induction to be used as a predictor of the likely length of induction; to determine whether plasma cortisol levels continued to decrease after o,p′-DDD was stopped, and whether the clinical parameters used to determine the endpoint were valid.

The results of the study showed that the plasma cortisol levels tended to drop in a somewhat linear fashion. Some dogs responded very rapidly (e.g. in 3 days). The laboratory endpoint was reached 1.5–2 days prior to the recognised clinical endpoint. The plasma cortisol levels continued to fall for 2 days after withdrawal of o,p′-DDD.

As a result of this trial, we now tend to test very early in the treatment protocol, somewhere between days 5 and 7. This is graphed and compared to the pretreatment values to see whether the induction period can be predicted.

Rosario Cerundolo *Italy* I will talk about the use of trilostane for the treatment of hyperadrenocorticism.

Trilostane is available as either a 60 mg or 120 mg capsule. It has been used in humans for the treatment of hyperadrenocorticism and postmenopausal breast cancer. After administration, it is rapidly absorbed and is concentrated in the adrenal, liver, lungs and kidney. It is metabolised by the liver and excreted by the kidney. Administration is recommended with food, as it is a gastric irritant. Trilostane inhibits steroidogenesis and, therefore, also interferes with the production of aldosterone and sex hormones. However, apparently this block is not as strong as its inhibition of cortisol synthesis.

The following trial was carried out. Twenty-two dogs with clinical signs and laboratory results consistent with hyperadrenocorticism were entered into the study. Three dogs had adrenal tumours and 19 had PDH. In four cases, there was concurrent disease: two had diabetes mellitus and two had mild renal failure.

Dogs were dosed with trilostane as follows: those less than 5 kg were given 30 mg/dog per day; 5–15 kg, 60 mg/dog per day; 15–40 kg, 120 mg/dog per day and greater than 40 kg, 240 mg/dog per day. Examinations were carried out at 10 days, and 4, 12, 24 and 48 weeks after beginning treatment. At each visit, a complete blood count (CBC), multiple biochemistry analysis (MBA), urine analysis (UA) and an ACTH stimulation test were performed.

All dogs treated showed reduction in polyuria, polydipsia, polyphagia and panting, increased activity and hair regrowth.

Three dogs with adrenal tumours were treated for 30 days. Two dogs had surgery at that time. The third owner refused surgery and elected to continue trilostane, and the dog continues to do well. Nineteen dogs with PDH have been treated. Eight have been on therapy for more than 24 weeks and 11 for more than 12 weeks.

On ACTH stimulation testing, occasionally an individual that was apparently well controlled clinically would show a high cortisol peak, which would be within the normal range when the dog was retested. The reason for this is not obvious. In one dog the plasma cortisol level was not controlled. Doubling the dose of trilostane for 1 month did not produce any improvement, at which time the owner elected for euthanasia. There was a progressive reduction in serum alkaline phosphatase (ALP), alanine aminotransferase (ALT), cholesterol and triglyceride concentrations, but no change in electrolyte values. No abnormalities were detected on UA. Side-effects observed were weakness in one dog (when the drug was slightly overdosed) and vomiting in one dog (when the drug was not given with food).

Overall, 17 of 22 dogs showed a good response to trilostane therapy. The owners of the two dogs with diabetes mellitus elected for euthanasia, as the diabetes was not controlled despite good reduction in cortisol levels. The two dogs with mild renal failure continued to deteriorate and died. In one dog, there was no change despite doubling the dose of the drug.

Thus, we can conclude that trilostane is effective in the treatment of hyperadrenocorticism. It has reversible side-effects, so even if hypoadrenocorticism is induced, drug withdrawal leads to resolution. Sex hormone status does not seem to be affected.

Ralf Mueller We will begin the round-table part of the forum by discussing the use of o,p′-DDD. At least 90–95% of my cases of PDH end up on o,p′-DDD. We would all agree that there is an induction dose and a maintenance dose. However, I have had a few clients who were not observant and I have ended up giving an intermediate maintenance dose that resulted in symptoms not being controlled for a year or two. For example, instead of giving 25 mg/kg every 12 h for 5–10 days, we have not used daily induction but rather used this dose twice weekly until the dog responds. The two cases in which I have used this did not control well. Is anyone else using no induction but rather just twice-weekly maintenance?

Dominique Heripret I believe that the goal of treatment of o,p′-DDD is adrenal destruction. If this is not done, then control will not be achieved. [No one else in the audience had used this approach.]

Cecilia Friberg *USA* Does anyone adjust their maintenance dose based on the level of cortisol that is achieved after ACTH stimulation, e.g. using a higher dose if there are high stimulation results?

Ralf Mueller I just use a standard 25 mg/kg every 12 h regardless of the stimulation results.

Dominique Heripret I do not believe that the ACTH stimulation test is a criterion to select the induction dose. I do not believe that I have seen any difference in the ease of induction based on the stimulation results.

Ralf Mueller I even believe that the length of induction is independent of the stimulation results.

Joe Bruner *USA* Dr Burton's results did not show any correlation between the initial ACTH stimulation results and the induction dosage.

Claire Seifert *USA* Has anybody noticed any breed sensitivity with respect to the induction dosage? [No one in the group had seen this.]

Ralf Mueller What do we recommend for owners to monitor during induction? I think we all agree that food and water intake is necessary. I believe that we all agree that if water intake drops below 60 mg/kg per day, induction is stopped. I think that what is more controversial is, how do you look at food intake? For example, some people feel that the dog must be anorexic before stopping the induction dosage. Others believe any reduction in the amount of food consumed or increase in the length of time in eating are indicators of the end-point. What are the group's criteria and do you recommend giving less food during the induction phase?

Giovanni Ghibaudo *Italy* I have the owners monitor food intake for at least 7 days prior to the start of induction. I also have them monitor for lethargy, a decrease in the amount of food eaten, an increase in the time to eat and a decrease in water intake.

Ralf Mueller I think that that is a very good point: we should have the average of at least a week of these various parameters pretreatment on which to judge subsequent changes.

Michael Shipstone *Australia* One point that should also be considered is that some of these animals may be suffering from renal medullary washout. So, reliance on water intake should not be overemphasised, as it may not fall, even though induction therapy may have been successfully completed. I have had one case where polyuria/polydipsia remained at the end of the loading dose, which was then judged by change in the appetite.

Ralf Mueller I instruct the owners to watch for changes in any of the parameters as an indicator of successful loading. From a practical viewpoint, we normally see any adverse effects or expected side-effects of induction approximately 3–7 days after starting. Thus, we have the owners start induction on Saturday so that these signs are generally seen between Tuesday and Saturday, when I am available immediately.

Cecilia Friberg I would like to discuss what might be a different subgroup of Cushing's dogs: those that present with recurrent pyoderma and that do not necessarily have polyuria/polydipsia. Thus, monitoring these animals using changes in clinical signs is very difficult. In these dogs, I use a lower induction dose (12.5 mg/kg every 12 h) and carry out ACTH stimulation testing much sooner (in the 5–7 day range). I have had reluctance from referring veterinarians to treat these dogs. So the next question is, should we treat these dogs?

Ralf Mueller I would treat these dogs because I believe I can achieve better control when they are in their early stages of disease. I monitor these dogs by food intake and feed a little less than normal, because in my experience even dogs that just present with pyoderma are very good eaters.

Dominique Heripret I don't agree. In my experience, it is very rare to have an animal with just pyoderma with hyperadrenocorticism without polyuria/polydipsia. It may be that these animals have adrenal hyperplasia causing abnormal ACTH stimulation results. I would wait for these dogs to develop polyuria/polydipsia before treating with o,p′-DDD. For me, recurrent pyoderma is not a sign of hyperadrenocorticism.

Joe Bruner *USA* I do not agree. I am an internist and my wife is a dermatologist. We each see a different population of Cushing's syndrome dogs. The ones referred to me are those with classic polyuria/polydipsia/polyphagia, pot-belly, poor joints, etc. The ones referred to my wife are those with recurrent pyoderma, alopecia, etc. I believe those dogs are truly cushingoid. They have more than just adrenal hyperplasia. They respond to o,p′-DDD, they have appropriate response to ACTH stimulation as part of normal induction protocols and get resolution of their recurrent pyoderma off antibiotics once the Cushing's syndrome has been controlled. I do not believe that there is one classic appearance of a cushingoid dog.

Ralf Mueller I would also disagree with Dominique. I rarely see the pot-bellied, polydipsic dogs. I see dogs with recurrent pyoderma. Possibly it is a reflection of the type of practice, having been working in a skin-only clinic for a long time. I see those cases with primarily skin abnormalities. Anything more classic is seen by the internists. I would expect that without treatment for Cushing's syndrome, the more classic signs would subsequently be seen.

Does anyone send cortisone home with clients when starting induction therapy. [No one in the group did.] What does the group use as a loading dose of o,p′-DDD?

Dominique Heripret I have had one case with PDH where initially I had to increase to 75 mg/kg per day and finally ended up using 100 mg/kg per day to successfully load the dog. This same dog was then maintained on 100 mg/kg twice weekly. I have also had an occasional case where a higher dose was required.

Does anyone use urine cortisol creatinine ratios (UCCR) in the diagnosis of Cushing's syndrome?

Ralf Mueller I use this test as a rule-out. For example, if I have a case of recurrent pyoderma and want to rule out the possibility of Cushing's syndrome, I will do the test. If it is negative, I believe that Cushing's syndrome has been completely ruled out. If it is positive and there is no other abnormality, e.g. liver or renal disease, I may investigate Cushing's syndrome a little further. I never diagnose Cushing's syndrome based on my UCCR. I will sometimes do a low-dose dexamethasone suppression test based on the UCCR.

Joe Bruner This is not a good screening test but is rather used for ruling out the disease.

Ralf Mueller Once induction has been achieved we move to maintenance. Do most people use a weekly dose? [Most people agreed they use 25 mg/kg twice daily on one day of the week.]

Diana Brown *UK* I use twice-weekly administration but still see relapses.

Dominique Heripret I generally use 25 mg/kg twice daily on one day of the week, but will use it twice a week if induction has taken longer than 15 days.

Ralf Mueller Once on maintenance, what percentage can be left at the same dose without adjustment and without relapse?

Dominique Heripret Between 0 and 10%. [There was general agreement in the group.]

Ralf Mueller Dominique, I was very interested in your earlier presentation in which you stated that animals absorb less and less o,p′-DDD as they come under control, and this was a very nice way to remind me that I may need to increase the dose to maintain control. How often do we monitor cases with an ACTH stimulation test?

Dominique Heripret I monitor at 4 and 8 weeks postinduction and if these results are satisfactory I repeat this test every 4 months.

Diana Brown I like to repeat the test every 3 months for the first year and if all is still going well I may reduce to every 4 months in the second year.

Teodora Muret *Switzerland* Is anyone aware of a potential for cardiotoxicity using o,p′-DDD?

Joe Bruner The original investigation showed direct neurotoxicity but I am not aware of any evidence of cardiotoxicity.

Ralf Mueller I would now like to discuss L-Deprenyl. I agree with Dominique: I have not found it to be effective. I have talked to David Church, who agrees with you that L-Deprenyl may appear to the owner to alleviate some of the symptoms of Cushing's disease, but there is no evidence that the disease is controlled.

Rosario Cerundolo As L-Deprenyl works only on tumours of the pars intermedia, the chance for it to be effective in most cases of Cushing's syndrome is very low.

Dominique Heripret I believe that it could only work very early in the disease. Once a tumour has formed, I do not believe that it would be able to exert control. We know that from the studies of Curtis and others that the incidence of pars intermedia tumours is 25–30% so that at the most, it could only work in 25% of case, if it works at all. I do not think that this is a drug for the treatment of Cushing's disease in the dog. However, it may be interesting for possible use in the cat.

Mike Wallace *USA* (Technical Services, Pfizer) It is my impression that improvement rates that can be expected are as previously mentioned: 25–30%, but this improvement is only transitory (6–12 months). I have heard people say they that use it as a bridge to o,p′-DDD. Furthermore, it should not affect the ACTH stimulation test and in fact very rarely affects the plasma cortisol level to any great degree.

Ralf Mueller I know that some dermatologists will use the drug in some very early Cushing's syndrome cases where, for whatever reason, o,p′-DDD is not being used, and then switch to o,p′-DDD subsequently.

Claire Seifert My impression is that there is some delay at the start of therapy before any benefits are seen.

Rosario Cerundolo How long do you wait before doubling the dose? It is suggested to use 1 mg/kg and if this is not effective to increase to 2 mg/kg.

Dominique Heipret Statistically, there was no difference between the 1 and 2 mg/kg dose rate in the first or second studies.

Mike Wallace The confusion may be being caused by the dose rate for cognitive dysfunction syndrome (CDS), the treatment of which has a variable dose range. So, if an improvement is not seen at the low dose after 1 month or so, the dose may then be increased.

Ralf Mueller We will now move to ketoconazole. I use this drug as a preparation for adrenalectomy, so I don't have much experience of its use in PDH dogs. The problem I have with ketoconazole is its side-effects. If you read Feldman, the side-effects are not a problem. Dogs presented to my skin clinic vomit severely if dosed at 20 mg/kg. I see nausea and vomiting even if I increase the dose slowly in a significant percentage of cases. In the 10–20 mg/kg range, I would see 30% adverse reactions.

Hui-P Haung *Taiwan* It is difficult to access o,p′-DDD in Taiwan, so ketoconazole is the primary treatment there. I have a case of PDH that I have been treating for the past 3 years with ketoconazole. I think that 80% of my cases are doing well on it.

Joe Bruner What dose do you use? I very rarely use 30 mg/kg as recommended, but usually dose at around 15–20 mg/kg and use an ACTH stimulation to assess control.

Hui-P Haung I usually use 2–3 weeks of 5 mg/kg every 12 h and then increase to 10–15 mg/kg every 12 h. The most common side-effect seen is vomiting. I would estimate that we are able to successfully control 80% of affected dogs using this drug, but will continue therapy for at least 2 months before considering it ineffective.

5.6

Teaching veterinary dermatology to students and residents

Donna W. Angarano[1] (Chairperson) and Karen L. Campbell[2] (Secretary)

[1] College of Veterinary Medicine, Auburn University, Auburn, Alabama, USA
[2] Department of Veterinary Clinical Medicine, College of Veterinary Medicine, University of Illinois, Urbana, Illinois, USA

Donna Angarano *USA* The goals of this workshop are to have an open discussion and to share methods of teaching veterinary dermatology to students and residents. We will also ask practitioners in the group to help us identify how well we are doing in preparing new graduates for clinical practice.

The first topic for discussion will be what techniques have we found helpful in teaching didactic courses to veterinary students. For example, I utilize unannounced three to four point quizzes in my lectures to help maintain student attention. We also give homework assignments that are worth three to four points per assignment. I have also obtained feedback on what students are learning by asking them to identify three things they learned in the lecture that day, write them down and return the list to me.

Gene Nesbitt *USA* Perhaps homework assignments could be completed and submitted online.

Sandra Merchant *USA* I use e-mail to communicate with students. A portion of our curriculum is problem-based case work-ups. Students work in groups of six to eight students. I provide a basic history. The student groups then contact me via e-mail with any additional questions they want to ask. Later I send them physical examination findings and they contact me with their problem list and the diagnostic tests they want. I require them to provide me with specific information on how they will perform the tests. The work-up of a case may continue over several weeks. Cases selected for first-year students are textbook examples, cases for second-year students will include some unexpected findings and cases for third-year students are real-life with findings that may not be classical or fit the diagnosis. Grading is done with one examination on content (approximately 30%), a self-review (5%), peer review by other group members (10%), facilitator grade (20%) and a group grade on how well they did with major learner issues (problem list, differentials, etc.) (approximately 30%).

Gila Zur *Israel* I use a similar case-based teaching method with small groups of students working together. The students present their findings to the entire class at the end of their dermatology section.

Michael Goldschmidt *USA* We also teach dermatopathology using student groups. Each group discusses changes and abnormalities on the case material (glass slides) assigned to them. They then present the case to the entire class. I encourage ways to liven things up. I invite the clinical dermatologists to present a short summary of the clinical findings of the diseases the students have been studying.

Terry Grieshaber *USA* One comment regarding teaching students problem-based learning in groups is that some students have difficulty in making the transition to independent thought and solo case management. I see this in some of the students who come to my practice for externships.

Geneviève Marignac *France* I have third-year students use a digital camera to photograph a case and prepare Power Point® presentations of the case for their peers.

Hilary Jackson *USA* I have rewritten learning objectives to be more concept oriented and thought provoking by encouraging comparing, contrasting and explaining rather than listing type answers.

Michael Goldschmidt I have found it helpful for instructors to review the notes taken by assigned note-takers.

Donna Angarano Our next topic for discussion is on methods of testing. I have provided you with samples of test questions submitted to me by faculty from several universities. A variety of testing methods are being used, including multiple choice, kodachrome-based, fill-in-the blank, short-answer and essay questions.

Karen Moriello *USA* I have provided samples of case-based examinations. Grading is based on how well the students meet six criteria: (1) identifying major clinical abnormalities and problems from the history and physical examination; (2) formulating a list of appropriate differential diagnoses for each problem; (3) formulating a list of appropriate diagnostic tests and procedures for the listed problems; (4) appropriate interpretation of laboratory data and diagnostic tests; (5) integration of history, physical examination findings and laboratory data in diagnosing the patient's problem; and (6) the treatment plan appropriate for the diagnoses. Students are required to pass one small-animal and one large-animal case to pass the course.

Donna Angarano The next topic for discussion is sharing of ideas that have been successfully used in clinical rotations. One that I have used is 'Dermatology Jeopardy'. We have two or three teams of two or three students. Teams can select from categories of questions with varying point values (e.g. large animals, parasitology, endocrinology, name that breed, starts with 'A', infectious agents, neoplasia, stop that itch, name that drug, immune-mediated, starts with 'P', stop that flea, etc.). We use regular jeopardy with five questions in each category worth one to five points, double jeopardy with five questions per category worth two to 10 points, and final jeopardy with students' wagers based on current points. We give candy as prizes for the winning team.

Gregory Campbell *USA* We have found it helpful when pathologists are called into the clinics to see cases with the clinicians.

Karen Moriello We send students out on two field trips. The first is to a specialty pet store to investigate a category of products (e.g. shampoos, flea control products, diets). The second is to a university garden with a list of plants to find and identify (e.g. pollinating plants associated with aeroallergens). Another teaching technique we are now using is having students investigate reviewing and responding to consultation requests submitted to the university using a faxed consultation request form.

Gene Nesbitt I require students to review several programs that are available through the World Wide Web (e.g. cases posted by Michael Lorenz from Oklahoma State University, structure and function schematics from the Ohio State University, cases from Georgia) and as interactive CDs

Richard Halliwell *UK* We are also working on interactive CDs.

Sandra Merchant Louisiana State University has an elective course for first-year students in which the students go to a local animal control facility and are able to do skin scrapings, cytology and skin biopsies using recently euthanized animals.

Michael Goldschmidt The University of Pennsylvania has a digitalized network drive, with photographs posted by the clinical dermatologists, available for students to view when studying dermatohistopathology. We used to have more regular rounds involving clinicians and pathologists as we reviewed recent surgical biopsy submissions.

Donna Angarano On to another topic: what are some of the advantages and disadvantages of non-degree and concurrent degree-based residency training programs?

Richard Halliwell A problem with combined programs has been participants dropping out of the programs after the clinical years. It is extremely difficult for an individual to complete a PhD program when 3–6 month clinical service blocks are interspersed with research blocks. It is probably best to have separate clinical training and research training segments to education. In the UK, thesis papers cannot be used to fulfill publication requirements for the specialty boards.

Hilary Jackson The combined programs have difficulty in attracting candidates. Combined PhD and residency programs require a structured program and a disciplined individual.

Peter Hill *UK* A 3 year combined program is often not enough time to complete writing a thesis. Following completion of 2 years of clinical training, many residents have lost interest in doing graduate work and research.

Karen Campbell *USA* The combined master's degree and residency training program at the University of Illinois has been successful. Courses taken in the graduate-training program are directly applicable in preparation for the dermatology certification examination. Having assigned courses provides the program with structure and the opportunity for sharing of ideas with graduate students in ancillary areas (pathology, food animal, equine, oncology, internal medicine, etc.).

Karen Moriello The time demands of clinics and cases can greatly interfere with graduate training.

Donna Angarano The 3 year combined master's degree and residency has been successful at Auburn University. Structured classes are a valuable addition to the training program.

Sandra Merchant If the residents and mentors are committed to protecting time set aside for training in the precepts of dermatology, 2 years of training can achieve all the requirements to be an excellent program. The faculty and residents at Louisiana State University like their 2 year programs.

Donna Angarano We are nearing the end of our time for this workshop. The final topic is to discuss what we are doing well in training students and to identify any shortcomings.

Chris Chesney *UK* Too many recent graduates and practitioners try to make diagnoses by response to treatment. They also do not know when and where to take skin biopsies, they misinterpret test results, and have a lack of fundamental training in the basic structure and function of the skin.

Sandra Merchant Students often do not recognize the relevance of the material they are being taught.

Hilary Jackson It is important for us to integrate information from the first 2 years of basic science coursework into our clinical courses.

Terry Grieshaber Another problem comes from clinical instructors in general practice or community practice at a university who are teaching inappropriate approaches to case management in a university setting. Referring veterinarians have often failed to do basics such as skin scrapings and dermatophyte cultures.

Mona Boord *USA* It is disheartening that many students do not seem interested in learning when an instructor takes extra time in trying to teach them about such basics as selecting otic preparations.

Sandra Merchant Universities that do not have enough teaching time for dermatology may find it helpful to do surveys documenting the importance of dermatology in clinical practice. This can help to convince administrators of the need to increase student contact time with dermatologists.

5.7

Novel and non-traditional therapies in veterinary dermatology

Hans-Joachim Koch (Chairperson) and Stefanie Peters (Secretary)

Tierärztliche Klinik, Am Schönenwald, Birkenfeld, Germany

Hans Koch *Germany* Let me first give a short introduction to this workshop. We are going to be talking about a difficult topic: novel and non-traditional therapies. It was not easy to get formal short contributions from colleagues. It seems that in the eyes of many people, 'new' or 'novel' means 'not yet explored' and makes people reluctant to present new material. So I am very grateful to the following colleagues who will present some of their work: Regina Wagner, Mona Boord, Stephen White and Jacques Fontaine.

We plan four short presentations, of about 10 min each, so hopefully we will have enough time for a detailed discussion of all topics. I want to encourage everybody in this room to participate and share his or her experiences with us.

Regina Wagner *Austria* spoke about the use of oral terbinafine in treating cats with *Microsporum canis* infection. Terbinafine (Lamisil®, Novartis) is an antimycotic drug that has been used in Europe since 1991 against fungal infections in humans, especially nail mycoses. Its mode of action is unique: terbinafine works by selective inhibition of the fungal enzyme squalene epoxidase (thus working one step earlier than the azoles), leading to an accumulation of squalene in fungal cells, subsequent cell membrane damage and cell death.

Terbinafine is highly lipophilic. After absorption, it diffuses from the blood to the dermis, epidermis and sebum, but not to sweat. In nails, it reaches therapeutic concentrations after 4 weeks of therapy and remains for up to 36 weeks after its cessation. The drug is eliminated in the faeces and urine. Terbinafine shows only a mild inhibition of the cytochrome P-450 enzymes.

There are some important drug interactions to consider. If combined with cimetidine, the dose of terbinafine should be decreased, whereas it needs to be increased when used in combination with rifampicin. The currently recommended dose for dogs and cats (extrapolated from the human dose) is 10–25 mg/kg per day, divided into two or three doses.

In the study I will present (carried out at the University of Vienna), two doses of terbinafine (12.5 and 25 mg/kg per day) were compared with standard griseofulvin therapy (60 mg/kg per day) in 58 cats with dermatophytosis due to *Microsporum canis*. The duration of therapy required to reach two consecutive negative fungal cultures was compared.

Group 1 (seven cats) received 12.5 mg/kg terbinafine per day and required 54 days of therapy, group 2 (26 cats) received 25 kg/kg terbinafine per day and required 56 days, and group 3 (25 cats, control group) received 60 mg/kg griseofulvin per day and required 63 days. Based on these results, it was concluded that terbinafine is effective in the therapy of feline dermatophytosis. Fewer days of therapy were required compared to griseofulvin and no changes in liver enzymes were observed.

Tiffany Tapp *USA* Do you have experience with pulse therapy?

Regina Wagner No.

Hans Koch Against which fungi is terbinafine not effective?

Stephen White *USA* I have no personal experience but, as far as I know, it is not effective against *Malassezia*.

Regina Wagner This is a rather controversial area.

Luc Beco *Belgium* From which species are the kinetics derived?

Regina Wagner From humans.

Hans Koch How effective is terbinafine in aspergillosis?

Regina Wagner There are no reports in animals. In humans it seems to work.

Mona Boord *USA* spoke about carbon dioxide (CO_2) laser surgery in veterinary dermatology. CO_2 lasers produce a wavelength of 10 600 nm, so they are well absorbed by water and do not penetrate tissue deeply. Major advantages of their use are the vaporisation of bacteria and viruses (thus sterilizing the surgical field, but requiring the protection of the surgeon, e.g. by wearing a protective mask), minimal bleeding and a marked decrease in pain by capping of free nerve endings. The latter is especially important in the surgical removal of squamous cell carcinomas of the planum nasale. CO_2 lasers can damage unprotected skin and the cornea and can also be reflected by high gloss surfaces such as scissors or forceps, so special care must be taken during surgery. The endotracheal tube must be covered to prevent its destruction.

The main indications for laser surgery compared to classical surgery are highly vascular areas, neoplasia and infective tissue such as sarcoids. In sarcoids in horses, this technique reduces the recurrence rate significantly (18% compared with 60% after standard removal) and also speeds wound healing. In squamous cell carcinomas in cats, this technique is also highly recommended, especially if they occur on the ear base, planum nasale or upper lip. Besides a marked decrease in postsurgical pain, the patients recover much faster and excellent cosmetic results can be achieved.

Other indications where I perform this technique with very good results are acral pruritic nodules, interdigital nodules, multiple lesions like sebaceous adenomas/haemangiomas that can be removed very quickly and allowed to heal by secondary intention, multiple cystadenomas in the ear canals of cats and the removal of proliferative changes in ears, especially of cocker spaniels.

Hans Koch How do you see the future for this technique? Will it become established in non-specialist practices?

Mona Boord I don't know. People at the universities seem to be reluctant to use CO_2 lasers, even after donation. Are they afraid of this new technique? I see more benefits for the general practitioner, but of course it depends on the number of cases that are seen or the indications you use it for.

Hans Koch What are the indications for laser surgery in human medicine?

Mona Boord The same. Other lasers are also used for the removal of tattoos, for facial peelings, etc.

Susan Wells *USA* Do you use laser surgery as monotherapy in cats with squamous cell carcinomas?

Mona Boord Yes. Surgery takes only about 15 min.

Stephen White spoke about the use of niacinamide and tetracycline in a number of canine skin conditions. Niacinamide (in Europe, nicotinamide) is one of the B group of vitamins. It does not have the vasoactive or the anticholinergic effects of niacin. The combination of niacinamide and tetracycline has been used in humans for approximately 15 years to treat autoimmune diseases. The mode of action is still unknown. A delay or a prevention of neutrophil migration and a reduction in histamine release from mast cells has been observed. However, this therapy is not very effective in canine atopic dermatitis, where it fails to reduce pruritus, or in canine pemphigus foliaceus, where significant neutrophil migration still occurs.

Niacinamide and tetracycline together have been effective in controlling approximately two-thirds of dogs with discoid lupus erythematosus (DLE). The dosage is 500 mg of each drug every 8 h for dogs weighing more than 10 kg and 250 mg of each drug for dogs less than 10 kg. There is a lag phase of usually 4–8 weeks before the full effect occurs. However, these drugs will induce as well as maintain remission. Once good control of the disease is achieved (usually noted by a decrease in ulceration and by repigmentation), drug administration may be reduced in some dogs to twice daily or even once daily. Some dogs may need low doses (e.g. 0.25 mg/kg every other day) of prednisone, or topical corticosteroids, for maximum control. This combination is not effective in the therapy of DLE of Australian shepherd dogs where there is also ulceration and involvement of the nasal cartilage. Approximately 15–20% of dogs with pemphigus foliaceus (PF) will also respond favourably to niacinamide and tetracycline. In cocker spaniels with PF which develop lots of crusts on the dorsum, the response rate seems to be higher. This drug combination may also be helpful in sterile pyogranulomas and idiopathic onychodystrophy. Side-effects are uncommon, but anorexia and lethargy have been noted. Vomiting may rarely occur due to the niacinamide and in very rare cases blood dyscrasias (autoimmune haemolytic anaemia, autoimmune thrombcytopenia) have been reported.

If there is a problem with owner compliance (not all owners are able to administer these drugs three times a day) my recommendation is to give 1000 mg tetracycline and 500 mg niacinamide in the morning and 500 mg tetracycline and 1000 mg niacinamide in the evening.

Fabia Scarampella *Italy* Do you have experience in combining this therapy with vitamin E?

Stephen White I have only used it a few times. My impression is that vitamin E is not effective in DLE.

Norma White *USA* In my opinion, this combination works well in DLE but not in pemphigus erythematosus (PE).

Stephen White Are we really sure what PE is? I think it is effective in approximately 30% of cases.

Tiffany Tapp Have you ever substituted tetracycline with doxycycline?

Stephen White I haven't but my resident has. I am not sure about the dose. Was it 5 mg/kg once or twice a day? It might also be effective in dogs with mild pyoderma.

Kim Larnree *USA* Have you used minocycline?

Stephen White No, but it has been used in the treatment of bullous pemphigoid in humans.

Susan Wells Rosychuk first described it in 1994. He combined tetracycline and niacinamide three times a day in German shepherd dogs which also had pannus and bleeding from the nose and mouth. He also tried it in other unusual skin cases. He had problems with administration three times a day.

Stephen White I am in a referral practice at the university. It may be that compliance is better there. When my owners do not allow skin biopsy in these cases, I try this therapy for 1–2 months. If no improvement is seen, biopsies must be performed.

Tiffany Tapp Have you used this combination in cats?

Stephen White I have never seen DLE in a cat. I tried it in another skin problem in a cat but the cat developed severe vomiting. So next time, I will either cut down the dose or use doxycycline.

Karen Kuhl *USA* I treated a cat with DLE with a good response, despite it being a bad case. The dose I use is 100 mg of each drug three times daily.

Harold Richardson *USA* I used the combination together with safflower oil in a case of mycosis fungoides. Also, one patient with cutaneous histiocytosis has been doing well with this combination for more than 2 years now.

Luc Nagels *Belgium* I treated a dog with chronic gingivitis (biopsy revealed a plasmacytic infiltration of unknown cause) with this combination. The patient did well for 1 year, than developed lymphoma that was refractory to chemotherapy.

Stephen White There are two reports of human mycosis fungoides treated with niacinamide and tetracycline. The symptoms resolved and stayed in remission for more than 1 year, perhaps due to the anti-inflammatory effect of therapy. Has anybody rebiopsed a dog with mycosis fungoides during this type of therapy? [Nobody in the group had done this.]

Harold Richardson I suspect the inflammation associated with the tumour may have resolved but that the tumour itself may still be present.

Fabia Scarampella I treated three cats with plasma cell pododermatitis with 5 mg/kg doxycycline twice daily initially, reducing after 10 days to once daily, and achieved complete remission in all cases.

Stephen White Were they feline immunodeficiency virus (FIV) positive?

Fabia Scarampella Two of the three were.

Jacques Fontaine *Belgium* spoke about the use of cyclosporin A (CsA) in veterinary dermatology. CsA, produced by *Tolypocladium inflatum gams*, was reported as being effective in the treatment of human atopic dermatitis in 1995, at the 4th Congress of the European Society of Dermatology and Venerology, Brussels. In humans, the initial dose is 3–5 mg/kg CsA (Sandimmun®, Novartis). It was reported to work well but slowly.

In dogs, there are only a few reports of its use. CsA has been used in immune-mediated diseases, epitheliotropic lymphoma, immune-mediated haemolytic anaemia, granulomatous sebaceous adenitis and perianal fistulae.

In this clinical study, 14 dogs with severe atopic dermatitis were included. Besides flea control and non-medicated shampoos, no other treatment was allowed. A subjective clinical score was performed on day 0 (before initiation of therapy) and days 15–20. Criteria assessed were pruritus (clinical score 0–3, with 3 being the maximum) and both severity and extent of lesions (clinical score 0–5, with 5 being the maximum). The results showed an improvement of both pruritus and lesions. Based on this study, it was concluded that CsA is very effective in treating allergic skin disorders, especially atopic dermatitis, in dogs. The tolerance to the drug was excellent.

Other indications for CsA, in my experience, are atopic dermatitis in cats, food hypersensitivity in cats, immune-mediated dermatitis, systemic lupus erythematosus, idiopathic nodular pannuculitis and perianal fistulae. Idiopathic cellulitis of the German shepherd dog and feline idiopathic ulceration may also respond.

The recommended starting dosage is 5 mg/kg per day. CsA can be combined with ketoconazole or steroids to increase the effect.

Eric Florant *France* I have used CsA for 18 months for different problems. It can be helpful in pyoderma and *Malassezia* dermatitis. It works well in atopic dermatitis, particularly in those cases with a more marked inflammatory response. Combining it with ketoconazole seems more efficacious, but in dogs with pyoderma it is less efficacious.

Jacques Fontaine I think it is dangerous in deep infections. I have never seen relapses of superficial infections in atopic dermatitis and I have treated betweeen 80 and 100 atopic dogs with CsA.

Eric Florant Atopic dogs have skin problems that favour the penetration of bacteria and thus they will develop a greater degree of pyoderma than others. Even when antibiotics or ketoconazole are given 1 month prior to CsA, success is not as good.

Luc Beco You showed good results in the two dogs with German shepherd dog pyoderma. Did these receive other simultaneous treatments?

Jacques Fontaine The German shepherd dog pyoderma was a concurrent problem. The patients presented because of perianal fistulae. There was no concurrent antibiotic therapy.

Hans Koch Eighteen years ago, a Belgian colleague presented information about German shepherd dogs with German shepherd dog pyoderma that he treated with steroids alone. CsA has anti-inflammatory effects also. Do we know the mechanism of action in German shepherd dog pyoderma? I think we have to be very cautious with our interpretation and I think we should be very careful in using CsA in cases where we do not yet know the exact pathogenesis of the disease we are trying to treat.

Louis Anzet *France* Do you have experience of treating feline plasmacytic stomatitis with CsA?

Jacques Fontaine No.

Louis Anzet I have used chlorambucil with good effect.

Jacques Fontaine Steroids are also helpful in some cases.

Ulla Bjornehammer *Sweden* You mentioned good results in your cats with food hypersensitivity. Did you give CsA with or without changing the diet?

Jacques Fontaine The diet was changed as well.

Olivier Elgassy *France* Were you able to reduce the dose of CsA in the long term in the atopic dogs you treated?

Jacques Fontaine That is an excellent question! In fact, there are two protocols in a current Novartis study. One gives CsA every other day and then twice weekly, and one reduces the daily dose. I cannot tell you so far which protocol is better. We certainly see relapses weeks or months after the therapy is stopped.

Luc Beco Could one reduce the dose to the lowest effective level, in a similar way to steroids?

Tiffany Tapp I think it would be a question of client education. In my experience it works very well, with no side-effects. How long, in your experience, can dogs stay on this drug and what kind of side-effects would you expect on this kind of therapy?

Luc Beco I have seen vomiting and diarrhoea that stopped within days of cessation of therapy.

Jacques Fontaine I have also seen hyperplasia of the gingiva, but only at higher dosages.

Luc Beco I think there are two kind of reaction: soft stools for days or months, or vomiting once or twice initially.

Hans Koch I feel that we have to be cautious. CsA has side-effects, although they are probably dose dependent and the dose has to be correct, especially in small dogs. I have seen one Yorkshire terrier treated with a dose of 7.5 mg/kg per day. However, the owner might have used a higher dose. This dog developed nasal bleeding and swelling of the mucous membranes of the mouth. But there is no doubt that side-effects are seen more commonly in humans.

Thank you very much for all your contributions and for the excellent discussion.

5.8

Clinical pearls of wisdom: practice tips for skin cases

Kenneth Mason[1] (Chairperson) and David C. Robson[2] (Secretary)

[1] Animal Allergy and Dermatology Service, Springwood, Queensland, Australia
[2] Melbourne Veterinary Specialist Centre, Mt Waverley, Victoria, Australia

Ken Mason *Australia* In this session, Ernie Smith will talk about the use of fluoroscein in intradermal skin testing (IDST). I will then give a short talk on the differential diagnosis of neck ulceration in the cat. We are going to have Greg Burton talking about his experiences with cyclosporine (Neoral®, Novartis), Mandy Burrows will talk about the treatment she is using for mycosis fungoides, Michele Rosenbaum will talk about Sweet's disease and carprofen (Rimadyl®, Pfizer) and Sonya Bettenay will follow up with nose and nail biopsy tips.

Ernie Smith *USA* As a practitioner, I really look for four items in a technique. Is it fast, is it cheap, is it easy and does it work? And those four things are the criteria I have used to put together this technique. When we do IDST, there are a number of things we look for to measure the reaction. These are the amount of redness or erythema, the size of the weal, the turgor that you feel with the tip of your finger and also the steepness of the elevation of the side of the weal. But sometimes it is difficult to measure that reaction if the skin is already erythematous, if there are already excoriations on the side, if the skin has chronic changes, if there is hyperpigmentation or if the animal is dark-coated and pigmented. Also, almost 8% of men world-wide are colour-blind (and less than 1% of women) and it is difficult for a colour-blind person to see reds and greens. This technique has value for these people also, as it gets rid of red as part of the test that has to be evaluated, and introduces yellow, which is much easier to see.

In cats, the skin is thinner than in dogs so with IDST there is physically not much room for the expansion and oedema to produce the weal. So cats are more difficult than dogs to read and this technique can be used in either species.

The first item you need is 10% sodium fluoroscein. It is used extensively in human ophthalmology for retinal angiography and, speaking with human ophthalmologists in my home area, they do not see anaphylactic reactions in people, and they will use a full vial. It also comes in tank vials. In the USA, there is a catalogue company called Henry Schein[a] and you can get it from them or your pharmacy can order it especially for you. The vial costs about US$8, which comes down to about US$0.20 per use for a 4.5 kg animal. It fulfils that cheap category in my criteria.

The second item you need is an ultraviolet light. There is a particular light I like which is made by the Burton company, which has two fluorescent tubes and two ultraviolet tubes with a magnifier in the centre. It may be handheld or you can put it on a stand if you want to have both your hands free.

When I do the skin test I use my usual technique using the same antigens, the same number of antigens and the same sedative. Immediately after administering the last intradermal skin test injection, 4.4 mg/kg of sodium fluorescein for a cat and 2.2 mg/kg for a dog is injected intravenously. The tests can be read in 5–10 minutes and again in 10–15 minutes. Before using this technique, I used to extend my reading times to 30 min. However, now I find I get the results much quicker, and even if I wait for 30 min there is never a change.

The yellowish colour by itself is easier to read than just looking for the erythema alone and the other

[a] Henry Schein: http:/www.henryschein.com

criteria are still there: the size of the weal, the steepness of the edges and the turgor. Under ultraviolet fluorescence, I think that you can appreciate how much easier this is to read.[b]

Birget Holm *Sweden* Have you tried a lower dosage of fluorescein?

Ernie Smith This is so low I don't really see it's necessary to go much lower. Have you tried lower doses and have it work just as clearly?

Birget Holm Yes we have and it does. We use a lower dose because we had side-effects in one cat.

Ernie Smith What kind of side-effects?

Birget Holm Ataxia.

Unknown participant How long did the ataxia last?

Birget Holm Just as the cat woke up; it was ataxic for a couple of hours.

Ernie Smith What have you managed to reduce the fluorescein dose to?

Birget Holm 2 mg/kg. Has anyone else seen any side-effects?

Daniela Delius *Germany* It's not really a side-effect but I have seen some cats getting very green mucous membranes.

Birget Holm I have also heard of cats getting green mucous membranes, which is worrying to the owners.

Ernie Smith Certainly the material stays within the bloodstream for up to 48 h, so the pet will pass urine that is a yellow–green colour. If it happens to urinate in the car on the way home, that dye will stay there forever. Certainly, cats go home in carriers with towels in them and dogs get walked as soon as they leave the clinic so they don't have any accidents in the car on the way home. So you should warn the client that the green mucous membranes are going to be there, but the biggest warning should be about not allowing the animal to urinate in the car on the way home or on the carpet at home.

Ken Mason I am going to talk about ulcerative dermatoses in the cat. In looking at skin biopsies from a number of cats, I have seen a linear ulcerative lesion histologically and I am reminded that the cat and the horse have an extra fibrous layer at this level in the skin. Presumably with chronic ulceration it proliferates and produces a classic linear fibrosis lesion. So this talk covers a number of diseases where I found this particular lesion and worked out the aetiology.

Cat 1 had a chronic, pruritic, ulcerative neck lesion as the only clinical sign. This cat was atopic and reacted to skin testing very clearly. It partially responded to desensitisation, allowing reduction of the prednisolone dosage from somewhere around 10–15 mg every 12 h to 5 mg every 48 h.

Cat 2 had had a neck ulcer for a long period. The cat was normally kept in a protective coat to stop the self-trauma. Skin testing showed the cat was atopic and flea allergic. Perfect flea control did not completely control the pruritus. There was intermittent erythema of the ears and papules in front of the ears, as well as the neck ulceration, which had become less severe. The cat periodically scratched at the ulceration but did not need to wear the protective coat. Desensitisation and intermittent cyclosporin resulted in complete remission. But before I did that, I was able to correlate the intense periods of pruritus at the shoulder lesion with pollination of the plants to which the cat was allergic.

Cat 3 had a very severe ulcerative neck lesion. Before I skin tested it, it had been given 2 mg/kg of dexamethasone on a Saturday. I skin tested it on Monday. While it was going into anaphylaxis, the lesions on the skin were growing and joining together. I have seen some very large skin reactions in the dog, but this was the biggest I have ever seen. We had to give it prednisolone sodium succinate because it was going pale and its head was swelling up. This was a severely atopic cat.

Cat 4 had a food allergy only. The cat had a subdermal fibrotic lesion on biopsy. Cat 5 was flea allergic. I did not find the subdermal linear lesion in this biopsy but I have seen it in other chronic ulcerative neck lesions in cats with flea allergy dermatitis. Cat 6 had a contact allergy due to a flea collar. I biopsied this lesion and found a linear sclerotic lesion.

Cat 7 has a disease in which I haven't found the linear fibrosis yet. It is a reaction to imidacloprid (Advantage®, Bayer). Some of these can become necrotic and quite ulcerative and I know of other colleagues who have seen these cases become quite severe. As I understand it, it can occur with fipronyl (Frontline TopSpot®, Merial) also. I suspect these cats are atopic as well, so it is not just a drug eruption. If it were a pure

[b] Dr Smith can be contacted at eksdvm@aol.com

drug reaction or drug toxicity then it would occur in all animals. The cat I have shown became clinically atopic a year later and was pruritic in the neck area at that time, but was much more so initially following the imidacloprid reaction.

Cats 8–10 are cats with the Ehlers–Danlos syndrome (dermatosparaxis), which we see a lot of, presenting with neck ulceration as the only sign. All are Burmese cats in Brisbane. They have a linear fibrotic lesion in the deep dermal tissue. They often present as neck ulceration, and are not that obvious as a cat with Ehlers–Danlos syndrome initially. They may be itchy, especially if they ulcerate. Others just have a necrotic eschar on the neck, which is an avascular necrosis resulting from damage to, and rupture of, the arteries and the blood vessels of the skin as it is stretched. Histologically, they are often read as toxic epidermal necrolysis because there is full-thickness epidermal death. The necrosis is caused by a vascular obstruction after rupture. The collagen looks normal on histology, which is confusing, but defective collagen is present.

The following cases are ones that look alike but histologically do not show subepidermal sclerosis. Case 11 is a cat with ear mites that have caused ulceration on the neck behind the ear.

The next two cases are of demodicosis in cats that had neck lesions. The first also had hyperthyroidism and follicular *Demodex* was isolated from the pruritic neck lesions. The second I don't have a good neck slide of, but it is a case of the short-bodied *Demodex*. Short-bodied *Demodex* can be incredibly pruritic in some animals.

This is a case of cryptococcosis with ulcerated nodules on the neck. It was diagnosed by a general practitioner as idiopathic ulcerative dermatitis of the cat and initially put on megoestrol acetate, then put on cortisone, which allowed us a very quick diagnosis. However, the cat died at the time I was staining the cytology.

These are getting a little bit less characteristic. This is a basal cell tumour in a cat. I'll stop at this point and take questions.

Kathleen O'Conner *Canada* Why do these lesions normally occur at the back of the head region? What is the rationale for that?

Ken Mason I believe that different animals find different methods of relieving pruritus. Dogs may 'swim' along, rub backwards and forwards on the carpet, roll on their backs on the lawn, scratch themselves or chew their feet. Every one of these dogs may have the same disease: atopy or food allergy. I just think that a group of cats scratch. Other cats hair pluck and get symmetrical alopecia. It's just the method that cat chooses to exhibit its pruritus. This is a subgroup of neck-ulcerating cats that are pruritic.

Kathleen O'Conner So they are itchy all over but that's only where they actually cause self-trauma?

Ken Mason I think that this is the case: they are probably itchy all over. However, once they damage that spot it becomes a recurrent problem.

Peter Lemmens *Belgium* Have you found similar lesions with injection reactions?

Ken Mason Certainly long-acting penicillins and vaccines in the interscapular region can induce the same disease.

Peter Lemmens How about steroid injections?

Ken Mason I agree that steroid injections may cause a similar response. Triamcinolone is one glucocorticoid which I have seen cause such problems. I wonder if these cats are partially atopic as well. I do not have proof in terms of personal cases but the interscapular region in the cat is very different to that of some other species. For example, it is the common site for vaccine fibrosarcomas. I think that it is very different in a number of ways.

Leigh Stevens *USA* Do secondary bacterial infections occur with ulcerative neck lesions?

Ken Mason Yes they do and, in fact, on histology one often sees large numbers of bacteria. However, antibiotics only partially resolve some cases. I frequently use antibiotics in cats with these lesions.

Michele Rosenbaum *USA* I'd like to speak about a new immune-mediated disease that I've been recognising, Sweet's-like disease in the dog. I've been hearing anecdotally that other people have been seeing these cases as well, including my pathologist, Dr Julie Yager. What it is, is an acute dermatosis in three dogs resembling Sweet's syndrome in people. Sweet's syndrome is an acute febrile neutrophilic dermatosis. It was first described in people in 1964 by Dr Sweet and it is characterised by painful erythematous papules, pustules and plaques. It is also associated with systemic signs such as fever, arthralgia, lymphadenopathy and a peripheral leukocytosis. In people, in about 20% of cases the disease is associated with an initial underlying upper respiratory infection or influenza and the disease comes on about 2–3 weeks later. It has also been associated with haematological malignancies such as acute myeloid leukaemia. Most cases, however, are idiopathic and that seems to be the case in the dog as well. It's thought to be a hypersensitivity reaction to a bacterial, viral or tumour antigen and it's more common in middle-aged women.

It usually occurs on the face, the neck and the upper extremities, and is associated with headache, arthralgia, myalgia and malaise. Histopathologically, there is a dense neutrophilic infiltrate that is primarily in the dermis. In people, the treatment is systemic corticosteroids that are tapered over 4–12 weeks. However, recurrences are very common and I have found that that has been the case in the dogs I've diagnosed with the disease as well. Other treatments include potassium iodide, clofazamine, dapsone and isotretinoin.

This disease was first reported in two dogs in 1999 at the American College of Veterinary Dermatology Conference in Hawaii by Dr Carlo Vitali in two cases that were associated with carprofen administration. One was a terrier mix dog and one was a Labrador mix. These dogs both had a pustular crusting and ulcerative dermatitis, as well as fever and non-septic arthritis, lethargy and lymphadenopathy. They also developed respiratory signs with alveolitis and broncheolitis and unfortunately both dogs died despite immunosuppressive therapy. There was some controversy at that meeting as to whether this was the same thing as people have or whether this was a unique entity. I'd like to present three cases that I've seen recently that were not on carprofen and are still alive.

The first case is a 4-year-old, castrated, wire-haired fox terrier with a history of atopy and beef allergy that was well controlled with dietary restriction and intermittent use of antihistamines and essential fatty acid therapy. The dog had not been on any medications for 2 months prior to this episode and had not had any vaccines for 6 months. It presented acutely to his local veterinarian for a supposed bee sting on the right side of the muzzle. It was treated with grape-flavoured children's Benedryl® (Warner Lambert), and within 24 h, developed very florid, ulcerative lesions around the muzzle and the eyes, along with swelling of the muzzle. The dog also had some ulcerations interdigitally and became very lethargic, anorexic and seemed reluctant to move. There were haemorrhagic, raised, red to violaceous plaques and papules over the right side of the muzzle. All his lesions seemed to be on the right side of the body, which I thought was very interesting. The dog had a habit of snapping at bees, so whether it really was stung we don't know. The right paw, the right side of the shoulder and the right side of the thorax were all affected with ulcerative lesions. Histopathological examination showed a severe neutrophilic dermatitis extending to the epidermis.

We treated the dog for dehydration and the swelling with intravenous fluids, intravenous dexamethasone initially followed by 0.5–1 mg/kg per day of prednisone together with cephalexin. It responded very well to therapy and was slowly tapered off prednisone over a period of 3–4 weeks. It had not responded to antibiotics alone by the local veterinarian. About 2 weeks later, the dog re-presented with similar lesions again affecting the right side of the muzzle, right mucocutaneous junctions, right pinna and right dorsal paw, and now is on a more slowly tapering dose of prednisone starting at anti-inflammatory doses of approximately 1 mg/kg per day. It is now down to approximately 0.25 mg/kg every other day and is doing well.

The next case I would like to describe is a 12-year-old English springer spaniel that presented with a fairly acute onset of a crusting dermatosis primarily affecting the periocular region, pinnae, the perioral region and around the planum nasale. The dog had some ulceration interdigitally. It also had submandibular lymphadenopathy, lethargy and fever. It had been treated with numerous antibiotics, including cephalexin, amoxicillin–clavulanic acid and quinolones such as enrofloxacin, and had shown no response. The dog also had some very deep lesions on the trunk that were ulcerative. The histopathology was similar to the first case. We saw a severe neutrophilic dermatosis affecting the upper and deep dermis. There were no acantholytic cells, no organisms and no other abnormalities. It responded very well to tapering doses of prednisone, enrofloxacin, medicated shampoos and intravenous fluids for the dehydration, depression and anorexia.

My third case is a 5-year-old German shepherd dog that presented with an acute onset of an ulcerative dermatosis around the tail base, the muzzle, the periocular region and the tongue, soft palate and planum nasale. The dog had fever, dehydration, submandibular lymphadenopathy, lethargy and anorexia similar to the previous cases but also distinct weight loss of approximately 4.5–5.8 kg. There was no history of recent vaccination or medication. The dog had previously had a very good medical work-up by the local veterinarian, with chest and abdominal radiographs and abdominal ultrasound, and nothing abnormal was found. Blood work-up was normal and I found this on the other two cases as well. Again, biopsy showed a severe neutrophilic dermatosis of the upper and deep dermis and the dog responded very well to intravenous fluids, whirlpool therapy and tapering doses of corticosteroids.

All three dogs have done very well on continuous low-dose corticosteroids, and this last one, my most recent case, is currently on about 0.32 mg/kg of prednisone every third day and is doing well. I am afraid to take them off the prednisone because of my experience with the first case that relapsed severely when I discontinued it. My questions are: has anyone else seen these cases, how are you managing them, has anyone been able to stop the corticosteroids for a long period of time and not have them relapse, and for how long should I continue the corticosteroids?

I think that this condition is similar to what we see in people. It may be clinically a little bit different and histologically it is slightly different. In people the neutrophilic infiltrate is seen basically just in the deep dermis and the panniculus, but in dogs you see it in the epidermis and the dermis as well. However, it is interesting to see that the condition is not just associated with carprofen and they don't necessarily die.

Does anyone have any questions or comments? Has anyone else seen this disease, or thought that they might have seen it?

Marilyn Stiff *USA* Do you think that the grape-flavoured Benedryl in the first case may have initiated the condition?

Michele Rosenbaum I think it's possible. I did question the owner about whether the dog had had Benedryl before. It had had Benedryl, but never the grape-flavoured variety, so whether it was the flavouring that did it I don't know. This is the same dog that was stung by the bee so it's hard to say.

Marilyn Stiff What about the other two cases?

Michele Rosenbaum The others had no medications at all. I questioned the owners repeatedly about that.

Ken Mason I have seen three cases. Two were in Chinese shar peis of 16–20 weeks of age soon after their vaccinations for distemper, hepatitis and parvovirus, and they were somewhat similar. Ultimately, there were large ulcerated areas of skin on the face and down the front of the legs, but they did respond to prednisolone given for a long period of time and, 3 months later, we were able to stop the glucocorticoid. I've had one idiopathic case in a Maltese terrier of 8 years of age for which I could not find any initiating drug history. It partially responded to therapy but required some skin grafts for ulcerations on the chest wall as well. Eventually, the tongue infarcted and the dog was ultimately euthanised. I don't know what triggered the disease but it did come in cycles, possibly when the prednisolone dose was being reduced.

Michele Rosenbaum I think that it is important in this condition to taper the prednisone slowly, as you would with other autoimmune diseases like pemphigus foliaceus, and not to stop it too soon.

David Robson *Australia* Dr Burton and I are going to talk about our experiences using cyclosporine in practice. We have used a reasonable amount of cyclosporine in practice and have found it useful in a couple of different conditions. The condition we use it for most is the recalcitrant atopics. We still prefer, and will always try, to get these animals onto hyposensitising vaccines first, so the ones that we are tending to use it for are the vaccine failures.

On that note, I don't think that cyclosporine therapy is compatible with either skin testing and/or concurrent allergy vaccination. The reason why I don't think it's compatible with skin testing is because it blocks mast cell mediator release and it also blocks interleukin-4 (IL-4) with the late phase reaction. So I can't see why it should not interfere with skin testing. Having said that, there have been a couple of studies in humans showing that it doesn't interfere with either prick or intradermal skin testing, but then neither do short-course corticosteroids in humans, so it is difficult to extrapolate too much from that. Has anyone had any experience skin testing or even serum testing in dogs or cats that have been on cyclosporine? [No-one in the group had experience of this.]

Hopefully it's something we may have at least a brief answer to over the coming weeks, as we are currently conducting a trial skin testing some dogs before and after 6 weeks on cyclosporine.

Our experiences with cyclosporine in the treatment of atopic dermatitis have been almost universally good in a limited number of cases. In dogs we frequently use it in combination with ketoconazole, usually at a 5–10 mg/kg/day dosage, to minimise the amount of cyclosporine we have to use. Obviously it's a fairly expensive medication and most of the dogs and cats we are using it in weigh less than 10 kg and often less than 5 kg. Success rates for getting these animals under control with cyclosporine or cyclosporine and ketoconazole without any other drugs are approximately 75–80%. It's not 100%: we have had the occasional failures at the lower dosage rate, and we don't like increasing it too much, for both safety and economic reasons.

In cats, we've had a good success rate. We tend to use the 25 mg capsules in most cases. We've had some palatability problems with the liquid in some cats but not all. The dose of 25 mg/cat seems to work well.

We have not had a lot of success in getting many of these animals onto every second day or every third day dosing. Most of them end up remaining on low-dose daily dosing, but there have been some exceptions where we have managed every second day dosing. Has anyone had any experiences in getting atopic dogs or cats down to every second or every third day dosing using cyclosporine?

Michele Rosenbaum I've had one dog that I've got down to a twice-weekly dose, and numerous other dogs which I have got down to a low daily dose but subsequently relapsed and were then again controlled by the 5 mg/kg per day dosage.

David Robson Have you used it in combination with ketoconazole?

Michele Rosenbaum I tried it once in a Great Dane on 5 mg/kg per day cyclosporine and 5 mg/kg per day ketoconazole and the dog had such bad gastrointestinal signs (vomiting and diarrhoea) that I stopped it.

David Robson I've not seen many adverse effects: diarrhoea has been the main one and some other gastrointestinal signs. They occur more often in cats than dogs. Has anyone in the group had any other experiences with adverse reactions to cyclosporine?

Peter Lemmens I had a small dog that was very nervous after dosing with the medication.

David Robson There have been limited neurological signs noted in humans at least. Paraesthesia, a burning sensation in the fingers and extremities, is the classical one but there have been a variety of other neurological side-effects noted uncommonly. It is very difficult for us to interpret that with dogs and cats.

Michele Rosenbaum I've seen severe haemorrhagic vomiting and diarrhoea in two small dogs less than 10 kg that were on just cyclosporine for refractory atopy. Both dogs got very dehydrated.

David Robson What dose rate did this occur on?

Michele Rosenbaum 5 mg/kg per day.

David Robson Atopy is the main indication that we are using it for at this stage. However, there have been a couple of cases of chronic pododermatitis in dogs that have not done well on other medications, such as combinations of antibiotics and immunosuppressive agents, that have come under control on 5 mg/kg per day or less of cyclosporine, usually in combination with ketoconazole and also often in combination with dimethylsulfoxide (DMSO) and enrofloxacin (Baytril®, Bayer) topically to keep the infection under control. Although the numbers are very low, it is something I would consider for these dogs where nothing else seems to have worked. Has anyone else had any other uses for cyclosporine?

Michele Rosenbaum I have not had severely atopic dogs that could get down to twice weekly dosing with cyclosporine therapy. Mine have all needed close to 5 mg/kg per day or they developed severe pruritus again. I have also used cyclosporine for the therapy of perianal fistulae and the two cases I have treated have needed 5 mg/kg every 12 h for 6–8 weeks to bring them into remission. They have then been maintained on twice-weekly therapy at the 3–5 mg/kg dose. Dogs with perianal fistulae seem to need lower doses for maintenance than do severe chronic atopics.

Greg Burton *Australia* One of the last things I did before coming over here was to sit down at the computer and print out the number of cases that we have treated with cyclosporine. We have 26 dogs that have been on cyclosporine for longer than a 6 week period and there have only been three of those (12%) that have failed to improve by more than approximately 80%. Here, I am using 80% improvement as a level where most clients and pets are happy and we have a clinically better dog, which is not necessarily perfect but which is having a very comfortable life. So I think that cyclosporine is a very valuable drug for dogs that have recalcitrant atopic dermatitis. Of the three dogs that didn't achieve this, subsequent to the 6 week trial of cyclosporine, two managed to the point where the owners were comfortable with them, using cyclosporine with or without ketoconazole in combination with low doses of prednisolone (approximately 0.25 mg/kg twice weekly). The doses of prednisolone used were much reduced compared with the level of corticosteroid that they had previously required.

Of the adverse reactions, vomiting is something that we have seen in cats, not in dogs. We've seen diarrhoea in dogs which has responded to lowering the dose of the ketoconazole (Nizoral®, Janssen-Cilag) rather than having to take them off the cyclosporine itself, and we have had one dog that, according to the owners, experienced gastrointestinal pain after having cyclosporine. She discontinued cyclosporine because every time the dog had a cyclosporine capsule it experienced what she described as abdominal cramping. It was a small dog.

Regarding the speed of response to cyclosporine in the treatment of atopy, the majority of dogs we see respond between the second and third week. It is very important when you are having discussions with clients that you give them an appreciation of when the drug should start making a difference. There were very few dogs of the 26 that improved dramatically in the first week and there were very few that took longer than 3 weeks before the owners contacted us saying that they were comfortable. In fact, in a lot of dogs, we were starting to reduce the dose prior to getting to 6 weeks on the drug.

So, regarding long-term maintenance, in my experience, the majority of dogs seem to do better on everyday therapy, but we certainly have some dogs that will adapt to alternate-day therapy. I've tended to use the liquid cyclosporine for dogs as it gives you flexibility of dosing and my standard protocol is that when the dog reaches 80% improvement, we reduce the daily dose by 25%. We use that dose for a 14 day period, and if they've remained stable on the lower dose, we will reduce the dose again by 25%. If we get down to 50% of the original dose and they are still doing well, then we'll try and go to therapy every second day or every third day. We have some dogs that are doing tremendously well having the drug just twice weekly, and some having it every second day. However, the majority of the dogs that I have seen are still requiring daily cyclosporine but at a lower dose than that on which we began.

Dr Robson spoke to you briefly about the pododermatitis cases, and that was an idea that for us came from Dr Mandy Burrows. The cases we are talking about are the chronic short-coated atopic dogs with pododermatitis, furunculosis and pyoderma. The two dogs that were treated were a cattle dog and a bull terrier. After biopsies and cultures, we treated with antibiotics and these dogs got somewhere between 40 to 60% better at maximum. We tried them on steroids and pentoxifylline (Trental®, Hoechst Marion Roussel) together, with no response, and we tried one on interferon, also without any response. These two dogs have done extremely well on cyclosporine at the same dose as used to treat atopics (3.5 mg/kg per day with 10 mg/kg per day of ketoconazole), which was then reduced. I'm very excited about the use of cyclosporine in pododermatitis cases, as we all see a lot of dogs with chronic, severe disease where there is hyperplasia of the tissue between the pads to a point where a fusion podoplasty may be considered. I know two cases is not very many, although Mandy Burrows has had a third case which has done extremely well, but I think cyclosporine is a potentially a very novel and effective drug for these cases. I'm not sure how much we can lower the dose in the long term, but our dogs have been on therapy for 12 and 8 weeks, respectively, and are doing extremely well. We are still reducing the doses at present.

We've had two cases of perianal furunculosis, one in a bull terrier and one in a German shepherd dog. My understanding is that the original publications reporting treating that syndrome with cyclosporine used a dose of 15 mg/kg and they treated these dogs for 16 weeks. However, we treated our two cases at the atopic dose of 3.5 mg/kg per day together with ketoconazole at 10 mg/kg per day, and lesions resolved in 4–6 weeks. Both dogs are now currently off therapy, one for 6 weeks and the other for a couple of months and, at present, there has been no relapse. Perianal furunculosis is something that people are referring to dermatologists rather than sending to surgeons. I think that's a disease we can probably help with a lot at a lower dose of cyclosporine.

We have also used it in cats. There is not a lot in the literature about its use in this species. We've used cyclosporine in seven cats with very severe chronic eosinophilic plaque syndrome and very severe miliary dermatitis. These are cats that have all been through a fairly rigid work-up, including food trials, flea trials, fungal cultures and antibiotic therapy, and were non-responsive. Two of the cats were skin-test positive but failed to respond to immunotherapy. Two more cats had fairly inconclusive results from skin testing and three we couldn't skin test because of the severity of their skin disease. Cyclosporine at 25 mg/cat has worked extremely well in these cases. One of the cats that I saw on the last day before I came away was a cat which had large reactions to fleas, large reactions to dust mites and three pollens on skin testing. The cat had been doing extremely well on cyclosporine until the owners moved house and it had a severe flea challenge. While still on 25 mg of cyclosporine daily, there was a relapse of its eosinophilic plaque. So cyclosporine is clearly not a drug which is necessarily going to work if you are not doing other things.

We have recently used it in a Persian cat with a severe idiopathic facial dermatitis. It had been on high doses of steroids, tetracycline and vitamin B_3 together with steroids, and interferon together with antibiotics, all of which, apart from very high doses of steroids, did not result in any improvement. This cat has also done extremely well on cyclosporine. It still had some clinical disease when I saw it last but the area of involvement has reduced from involving essentially the whole face to a very small 3–4 mm lesion under the right eye. Initially, after finishing cyclosporine, there was a remission of between 4 and 6 weeks and then the disease started to relapse. The cat went back onto cyclosporine and again the disease resolved. Whilst not common, it is a difficult disease to manage and it's something for which cyclosporine may prove to be a useful therapy.

Daniela Delius Have you any experience with the topical use of cyclosporine for perianal fistulae in the German shepherd dog?

Greg Burton We haven't used topical cyclosporine in any of these cases. We have, however, used topical cyclosporine in two situations. First, we have used it topically in a 1% solution in chronic recurrent atopic otitis. These are cases in the early stages of immunotherapy where the predominant symptom is recurrent otitis. They have been treated with antibiotics and are cytologically clear but still have inflamed pinnae and intermittent head shaking. In the past we would have used a 1% dexamethasone solution in Ear Clean® (Bayer) or Epi-Otic® (Virbac) as a vehicle and flushed their ears a couple of times a week. We have used 1% cyclosporine in a propylene glycol base rather than an oil base in a few of these cases, with moderately good results.

Secondly, we have used it topically in discoid lupus erythematosus cases as adjunctive therapy where the animals are already on azathioprine or tetracycline and niacinamide. I don't think that I've had any cases where I've used it as sole therapy. I think it has a role in the treatment of this disease. Ken might have a comment on this because I got the idea from him.

Ken Mason I get a lot of atopic dogs that then develop recurrent pyoderma and when they are investigated I find they've got Cushing's syndrome. If I treat the hyperadrenocorticism with mitotane (Lysodren®, Bristol Myers) the atopy becomes uncontrollable, so then it may be necessary to consider putting them back on steroids. I've had 10 cases that were totally uncontrolled. Recently, however, I've started putting them on ketoconazole and cyclosporine. The ketoconazole dose is 10–15 mg/kg and a side-effect of ketoconazole is that it blocks cortisone production, so then I'm able to use 2 mg/kg of cyclosporine with that and these dogs just look like they are puppies.

Michele Rosenbaum Do you have them on mitotane as well?

Ken Mason No, I do not. I use ketoconazole only at 10–15 mg/kg per day. I start at 10 mg/kg per day, then perform an adrenocorticotropic hormone (ACTH) stimulation test and aim for a post-ACTH stimulation cortisol level of 50–80 nmol/l, at which they do very well. I've now had some on 2 years of this treatment. I do find that they may get tail-base alopecia like a Cushing's syndrome case, but their atopy is perfectly controlled. After the atopy is under control, which takes 2–4 weeks (I agree with the period that Greg was saying), I reduce the frequency of cyclosporine administration to every second or third day. I don't lower the dose, I lower the frequency of administration. I keep the ketoconazole at 10 mg/kg per day or the dose required to control the Cushing's syndrome and I give that once daily every day. I have one dog on once-a-week cyclosporine, but it's on ketoconazole every day. If you look at the way ketoconazole works, you really should be giving it twice daily to control hyperadrenocorticism. I'm only giving it once a day, so I still have residual Cushing's syndrome in these cases, but the dogs are doing so well, I can't convince the clients to increase the dosage. So I believe half the day the cortisol levels may be out of control but the other half of the day they are fine.

As far as perianal fistulae are concerned, I use azathioprine (Imuran®, GlaxoWellcome) and metronidazole. It's a lot cheaper (written up by Tisdall *et al.*, 1999) and it works fine.

Clifford Alderman *UK* What are your selection criteria for cyclosporine therapy?

Greg Burton The dogs that we are putting on cyclosporine are dogs that are having steroid side-effects or are requiring high-dose steroids to control their signs. So we are talking of dogs that are on more than 0.5 mg/kg alternate-day therapy, or those dogs that seem to be supersensitive to corticosteroids. I'm not advocating cyclosporine as a Rolls Royce treatment for atopy. I actually think immunotherapy is the Rolls Royce treatment for atopy. Of the dogs where immunotherapy appears to be inadequate, which for us is probably about 25% of cases, about half will be able to be managed with a combination of fatty acids, antihistamines, shampoos, low-dose steroids or pulse steroids (preferably approximately 1 mg/kg prednisolone once a week). The other half are the recalcitrant ones in which, in the past, we would have probably used things like prednisolone and azathioprine together. I think that cyclosporine has a role for those dogs, but I don't think that it's a first-line choice for atopy. Regarding long-term safety, I don't know whether we can say to the owner of a 2-year-old dog walking through your door with a pruritic skin disease, 'I'm going to give you cyclosporine for the next 10 years' and know that we can do it safely.

Something that I forgot to mention before is the West Highland white terriers that exhibit classical atopic symptoms. We work them up for everything, but often I find they are a breed which have either spectacular skin tests or very flat skin tests, and some of those dogs also have very flat enzyme-linked immunosorbent assays (ELISA). They present with recurrent *Malassezia* disease and massive lichenification of their lower limbs. Some of these dogs do not respond totally to antimicrobial therapy and they are still left with pruritus and very severe lichenification of their lower limbs. Cyclosporine is like a magic wand in reducing the epidermal hyperplasia of these dogs. It has an antiproliferative effect on keratinocytes, and not only does it do that, it often makes them grow hair.

Ken Mason I agree. It does produce good improvements in West Highland white terriers that are very severely atopic. I use ketoconazole and cyclosporine.

Marilyn Stiff I use cyclosporine in alopecia areata and it does seem quite useful.

Unknown participant Are there any reports of long-term bone marrow suppression in the literature?

David Robson Bone marrow suppression has not been commonly reported. I think out of the cases reported in dogs, only one described a normocytic, normochromic anaemia, and two an unspecified anaemia. It seems very safe with respect to the bone marrow.

Michele Rosenbaum I have had one dog with severe refractory atopy that has been on cyclosporine at 5 mg/kg per day for 3 years with complete blood counts, chemistry screens and urinalyses done every 6–12 weeks with no clinical or laboratory abnormalities seen. I have also used cyclosporine at 5 mg/kg per day with ketoconazole at the same dose as described for West Highland white terriers with epidermal dysplasia with excellent results. In a few cases I was able to taper both drugs to every 48–72 h, while in others, daily dosing with cyclosporine, with twice-weekly ketoconazole, has been needed.

Mandy Burrows *Australia* I would like to talk about the therapy of the erythematous plaque/patch stage of confirmed epitheliotrophic lymphoma. We have two dogs that we have begun on lomustine at 90 mg/m^2 once every 3 weeks. Lomustine is a nitrogen mustard derivative and the idea for this came from this drug being used successfully in the rescue therapy of dogs with multicentric lymphoma. There was a paper that was published in the *Journal of Veterinary Internal Medicine* and there's an abstract that was presented at the American College of Veterinary Internal Medicine Congress. These dogs have shown a marked and considerable cosmetic improvement on this particular drug.

The first dog was a dog that I treated initially with interferon. It did not tolerate the drug well, developing malaise, fever and depression. I used it on a second dog because my clinical impression was that the lomustine had been so effective in the first patient. This particular animal we monitored for a nadir in the neutrophil count at day 7 after starting therapy. It is essential to be particularly careful with respect to the development of neutropenia. We monitor them again at day 20 prior to giving them the next dose of lomustine. If the neutrophil count decreases to less than 2×10^9/l then I would reduce the dose by 50% and if less than 0.5×10^9/l, I would withdraw the drug.

The reported side-effects of lomustine include gastrointestinal problems and myelosuppression. We have not had any problems with side-effects in any of our patients. Does anyone have any comments?

Greg Burton We started using this drug after discussion with Helen Power, who has been using it for a while. In the last year, we have seen a rather large number of cases of mycosis fungoides (approximately 10), on which we've used various things. On the last six cases, we've used lomustine. We started using lomustine initially for a dog that came in with quite advanced tumour-stage mycosis fungoides. Conservatively, that dog would have had approximately 50–100 small nodular lesions over the entire body. The response to lomustine was very dramatic and so since then we've used it in a number of other dogs. The dogs that we're treating are certainly improving clinically. The dose that we're using is a little lower than the dose that Dr Burrows is using. We're using a 60 mg/m^2 dose, and we're using it in conjunction with prednisolone, because of an anecdotal comment that there is more toxicity with higher doses and that using lomustine and prednisolone together would allow a good response on a lower dose.

None of these six dogs has gone into clinical remission. All have clinically improved on this therapy, particularly the dog with the multiple nodules. The number and size of the nodules have reduced dramatically, but the dog still has tumour-stage disease. This dog has been on therapy now for five treatments at 3 weekly intervals. The other dogs we have used it on have had lesions, which included plaques on the muzzle and ulcerative disease on the ventral abdomen. The ulcerative disease has resolved with lomustine therapy and the plaque lesion on the muzzle has reduced in size but has not gone away. So, at this point, I think the dogs' quality of life is improved by being on lomustine therapy. I think that the tumours have taken backward steps while being on lomustine, but we are still a fair way away from having any dogs go into full clinical remission.

Sonya Bettenay *USA* What's the cost difference between treatment using lomustine and other therapies? Is it more expensive?

Greg Burton No, lomustine for us is quite a lot cheaper. The retinoids are extremely expensive for most of the dogs that we are treating (golden retrievers being the number one dog that we see). For a golden retriever-sized dog it probably works out for us at about AUS$80–85 for every 3 week lomustine treatment (which does not include monitoring blood work). We haven't been monitoring at day 7 (which is ideal), for the convenience of the clients. We start at very low doses and work up, and we feel comfortable that the drug is very well tolerated. So we were monitoring them at the 3 week mark before giving the subsequent dose, and the six dogs we have treated have had no adverse reactions.

Michele Rosenbaum At what frequency are you using the lomustine?

Greg Burton We are using it every 21 days.

Sonya Bettenay I would like to talk about biopsy technique, including that of the nose and nails. My topic today is how you can take the best samples so your dermatopathologist can give you the best chance of a diagnosis.

Skin biopsies can be a waste of time, but they can also be a very valuable tool and very often this is a reflection on where, how and why the samples were taken. First, I recommend that you use micro-instruments. These are all ophthalmic surgery instruments and they're just a little bit more delicate, a little less likely to cause tissue damage when you are sampling. We like using biopsy punches. Biopsy punches are particularly sharp and are very good at delivering even pressure when you take the sample. So if you can choose to take a sample using a punch you may actually get less tissue trauma. If you're going to use a punch, you position the skin by holding it firmly, hold the biopsy punch at a 90-degree angle and rotate in one direction. How you remove the sample depends on whether you're sampling for deep disease (draining tracts, holes and ulcers) or superficial disease (depigmentation, superficial crusting and minor erosion). If you suspect a deep lesion you should pick it up by the edge of the epidermis. If you think you have a superficial lesion you should try to pick it up by the panniculus. Curved iris scissors are useful to slide and snip underneath the biopsy, as there are not usually major vessels if we're not biopsying noses and feet. Just snip underneath and you don't even have to hold the biopsy: you're not going to crush anything. When we look under the microscope at a crushed biopsy, all of the cells get squashed and it may be impossible to differentiate between cells.

The first practice tip is: when you're taking a skin biopsy use special instruments and be gentle.

One of the things that I'd like to run through is selecting biopsy sites on noses. They are difficult areas to biopsy. They bleed significantly and you have to just about have a general anaesthetic. In selecting the site, we like to have it immobile and we are usually choosing depigmented and/or ulcerated areas. Remember that the definition of an ulcer is that the epidermis is gone. The lesions in discoid lupus erythematosus and in pemphigus foliaceus (which are the most frequent suspect diseases for which noses are biopsied) are in the epidermis. So if we biopsy an ulcer, we're actually not going to be biopsying the affected part. What we want to do is to biopsy the intact skin.

The second thing we want to think about is what has actually happened if the skin has gone white. What has happened is that the disease has been there, the antibodies have gone in and attacked the skin, the skin has lost all its pigment and probably the immune cells have gone off to another area. So, the white areas are probably past the diagnostic stage. Please try to avoid biopsying the white areas. If it's already depigmented, we're probably not going to be able to give you an answer.

Crusts may or may not be diagnostic. Sometimes a crust is forming over a healing ulcer and is not useful. If you think you can differentiate these then don't biopsy them but do pick the crusts that are still 'growing up'. The best part to biopsy is the part where it is going grey. So it's not white yet, but it's not black and healthy. The skin has active disease there.

In selecting the site for a nose biopsy, do not biopsy ulcers or white areas. Choose the grey areas and also proliferative crusts if they are present.

Selection of site, then, depends on how the sample is to be taken: by excision or by punch biopsy. Now I've already said I prefer punches because they produce even pressure and nice sharp edges. It is important, however, to understand what happens in the pathology laboratory. If the technicians get an elliptical biopsy, they always section it lengthways, but if they get it in a circle they won't care which way it is sectioned. It is also important to remember that to them your biopsy sample looks like a little grey blob with, possibly, a couple of hairs sticking out of it. Very often they don't even see the pustules that you gave them. So if you take a round biopsy, half of which is normal and half abnormal tissue, the technician may section it so that all normal tissue is given to the pathologist.

If you're using a punch, try and have 100% of the same tissue in the biopsy, so whichever which way it is cut, the pathologist is going to see what you wanted to be seen.

Next, what should you do you with a crusty dog? Just go straight through the crusts with your scalpel or biopsy punch without any preparation, not even alcohol. It is then very important to write in big letters on the front of the request form 'Cut in crusts please'. What we used to do was to have a piece of pink paper stuck on the request form with this on it. If the technicians know that there are crusts, they will go looking for them. However, if you don't tell them then they might just throw them out, because that's what happens to the leftover formalin, with possible loss of diagnostic clues.

When biopsying crusted lesions, do not prepare the site at all and do not forget to write in large letters on the request form to 'cut in crusts'.

Now, what's the tip about biopsying pustules? When we biopsy a pustule, what we're hoping to do is to allow the pathologist to see whether there are acantholytic cells, neutrophils with cocci or whatever else is in there. If I used a biopsy punch and by my surgical technique lost the top of the pustule, then the pathologist would get almost an ulcer and would be unable to make a diagnosis of pemphigus.

If you have pustules, do not biopsy using a punch; use an excisional technique.

Three words with respect to alopecia: 'baldest is best'. You want to give the most representative bald sample to the pathologist so they can see the worst affected follicles. You don't want to give them partially affected lesions so they can see some good ones and some bad ones. They want all the bad ones they can get.

Practice tip for biopsying alopecias: sample the worst affected areas that you can.

The last thing I just want to run through is toenails. These are slides borrowed from Dr Mueller's presentation, so apologies to those who have already seen it. This is a toenail biopsy technique that saves the dog's toe and that can be very important because sometimes that can be the difference between being able to get a diagnosis and not. Some owners will not let you amputate a toe but they might let you take a toenail biopsy. The thing about this new technique is that it only works on diseased toenails. If you try to do this with a healthy toenail, you'll just end up with broken fingers and broken biopsy punches. It won't work on a normal healthy toenail. A biopsy punch is used and orientated so it is running parallel to the toenail. What you are hoping to do is to go in the lateral quadrant and take the side edge of it. The technique does require some brute strength. When you feel like you have pushed so hard that you feel like you are digging into bone then you probably are and you must stop. So what you do, in summary, is get the toenail, get the punch and rotate as you would do when taking a normal biopsy, pushing very hard along the edge corner of the toenail until the punch stops. Then a little blade is used to cut across the bottom of the biopsy punch. So, you actually have to push it and then cut the back end off and then you have to get the bit out from inside the biopsy punch with a needle or something similar. You then can put a stitch or two in (you don't need to stitch too much) and bandage it very firmly. You do need a firm pressure bandage with these things: they bleed a lot after surgery. Using this technique, there is considerable bleeding and so we use a tourniquet.

The other thing that we have started doing recently is digital nerve blocks for anaesthesia. This procedure is very painful and we always premedicated animals with heavy-duty painkillers, but some of them were still very uncomfortable after recovering from anaesthesia and the digital nerve blocks really have reduced this problem. Postoperative analgesia is terribly important.

Approximately half of the dogs chew the sutures out themselves, while the others come back in 2 weeks. They heal up without having deformed toenails. I don't understand how we get away with this but it's a very nice procedure. The cosmetic side of it is really acceptable.

It is very important to put India ink on the skin so that the technician can orientate the biopsy. Normal fixation is used and, as there is not a lot of bone in the biopsy, it doesn't need a week to be decalcified before the sections can be cut. Usually these biopsies can be processed within 1–2 days. We'll often take two biopsies from the one foot if they have multiple toenails affected, so that they are only lame on one foot for a few days.

Practice tip: consider onychobiopsy rather than onychectomy for nail biopsies.

Finally, some additional comments borrowed from Dr Mueller's lecture. If you have a client who has limited funds, the most important test to carry out is a nail biopsy. Always do an elimination diet trial because a significant percentage of these dogs have food hypersensitivity, as shown in Dr Mueller's work. If you are going to perform any other test carry out a bacterial culture and sensitivity because this has been one of the most useful tests. He did other tests, including serum antinuclear antibody titres, complete blood counts, serum biochemistry analyses and other tests including fungal cultures.

The last practice tip is that if you have a client with limited funds when working up a dog with only toenail disease, then the three highest yield tests are toenail biopsy, an elimination diet trial, and bacterial culture and sensitivity.

Further reading

Graham, J. C. & Myers, R. K. (1999) Pilot study on the use of lomustine (CCNU) for the treatment of cutaneous lymphoma in dogs. In: *Proceedings of the 17th Forum of the American College of Veterinary Internal Medicine*, Chicago, USA, p. 723.

Griffiths, L. G., Sullivan, M. & Borland W. W. (1999) Cyclosporin as the sole treatment for anal furunculosis: preliminary results. *Journal of Small Animal Practice,* **40**, 569–572.

Honigsmann, H. & Wolff, K. (1993) Acute febrile neutrophilic dermatosis (Sweet's syndrome). In: *Dermatology in General Medicine*, 4th edn (Eds T. B. Fitzpatrick, A. Z. Eisen, K. Wolff, I. M. Freedberg & K. F. Austen), pp. 1152–1155. McGraw-Hill, New York.

Mathews, K. A. & Sukhiani H. R. (1997) Randomized controlled trial of cyclosporin for treatment of perianal fistulas in dogs. *Journal of the American Veterinary Medical Association,* **211**, 1249–1253.

Mathews, K. A., Ayres, S. A., Tano, C. A. Riley, S. M., Sukhiani, H. R. & Adams, C. (1997) Cyclosporin treatment of perianal fistulas in dogs. *Canadian Veterinary Journal,* **38**, 39–41.

Moore, A. S., London, C. A., Wood, C. A. Williams, L. E., Cotter, S. M., L'Heureux, D. A. & Frimberger, A. E. (1999) Lomustine (CCNU) for the treatment of resistant lymphoma in dogs. *Journal of Veterinary Internal Medicine,* **13**, 395–398.

Mueller, R. S. & Olivry, T. (1999) Onychobiopsy without onychectomy: description of a new biopsy technique for canine claws. *Veterinary Dermatology,* **10**, 55–59.

Mueller, R. S., Friend, S., Shipstone, M. A. & Burton, G. (2000) Diagnosis of canine claw disease – a prospective study of 24 dogs. *Veterinary Dermatology,* **11**, 133–141.

Munro, C. S., Higgins, E. M., Marks, J. M., Daly, B. M., Friedmann, P. S. & Shuster, S. (1991) Cyclosporin A in atopic dermatitis: therapeutic response is dissociated from effects on allergic reactions. *British Journal of Dermatology,* **124**, 43–48.

Remitz, A., Lauerma, A. I., Erkko, P. & Reitamo, S. (1996) Delayed-type hypersensitivity in palmoplantar pustulosis: effect of cyclosporin A treatment on skin testing with recall antigens. *Acta Dermato-Venereologica,* **76**, 310–313.

Rosenkrantz, W. S., Griffin, C. E. & Barr, R. J. (1989) Clinical evaluation of cyclosporin in animal models with cutaneous immune-mediated disease and epitheliotropic lymphoma. *Journal of the American Animal Hospital Association*, **250**, 377–384.

Ryffel, B. (1982) Experimental toxicological studies with cyclosporin A. In: *Cyclosporin A* (Ed. D. J. G. White), pp. 45–75. Elsevier Biomedical Press, Amsterdam.

Tisdall, P. L. C., Hunt, G. B., Beck, J. A. & Malik, R. (1999) Management of perianal fistulae in five dogs using azathioprine and metronidazole prior to surgery. *Australian Veterinary Journal*, **77**, 374–378.

Vitale, C. B., Zenger, E. & Hill, J. (1999) Putative Rimadyl-induced neutrophilic dermatosis resembling Sweet's syndrome in 2 dogs. In: *Proceedings of the 15th American Academy of Veterinary Dermatology/American College of Veterinary Dermatology Annual Meeting*, Maui, pp. 69–70.

5.9

New treatments for canine atopic dermatitis

Thierry Olivry[1] (Chairperson) and Rosanna Marsella[2] (Secretary)

[1] North Carolina State University, Raleigh, North Carolina, USA
[2] University of Florida, Gainesville, Florida, USA

The workshop began with a brief introduction and the acknowledgement of support from Novartis Animal Health by Dr Olivry. Available treatments for canine atopic dermatitis (AD) were briefly reviewed, including symptomatic therapy commonly used (e.g. glucocorticoid therapy), immunotherapy and the importance of secondary skin infections as flare factors causing pruritus and skin lesions in affected dogs. As the focus of this workshop was alternative treatments for canine AD, Dr Olivry proceeded to list the drugs that would be discussed. They included cyclosporine, pentoxifylline, canine γ-interferon, capsaicin and zileuton. Results of both open and double-blinded clinical trials were presented.

Use of cyclosporine for management of atopic dermatitis in dogs: a pilot trial (J. Fontaine)

Jacques Fontaine *Belgium* Cyclosporine A (CsA) is a polypeptide antibiotic with unique immunosuppressive properties. Initially designed for the prevention of organ transplant rejection, it has been shown recently to be effective for the treatment of AD in humans. Because of the similarities existing between this disease in both the canine and human species, we decided to evaluate whether CsA would alleviate the clinical signs of AD in dogs. This pilot trial was designed as an open, uncontrolled experiment. Fourteen dogs with chronic AD were selected and were given CsA monotherapy at the dosage of 5 mg/kg once daily for 2 weeks. Subjective scores were assessed before and after treatment based on the extent and severity of both pruritus and skin lesions. At the end of the trial, median pruritus and lesional scores had decreased by 100% and 60%, respectively, compared with baseline scores (Wilcoxon test, $p < 0.002$). Adverse drug reactions were not observed during this study.

The results of this pilot study suggest that CsA is very effective for the management of AD lesions in dogs, as in humans. The efficacy of CsA to decrease skin lesions was less spectacular than for the reduction of pruritus. Unfortunately, our trial lasted only 2 weeks, which might be too short for a marked decrease in lesional scores evaluating chronic AD skin lesions. In spite of the non-blinded and uncontrolled design of this experimental trial, we believe that the marked reduction in clinical signs as well as chronicity of the skin lesions preclude the assumption that the benefit was merely due to a placebo effect. Nevertheless, recommendation of CsA administration to treat dogs with chronic AD should await confirmation of these favorable results in larger blinded and controlled studies.

Cyclosporine A for treatment of canine atopic dermatitis: a prednisolone-controlled blinded trial (T. Olivry)

Thierry Olivry *USA* The purpose of this study was to determine, in a blinded and controlled design, whether cyclosporine would be successful in treating clinical signs of AD in dogs. Thirty dogs with AD were randomly allocated to receive once-daily oral solutions of either Neoral® cyclosporine (5 mg/kg) or prednisolone (0.5 mg/kg) for 6 weeks. Before, and 3 and 6 weeks after therapy, skin lesions were graded by the investigators using the Canine AD Extent and Severity Index (CADESI). Pruritus was assessed by the owners using a visual analog scale (PVAS). In both groups, CADESI and PVAS values were significantly lower at 6 weeks post-treatment than before the initiation of therapy (Friedman test, $p < 0.0004$). The median percentage reduction in the baseline clinical score at 6 weeks was 68–70% in the prednisolone group and 58% in the cyclosporine group. In the cyclosporine group, three of 15 dogs improved more than 75% and nine of 15 dogs improved more than 50%. The median percentage reduction in pruritus was 78% in the cyclosporine group and 81% in the prednisolone group. The percentage reductions in CADESI and PVAS values were not statistically different between groups (Mann–Whitney test, $p > 0.3$). Thus, we did not detect a difference in clinical efficacy between treatments.

Three dogs did not complete the study. One dog, treated with prednisolone, developed superficial pyoderma. In the cyclosporine group, one dog developed angioedema after 2 days of treatment and the drug may have worsened pre-existing regurgitation in another patient. One dog completed the trial but developed generalized papillomatous dermatitis, which resolved upon antibiotic therapy and discontinuation of the drug. The adverse effects reported in this study have been documented before with high doses and prolonged treatment. More specifically, it seems that the papillomatous dermatitis may be related to increased epidermal proliferation and not to papilloma virus. Our study provides evidence that, in dogs with AD, the effect of cyclosporine is similar to that of prednisolone. We propose that Neoral® cyclosporine could be considered as a valuable alternative to corticosteroid therapy in atopic dogs.

David Duclos *USA* In humans, there seems to be a difference between Neoral® and Sandimmune®. Did you notice that in dogs?

Thierry Olivry Neoral is microemulsified and has increased bioavailability. I do not have a lot of data regarding the difference in bioavailability. However, I had one dog in the pilot study whose lesions were not controlled with Sandimmune but improved dramatically when switched to Neoral. This led me to believe that absorption and bioavailability are better with Neoral. I did not measure blood levels in this case, but the pharmacological data suggest an increased and more consistent bioavailability of cyclosporine with Neoral.

David Duclos Do you have any experience with cats and cyclosporine?

Thierry Olivry I do not have much experience with cyclosporine use in cats but Pascal Prelaud recently completed a trial using cyclosporine in 12 cases of eosinophilic granuloma complex (25 mg of cyclosporine/cat 2 h before a meal). Cats were treated for 60 days. In this study, cyclosporine was not effective for indolent ulcers but was useful in cases of eosinophilic plaque and oral eosinophilic granuloma.

Jacques Fontaine I have noticed good responses in eosinophilic plaque, but not in miliary dermatitis and in cases of indolent ulcer. I have also had some success in cases of eosinophilic granuloma and head and neck pruritus. I have used higher dosages in cats than in dogs (15 mg/cat).

Monika Linek *Germany* Did you notice whether different breeds responded differently to cyclosporine therapy?

Thierry Olivry It is too early to say. I do not have enough experience to draw any conclusions.

Nina Shoulberg *USA* Have you seen any long-term side-effects with cyclosporine therapy (e.g. demodicosis) due to immunosuppression?

Thierry Olivry So far we have treated almost 75 dogs with cyclosporine and I have not seen demodicosis as a side-effect. I am sure that we will in the future. However, it seems that we do not have a problem with recurrent bacterial infections. I had a couple of dogs that were treated with cyclosporine and developed bacterial folliculitis, and with the owner's approval we decided not to treat the infection and see if it would go away on its own. In both dogs, lesions of bacterial folliculitis improved spontaneously. So it seems that we may not have any problem with immunosuppression of neutrophils with cyclosporine therapy. However, since cyclosporine suppresses lymphocyte function, it is logical to expect development of demodicosis in some dogs.

Betsy Willis *USA* How quickly does cyclosporine act?

Thierry Olivry Cyclosporine seems to work within a couple of weeks in some dogs, whilst in others it may need longer. If no improvement is seen within a month you may need to change drug. Cyclosporine does not work as quickly as prednisone.

Pascal Prelaud *France* I agree. Cyclosporine is quite expensive, so if no response is seen in a month it is likely that it will not work.

David Duclos What happens with the withdrawal of the drug?

Thierry Olivry As the drug is tapered, there is a progressive worsening. There is no rebound effect, but lesions and pruritus just return to previous levels. Human patients may have remission of the disease for months after discontinuation, but in dogs the improvement does not last very long once the drug is discontinued. I have only one case that stayed symptom free after discontinuation, but that dog had been on cyclosporine for 3 years. The vast majority of dogs will need continuous use of the drug.

David Duclos I had a case that was on daily prednisone and that responded to cyclosporine after 6 months of therapy, but no improvement was seen in the first month.

Patrick Nichols *USA* Are you initially using cyclosporine with steroids?

Thierry Olivry No. There is no reason for concurrent use of steroids and cyclosporine.

Mitch Song *USA* I have one dog in which cyclosporine helped somewhat but not sufficiently. In that dog, adding low doses of steroids was helpful to control the disease.

Preliminary investigations on recombinant canine gamma-interferon for treatment of canine atopic dermatitis (T. Iwasaki, S.-J. Park, N. Kanazawa, K. Ohno, T. Kubo and T. Mori)

Toshiroh Iwasaki *Japan* In this report, we evaluated the effect of canine recombinant γ-interferon (rcIFN-γ) on canine AD clinically and immunologically. Ten dogs with AD were enrolled in this study. No parasite infection, pyoderma, *Malassezia* infection or seborrhea was found in these dogs. There were nine shih tzus and one basset hound. rcIFN-γ 10 000 U/kg was administered subcutaneously once a day, three times each week for 2 weeks. A total of 60 000 U/kg of rcIFN-γ was injected.

The evaluation of clinical symptoms was performed pretreatment, 1 week and 2 weeks after treatment according to the degree of pruritus, distribution and severity of lesions. Cytokine levels in peripheral blood mononuclear cells (PBMC) were determined by quantitative competitive reverse transcription–polymerase chain reaction (RT-PCR) at pretreatment and 2 weeks after treatment. IFN-γ was measured as a T-helper-1 (Th_1) cytokine and interleukin 4 (IL-4) as a Th_2 cytokine.

At 2 week evaluation, the efficacy was considered excellent in two patients, fair in four and poor in the remaining four. The IL-4/IFN-γ ratio was decreased in seven out of 10 dogs. In two excellent cases the IL-4/IFN-γ ratio decreased, and in the poor cases three out of four cases showed increased IL-4/IFN-γ. These results suggest that canine rcIFN-γ might be effective in canine AD and the mode of action may relate to the change in IL-4/IFN-γ ratios.

Thierry Olivry Did you produce the recombinant in your laboratory?

Toshiroh Iwasaki Yes, the sequence for canine IFN-γ has been published.

Thierry Olivry Did you see any of the side-effects that are observed in humans receiving IFN-γ, such as fever and lethargy?

Toshiroh Iwasaki No, we did not see any adverse effects.

Thierry Olivry Was the dosage that you used similar to the one that appears to be effective in people?

Toshiroh Iwasaki No, the dose that we used is the one recommended in cats. According to a Japanese company, the recommended dose is 10 000 U/kg.

Rosanna Marsella *USA* Could you comment about the duration of improvement once therapy is discontinued? In humans it appears that clinical improvement does not last very long once injections are stopped and there is a progressive worsening of clinical signs. Did you notice this in dogs?

Toshiroh Iwasaki Dogs also need continuous injections. We will need to formulate a maintenance protocol or use a longer lasting product to have more prolonged beneficial effects.

Double-blinded placebo-controlled cross-over study on the effects of pentoxifylline in canine atopic dermatitis (R. Marsella)

Rosanna Marsella The pathogenesis of canine AD has not been completely established. It has been hypothesized that increased phosphodiesterase (PDE) activity may play a role in atopic disease in both dogs and humans. Recent studies also have shown that tumor necrosis factor-α (TNF-α), IL-1 and IL-6 may play an important role in allergic reactions in both humans and mice. Pentoxifylline (PTX) is a PDE inhibitor that has multiple immunomodulatory properties, including suppression of TNF-α, IL-1 and IL-6 production in rodents and humans. PTX also suppresses *in vitro* production of TNF-α by canine neutrophils and macrophages and may represent a useful anti-inflammatory drug for management of canine AD. The objectives of the present study were to investigate the effects of PTX on clinical signs (erythema and pruritus) in dogs with AD.

The study was designed as double-blind, placebo-controlled, cross-over clinical trial. Diagnosis of AD was based on suggestive clinical signs, compatible history, exclusion of other diseases and three or more positive reactions from an intradermal skin test using 57 allergens. Reactions were scored on a scale from 0 to 4, where 0 was the score of the negative control (saline) and 4 the score of the positive control (histamine). House dust mite (HDM, *Dermatophagoides farinae* at 25 PNU/ml) was the reference allergen, as all dogs had positive (4+) reactions to it. Food allergy was excluded by appropriate food trials and secondary skin infections were treated before beginning the study. Glucocorticoids were discontinued 2 months prior to inclusion in this study and antihistamines 2 weeks before. Selected dogs were divided into two groups. Division was blinded and randomized. One group received oral PTX at 10 mg/kg twice daily for 4 weeks, while the other group received a sugar tablet twice daily for 4 weeks. After a washout period of 2 weeks the groups were switched. Clinical signs (erythema and pruritus) were scored on a scale from 0 to 5 (higher values meaning more severe manifestations), by both the owners and the investigator (R.M.) pre- and post-treatment (day 0 and day 28). The total score for each dog was the sum of its score for pruritus and erythema.

Ten dogs with AD were selected and completed the study. During PTX treatment, the scores given for pruritus decreased significantly from both owners ($p = 0.007$) and investigator ($p = 0.0002$). Erythema was significantly decreased during PTX treatment ($p = 0.05$). When placebo and PTX groups were compared, there was no difference for any of the clinical signs on day 0. However, on day 28, the score for erythema was significantly higher in the placebo group than in the PTX group ($p = 0.0096$) and scores for pruritus were significantly higher in the placebo group for both owners ($p = 0.003$) and investigator ($p = 0.0001$).

In conclusion, although the number of dogs enrolled in this study is small ($n = 10$ per treatment), it suggests that PTX may be a useful adjunctive anti-inflammatory therapy for allergies in dogs. Most of the dogs had residual pruritus at recheck visits, but a decrease in the score was observed with PTX. PTX may be considered as an adjunctive treatment for canine AD, especially in animals that have combined contact allergy and AD.

Use of pentoxifylline in dogs with atopic dermatitis: clinical experience with 80 cases (I. Bleich)

Israel Bleich *Brazil* The objective of the present study was to determine the usefulness of PTX to control pruritus in dogs with AD during the induction phase of immunotherapy. Eighty dogs of various breeds and ages affected with AD were selected and treated with PTX (Trental®, Hoechst Marion Roussel) at dosages of 10–15 mg/kg, twice daily for at least 6 months. All patients were also given injections of allergen-specific immunotherapy based on results of IgE serology (*in vitro* allergy test). Antibiotics were also prescribed when dogs exhibited symptoms of superficial pyoderma. Corticosteroid administration was not allowed during this trial.

We evaluated response to treatment according to age groups. In dogs between 1 and 3 years of age, 30% had a good response within 30 days, 23% had a good response in 60 days and 47% did not respond. In dogs between 3 and 5 years of age, 40% had a good response in 30 days, 10% had a good response in 60 days and 50% did not respond. In dogs between 5 and 8 years of age, 35% had a good response within 30 days, 32% had a good response in 60 days and 42% did not respond. Finally, in dogs older than 8 years of age, 62% had a good response within 30 days, 19% had a good response within 60 days and 19% did not respond. When all dogs were evaluated together, 41% had a reduction of pruritus within 15–30 days after initiating PTX therapy and 20% of dogs had a good response after 60 days. In other dogs, pruritus began to improve after 4–6 months, probably reflecting the efficacy of immunotherapy rather than that of PTX. Animals with predominant hypersensitivity to grasses and plants appeared to respond faster than dogs allergic to molds and/or other indoor allergens. We also observed that older animals, above 8 years of age, seemed to respond better and faster to PTX administration than younger animals. An improvement in vitality, activity, cognitive function and hair growth was also seen in the majority of our patients. Adverse side-effects with PTX administration were not reported in any dogs.

Our clinical observations suggest that PTX can be used to relieve pruritus in dogs with AD during the induction phase of immunotherapy and could be a valuable addition to the pharmacotherapy of canine AD.

David Duclos Did you use the generic PTX or Trental®? There are some dermatologists that believe that switching from a brand name to a generic may result in worsening of the condition.

Israel Bleich I used the generic form of PTX.

Rosanna Marsella I have had dogs that were controlled on Trental and that experienced worsening of signs once switched to the generic form.

Mandy Burrows *Australia* I use PTX at 20–25 mg/kg twice daily in conjunction with antihistamines (especially chlorpheniramine at 0.5–2 mg/kg) and my clinical impression is that this regimen is quite effective. It appears to be more effective in dogs with reactions to pollen rather than the ones that are primarily HDM allergic.

Thierry Olivry Do you have any comments on using PTX alone and then topping it up with antihistamines?

Mandy Burrows No, I cannot comment on PTX as single therapy. I can comment that PTX at 20 mg/kg seems to be more effective than at 10 mg/kg.

Israel Bleich Did you notice any adverse effect when you used higher doses?

Mandy Burrows At 25 mg/kg, only one of 10 dogs developed nausea and vomiting, which resolved with administration of medication on a full stomach.

Nina Shoulberg Do you have any idea why older dogs respond better to PTX treatment?

Israel Bleich One possible explanation is that it may be related to improved microcirculation. In these dogs, there was also a dramatic improvement in cognitive function and activity level.

Use of misoprostol in the pharmacotherapy of canine atopic dermatitis (T. Olivry)

Thierry Olivry In a previous open pilot study, misoprostol monotherapy was shown to decrease clinical signs of canine AD (Olivry *et al.*, 1997). The current study, using a blinded, placebo-controlled design, was performed to confirm earlier results and to determine whether the efficacy of misoprostol was due to decreased dermal cellularity and TNF-α gene transcription and secretion. Twenty dogs with AD were given 3 weeks of either placebo or misoprostol (5 μg/kg by mouth every 8 h). Skin lesions were graded by the investigators using the CADESI before and after therapy. Pruritus was assessed by the owners using a visual analog scale. Before and after treatment, skin biopsies were obtained from lesional skin at similar body sites. Specimens were processed for histopathology and dermal cell counts were estimated using a visual analog scale. Messenger RNA was extracted from frozen sections of each sample and the number of skin TNF-α mRNA copies was obtained from a quantitative-competitive RT-PCR using canine-specific primers. Cutaneous TNF-α protein expression was assessed using a semiquantitative evaluation of epidermal and dermal fluorescence score using an indirect immunofluorescence method and an anti-feline TNF-α monoclonal antibody.

Both pruritus and clinical scores were significantly decreased after misoprostol therapy but not after placebo administration. During misoprostol therapy, the median decrease in pruritus and clinical scores was approximately 30%. In the misoprostol treatment group, two dogs worsened while on misoprostol, five of 12 dogs had more than 50% improvement in clinical score and the pruritus of four of 12 improved more than 50%. Both dermal cellularity and number of cutaneous TNF-α mRNA copies were lower in biopsies from dogs receiving misoprostol, but were not significantly different from those of placebo-treated animals. Cutaneous TNF-α fluorescence scores were lower in skin biopsies from dogs treated with misoprostol compared with those receiving placebo.

These observations confirm the modest efficacy of misoprostol for treatment of canine AD. It is reasonable to hypothesize that increased efficacy may be achieved by combining misoprostol with antihistamines in order to block both the immediate and the late phase reaction. These studies also suggest that the effects of misoprostol were not due to an inhibition of inflammatory cell emigration or to transcription of the TNF-α gene. However, misoprostol administration was associated with a decrease in cutaneous TNF-α protein expression.

Nina Shoulberg After the first open study was presented, I tried misoprostol but it did not work very well. I had a couple of cases that had an excellent response and have been well controlled for a long time without any other medication, but overall it was not very effective. It is quite expensive so I do not use it much.

David Duclos I used it once and it did not work.

Pascal Prelaud Did you use other drugs in those cases?

Nina Shoulberg Yes, we had tried antihistamines without success and we were looking for an alternative to prednisone. So it was a selected population of dogs that was hard to control. Possibly in a general population it would be more successful.

Thierry Olivry When we did the study, we tried to avoid recruiting all the difficult cases. In some cases the response is excellent. We did not see any side-effects in the controlled study. It is not nearly as effective as cyclosporine. Adding an antihistamine may increase the efficacy of misoprostol. Possibly combination is the key.

Preliminary results of a double-blinded, placebo-controlled clinical trial to evaluate the efficacy of 0.025% capsaicin lotion for canine atopic dermatitis (R. Marsella)

Rosanna Marsella In humans there is increasing evidence that neuropeptides, such as substance P (SP), are involved in the pathogenesis of AD. In humans, SP release is triggered by various stimuli, including histamine. In humans, receptors for SP have been identified on a variety of cells, including mast cells. Stimulation of mast cell SP receptors leads to cell degranulation and histamine release. SP also has numerous proinflammatory actions. It is chemotactic for neutrophils, monocytes, T-cells and eosinophils. It induces the expression of adhesion molecules by postcapillary venules of the skin. It induces proliferation of T-lymphocytes (especially of the helper phenotype) and of keratinocytes. It stimulates the secretion of proinflammatory cytokines from monocytes and keratinocytes. Cytokines or second messenger signaling mediate some of SP's actions. SP is released after allergen challenge in humans with atopic disease and significantly contributes to the recruitment of eosinophils in allergic rhinitis. Abnormal reactivity to injections of SP has been reported in human patients with AD.

Capsaicin is an alkaloid derived from the seed and membranes of plants of the nightshade family (active principle of chili pepper). Repeated application of topical capsaicin causes depletion of SP from sensory nerve endings and abolishes pain and itch. Relief is usually noted within 14 days and persists for a few weeks. The effects of capsaicin on SP appear to be principally on type C sensory neurons. The purpose of this study is to investigate the role of SP and the efficacy of capsaicin therapy in canine AD. The results that I will present today are preliminary and to date only eight dogs have completed the study. As more dogs will be enrolled in the next months the results of this trial may change over time.

Eight privately owned dogs with non-seasonal AD were selected. The diagnosis of AD was based on a suggestive history, compatible clinical signs, exclusion of other diseases and at least three positive reactions in an intradermal skin test using the 57 most common allergens of the region. All secondary skin infections were treated prior to entering the study. All drugs were discontinued 2 weeks prior to the beginning of the study. During the study, only heartworm prevention and flea control (monthly application of Frontline®, Merial) were allowed.

Once selected, dogs were randomly divided into two groups (A and B). Division was blinded to the investigator and owners. Group A received applications of capsaicin lotion (0.025%) to the affected areas twice daily for 6 weeks, while group B received a lotion containing the vehicle. After the first 6 weeks, there was a washout period of 4 weeks and then the groups were crossed over. Concentration, frequency of application, duration of treatment and washout periods were decided based on studies in people. Systemic absorption and maximum dose of capsaicin allowed are not a concern in people. In this study a maximum daily amount of 2.5 mg (10 ml) of capsaicin for a 30 kg dog

(0.08 mg/kg) was used, based on clinical experience. Dogs were distracted after lotion application or an Elizabethan collar was used to prevent licking until the lotion was absorbed.

Both owner and investigator were blinded and scored pruritus on a scale from 0 to 5, where a higher number means more severe clinical signs. The investigator evaluated pruritus at the beginning and at the end of each treatment, while the owners were required to score pruritus on a weekly basis. According to investigator evaluation, there was no significant difference in scores on day 0 between the two groups. A decrease in pruritus was found on day 42 with lower scores assigned to the capsaicin group, although this difference was not statistically significant. It is possible that such a difference may reach significance with a larger group of dogs.

According to the owners' evaluation, there was no difference in scores between treatment groups on day 0. In the capsaicin-treated dogs, there was a significant worsening at week 1 and a significant improvement at week 6. In the placebo group there was a significant worsening at week 6 when compared to the beginning of the trial.

In conclusion, these preliminary results support the use of topical capsaicin as a potential adjunctive symptomatic therapy for dogs with AD. A larger number of dogs is necessary, though, before final conclusions can be made.

Thierry Olivry How did you select the concentration you used in this trial? On the market there is a variety of concentrations available.

Rosanna Marsella The selection of concentration was based on the information available in the human literature when clinical trials were done using capsaicin for a variety of pruritic skin conditions. In published studies, there is no information on the maximum amount allowed on a daily basis and I decided to establish a maximum amount of lotion that could be used per day and per kilogram.

Thierry Olivry How did you apply it?

Rosanna Marsella Owners were instructed to apply it only on pruritic areas, before taking their dogs for walks so that the animal was distracted and would not lick it off.

Al Sears *USA* We have used capsaicin for quite a while, especially on lick granulomas, with good success. We use 0.075% concentration. Lesions seem to dry out in 4–5 days. If they recur, we treat them again.

Mitch Song We use higher concentrations of capsaicin for AD, but with pretreatment with topical anesthetic because of the burning sensation.

Pilot double-blinded placebo-controlled cross-over clinical trial to evaluate the efficacy of zileuton for canine atopic dermatitis (D. Crow and R. Marsella)

Dennis Crow *USA* In humans leukotrienes (LT) have been proven to play key roles in allergic mediated inflammation. Specifically, several studies suggest that LT play an important role in AD in both people and dogs. Leukotriene receptor antagonists and inhibitors have been used successfully in the management of asthma and allergic rhinitis in humans. Zileuton is a 5-lipoxygenase inhibitor, which in turn inhibits LT (LTB_4, LTC_4, LTD_4 and LTE_4) formation. Pharmacokinetic data for zileuton in the dog are available. Zileuton is extremely rapidly absorbed in the dog (peak levels being achieved within 1 h of oral administration), with a half-life of approximately 7.5 h. The goals of this project were to evaluate the effects of zileuton on the clinical signs (pruritus and erythema) of canine AD. As zileuton has been reported to cause alanine aminotransferase (ALT) elevation in people, this liver enzyme was monitored in this pilot study.

Nine dogs with AD were selected and randomly divided into two groups. All dogs completed the study. Treatment allocation was blinded to the investigator and the owner. Group A received zileuton (Zyflo®, Abbot Pharmaceuticals) suspension orally at 2 mg/kg three times daily for 30 days. Group B received placebo carrier suspension three times daily for 30 days. After a washout period of 5 days, the groups were crossed over and group A received the placebo while group B received zileuton at 2 mg/kg three times daily.

Clinical signs (erythema and pruritus) were evaluated and scored at the beginning and at the end of each treatment (days 0 and 30). Peripheral blood (3 ml) was drawn from all dogs on days 0 and 30, 1 h after drug administration, for ALT assays. Tubes were centrifuged at 2400 rpm at room temperature for 15 min to obtain serum. The ALT assays were performed using a commercial chemistry analyzer.

There was no difference between treatment groups in the investigator score of erythema at the beginning of the study. At day 30, erythema had significantly decreased following zileuton treatment. Erythema did not change over time during placebo treatment. At day 30, zileuton-treated dogs had significantly lower investigator scores of erythema than the placebo-treated dogs.

At the start of the study, there was no difference in the investigator clinical scores of pruritus between zileuton- and placebo-treated dogs. Investigator scores of pruritus did not change over time between treatment groups or within each group. No secondary infections were noted with zileuton or placebo throughout the study. The owners' perception of their dogs' pruritus did not change significantly over time in either group. However, the zileuton-treated dogs had a significantly lower owner pruritus score than the placebo-treated dogs at weeks 1 and 2. Zileuton administration for 30 days did not produce adverse clinical effects. One dog developed mild ALT elevation by day 30. A full biochemical profile was performed which did not show elevation in any other parameters. The ALT elevation decreased into the normal range 1 week after cessation of zileuton therapy.

In conclusion, zileuton had no effect on pruritus in this limited pilot study. It is reasonable to hypothesize that the excess free arachidonic acid may be available for prostaglandin synthesis and prostaglandins are known mediators of pruritus. Zileuton significantly decreased erythema at 2 mg/kg and in 30 days of therapy did not produce adverse clinical effects. Monitoring of ALT is recommended in dogs receiving this drug. Further studies are needed to evaluate the potential of this treatment for canine AD.

Thierry Olivry Has anybody used the latest leukotriene receptor inhibitor Zafirlukast?

Liora Waldman *Israel* I have used it for AD for 30 days without clinical response.

Bob Shick *USA* I have used Zafirlukast in several atopic dogs and this medication did not appear to be helpful.

Further reading

Olivry, T., Guaguère, E. & Héripret, D. (1997) Treatment of canine atopic dermatitis with misoprostol, a prostaglandin E_1 analogue: an open study. *Journal of Dermatological Treatment*, **8**, 243–247.

5.10

Flea control and flea allergy dermatitis

John MacDonald[1] (Chairperson) and Keith A. Hnilica[2] (Secretary)

[1] Auburn University, College of Veterinary Medicine, Auburn, Alabama, USA
[2] University of Tennessee, College of Veterinary Medicine, Knoxville, Tennessee, USA

John MacDonald *USA* The treatment of flea infestations has changed dramatically over the past decade with the use of dips, biological agents, sprays, electronic flea collars and other alternative products.

There seems to be a decrease in cases of flea allergy dermatitis, based not only on clinical impression, but also on the number of dogs that are positive on intradermal allergy testing. We normally expect 60–70% of our atopic dogs to react to flea allergen, but this seems to be decreasing.

If we more successfully control flea infestations is there likely to be an increase in the number of animals susceptible to developing flea allergy dermatitis? Richard Halliwell demonstrated that fewer numbers of fleas and repeated exposure were associated with increased symptoms of flea allergy. We don't fully understand the relationship with flea exposure but it is definitely a component in the development of flea allergy dermatitis.

Concerning the diagnosis of flea allergy dermatitis, intradermal allergy testing is used to document the allergy and to help convince the pet owner that the flea infestation is the cause of the dermatological disorder. [Only four of the 20 people present reported using intradermal allergy testing to diagnose flea allergy dermatitis.] The serological tests commercially available may also provide an accurate method for the diagnosis of flea allergy dermatitis. [None of the individuals present reported using serological testing for the diagnosis of flea allergy dermatitis.] The intradermal allergy skin test can be used to show the owner the reaction caused by flea extract. Serological testing does not always correlate with intradermal allergy testing. Is it more reliable for the diagnosis of flea allergy dermatitis?

Keith Hnilica *USA* I have been trying to compare several commercially available blood allergy tests and intradermal allergy testing. There seems to be little correlation between the serological tests. The most recent patient I tested had positive flea-test results from Heska and Veterinary Allergy Reference Laboratories but negative test results from Greer Laboratories.

Albert Ahn *USA* (Merial) Why does this occur?

Keith Hnilica All three tests measure immunoglobulin E (IgE) levels, although they use different methods. The mixed test results raise questions concerning the reliability of the different serological tests.

Dunbar Gram *USA* It may be related to the timing of exposure and the degradation of IgE.

John MacDonald The degradation of IgE could certainly cause fluctuations in the serum levels. The immunological memory is also a component.

Albert Ahn What is the correlation of IgE levels in flea allergic dogs and cats?

Keith Hnilica In a recent study in flea allergic cats, we verified the flea allergy dermatitis using Heska's serological test for flea-specific IgE. There seemed to be a good correlation with the severity of clinical signs and even the number of fleas and the serum IgE levels.

John MacDonald The complexity of the immunological reaction involved in flea allergy dermatitis and the late phase reactions make intradermal allergy testing only about 90% diagnostic if only immediate reactions are evaluated.

Flea control

John MacDonald The use of the new highly effective adulticides and insect growth regulators seems to have decreased the environmental flea load. [However, only two of the 20 people present reported using environmental flea-control products routinely.] There seems to be a general preference for the use of treatments that can be applied to the animal to control the adult flea population and prevent the infestation of the environment rather than trying to treat the entire environment, which may be very large.

The use of concentrated permethrin products (65% spot-on treatments) continues to raise many concerns regarding the efficacy and toxicity of these over-the-counter (OTC) products. There is a perception among some pet owners that the concentrated permethrin products are comparable to the fipronil or imidacloprid products. This is largely due to the marketing of these permethrin concentrate products to fill a niche in the market.

Paul Overgaauw *The Netherlands* The use of these products was reported to be decreasing in The Netherlands with the availability of the newer, less toxic, more effective treatments.

Juliet Penaliggon *USA* (Merial) The OTC products are marketed very heavily by the product manufacturers. So there is a move towards the use of the OTC products.

David Stansfield *USA* (Novartis) The trend in the USA has been away from the pet stores and to the veterinarians, with a dramatic decline in the permethrin spot-ons. This year there was a new permethrin compound launched with a big marketing effort that may cause a swing back towards the pet stores. However, data are not available for this year.

Keith Hnilica What do you think about the efficacy of the permethrin concentrate products? I typically use the Advantage®/Frontline® type products, but I have been able to use a 65% permethrin product as a repellant (weekly) and had success. My concern has been regarding the toxicity of these products, especially for cats. They could develop a toxic reaction from close contact with a dog that has been treated with a permethrin concentrate. Is anyone else using concentrated permethrins and have you found them successful or dangerous?

Dunbar Gram I have seen a shift back towards OTC products in Virginia. In general, when pets have been on an effective therapy beforehand, they have eliminated the infestation in their environment. They can then use the OTC products more as a preventive, and as long as the product contains an insect growth regulator (IGR), they seem to work satisfactorily. When there is a recurrence, the flea allergic pet often gets treated with the prescription product and the co-inhabitants will often get treated with the cheaper OTC product and that helps with the cost.

John MacDonald The perception is that if the clients don't have a problem, then these less effective products demonstrate good efficacy. I can say for sure that when they were used before imidacloprid and fipronil became available, they were not effective drugs. When put under pressure in a flea-endemic area, they are not effective. The trend has been to keep a product on an even keel, even though the product may not have as much of a reputation under severe conditions.

Albert Ahn As a veterinarian, I recently took exception to comments made by Harts, one of the largest OTC purveyors of flea and tick products, specifically regarding the launch of their new product Harts Drops for dogs and cats. They were saying that you could go to a pet store and obtain the products in the USA at one-third of the cost of veterinary products. Additionally, they were saying that you could cut the veterinarian out of the picture. First, as a veterinarian I was offended, and as a Merial employee I was troubled because my pharmaceutical company has tried very hard to build a partnership and alliance to provide important information about the products and their proper use for flea and tick control. I looked at the comments as a legitimate safety threat but also an economic threat to practicing veterinarians.

John MacDonald I went through the courses to become a certified pest control operator, which was an experience. During a continuing education program, the representative of the chemical company gave a slide presentation that was based on the concept of 'No More Vets'. During the talk, he stated that vets did not know about flea control.

Paul Overgaauw Are these veterinary products sold through pet shops and which molecules are being used?

Albert Ahn These are products developed for pet shops and are generally permethrin-based products. Some are combined with IGRs.

Paul Overgaauw As long as it is legal for the pet owner to go to the pet shop instead of the veterinarian, this is appropriate.

Albert Ahn The concern is that the veterinarian is the resource for the pet owner concerning ectoparasites and endoparasites, zoonoses and toxicity. A clerk in a pet shop is not able to counsel pet owners, so it is irresponsible for any company to encourage bypassing the veterinarian.

Paul Overgaauw As the products become available OTC, veterinary sales decrease and veterinarians do not want to carry the products anymore. That is a problem that we just have to deal with.

Keith Hnilica One of my concerns is that the products that are being marketed through pet shops are actually more toxic to the pet, humans and the environment compared with products available through veterinarians.

John MacDonald The marketing of permethrins without discrimination of species has led to toxicities. We are caught in the middle between the legal appropriateness of OTC products and the perception of the ideal client–vet relationship. There are issues regarding proper pet care that are missing from the marketing of OTC products.

David Bledsoe *USA* (Bayer) This issue is similar to vaccines. The veterinarian should not be in the position of just dispensing products, but rather should rely on their unique services. The way to counter the OTC marketing is with service. Clients don't understand that all of the new veterinary flea-control products are superior to OTC brands and the way to fight that is with service.

Dunbar Gram I do not dispense any flea products, but make recommendations, so they listen to what I say because they know that I do not have a financial interest in selling them products. [Dr Gram works in a 100% referral practice.]

John MacDonald There are also issues about the longevity of these products, especially if we are aggressively shampooing the patient. There does seem to be some product variability based on published information.

The efficacy of selamectin (Revolution®, Stronghold®) in the treatment and control of flea allergic dermatitis in dogs and cats exposed to infestations of *Ctenocephalides felis* (S. K. Dickin, M. G. Murphy, R. Bond, I. S. Mason, M. Payne-Johnson, D. G. Smith, A. D. Jernigan and T. G. Rowan)

Sandi Dickin *UK* (Pfizer) The efficacy of selamectin was evaluated in the treatment and control of flea allergic dermatitis (FAD) in two well-controlled studies. Twenty-two dogs and 24 cats with FAD (confirmed by intradermal testing, serum IgE concentrations or provocative flea challenge and clinical signs) were allocated randomly to treatment with placebo or selamectin administered topically at a minimum dosage of 6 mg/kg. Dogs were treated on days 0 and 30, and cats on days 0, 30 and 60. Animals were housed in simulated flea-infested home environments and were infested with unfed viable adult fleas on days −13, −2, 14, 28 and 42; cats were also infested on days 56 and 70. Efficacy was assessed by comparing the clinical signs of FAD, including the duration of pruritic behavior per day in dogs, within and between treatments and by comparing the number of therapeutic interventions per animal between treatments.

There were no mortalities or suspected adverse drug experiences during the studies. The mean number of therapeutic interventions per animal for selamectin compared with placebo was significantly lower in dogs (0.0 vs 10.1, $p = 0.0001$) and cats (1.0 vs 13.5, $p = 0.001$); no interventions were required in selamectin-treated cats after day 27. In dogs and cats, selamectin significantly reduced the incidence (dogs, $p = 0.0158$; cats, $p = 0.0029$) and severity (dogs, $p = 0.0042$; cats, $p = 0.0241$) of clinical signs of FAD and the daily duration of pruritic behavior in dogs ($p = 0.0164$). Thus, selamectin was highly effective in the treatment and control of FAD in dogs and cats. Selamectin is available in Europe and North America.

Paul Overgaauw Would anyone expect any differences between the systemic and topical products with regard to preventing the flea from sticking on the pet?

Byron Blagburn *USA* Certainly products that can prevent the flea from biting the animal are ideal, but even with products that do not work by contact, once the flea burden is pushed below the threshold that causes severe clinical signs, the animal is much better, with a remarkable decrease in FAD.

Dan Domingo *USA* I think all products work on FAD by decreasing the overall load, not by preventing the flea from biting.

John MacDonald As long as we can keep the flea load below the allergic threshold for a dog, it is going to have beneficial effects on control. Michael Dryden showed with his work in Tampa, Florida, that 18–21 days after treatment with imidacloprid or fipronil there were fleas feeding but minimal clinical signs by keeping the flea burden low enough to avoid that threshold.

David Bledsoe (Bayer) Given the nature of flea biology, there isn't any product (including Advantage®) that can prevent fleas from initially feeding, so the key is reducing the antigen load. Product X is not necessarily better than product Y but, instead, the key is getting rid of the fleas to decrease the antigen load in the long run and then preventing reinfestation.

Dunbar Gram I still see a number of clinical flea allergic cases where the client or I never see fleas but if we step up our flea control the animal improves. This is more often a problem of cats compared to dogs.

John MacDonald That is a key factor in flea denial. Some animals are so sensitive to fleas that we or the owner never see the fleas. We use a flea comb to demonstrate any fleas to the owner. In flea studies, once a cat becomes flea allergic, it is very difficult to maintain a flea infestation on the cat because of its ability to remove the fleas.

Frontline Plus® (fipronil with *S*-methoprene) (A. Ahn)

Albert Ahn (Merial) Frontline has proven itself to be effective against fleas and four species of ticks. How could flea control be improved? Owner compliance, biological and environmental variation (from house to house) and current integrated pest management strategies have provided the reasons and methods to help provide added assurance in a single product. During the development phase, three IGRs were considered, *S*-methoprene, pyriproxyfen and lufenuron. *S*-methoprene was chosen for three reasons. The efficacy and safety information is readily available, providing the product with a long history. The World Health Organization has approved *S*-methoprene as an additive to human drinking water to help reduce mosquito populations. Additionally, the translocation properties make this an effective agent in dogs and cats. Finally, there is the ability of this product (as a mimic of the natural juvenile hormone) to affect the flea life cycle at several points. The adult flea comes into contact with the product and incorporates the *S*-methoprene into its ovaries, causing an ovicidal effect. If larvae are hatched, they are not viable. Additionally, any larvae that contact the product will be unable to mature and eventually die. The combination of fipronil with *S*-methoprene allows attack of the flea life cycle at three different points, adulticidal, ovicidal and larvicidal, in a single product.

Dunbar Gram Is the ultraviolet stability of *S*-methoprene a concern?

Albert Ahn The scientific data suggest that if *S*-methoprene is painted on glass and exposed to sunlight it will break down. However, other work suggests that clinically there is no compromise of *S*-methoprene. In the Frontline Plus® product, the concentration of *S*-methoprene has been increased to ensure that the product will perform well.

Nitenpyram (D. Stansfield)

David Stansfield (Novartis) Nitenpyram, a neonicotinoid, affects the insect-specific nicotinic acetylcholine receptors in postsynaptic membranes and does not inhibit acetylcholinesterase. It is in the same class as imidacloprid. It has been formulated as an oral (systemic) flea adulticide. Maximum blood levels are reached in a few hours and it is eliminated within 24 h. It starts to kill fleas in 15–20 min with rapid gastro-intestinal absorption and low toxicity. The product is formulated as a flavored tablet designed to be given every other day. Studies alone, or in combination with Program® (lufenuron), on dogs and cats in natural environments conducive to the flea life cycle demonstrated a rapid decline in the flea population by day 14 (90%), with the flea population being eliminated by day 28. With Program® alone, the flea population was reduced by day 42. Nitenpyram was able to significantly reduce the flea populations.

Margaret Swartout *USA* How is this compound excreted?

David Stansfield The agent is excreted primarily through the kidneys.

Advantage® (imidacloprid) (D. Bledsoe)

David Bledsoe (Bayer) Advantage (imidacloprid) Topical Solution has proven to be an effective method of flea control on dogs and cats. To date, no evidence exists of imidacloprid resistance in field flea populations. However, to fully investigate this issue, and its potential ramifications, Bayer has initiated a unique effort to monitor the susceptibility of field flea populations to Advantage, both in the USA and internationally. The program involves collecting flea eggs from client-owned pets, analysis of imidacloprid susceptibility of these flea isolates and characterization of the mechanism(s) of resistance should it be found. If resistance is found and its mechanism(s) elucidated, strategies can then be devised to combat it. It is anticipated that this international susceptibility-monitoring program will add a great deal to the scientific knowledge base regarding fleas and resistance, and will allow the veterinarian and pet owner to continue using Advantage with confidence.

The future of flea control (B. Blagburn)

Byron Blagburn Most of the flea-control chemistry comes from crop protection data. This is likely to continue in the future. The spinosins and pyroles show promise and there is some interest in developing these compounds. We will see a merging in parasite control with the external and internal products. This has already started to happen and is likely to continue. We will see some new chemistry being developed, but also new applications of old reliable chemistries. We will also see new formulations such as microsphere technologies. We are on the verge of having a microsphere-based moxidectin product. Increasing competition from smaller corporations will continue to grow. There are many opportunities and threats out there. The biggest threat may be complacency.

5.11

Diagnosing and treating psychogenic alopecia

Alexander H. Werner[1] (Chairperson) and Guillermina A. Manigot[2] (Secretary)

[1] Valley Veterinary Specialty Services, Studio City, California, USA
[2] Dermlink Buenos Aires, Ciudad de Buenos Aires, Argentina

This workshop was entitled 'Diagnosing and treating psychogenic alopecia'. However, in the audience, there were colleagues with a strong interest in behavioral medicine, including dermatologists and behaviorists and general practitioners with an interest in dermatology, and it was agreed that these conditions might be better considered as psychodermatoses, as alopecia is not always the only presenting sign.

Alexander Werner *USA* conducted the first discussion, defining which skin conditions might be included in the psychodermatoses group (see below), as well as discussing various differential diagnoses and the necessary investigative procedures. The audience felt that distinguishing between true psychodermatoses and those with primary organic causes is difficult.

Some attendees stated that many psychodermatosis cases are examined only by behaviorists and, therefore, dermatoses related to behavioral problems are more frequent than the dermatological literature reflects.

The audience agreed that all the conditions described by Dr Werner might not be entirely related to a behavioral disorder as their etiologies remain obscure. Keeping this in mind, Dr Werner described briefly each of the conditions usually considered as psychodermatoses and participants gave their personal opinions and experiences to the forum. The following were conditions considered by the workshop to be psychodermatoses: acral lick dermatitis, flank sucking, tail biting/chasing, anal licking/checking of the rear, foot licking/nail biting, hair pulling/overgrooming/barbering, cutaneous hyperesthesia and nursing.

Participants felt that the cornerstone of diagnosing psychodermatoses was the work-up, which should include a thorough physical examination, complete laboratory testing including endocrine profiles (most importantly thyroid and adrenal function tests), complete blood count and routine biochemistry panels, urine analysis, allergy testing (if pruritus is present), fecal examination, bacterial and fungal cultures from lesions, trichograms, skin scrapings, Wood's lamp examination, cytology (especially examining for *Malasezzia*), examination for ectoparasites and radiographs of joints near the affected areas (checking for evidence of osteoarthritis, periostitis, spondylitis or intervertebral disk disease). Some of the group emphasized the importance of food trials, response to corticosteroids, identification of pain and diagnosis of urinary tract infections (feline lower urinary tract disease, especially for licking of the perianal area in cats). Two additional causes of classic 'psychogenic' alopecia in cats that were mentioned included nephritis and anal sacculitis. The expression of anal sacs in all cases in affected cats was strongly suggested.

Neurological conditions or neurotransmitter/neurochemistry impairment or imbalance were also considered a possible cause of clinical signs. Recommendations for investigation of these diseases included watching for seizures, cognitive dysfunction tests and examination for hyperkinesia.

Participants agreed that a behavioral history was very important and that breed, age, sex, presence of other pets, presence of children, origin of the pet, reproductive status, territorial stress, human–animal bond changes and changes in the animal's daily schedule had to be considered in a complete investigation (as indications for the onset of conflict, frustration or displacement activity).

It was stated that the most frequent causes of supposedly behaviorally related dermatoses could be discovered after a complete investigation, following a list of differential diagnoses.

Stephen Waissglass *USA* commented on a study that he is initiating, which will try to identify the potential organic causes for psychodermatoses in cats.

Leslie Larson Cooper *USA* was an invited speaker and is a board-certified behaviorist. She discussed the importance of identifying and treating any underlying organic disease and then treating for pain and pruritus, prior to initiating treatment with psychoactive drugs. Investigations should thoroughly explore the environment, as a way of identifying triggering situations. She explained the neuropsychiatric mechanisms of compulsive disorders, as well as repetitive or ritualized behaviors. It was her opinion that many of these animals may have anxiety or phobias, or are under-exercised, but a small group of them might indeed have a true neurotransmitter alteration as an organic cause for the behavior.

Guillermina Manigot *Argentina* described the groups of drugs used to treat psychodermatoses and emphasized those that she felt were most effective. These were fluoxetine, amitriptyline, selegiline, alprazolam and diazepam. It was her opinion that if standard drug therapy was ineffective, an increase in dosage (two to three times the initial dosage) might result in an adequate response. The participants also contributed personal experiences and opinions.

The participants concurred that the most useful drugs were fluoxetine, alprazolam, amitriptyline, clomipramine and selegiline. Clomipramine was felt to be as safe as amitriptyline but had a more rapid response. Fluoxetine was also considered to be safe, as well as having anticompulsive effects. Interference with learning was not noted, but a higher dose than typically reported might be required to effect a response. Most participants felt that fluoxetine's benefits made it worth its cost. Alprazolam was found to be useful for those cats with territorial stress and anxiety-related conditions. It was also considered safe in dogs with mixed behavioral disorders that included phobias and skin conditions. Doxepin was considered to be more of an antipruritic drug than an anticompulsive medication.

Leslie Larson Cooper and Alexander Werner added that buspirone could be useful in many feline cases.

Guillermina Manigot thought that it may be necessary to consider using combinations of behavioral drugs.

Finally, newer drugs that might be considered for study in patients with psychodermatoses were discussed. They include other selective serotonin reuptake inhibitors (sertraline, paroxetine), opioid receptor effectors (naltrexone), haloperidol and fluvoxamine. Experience with these medications was lacking.

Participants concluded that behavioral modification, conducted at home under supervision of a behaviorist, is mandatory in difficult cases, because drug therapy alone may not always resolve the situation.

5.12

Acariasis: biology and treatment

Patrick Bourdeau[1] (Chairperson) and Andrea G. Cannon[2] (Secretary)

[1] Ecole Nationale Veterinaire de Nantes, Nantes, France
[2] Animal Dermatology and Allergy, Sacramento, California, USA

Patrick Bourdeau *France* commented on the definition of 'commensal' from a book *Commensal et Parasites* by Van Beneden. Commensal comes from the Latin, meaning 'at the same table', which differs from parasites that use everything for themselves and there is no benefit for the host. So, *Demodex* is not a commensal but a perfect parasite. If the host does not maintain the equilibrium, then we see disease. Approximately 30 000 mite species are known but there are probably half a million species.

Comments were made on the life cycles of parasites (typically egg, larvae, three nymphal stages and adult). Many species have adapted and reduced the number of nymphal stages. Some situations are unique, as in two cases of dermatitis caused by a cheyletid butterfly parasite. Life cycles may differ. Permanent parasites are those in which all the life cycles occur on the host life, e.g. *Sarcoptes*. Sessile parasites have long periods of parasitism, e.g. *Ctenocephalides felis and Ixodes* spp. Intermittent parasites only feed on the host, e.g. mosquitoes. In general, the more permanent the parasite, the more specific it is and environmental resistance increases with decreased host specificity. We need to keep all these factors in mind to develop efficient strategies to treat acariasis.

Parasites stimulate immune responses in the host. For example, cross-reactivity between house dust mite antigens and *Sarcoptes* antigen has been demonstrated. Cross-reactivity was also observed with *Otodectes* and *Cheyletiella* and other mites such as *Trombicula*.

Why do we see severe disease in one host and not another? Host response to the parasite is very important. Host response limits the numbers of parasites. Increased reaction to the parasite will lead to decreased numbers of parasites. Sheep with severe psoroptic mange have few parasites and these are very difficult to demonstrate on skin scrapings. In contrast, in Norwegian scabies, immunodeficiency of the host and absence of a response are associated with large numbers of mites.

Several possibilities exist in treated acariasis, including clinical cure and parasitological cure and/or a persistence of low numbers of parasites in apparently cured animals. This latter situation may be the case in demodicosis. In the case of a persistent infestation, if the immune system is compromised, then a recurrence may occur. Subclinical infestations can also occur and could be common in some diseases (e.g. *Otodectes*). The clinical disease is just the tip of the iceberg.

Jan Hall *Canada* Asymptomatic carriers of *Sarcoptes* are a large problem in Ontario.

Patrick Bourdeau had had one dog from the nutrition department that kept having recurrence of suspected scabies (skin scraping negative) which temporarily responded to treatments. This dog had contact with another dog through a fence. The other dog was not pruritic but the dog was skin scraping positive.

Pneumonyssoides caninum, the canine nasal mite (L. Gunnarsson)

Lotta Gunnarsson *Sweden* *Pneumonyssoides caninum* is a parasite that was first reported in the USA in 1940 and which lives in the canine nasal cavity and sinuses. Subsequently, it has been reported in other countries in Europe (1971), and world-wide. The female mite is 1–1.5 mm by 0.6–0.9 mm and the male is smaller. The parasite is ovoid and light yellow in colour, and can move at 1 cm/s. In Sweden, the prevalence of

P. caninum from June 1992 to November 1999 was 21% (111 of 534) in dogs presenting for necropsy. The dogs had between one and 250 mites, with a median count of 13. Of the 1267 mites counted, 83.5% (1058) were female, 3.5% (45) were male and 13% (164) were larvae. In a dry Petri dish the mites died in 24 h. In a moist Petri dish the mites survived for 3 weeks, whether kept refrigerated or at room temperature. In an experiment inoculating 13 dogs with *P. caninum* and counting mites at necropsy, 12 of the 13 dogs had live mites at 6–42 weeks postinoculation. Clinical signs included sneezing, reverse sneezing and decreased ability to smell.

A definitive diagnosis of *P. caninum* infection is difficult to achieve. Mites can be directly visualized or the nasal cavity can be flushed and retrieved fluid examined for mites. At present, many dogs with clinical signs compatible with *P. caninum* are often given diagnostic treatments. Antibodies were detected using an indirect *P. caninum* enzyme-linked immunosorbent assay (ELISA) in four experimentally and 77 naturally infected dogs.

Robert Alva *Italy* (Merial) How do you propagate *P. caninum*?

Lotta Gunnarsson Mites were collected from dogs at necropsy.

Patrick Bourdeau Do Swedish dogs receive routine anthelmintics?

Lotta Gunnarsson No, it's unusual for them to receive routine anthelmintics except in summer for ticks.

Patrick Bourdeau They must not have received ivermectin. This could explain the high prevalence in your country.

Lotta Gunnarsson That is correct.

Mike Wallace *USA* How long do dogs remain positive on the ELISA?

Lotta Gunnarsson There are not enough dogs to say definitively, but it takes about 2 months before they are negative on ELISA. I would be happy to analyse serum samples from dogs.

Efficacy of fipronil against the mite *Sarcoptes scabiei* var. *canis* on dogs (R. Alva)

Robert Alva (Merial) The goal of this study was to confirm the efficacy of fipronil in treating induced cases of scabies. Eighteen mixed-breed dogs (eight females, 10 males) were divided into three groups. Group 1 was a control group, group 2 was sprayed with Frontline® Spray at 6 ml/kg on days 0 and 28, and group 3 was treated with the Spot-On formulation of fipronil as per label instructions on days 0 and 28. Skin scrapings were performed from four areas on each dog and were counted on days 7, 21, 35, 49 and 63. *Sarcoptes* lesion scores (on a 1–5 scale) and body weights were recorded on days −1, 7 and weekly to day 63. Live mites were found on control animals throughout the study, except for one dog on days 49 and 63. The Frontline-treated group had significantly ($p < 0.05$) fewer mites than the controls at each count. No live mites were found in this group on days 7, 49 and 63. The Spot-On-treated group had significantly fewer mites than the control group ($p < 0.05$) on days 21–63. No live mites were found on these dogs on days 35, 49 and 63. Lesion scores were significantly ($p < 0.05$) reduced in both treated groups at several time points after day 28. It was concluded that fipronil in both formulations is effective against *Sarcoptes scabiei* var. *canis* infestation in dogs. It is recognized that further studies are still needed.

Avermectins and milbemycins in the treatment of acariasis (W. Ryan)

Bill Ryan *USA (Merial)* This discussion will focus on the use of ivermectin for the treatment of mites not ticks. Ivermectin works well on livestock for the prevention of ticks, but efficacy is decreased in companion animals. There is a wide safety margin for the avermectins and milbemycins in dogs. Ivermectin is a macrocyclic lactone that is highly lipophilic with wide tissue distribution. Increased concentrations are found in the gut, lung and skin of cattle, ear wax of swine and in the bile and feces. Ivermectins block the glutamate-gated chloride channels and the γ-aminobutyric acid (GABA) gated channels. They do not usually cross the blood–brain barrier due to p-glycoproteins. So why are some collies sensitive to ivermectin? In a mouse model (CF-1), where the mice have an absence of p-glycoproteins, ivermectin toxicity is seen.

Ivermectin used at 200–400 μg/kg will eliminate all mites in one or two doses. For *Demodex*, 600 μg/kg daily has been reported to be effective. Milbemycin is used at 2–4 mg/kg with two doses per month, or more often if needed. Selamectin is used at 6–12 mg/kg for

Sarcoptes or *Otodectes*. Moxidectin is used in the same way as ivermectin.

Helen Power *USA* noted that the original published dose of ivermectin for demodicosis (600 μg/kg) was a mathematical error.

Jan Hall concurred with Helen Power's comment and added that she has had success with 300 μg/kg by mouth daily for demodicosis, but that the 600 μg/kg dose may give a faster improvement. She asked whether Dr Ryan could comment on the oral versus the subcutaneous route.

Bill Ryan I have no definite answer. Subcutaneous reactions are a good indication to use the oral route but there are no studies.

Patrick Bourdeau So, the speed of response may be dose related. The same is seen with milbemycin oxime, where an every-other-day dose doubled the response time. Moreover, molecules have different kinetics. For example, in cats, doramectin was compared to ivermectin for the treatment of *Notoedres*. The results were that several injections of ivermectin were required whilst a single dose of doramectin was successful.

Dan Domingo *USA* (Pfizer Animal Health) I am not surprised by these results. Doramectin is similar to selamectin. Selamectin is very efficacious in treating infestation with *Otodectes* in dogs and cats. To treat scabies, how many of you use: ivermectin [six people in the group did], selamectin [four people], moxidectin [no one did and it was noted that moxidectin is approved for use in cattle and not dogs] or milbemycin [it was stated that it was very expensive]?

Control of *Otodectes cynotis* infestations by selamectin in dogs and cats (D. Domingo)

Dan Domingo (Pfizer Animal Health) Selamectin is a novel avermectin developed for use in dogs and cats. The recommended dose is 6 mg/kg in dogs and cats that are at least 6 weeks old. Selamectin is an endectocide controlling fleas, ear mites and nematodes. The efficacy of selamectin dosed either once or twice at monthly intervals in treating natural infestations of *Otodectes* in dogs and cats was examined. In dogs, naturally infected dogs were treated with either selamectin or a placebo on day 0 or days 0 and 30. Cats were treated with either placebo or selamectin on day 0 only. No mites were found in any of the selamectin-treated animals on day 30 or 60 after the last treatment.

Field studies were conducted in the USA and Europe. In total, 135 dogs were enrolled: 45 dogs received ear cleaning and treatment with pyrethrin and piperonyl butoxide and the other 90 dogs received selamectin with no ear cleaning. The proportion of dogs with viable mites in the selamectin group was 47%, 23% and 10% at days 14, 30 and 60, respectively. In the pyrethrin group, the proportion of dogs with viable mites remained at 35% at day 60.

Sixty-eight cats with naturally occurring ear mite infestations were treated with a single dose of selamectin and another 35 cats were treated with pyrethrin and piperonyl butoxide on day 0. The presence of viable mites was reduced to 5% and 0% on days 14 and 30, respectively, in the selamectin group. In the pyrethrin group at day 30, the viable mites remained at 12%. Again, ear cleaning was allowed only in the pyrethrin group.

Although mites were significantly reduced, and clinical signs such as head shaking, pruritus and debris improved, these signs were observed in both groups until the end of the study at day 90. This reinforces the need to clean the ears prior to treatment to resolve clinical signs.

Patrick Bourdeau Why do cats differ from dogs?

Dan Domingo Pharmacokinetics differ between cats and dogs. There is increased bioavailability in cats and therefore quicker control. This is also true with other ectoparasites such as *Sarcoptes* and fleas. In the pyrethrin-treated group, the veterinarians were allowed to treat other pets in the households and to clean the ears, but not in the selamectin group. In the positive control group there was no other antiparasitic used.

Patrick Bourdeau It may be necessary to treat the entire coat in severe *Otodectes* infestation. With selamectin, you may get systemic effects and there may be a need to treat topically as well as in the ears with other products.

Jan Hall It works well but owners are frustrated by the continuation of clinical signs.

Bill Ryan At the heartworm society meeting it was said that the increased effectiveness in cats compared with dogs may be due to cats grooming and not to bioavailability.

Dan Domingo The grooming activity may contribute but there are actual bioavailability differences between cats and dogs.

Patrick Bourdeau Since there are still clinical signs present when we cannot find the mites, perhaps there are a small number of mites remaining.

Dan Domingo In our studies, we looked at viable mites but not eggs, which may also be a factor.

Amitraz collars in the prevention of Lyme borreliosis (O. Elfassy)

Oliver Elfassy *France* (Virbac Animal Health) Amitraz is an acaricide that causes detachment and repels ticks. The iron content is used as a measure of feeding in ticks. In dogs with an amitraz collar, the iron content of the ticks is almost the same as in unfed, laboratory-reared ticks. The purpose of this study was to evaluate the effectiveness of the amitraz collar in preventing Lyme disease in dogs.

Eight beagle dogs were divided into two groups of four dogs each. Dogs were unvaccinated for *Borrelia burgdorferi* and had had no tick exposure. An ELISA was used to follow infection rate. On days −15 and −1, all dogs had negative ELISA for *B. burgdorferi* and on days −15 and 56, all dogs were negative for *Ehrlichia canis, Babesia canis* and *Rickettsia rickettsii*. On day 0, one group had amitraz collars while the other group served as the control group. On day 7, *Ixodes* ticks that were captured in Connecticut with a 39.4% infection rate were placed on each dog along the dorsal midline in a 1:1 ratio of males to females. All untreated dogs developed anti-borrelia antibody in the high to very high range. The antibody pattern followed the typical pattern described in the literature. *Ehrlichia canis, B. canis* and *R. rickettsii* were ruled out as a cause of the antibody response by Western blot analysis and serology. None of the treated dogs developed an antibody response to *B. burgdorferi, E. canis, B. canis* or *R. rickettsii*. Poststudy polymerase chain reaction studies confirmed the infectivity of the ticks. Our conclusions were that amitraz collars are effective in preventing the attachment and feeding of ticks and are effective in preventing *B. burgdorferi* transmission.

Dan Domingo What is the transmission time of tick-borne diseases?

Olivier Elfassy It is variable depending on the disease, but it seems that the transmission of *B. burgdorferi* increases at 24–48 h.

Patrick Bourdeau Experimental transmission with infected ticks to rodents is rapid. It is dependent on the number of ticks and the percentage of infected ticks. A study in rabbits looked at time to blood meal in relation to their size. In a human hospital, the size of ticks extracted was analyzed. The results suggest that the delay of infection is relatively long in humans. Natural infection probably takes longer than in the laboratory.

Bill Ryan Gary Malfordis's model of ticks in rodents showed that Lyme disease increased exponentially 48 h from attachment.

Patrick Bourdeau Viral transmission is quicker. Thank you to all contributors for their intellect and for attending this session. It has been very interesting, but we have only started on this topic. Hopefully this should start us thinking and developing new ideas.

5.13

Equine dermatology

Marianne M. Sloet van Oldruitenborgh-Oosterbaan[1] (Chairperson) and
Mona J. Boord[2] (Secretary)

[1] Department of Equine Sciences, Faculty of Veterinary Medicine, Utrecht University, The Netherlands
[2] Animal Dermatology Clinic, San Diego, California, USA

Marianne Sloet *The Netherlands* Ladies and gentlemen, I am very honored to be chairing this workshop and I am very glad that Mona Boord is helping me with this job. I am a specialist in equine internal medicine. Equine dermatology is my hobby but I am not a dermatologist, nor a pathologist. At Utrecht, Jan Koeman is our pathologist and he has helped me to prepare the cases we will discuss. We hope today to present some unusual cases. The cases are from Utrecht. I hope we will have as much discussion as possible to get a better understanding of some equine dermatology problems and we may find some solutions.

Today's first subject will be pruritus. Some causes of pruritus in the horse are very common, like this Friesian mare with severe pruritus of the lower limbs. Skin scrapings revealed *Chorioptes equi*. Here is another case, a pony gelding with some pruritus at the neck. You can see the nits easily. The results of skin scrapings revealed *Damalinia equi*. Also shown is a pony with sweet itch, or, more accurately, insect hypersensitivity, which is a big problem in many places in the world and also in The Netherlands, in both ponies and horses. *Culicoides* spp. are the most common cause. Insect hypersensitivity is relatively easy to diagnose. Much more difficult to diagnose are horses with pruritus as a result of food allergy or atopy, but this is not what I would like to cover today.

So, we understand the common causes for pruritus in horses, the parasitic and allergic dermatoses, but there is more. If we look in Danny Scott's book, we will find the following important questions related to equine pruritus. Was pruritus the first thing noted? How severe is the pruritus? Is it intermittent, seasonal or constant? What is the response to glucocorticoid therapy?

The first case I want to present is Harrie, a 23-year-old fjord gelding. He was referred in March with the complaint of severe pruritus of the neck and trunk for the previous 5 months. Harrie was at pasture during the day and stabled during the evening. A dexamethasone injection had given only a short improvement. At the clinic, Harrie showed typical lesions resulting from scratching and rubbing, but during his 14 day stay with us he did not show any pruritus. As it was March, insect hypersensitivity was not likely. We could not find any ectoparasites and a bacterial culture was negative. Histopathological examination of a skin biopsy revealed only non-specific perivascular dermatitis resulting from rubbing. Harrie was sent home but within a few days the rubbing returned and so did Harrie. Again, we could not find any ectoparasites or other cause. We discussed an elimination diet, as Harrie did not show any symptoms while with us. Harrie went home again and again the pruritus returned. Three days later the mail delivered a little packet from Harrie's owner, an old farmer. Immediately after he had put Harrie in his stable, he had seen in the evening sun that dust from the roof was filtering down. He had collected this dust from Harrie's back and asked us to look whether this could cause an allergic reaction. The dust was full of mites: *Dermanyssus gallinae*. The explanation was that Harrie's owner was an old-fashioned farmer and before going to our clinic he took a bath and he washed Harrie also, but had never told us. This teaches us to be very thorough in getting our histories and to be clear in our instructions not to bathe the horse prior to examination.

The next case is Tom, an 18-year-old Dutch warmblood gelding with a 2 month history of severe pruritus over his entire body. We could not detect any ectoparasites or dermatophytes. Tom also had severe weight loss and on rectal palpation (we internists always want to do a rectal examination) there was enlargement of the left kidney. Tom had areas of partial and almost complete alopecia in the areas of pruritus. We did hematology and blood biochemistry. The packed cell volume (PCV) was low at 30% and decreased during his stay with us to 23%. The urea was normal. We had been concerned about uremia being a possible cause of the pruritus. The total protein was increased at 81 g/l and electrophoresis showed an increased percentage of β-globulins at 30%. Does anyone have any thoughts?

Danny Scott *USA* We have certainly seen generalized pruritus associated with internal malignancy and I would pursue the renal enlargement.

Wayne Rosenkrantz *USA* Another possibility would be generalized granulomatous disease.

Marianne Sloet Here is the histopathology of the skin biopsy. This appears to have similarities to the French flag sign. I am not a pathologist but I am told there is epidermal pallor and, on higher magnification, we can see the necrotic keratinocytes and possible toxic epidermal necrolysis.

Wayne Rosenkrantz It is difficult to tell without the glass slide to view the other sections for comparison, but we don't have the classic parakeratosis associated with superficial necrolytic dermatitis and there is epidermal pallor associated with keratinocyte necrosis.

Danny Scott I agree.

Marianne Sloet The horse was not doing well and was continuing to lose weight and was euthanized. Here you see a specimen of the kidney diagnosed as an anaplastic malignant tumor. There were also metastases in the spleen and the regional lymph nodes. Why do we see pruritus with malignancy? I do not know but I have seen several cases now.

The next case is Uran. He is a 13-year-old mini-Shetlander stallion. He had been bought 2 months before with skin problems. The pruritus was said to have been present for 5 years. Uran showed some ataxia and hypermetria of the hind limbs. At home, Uran was at pasture with 13 other ponies. They were normal. He was only pruritic over the neck, more specifically at the cranial cervical area, bilaterally symmetrically. This pony was scratching with its rear hooves all the time except when walking, eating or sleeping. The right side was more severely affected with ulcerated lesions. Insect hypersensitivity was not likely as Uran was admitted in April. The skin biopsies showed a thickened epidermis with acanthosis and hyperkeratosis. The dermis was fibrotic, showing hardly any inflammation. Does anyone have any ideas?

Danny Scott I would be concerned about a protozoal myelopathy.

Marianne Sloet But that is not present in The Netherlands. As there was ataxia, a cervical X-ray was taken. Here you see a lateral view of the cranial cervical vertebrae (C1–C3). The axis (C2) had a fracture. Our theory was that the pruritus was secondary to irritation of the local cervical nerve, innervating the dermatome where the pruritus was located. The professor of radiology, Kees Dik, was not convinced and wanted proof that compression of the cervical nerves was present. So a computed tomography (CT) scan was done. A suboccipital myelogram was made. The CT scan at the level of C2–C3 shows right-sided compression of the local cervical nerve and there may be some compression of the left side. This fits with the more severe lesions at the right side of the neck. Our advice to the owner was euthanasia. However, the owners wanted the pony home for breeding. At home his condition deteriorated and he was euthanized 2 months later.

Steven White *USA* This would appear similar to children with pain or pruritus associated with certain dermatomes.

Ken Mason *Australia* This would appear quite similar to seringomyelia of the King Charles spaniel, where they are incredibly pruritic between the ear and the shoulder.

Ralf Mueller *USA* Was it apparent that the horse had pain in the neck?

Marianne Sloet It was not possible to tell with this pony. He would not stop scratching to allow a good neurological examination.

The next case is Pablo, a 3-year-old Dutch warmblood gelding. Pablo had a 6 week history of severe skin lesions of the non-pigmented lower limbs. Over the past 2 weeks, the whole body had become involved. He had been seen by three previous veterinarians and had an extensive drug history with poor response. Our clinical findings revealed enlarged mandibular and prescapular lymph nodes. On rectal palpation, swellings were palpable in the mesenteric root region. Also, a systolic murmur of the aortic valve was heard. Slides of the horse showed patchy, diffuse to partial alopecia, with scale and crusting over most of the body. Histopathological examination revealed a crusted dermatitis with perivascular inflammation in the dermis. A higher power shows mononuclear infiltration with a lot of eosinophils. As we had no clear diagnosis, treatment with dexamethasone was started. He received 0.2 mg/kg daily for 14 days. This gave significant improvement. However, we were still looking for the primary cause of the problems. In the peritoneal fluid there were no tumor cells. An aspiration biopsy of an enlarged lymph node did not reveal any tumor cells. During the 2 weeks the horse stayed with us, it lost 60 kg. He also showed mild to moderate colic several times. On a biochemistry panel, Pablo had a decreased PCV of 28% and a low total protein concentration. Liver enzymes were normal. The horse's skin was clear at 14 days so the dexa- methasone was stopped. Within 3 days the pruritus returned and the skin lesions returned too, with oozing and erythema. Does anyone have any thoughts?

Harrold Schott *USA* I would still be concerned about peritonitis.

Wayne Rosenkrantz When were the steroids given?

Marianne Sloet We always give steroids in the morning, based on studies showing that the horse's natural peak is at that time. We have done this for 10 years and have very rarely had laminitis, and in the few cases that developed laminitis the owners had given the medication at other times. We had no idea with this case and the insurance company did not wish to spend any more money. The horse was euthanized. At necropsy a chronic adhesive peritonitis was found. The wall of the jejunum was chronically thickened but on histopathological examination had no tumor. The serosa of the jejunum was thickened with an increased amount of connective tissue. On histopathological examination there was a large number of macrophages containing iron. Histopathological examination of the skin of the tarsus revealed an acanthotic epidermis with perivascular inflammation and some eosinophils. When I showed these slides to Dr Claudia von Tscharner, she suspected a vasculitis.

Wayne Rosenkrantz These lesions were worse on the non-pigmented areas so I would also consider a photocontact component.

Danny Scott The histopathology shows well-demarcated inflammatory cells around the vessel. This is a possible vasculitis. We have seen cutaneous vasculitis with intestinal inflammatory disease.

Harrold Schott One could have done a glucose tolerance test. The horse may have had an earlier, more severe colic that caused the adhesions.

Alexander Werner *USA* In dogs with inflammatory bowel disease and pruritic skin disease, we are often concerned about a food allergy.

Harrold Schott We have associated an inflammatory bowel disease in the horse with eosinophilic enteritis and dermatitis.

Marianne Sloet I have one case of eosinophilic enteritis with a very grave prognosis that is still doing very well. Remember the aortic murmur of Pablo? The little nodules on the aortic valves are probably of parasitic origin and will have caused the murmur.

The next topic I would like to cover is 'crusted lower limb problems'. What do I mean? I have had cases with no pruritus, only one limb involved, scaling, crusting and hair loss, sometimes edema, no ectoparasites, no dermatophytes, no bacteria and some response to systemic glucocorticoids.

Dana is one of these cases. She is a 13-year-old, Dutch warmblood mare with a 2–3 year history of abnormal skin on the plantar metatarsus. It may have started with pastern dermatitis. It had been treated with several ointments and solutions without any effect. The lesions are seen here on the left hindlimb. Here is the histopathology of the lesion. There is a thickened epidermis with diffuse lymphohistiocytic infiltration in the upper dermis with a few giant cells. The conclusion of Jan Koeman was that this might be sarcoidosis. Now, 2 years later, the lesion is still there and the owner keeps it acceptable with local treatment with oil. The skin is very fragile and bleeds easily. When I showed this to Claudia von Tscharner she was not sure these were true giant cells. She was concerned about possible cholesterol clefts.

Wayne Rosenkrantz In the area pointed out, I don't see multiple nuclei. I would be more concerned about a localized keratinization disorder, especially with it only affecting this location and still being present 2.5 years later.

Danny Scott It appears not unlike lichenoid keratosis. We see a dense band of lymphohistiocytic inflammation.

Marianne Sloet The next case is Joyful Lady, a 9-year-old, Dutch warmblood mare bought 9 months previously with a skin problem. The first diagnosis at home was pastern dermatitis and the horse had been treated with different ointments and solutions with some effect. The hematology and blood biochemistry values were normal. Here you see the horse with the lesion over the left forelimb. The histopathology again shows a diffuse lymphohistiocytic infiltration in the upper dermis with some giant cells. The conclusion was sarcoidosis. The horse is doing well on a low glucocorticoid dose. From what I read about sarcoidosis, it is a systemic disease and has not been reported as a localized problem.

The last case of crusting limbs I will present is Ilando, a 6-year-old, Dutch warmblood gelding with a 1 year history of a severe dermatosis of the right hind lower limb. Local treatment with ointments or solutions was unsuccessful. Also, there was no response to systemic glucocorticoids and antibiotics in the history. The clinical photos show a crusting dermatosis of the right lower limb. Is there any discussion?

Wayne Rosenkrantz I don't know what has recently been used on the horse, but I would be concerned about an allergic or irritant contact dermatitis. Other differentials would include folliculitis, vasculitis and a keratinization disorder.

Marianne Sloet This slide shows the histopathology with some infiltration of the vessel wall by neutrophils. Here we see 'nuclear dust', which may indicate a leukocytoclastic vasculitis, but this was a pigmented limb. As I discussed earlier this week, leukocytoclastic pastern vasculitis described as a disease of the non-pigmented lower limb seems to occur in the pigmented limbs as well.

Danny Scott I don't see why it couldn't stay localized to one location and be a localized disease.

Marianne Sloet The next topic is, how important is leukotrichia, leukoderma or vitiligo? Is it really a disaster? Certainly it is not a problem in most cases. This horse was referred to Utrecht for colic and the owner asked why her horse had lost some color on the hairs of his face and hindquarters. She also wanted to know how to treat it. My answer was that there is no treatment. The owner was satisfied with this answer. Here is another example with vitiligo around the eye. This occurs often, especially in the offspring of certain stallions. Another slide here shows hypopigmentation of the muzzle. Here is a photo of leukotrichia that is most likely the result of a saddle sore. However, in Friesian horses, white hairs are not allowed and stallions with white hairs are excluded from breeding. A case presented to me was a 3-year-old Friesian stallion that had been at the central stallion training center for selection. Suddenly, some white hairs appeared on the thorax. The horse was referred to Utrecht with the question: is this congenital, acquired or hereditary? As a breeding stallion this horse is worth a lot of money. If he is not to be used for breeding, his value changes significantly and the financial consequences are enormous.

These cases need a very careful approach. The case is in litigation and they would not allow me to take a picture of the entire horse, but here are the photos of the places with a few white hairs. What is your answer to this question? The judge is asking me for a report. I was not allowed to biopsy the horse.

The question gets even more difficult if you look at this case. This is an 18-year-old, Friesian stallion referred for lameness. The horse was fully black until several years ago. The transparency shows large patches of leukotrichia extending over the hip and lateral left leg of the stallion. Where do these white hairs come from?

Danny Scott I would just consider this a cosmetic problem.

Marianne Sloet Be certain that leukotrichia in Friesian horses is a disaster!

Now as our final topic I would like to discuss some very rare cases. Komiek is an 8-year-old, Dutch warmblood gelding. The chief complaint was a 3 week history of abnormal tissue on the inside of the right upper lip and gingiva around the upper canine tooth. There were no problems with eating, but the owner considered that the horse was in pain during riding. Hematology and blood biochemistry values were unremarkable. Komiek is a big horse and here you see the lesions in his mouth. They were not painful on palpation. The transparency shows a papulated sessile mass affecting the right upper lip and gingiva. The histology of the lip lesion shows some inflammation in the upper dermis and the epidermis may be a little lichenified. Histology of the mucous membrane showed some hyperplastic epithelium with moderate subepithelial inflammation and a mononuclear infiltrate. The horse was treated systemically with prednisolone without any response. Three months later, it was treated with laser surgery with some response. One month postsurgery, the horse was referred to our clinic at the request of the insurance company, requesting an evaluation. The owner reported that the horse was still in pain. The company wished to know whether they should pay for the horse and slaughter it, or what other recommendation we had. At our clinic, riding and handling the horse was no problem at all. Are there any thoughts as to the primary cause of this lesion?

Wayne Rosenkrantz It clinically and histopathologically resembles a nevus.

Danny Scott I agree it could be a nevus but it could be re-evaluated with a repeat biopsy.

Marianne Sloet Now I would like to discuss Melik, a 2.5-week-old donkey stallion. Over the past 4 days he had developed lesions on the limbs. The owner said that an adult stallion had probably attacked the foal. The lesions had deteriorated quickly. I had seen a case similar to this in a calf and on admittance was concerned about the possibility of ergotism, zinc deficiency and dermatosparaxis. However, none of these diagnoses fitted well. Here you see the foal. There are large areas of epidermal ulceration on the distal extremities. The foal was otherwise bright, alert and responsive. He was eating and drinking. Histopathological examination was not diagnostic. Are there any comments?

Danny Scott This appears similar to foals reported with epidermolysis bullosa. Another differential would include vasculitis.

Marianne Sloet Here is the same foal 15 days later on treatment with non-steroidal anti-inflammatory drugs and antibiotics. The skin lesions improved a little, but the foal deteriorated and developed diarrhea. We can see that the ears were becoming involved and the ligaments were becoming very weak, with the joints hyperextending and bending in abnormal directions. The foal was euthanized. The zinc concentration was normal in blood, liver and kidney. Here, postmortem histology shows a thick cellular crust with fissures between the epidermis and the dermis. Here you see a place without a crust: there is chronic inflammation and loss of the epidermis, especially on the left. Here is an area with intact epidermis. At the dermoepidermal junction you see vacuolar degeneration just beneath the stratum basale. The final conclusion of Jan Koeman was epidermolysis bullosa.

I am finished with the cases I planned to discuss, but we have a little time left and I brought extra cases in case there was time remaining. [The group decided to continue with additional cases.]

Orvelle is a 3-year-old, Dutch warmblood mare. She had been at the central mare training center 3 weeks before, and 1 week before presentation developed multiple, 1–3 cm nodules on the hindlimbs. There was no pruritus and no pain. Our differential diagnoses included habronema, *Sporothrix schenckii*, botryomycosis and eosinophilic granuloma. Histopathological examination of the lesions showed extensive perivascular infiltration of eosinophils in the deep dermis. On higher magnification, we can see small areas of collagen degeneration and focal calcium deposition. This was diagnosed as eosinophilic granuloma.

The final case I would like to present is Jiri, an 8-year-old, Dutch warmblood gelding. He had a 1.5 year history of abnormal coronary bands on all four legs. He was not apparently in pain and there was no pruritus. On physical examination there were transverse cracks and separations in the hooves, and after scraping the coronary bands they start to bleed. The horse had never had any extra vitamin E and/or selenium.

Unknown participant There are occasions when a feed manufacturer can have a shipment of feed with large amounts of selenium. I would recommend checking selenium levels anyway.

Ralf Mueller I would think this horse may have active disease at the matrix or permanent damage to the matrix. This may be immune mediated, drug related or possibly nutritional.

Marianne Sloet I would like to finish by saying that equine dermatology world-wide needs much more attention and much more clinical research. I thank you for your attention and your contributions.

5.14

Thyroid and adrenal function testing

Keith L. Thoday[1] (Chairperson) and Carmel T. Mooney[2] (Secretary)

[1] The University of Edinburgh, Department of Veterinary Clinical Studies, The Royal (Dick) School of Veterinary Studies, Hospital for Small Animals, Roslin, Midlothian, UK
[2] University College Dublin, Ballsbridge, Dublin, Ireland

Keith Thoday *UK* opened the workshop with comments on the frequency with which thyroid and adrenal disorders occur in the dog, their association with skin disease and the difficulties often encountered in confirming a diagnosis.

Carmel Mooney *Ireland* addressed the topic of routine clinicopathological findings in canine hypothyroidism and which tests suggest pursuing the diagnosis.

Hypercholesterolaemia, anaemia and an increased circulating concentration of creatine kinase are the most common routine clinicopathological abnormalities associated with hypothyroidism. The hypercholesterolaemia results from reduced lipid degradation. The anaemia is usually mild, normocytic and normochromic, and is considered to be a physiological adaptation to the reduced metabolic rate and oxygen requirements. The aetiology of the increased creatine kinase is unclear and while it may be related to a hypothyroid myopathy in some individuals, it may simply reflect decreased plasma clearance of this analyte.

It was pointed out that these abnormalities lack both sensitivity and specificity for diagnosing hypothyroidism. Importantly, values are often compared with laboratory reference ranges, frequently derived from a narrow population of animals, and which are only capable of distinguishing health from ill health without indicating the underlying disease process. Thus, Dr Mooney and colleagues had evaluated data from 140 dogs with clinical signs suggestive of hypothyroidism in which the diagnosis was either confirmed ($n = 52$) or refuted ($n = 88$) by the results of a thyrotropin (thyroid stimulating hormone, TSH) response test.

Hypercholesterolaemia, hypertriglyceridaemia, anaemia and decreased fructosamine and increased creatine kinase concentrations were confirmed as common abnormalities in hypothyroidism. However, similar abnormalities were frequently found in the euthyroid sick dogs. Compared with a reference range derived from these dogs, a decreased red blood cell count, haemoglobin concentration, neutrophil count and elevations in γ-glutamyl transferase and cholesterol concentrations were the most common abnormalities indicative of hypothyroidism. The magnitude of the elevation in cholesterol was also helpful diagnostically, as 53% of hypothyroid dogs had a value exceeding 10 mmol/l (with 20% exceeding 15 mmol/l), whereas only 22% and 4% of euthyroid sick dogs had values exceeding these respective limits. Unfortunately, the data needed to generate such information are demanding in terms of clinical material, case classification and time, but the improved diagnostic specificity makes it highly desirable.

Keith Thoday agreed that the generation of reference ranges from animals with compatible clinical features, in which the diagnosis of a disorder was subsequently confirmed or refuted, was highly desirable.

Sarah Ambler *UK* said that for many cases, assessment of routine clinicopathological parameters was prohibitively expensive and if signs compatible with hypothyroidism were present, as much valuable information could be obtained from a plasma total thyroxine (TT_4) concentration determination alone.

Colleen Mendelsohn *USA* suggested that urinalysis was also important to eliminate other disorders with similar clinical features, particularly hyperadrenocorticism.

Dominique Heripret *France* commented that the anaemia associated with hypothyroidism was not usually clinically apparent and, in many cases, the parameters were within the respective reference ranges. It was also pointed out that circulating triglyceride and cholesterol concentrations are affected by feeding, a factor for which many practitioners do not allow.

Carmel Mooney argued that the magnitude of elevation in cholesterol in healthy dogs postprandially was mild.

Peter Graham *USA* suggested that a more reliable test for hypercholesterolaemia would be to measure it pre- and postfeeding.

Peter Graham then presented details on the common thyroid hormone tests used to confirm a diagnosis of hypothyroidism. Although overdiagnosis of hypothyroidism was considered a problem, using the tests simply to decide whether a dog was hypothyroid or euthyroid did not take into account the progression of thyroid disease through subclinical thyroiditis, subclinical hypothyroidism and overt thyroid hormone deficiency. In addition, he pointed out that several months could elapse between laboratory evidence of hypothyroidism and the development of overt clinical signs.

Determination of the plasma TT_4 concentration is widely available and is generally considered an inexpensive test and an effective indicator of normal thyroid function when values fall within the reference range. However, a significant proportion (18–25%) of euthyroid dogs also has low values. In addition, the presence of thyroxine (T_4) autoantibodies (T_4AA) may affect the interpretation of results. Of 16 250 canine blood samples sent to the Endocrine Laboratory at Michigan State University, 1093 were diagnosed as being indicative of hypothyroidism. T_4AA were present in 14.5% of these samples, resulting in spuriously normal and high values in 8.8 and 1.2% of samples, respectively. In addition, TT_4 analysis gives no indication of the presence of subclinical hypothyroidism. Free T_4 (FT_4) analysis is considered a better diagnostic test, providing equilibrium dialysis and not analogue methods are used. It is less susceptible to the effects of non-thyroidal illness and the presence of T_4AA, but its determination is more time-consuming and expensive, and the test sample is sensitive to changes during transit. As with TT_4, a FT_4 analysis alone cannot be used to diagnose subclinical hypothyroidism. Measurement of the plasma endogenous TSH concentration is considered to be a test of high specificity (82–100%) but with limited sensitivity. Therefore, a high TSH value invariably indicates thyroid dysfunction. If a TT_4 concentration is low, with a reference range TSH value, non-thyroidal disease is most likely, but it was pointed out that such a combination could occur in approximately 15% of hypothyroid dogs. If the plasma TT_4 or FT_4 concentration is within the reference range but the TSH value is high, partial or impending thyroid failure is likely.

Dominique Heripret commented that he did not use measurement of endogenous TSH concentration in the investigation of hypothyroidism because of its poor diagnostic performance.

Carmel Mooney asked whether all the methods available for TSH measurement gave similar results and whether any precautions were required.

Peter Graham replied that in comparative studies, enzyme-linked immunosorbent assays (ELISA), chemiluminescent and immunoradiometric (IRMA) assays all performed similarly, but that serum separator tubes should be avoided when using the chemiluminescence technique.

Jane Summers *UK* told the group that measurement of FT_4 by equilibrium dialysis was available in Cambridge, UK.

[After a question from the chair, approximately 25% of the audience said that they used a combination of endogenous TSH assays, with either FT_4 or TT_4 measurements, to diagnose hypothyroidism.]

Colleen Mendelsohn asked whether dogs with reference range T_4 and TSH concentrations should be treated with L-thyroxine.

Liora Waldman *Israel* commented that this would be prohibitively expensive.

Dominique Heripret suggested that because reference range TT_4 and TSH values could potentially occur in hypothyroidism, then therapy in such a dog could be contemplated providing that the dog appeared to be clinically hypothyroid.

Heidy Zenulila *Mexico* asked whether dogs with low normal T_4 and TSH concentrations warranted treatment. There was unanimous agreement that treatment was not warranted in such cases.

Carmel Mooney then addressed the current role of dynamic thyroid function testing in the diagnosis of hypothyroidism. Previous difficulties with the TSH and thyrotropin-releasing hormone (TRH) response tests related to the numerous protocols recommended, but these had recently become more standardised. Currently, the problem with the TSH response test primarily related to the limited availability of pharmaceutical grade TSH. Chemical grade bovine TSH remains available but it is expensive, unlicensed and associated with anaphylactic-type responses in a small number of individuals. In addition, while some workers consider it the gold standard of the currently available diagnostic tests, it can be argued that the supraphysiological concentrations administered could result in adequate stimulation, not only in secondary hypothyroidism, but also in early cases of primary hypothyroidism. Pharmaceutical grade TRH is widely available and was originally touted as a viable alternative to TSH stimulation, capable of diagnosing not only primary but also secondary hypothyroidism. Unfortunately, TRH administration results in a limited T_4 response, leading to a possible diagnosis of hypothyroidism in both healthy dogs and those with significant non-thyroidal disease. In addition, TRH can be associated with adverse reactions such as salivation and nausea. Despite these concerns, few studies have compared the tests, although in one the results from the TRH response test would have misclassified many euthyroid animals as hypothyroid compared with the TSH response test. This suggests that the TRH response test is the least useful dynamic test for diagnosing hypothyroidism.

An alternative is to measure the plasma TSH concentration 30 min after TRH administration. In humans, primary hypothyroidism is associated with a greater and more prolonged increase in TSH concentration, whereas in secondary hypothyroidism there is a minimal increase. However, in hypothyroid dogs, there is a minimal increase in TSH values after TRH administration, but the overall diagnostic accuracy is similar to a combined basal T_4 and TSH measurement. The consensus, therefore, appears to be that because a firm diagnosis of hypothyroidism cannot be achieved in all cases using a single basal sample, these tests may still have a role to play and of those available, the TSH stimulation test is the most valuable. The production of a human recombinant form of TSH may increase the availability of TSH, and this has recently been shown to produce a similar T4 response in healthy dogs to that obtained after administration of bovine TSH.

[After a question from the chair, approximately 10% of the audience responded that, diagnostically, they used the TSH response test but none used the TRH response test.]

Keith Thoday commented that the shelf-life of reconstituted TSH is significantly prolonged after freezing, reducing the cost of the test.

Sarah Ambler suggested that the TRH response test was useful to rule out hypothyroidism, as a normal response confirms euthyroidism.

Peter Graham finished the discussion on hypothyroidism with a presentation on alternative tests for its diagnosis, including thyroglobulin autoantibodies (TgAA), T_4AA and triiodothyronine (T_3) autoantibodies (T_3AA), total T_3 (TT_3), free T_3 (FT_3) and reverse T_3 (rT_3) concentrations and '*k*'-values. Therapeutic trials with L-thyroxine were not considered valuable because of its inherent pharmacological effects. Thyroglobulin autoantibodies were considered to be 100% sensitive and specific when compared with histopathological evidence of lymphocytic thyroiditis. Thyroglobulin autoantibodies also detect subclinical thyroiditis, although it remains unclear whether all these animals progress to subclinical or overt hypothyroidism. A current study is investigating 230 cases with positive TgAA and, thus far, only approximately 15% per year have developed hypothyroidism.

TgAA status is often also positive in thyroid carcinoma. The greatest prevalence of TgAA occurs in young to middle-aged dogs, with a slight rise in older dogs, reflecting the development of thyroid carcinoma in this age group. Some breeds are over- and some underrepresented. Over 30% of hypothyroid dogs have T_3AA, limiting the value of T_3 analysis for diagnosing hypothyroidism. Assays for rT_3 measurement are expensive, not easily available and of limited diagnostic value, particularly since measurement of canine TSH became possible. So-called *k*-values, obtained after mathematical manipulation of cholesterol and T_4 concentrations, were not considered useful because not all hypothyroid dogs have hypercholesterolaemia. Radionuclide imaging, although possible, was of no value in investigating hypothyroidism in adult dogs, but was considered useful in determining the site of the lesion in congenital cases. T_3 uptake and free thyroxine index measurements, although still occasionally encountered in human medicine, were of no value in investigating canine hypothyroidism. [Following a question from the chair, none of the audience had recognised T_4AA in their hypothyroid dogs.]

Dominique Heripret then addressed the topic of routine clinicopathological findings in canine hyperadrenocorticism. He pointed out that these tests could only be interpreted correctly in the light of clinical findings.

Hyperadrenocorticism is most commonly encountered in small breed dogs such as poodles, Boston terriers, Yorkshire terriers and dachshunds. Typical clinical signs include polyuria, polydipsia, polyphagia, alopecia, calcinosis cutis, panting and pseudomyotonia, which gives typical dive-bomb sounds on electromyelography. An elevated serum alkaline phosphatase (ALP) concentration was considered a sensitive but non-specific indicator of hyperadrenocorticism. Despite cortisol inducing a specific isoenzyme of ALP in dogs, it was not considered useful to measure this fraction. A stress leukogram was also considered a common finding. It consisted of a neutrophilia, resulting from capillary demargination, lymphopenia from lymphocyte destruction and eosinopenia from bone marrow sequestration. Erythrocytosis has also been reported. Other abnormalities encountered included an increased alanine aminotransferase concentration from excess glycogen and lipid deposition in the liver, hypercholesterolaemia, hypertriglyceridaemia, hyperglycaemia, mild changes in plasma sodium and potassium concentrations, a low TT_4 concentration and a low urine specific gravity. Typically, a diagnosis of hyperadrenocorticism was pursued in dogs with compatible clinical signs, a marked increase in ALP concentration, hypercholesterolaemia and a low urine specific gravity.

[Following a question from the chair, there was unanimous agreement that screening laboratory tests should be carried out prior to performing adrenal function tests in dogs suspected of hyperadrenocorticism.]

Colleen Mendelsohn voiced concern that using these criteria, hyperadrenocorticism would be missed in some dogs that did not have a high circulating ALP concentration.

Sarah Ambler asked whether it was correct to advise a low-dose dexamethasone suppression test in dogs with polyuria/polydipsia.

Peter Graham replied that false-positive results were common with this test and it should be used judiciously, taking into consideration signalment data and clinical signs.

Rosario Cerundolo *Italy* addressed the problem of which test was most suitable to confirm a diagnosis of hyperadrenocorticism. Those tests most frequently recommended were the adrenocorticotropic hormone (ACTH) stimulation test and the low-dose dexamethasone suppression test. The ACTH stimulation test often involves the intramuscular injection of 2.2 U/kg of ACTH gel with samples being taken for cortisol estimation at 0 and 2 h. As an alternative, tetracosactrin could be used at a dose of 1, 5 or 10 μg/kg intravenously with subsequent samples being taken at 0 and 1 or 1.5 h. This test was considered to be relatively specific but insensitive. For the low-dose dexamethasone suppression test, 0.01 mg/kg is injected intravenously and samples are taken for cortisol estimation at 0, 3 or 4 and 8 h. This test was considered to be relatively sensitive but non-specific. Endogenous ACTH determination could be used for ectopic ACTH-producing tumours and to differentiate pituitary-dependent hyperadrenocorticism (PDH) from functional adrenal tumours. Urine tests were, however, considered less stressful for the dog. The urine sample could be collected in the home environment and a urine cortisol: creatinine ratio calculated. High values were expected in hyperadrenocorticism but could also occur in patients with a high fluid intake and those undergoing significant stress. For this reason, a 3 day urine collection procedure at home during an oral low-dose dexamethasone suppression test had been adopted by some workers. A 10 day collection of urine was also advocated to diagnose cyclical hyperadrenocorticism. Gas chromatography and mass spectrophotometry to detect cortisol and its metabolites was routinely used in humans. In addition, cortisol measurement in human saliva was possible. A salivette is used to collect saliva at home with night-time sampling before and after oral dexamethasone suppression. Salivary analysis had been studied several years ago in dogs but, because the study had not been standardised, interpretation of the results was difficult.

[After a query from the chair, five members of the audience reported that they first used the ACTH stimulation test in the investigation of hyperadrenocorticism, seven used the low-dose dexamethasone suppression test and one used the urine cortisol: creatinine ratio, although more to rule in, rather than rule out, the disease.]

Dominique Heripret commented that the relatively low use of the urine test might simply be related to familiarity. Both he and Keith Thoday suggested using both the ACTH stimulation and low-dose dexamethasone suppression tests in all dogs.

Colleen Mendelsohn suggested that the ACTH stimulation test be used if there was any suspicion of exogenous steroid administration, as it is the only test capable of diagnosing iatrogenic hyperadrenocorticism. In other cases, a urine cortisol:creatinine ratio would suffice.

Heidy Zenulila asked whether the urine cortisol: creatinine ratio could be measured in a human laboratory.

Peter Graham replied that, although cortisol is preserved between species, the urine matrix differs. Thus, while the assay only measures cortisol in human urine, in dogs it may measure metabolites that cross-react with cortisol. The effect of this could be minimised by determining a reference range for the laboratory used.

Dominique Heripret discussed the tests used to differentiate PDH and functional adrenal tumours (ADH). This was considered important because the causal lesion affected the prognosis and treatment options. In the low-dose dexamethasone suppression test, approximately 30–50% of dogs with PDH exhibit cortisol suppression at 3–4 h, followed by escape. With a higher dose (0.1–1.0 mg/kg), 80–90% of dogs with PDH exhibit some cortisol suppression. However, there is a significant risk of adverse reactions, including death, with this test and its use should be carefully monitored. Oral administration of a high dose of dexamethasone and collection of urine for a cortisol:creatinine ratio determination may be helpful, but is highly dependent on good owner compliance for urine collection. Endogenous ACTH measurements are capable of distinguishing the site of the lesion, but such assays are not freely available and proper sample handling is crucial. Ultrasonography is extremely efficient in depicting adrenal tumours, particularly if short axis measurements of the adrenal glands are obtained. Computed tomography (CT) scans, if available, are capable of depicting pituitary lesions.

The necessity for distinguishing the site of the lesion was pointed out and the conclusion was initially to use the results of the low-dose dexamethasone suppression test. If this was inconclusive, it was advised to select the easiest test for both the patient and owner with the least risk of adverse reactions. If the final diagnosis remained unclear, further tests, as necessary, should be selected.

[After a question from the chair, half of the audience reported that they used the high-dose dexamethasone suppression test as their first choice for discriminating PDH from ADH in cases in which the low-dose dexamethasone suppression test was inconclusive.]

Colleen Mendelsohn suggested that the use of ultrasound, and if inconclusive, an endogenous ACTH measurement, was more effective and safer.

Carmel Mooney pointed out that the values quoted for circulating endogenous ACTH above and below which PDH and ADH were confirmed, respectively, were extremely disparate. Values were often found within the 'equivocal' category. It was felt that the fault lay particularly with the value quoted for PDH, which was considered inappropriately high.

Rosario Cerundolo finished the discussion on hyperadrenocorticism with a brief presentation on alternative tests for its investigation. The major adrenal and gonadal steroidogenic pathways were highlighted for cortisol, aldosterone and the sex hormones. In humans, dehydroepiandrosterone sulphate tends to be decreased in adrenal adenomas whereas, by comparison, 17-hydroxyprogesterone, testosterone, androstenedione and dehydroepiandosterone are increased in adrenal carcinomas. In addition, pregnenolone and 11-deoxycortisol tend to be increased in adrenal carcinomas compared with healthy patients or those with adrenal adenomas. In dogs, preliminary work suggests that the plasma 17-hydroxyprogesterone concentration may be increased before and after ACTH stimulation, in functional adrenal tumours. In the future, urine steroid profiles may help to distinguish malignant from benign adrenal tumours.

Keith Thoday concluded the session by thanking the speakers, and particularly the audience, for their part in the discussions.

5.15

Dermatophytosis

Ann Robinson (Chairperson) and Aiden P. Foster (Secretary)

University of Bristol, Langford, North Somerset, UK

Ann Robinson *UK* Dermatophytosis is a fascinating cutaneous infection about which there is still a great deal to learn. It can be difficult to manage in clinical practice. The aim of this workshop is to provide an opportunity to share insights, problems and solutions. The invited speakers have been asked to give short presentations to stimulate group discussion. The topic areas to be covered are clinical presentation, pathogenesis, therapeutics and vaccine development.

Ljiljana Pinter *Croatia* presented a short review of the clinical manifestations of dermatophyte infections in the cat, dog, rabbit, chinchilla, guinea-pig, cow and goat.

Didier Carlotti *France* reviewed the clinical presentation of dermatophytosis due to *Microsporum persicolor* and *Microsporum gypseum* in the dog, as detailed by Carlotti & Bensignor (1999).

James Noxon *USA* Have tape strips or impression smears for hyphae, direct from the animal infected with *M. persicolor*, been helpful in making a diagnosis?

Didier Carlotti There has been no success using Scotch® tape routinely looking for *M. persicolor* hyphae.

Lynn Schmeitzel *USA* Who has seen *M. persicolor*? [A show of hands confirmed that most of the audience had seen this dermatophyte.]

Doug DeBoer *USA* Could the audience comment on unusual clinical presentations of dermatophyte infection, given that T. Olivry has seen pemphigus foliaceus in the cat with dermatophyte infection?

Ann Robinson had seen a cat with otitis externa and a black waxy discharge that was negative on cytology and grew *M. canis* and which responded to therapy.

Didier Carlotti had seen a Wood's lamp-positive, culture-positive dermatophyte infection with onychogryphosis.

James Noxon had seen a dog with 'collie nose' that was associated with a *Trichophyton* infection and a dog with hyperkeratotic footpads of all four feet with *M. gypseum* infection.

Karen Moriello *USA* described an 'atopic' cat, positive on intradermal skin testing, that presented with symmetrical alopecia. There was no fungal infection apparent histologically but there was a positive culture from a toothbrush sample.

Bernard Mignon *Belgium* presented a review of the role of virulence factors in dermatophyte infection. Dermatophytes may have a variety of effects on the host. Why, for example, is *T. rubrum* infection chronic in some humans? In cats, *M. canis* infections can be very inflammatory or chronic in some animals. In order to appreciate the pathogenesis of infection, we have to understand the host–fungus relationship in terms of the innate and specific immune responses of the host and the role of fungal virulence factors.

Dr Mignon summarised studies of a 31.5 kDa serine protease (keratinase) produced from a feline isolate of *M. canis*. Some of this work has been published (Mignon *et al.*, 1998). In other species of fungus, the proteases are important for tissue invasion, the provision of nutrients and the control of host defence mechanisms. The 31.5 kDa protein has been evaluated using serum IgG enzyme-linked immunosorbent assay (ELISA) immunohistochemistry in cats and guinea-pigs and delayed type skin-test reactivity in guinea-pigs. The protein did not appear to be immunogenic in infected cats or guinea-pigs compared with a crude antigen preparation from a cultured isolate of *M. canis*. A second keratinase protein is the subject of further studies reviewed in free communication FC-81 (Mignon *et al.*, 2000). Further studies are warranted to investigate the precise role of these keratinase proteins in terms of their pathogenicity and the nature of the host response.

Lynn Schmeitzel asked about distinguishing asymptomatic carriers from asymptomatic cases. The animal acting as a mechanical carrier may be culture positive on one occasion, while a symptomatic cat may be Wood's lamp positive and have clinical lesions, although they may be difficult to find. Asymptomatic carriers may be detected historically as they may cause highly contagious infections to other animals and humans.

Ken Mason *Australia* Robinson *et al.* (1998) and Paterson (1999) have reported two studies demonstrating the value of Malaseb® as a product for the reduction of both the clinical signs of cats with dermatophytosis and the environmental burden of contamination. A further study was presented in which a group of Persian cats was treated with griseofulvin and a topical product including either placebo shampoo base, 2% chlorhexidine, 2% miconazole in shampoo base or Malaseb shampoo. Mason *et al.* (2000) gives further details of the study. The conclusion of this study was that the most effective treatment regimen for the infected cats and the environment included both miconazole and chlorhexidine. A similar synergistic effect has been suggested for human *Candida* infections (Codd & Deasy, 1998). It is thought that this synergism may be due to cell wall damage by chlorhexidine, improving the penetration of miconazole.

The *in vitro* effect of Malaseb shampoo was measured against eight isolates of *M. canis* from the dog, cat and horse. The study was performed at a human hospital microbiology laboratory. The study demonstrated a synergistic effect of chlorhexidine and miconazole.

Charles Chen *Taiwan* The use of terbinafine was discussed in relation to the dog, in particular. Further details are given in Poster P-2 (Chen, 2000). At doses of 10–30 mg/kg, there were no side-effects noted and liver biochemical parameters were within normal limits. One animal that was difficult to treat was the Yorkshire terrier with dermatophytosis. Dr Chen wondered why this should be.

Carmel Taylor *Hong Kong* The treatment period for dermatophytes such as *M. persicolor* in Yorkshire terriers appeared to be longer before negative cultures were obtained. Why should this be?

Ken Mason regarded the Yorkshire terrier as a breed something akin to the Persian cat in terms of its susceptibility to chronic dermatophyte infection, and this may be due to some kind of innate immune deficiency.

Didier Carlotti commented that the clinical presentation of the Yorkshire terrier with *M. canis* infection was often more generalised and, therefore, in this breed treatment takes longer to resolve the infection.

Steve Young *USA* asked a question about the possible use of lufenuron in the management of dermatophytosis.

Charles Chen mentioned a case where he combined lufenuron and terbinafine therapy. It was not easy to draw a conclusion about efficacy based on one case, but the treatment period had possibly been shorter than expected.

Louis Ansay *France* reported improvement in a Yorkshire terrier and two poodles with dermatophytosis, a rabbit with *Trichophyton* infection and a poodle with *Malassezia* infection that all received an injection of lufenuron (Ansay, 2000). It was possible that the improvement could not be distinguished from spontaneous resolution in some cases. The use of lufenuron for dermatophytosis is off-label and there is very limited information to support its use for canine dermatophytosis.

Anna Marie Bratberg *Norway* reviewed the process of vaccine development, discussing the particular topic of the challenge test for efficacy, using a standardised target host species of animal and appropriate inoculum of a suitable challenge strain of dermatophyte.

There was general agreement that the cat is the main target species for the development of a safe, highly efficacious vaccine that provides protection to kittens and adult cats. The currently available product in North America (manufactured by Fort Dodge) is mainly used to support therapy, and may be associated with a reduction in the duration and extent of clinical signs.

The final discussion was about the treatment of the environment. Gross decontamination must be aggressive and the area may then be treated with enilconazole as a fogger (Clinafarm®, Janssen) developed for use in poultry houses, for effective spore kill.

Further reading

Ansay, L. Y. J. (2000) Lufenuron: a new concept in dermatophytosis therapy. Proceedings of the Fourth World Congress of Veterinary Dermatology, San Francisco. *Veterinary Dermatology*, **11** (Suppl. 1), P-49, 56.

Carlotti, D. N. & Bensignor, E. (1999) Dermatophytosis due to *Microsporum persicolor* (13 cases) or *Microsporum gypseum* (20 cases) in dogs. *Veterinary Dermatology*, **10**, 17–27.

Chen, C. (2000) The use of terbinafine for the treatment of dermatophytosis. Proceedings of the Fourth World Congress of Veterinary Dermatology, San Francisco. *Veterinary Dermatology* **11** (Suppl. 1), P-2, 41.

Codd, J. E. & Deasy P. B. (1998) Synergistic antifungal interaction between miconazole nitrate and chlorhexidine acetate. *International Journal of Pharmaceutics*, **173**, 3–11.

Mason, K. V., Frost, A., O'Boyle, D. & Connole, M. D. (2000) Treatment of a *Microsporum canis* infection in a colony of Persian cats with griseofulvin and a shampoo containing 2% miconazole, 2% chlorhexidine, 2% miconazole and chlorhexidine or placebo. Proceedings of the Fourth World Congress of Veterinary Dermatology, San Francisco. *Veterinary Dermatology*, **11** (Suppl. 1), P-43, 55.

Mignon, B., Swinnen, M., Bouchara, J. P., Hofinger, M., Nikkels, A., Pierard, G. *et al.* (1998) Purification and characterization of a 31.5 kDa keratinolytic subtilisin-like serine protease from *Microsporum canis* and evidence of its secretion in naturally infected cats. *Medical Mycology*, **36**, 395–404.

Mignon, B., Brouta, F., Descamps, F. & Losson, B. (2000) *Microsporum canis* virulence factors and immunogens: first purification and characterization of a 43.5 kDa keratinolytic metalloprotease. *Veterinary Dermatology*, **11** (Suppl. 1), 40.

Paterson, S. (1999) Miconazole/chlorhexidine shampoo as an adjunct to systemic therapy in controlling dermatophytosis in cats. *Journal of Small Animal Practice*, **40**, 163–166.

Robinson, A., Sparkes, A. H. & Shaw, S. E. (1998) *In vivo* efficacy of Malaseb® for feline *Microsporum canis* infections. In: *Proceedings of the 15th Congress of the European Society of Veterinary Dermatology–European College of Veterinary Dermatology*, Maastricht, The Netherlands, p. 168.

5.16
Hereditary and congenital skin diseases

Zeineb Alhaidari[1] (Chairperson) and Eric Guaguère[2] (Secretary)

[1] Clinique Vétérinaire, Roquefort Les Pins, France
[2] Clinique Vétérinaire Saint Bernard, Lomme, France

Dog genome maps: gene hunting for hereditary diseases (C. Renier)

Corinne Renier *France* Owing to the 300 well-established purebreeds, the canine species is a powerful resource for dissecting the molecular basis of genetic diseases and traits. To this aim, we have constructed a dog whole genome radiation hybrid panel made of 126 hybrid cell lines by fusing fibroblasts, irradiated at 5000 rads, with TK-hamster cells (RHDF5000). We also have identified 300 dog gene markers and 800 microsatellite markers. These tools allowed us to construct the first ever canine radiation hybrid map of the dog by positioning 400 markers.

Placing these genes allowed us to characterize conserved segments between canine, human, mouse and pig chromosomes. Then, through collaborative effort, an integrated linkage/radiation hybrid map containing 600 markers has been constructed and each of the 39 canine chromosomes (CFA1–38, X and Y) has been assigned to the radiation hybrid groups. A 1500 marker radiation hybrid map covering 95% of the dog genome has been produced. This map, harboring 1200 microsatellites and 300 genes, will be of great value in identifying diseases or phenotypic or behavioral traits through linkage of the trait with polymorphic markers and the candidate gene approach.

These data are available on: http://www.recomgen.univ.rennes1.fr/doggy.html

Dermatomyositis and ulcerative dermatosis (vesicular cutaneous lupus) in the shetland sheepdog and collie (H. A. Jackson)

Hilary Jackson *USA* A syndrome of ulcerative dermatitis, termed ulcerative dermatosis of the Shetland sheepdog and collie (UDSSC), has been described which is apparently unique to the Shetland sheepdog and rough collie. The pathogenesis of this disease is poorly understood and it has been suggested that it may be a variant of canine dermatomyositis that is also seen in these breeds. The author has collected clinical and historical data on a series of 17 dogs with UDSSC; follow-up information is available for 10 of these cases. In addition, the histological pattern present in cutaneous biopsies of UDSSC has been compared with dermatomyositis.

In Shetland sheepdogs and collies, dermatomyositis is typically a disease of young animals. Cutaneous lesions consist of erythema and ulceration, progressing to cicatricial alopecia and hypopigmentation. Lesions are distributed over pressure points of the face and limbs, and often involve the periocular and pinnal skin. Myositis is a common, but not consistent, development. Ulcerative dermatosis of the Shetland sheepdog and collie, however, invariably develops in adulthood and appears to have a seasonal onset, with most cases being seen in the summer months. This observation, and the distribution of lesions over sparsely haired areas, supports a role for ultraviolet radiation in the pathogenesis of the disease. The primary lesion is a transient vesicle or bulla that may only be appreciated in histological sections of lesions, as they rupture readily to manifest as annular, polycyclic or serpiginous ulceration. The lesions are typically distributed over the groin, axillae and ventral abdomen, and often involve the mucocutaneous junctions and concave aspects of the pinnae.

Histological features, in conjunction with the clinical presentation, are useful in differentiating these two diseases. Dermatomyositis is characterized by follicular atrophy and a cell-poor interface dermatitis and folliculitis, whereas UDSSC is characterized by a cell-rich interface dermatitis and folliculitis. Vesiculation at the dermoepidermal junction is a common feature and follicular atrophy is rare. The histological features of UDSSC are similar to cutaneous lupus in humans and distinct from those of dermatomyositis. Follow-up data on a small number of dogs with UDSSC suggest that this disease may be difficult to manage and a guarded prognosis should be given. By contrast, although dermatomyositis is a chronic relapsing disease, in the absence of severe myositis, the majority of dogs have a fair prognosis for long-term management.

Sebaceous adenitis in the akita: clinical and histological findings, management and inheritance (I. Reichler)

Iris Reichler *Switzerland* The akita is a breed with a high predisposition for sebaceous adenitis. This study describes the clinical and histopathological findings of 26 akitas for which the diagnosis of sebaceous adenitis was established histologically by showing an inflammatory reaction targeted against the sebaceous glands or a reduction in the number of glands. The first skin lesions occurred mainly on the dorsal midline. They were seen as small areas of scaling and alopecia and, with time, could be found over the entire body. The skin condition did not consistently deteriorate in all akitas. In some cases there was improvement. The progression of sebaceous gland destruction was also individually very variable and was not seen in all cases. Bud-like sebaceous gland proliferation could be identified. Therefore, it seems that regeneration of sebaceous glands may occur.

The different courses of sebaceous adenitis may be due to the different treatments used. It is difficult to assess the success of the various therapy combinations because of the limited numbers of cases and the immense differences in the appearance of symptoms. The owners were advised to wash the patients once or twice a week with antiseborrheic shampoos and rinses. A long-term improvement was seen in six dogs that additionally received fish oil. By analysing the pedigrees of 16 litters, an autosomal recessive inheritance appears to be possible. Apart from the genetic background, immune-mediated factors possibly influence the onset and the course of sebaceous adenitis.

Eric Guaègure *France* Is there any difference between dogs of American and Japanese origin?

Iris Reichler No, sebaceous adenitis was observed in both.

Zeineb Alhaidari *France* In France, sebaceous adenitis is described only in dogs of American origin.

Iris Reichler I have been discussing the condition with a Japanese breeder. Dogs from Japan also show this condition.

Identification of the genetic basis of canine junctional epidermolysis bullosa in the German shorthaired pointer (F. Spirito)

Flavia Spirito *France* We have studied the genetic background of families of inbred German shorthaired pointers with littermates suffering from a mild form of junctional epidermolysis bullosa (JEB). Junctional epidermolysis bullosa is a heterogeneous group of recessively inherited genodermatoses. In humans, these conditions are characterized by blistering of the skin and mucous membranes consequent to genetic mutations affecting either the major hemidesmosome components or the heterotrimeric (α_3, β_3, γ_2) protein laminin-5, the primary extracellular adhesion ligand of the basal keratinocytes.

The JEB dogs show a generalized fragility of the skin resulting in blistering, erosions and ulcers of the integument and oral mucosa. Dystrophic nails and pitted enamel are concurrently observed. In the involved skin, immunoepitope mapping of the dermoepidermal junction localized the cleavage plane of the blister within the lamina lucida of the basement membrane zone. Ultrastructural examination confirmed the junctional nature of the tissue separation and revealed the presence of well-formed hemidesmosomes.

Analysis of secondary cultures of keratinocytes isolated from the affected dogs showed that expression and secretion of the laminin α_3- and γ_2-chains is reduced. The altered expression of the α_3- and γ_2-polypeptides was confirmed by Western blotting and immunoprecipitation analysis of spent medium obtained from cultures of canine JEB keratinocytes. These observations suggested that the genes for the laminin α_3- and γ_2-chains are candidates for the disease. To identify possible genetic mutations associated with canine JEB, the full-length cDNA for the laminin α_3- and γ_2-chains was isolated by reverse transcription polymerase chain reaction (RT-PCR) amplification of total RNA purified from keratinocytes obtained from two JEB dogs and a healthy unrelated control. Sequence analysis of the laminin α_3 and γ_2 cDNAs showed 85% identity of the amino acid sequence between dogs and humans. Screening for genetic mutations excluded involvement of the laminin γ_2-chain in the disease, and detected a homozygous nucleotide change (1514C-to-T) in the laminin α_3- chain cDNA. The Mendelian inheritance of mutation 1514C-to-T was assessed by allele-specific oligonucleotide analysis (ASO) of the genomic DNA obtained from the members of the probands' families. The possibility that the C-to-T substitution represents a polymorphic variation in dogs was tested by screening of PCR-amplified genomic DNA from 50 unrelated individuals. The mutation was not found in any of these samples. Mutation 1514C-to-T predicts an amino-acid substitution (505T-to-I) within domain I of the laminin α_3-polypeptide that alters the hydrophobicity of a stretch of 14 amino acids highly conserved during evolution in humans, mouse and dog. Unstable binding of the aberrant laminin α_3-chain to the $\beta_3\gamma_2$ heterodimer, therefore, accounts for the secretion of reduced amounts of functional laminin-5 in the extracellular matrix produced by the canine JEB keratinocytes.

The identification of the causal mutation of canine JEB has allowed the development of a screening test to identify the healthy carriers. At present, the affected dogs serve as a model to study the pathomechanisms of JEB. Despite the differences between the human and canine integument, these animals constitute an invaluable genetically defined system to test gene replacement therapies.

Epidemiological and clinical aspects of a series of eighteen cases of canine junctional epidermolysis bullosa in the German shorthaired pointer (E. Guaguère)

Eric Guaguère Hereditary JEB is associated with defective hemidesmosome-anchoring filament proteins leading to cleavage in the lamina lucida of the epidermal basement membrane. In humans, these conditions are characterized by blistering of the skin and mucous membranes consequent on genetic mutations affecting either the major hemidesmosome components or the heterotrimeric protein laminin-5. In 1997, Olivry *et al.* demonstrated that German shorthaired pointers suffering from JEB had a lack of collagen XVII expression. Recently, Spirito *et al.* (1999) identified in other German shorthaired pointers another hemidesmosome component deficiency, a lack of expression and secretion of laminin-5 (α_3- and γ_2-chains).

I would like to present some epidemiological and clinical aspects of a series of 18 cases of JEB in the German shorthaired pointer breed, caused by a lack of expression and secretion of laminin-5 (α_3- and γ_2-chains).

In France, breeders have been aware of this disease for about the past 20 years. Between 1997 and 2000, we have observed 18 cases of JEB in the German shorthaired pointer belonging to six litters from different kennels. No sexual predisposition has been reported (eight females and 10 males). The analysis of pedigrees has shown that this JEB is transmitted as an autosomal recessive trait. Cutaneous signs develop in 50% of cases (nine dogs) within 3 weeks, in 28% of the cases (five dogs) within 6 weeks, in 17% of cases (three dogs) within 8 weeks and in 5% of cases (one dog) at the age of 16 weeks. At the age of 3 weeks, cutaneous lesions began as paronychia and onychomadesis affecting several digits. Rapidly, moderate and well-delineated ulcers appeared on some footpads and on the medial aspect of the pinnae. At 8 weeks, cutaneous lesions were similar, but 50% of the pups exhibited oral ulcers on the gingivae, lips and tongue. Nikolsky's sign was positive in all cases. Other ulcers progressively appeared on the pressure points of the extremities, causing lameness, and on the lateral aspects on the elbows. In most cases the aggravation of ulcers on the pressure points became so serious that the pups had to be euthanized.

We have seen two cases in adult dogs (although the first lesions appeared at the age of 8 weeks). These dogs exhibited less serious clinical forms that enabled the animals to lead almost normal lives. In adult dogs, small ulcers were observed on the footpads, the scrotum and teats. Premature wear of the teeth due to enamel hypoplasia was observed in both cases.

Eric Guaguère Do you observe JEB in the USA?

Robert Dunstan *USA* No, I haven't seen it.

Studies on the inheritance of alopecia in the Irish water spaniel (R. Cerundolo)

Rosario Cerundolo *UK* The Irish water spaniel (IWS) is a breed with peculiar coat characteristics. The breed standard states that an area of smooth hair forming a V-shaped patch should be present on the throat and the tail should be bare. For many years, dogs have been selected according to this coat pattern but, in recent years, various patterns of alopecia and/or hypotrichosis affecting variously the laterodorsal neck, flanks, dorsum, rump and the caudal part of the thighs have been anecdotally reported.

Since 1995 we have collaborated with the British IWS Association to characterize and investigate the causes of these coat problems. A survey was carried out among the members of the association and affected dogs were examined. When direct examination was not possible, a full history was provided by the attending veterinarian and photographs of the dogs were obtained. Routine dermatological investigations with skin biopsy, blood investigations, including hormonal tests, and dietary studies were carried out in the affected dogs. These studies are being reported elsewhere. They indicated that histopathological abnormalities of the hair follicle are common, but sex hormone and dietary factors also influence the severity of the condition.

In this study we investigated whether the coat problems affecting this breed have an inherited nature. The pedigree of affected dogs identified from the survey and also of others with similar lesions, of which we became aware during the study, were examined. Information on the clinical status of ancestors and littermates was collected, dogs being identified as affected, not affected or of unknown status where, for example, animals died prematurely, could not be traced or were too young for a definitive diagnosis. Pedigrees were also studied of Irish water spaniels without alopecia. A detailed study was made of four families.

Inspection of five generations of pedigrees of affected dogs indicated that consanguinity levels were relatively high. More stringent comparative analysis of the pedigrees of affected dogs and unaffected dogs is continuing. A composite pedigree showing the interrelationships of all affected cases and their family members was constructed. Examination of the pedigree showed a strongly familial pattern of transmission with, in most cases, affected animals having at least one affected parent, which in turn also had an affected dam, sire or both. Segregation analysis could not be carried out because of the unknown status of some dogs. In the four families studied, there were 37 dogs of which 15 were affected, seven were not affected, six died and nine were of unknown status. The data overall suggest that a single autosomal gene may play a major causal role in this abnormality, the familial incidence supporting, but not proving, a dominant transmission.

It would appear that this condition is subject to autosomal dominant inheritance. It is envisaged that the role of this gene would be to control genetic susceptibility to the alopecia, the clinical condition arising as a result of the interaction of genotype with hormonal status and diet.

Robert Kennis *USA* How early could the condition start?

Rosario Cerundolo In males, generally at 5–6 years, but the condition progresses. In females, oestrous cycles may give an indication earlier.

Robert Dunstan Portuguese water dogs have the same type of pattern hair loss. Could these two breeds be genetically related?

Rosario Cerundolo The first reports of Irish water spaniels speak of water spaniel dogs. They could have used Portuguese water dogs. However, the hair loss in Portuguese water spaniels is more cyclical and this is not the case in Irish water spaniels.

Hilary Jackson What are the histopathological aspects of non-lesional skin in affected dogs and in normal Irish water spaniels?

Rosario Cerundolo Biopsies of non-lesional skin sometimes demonstrated abnormalities. No normal dogs were sampled.

Some cases of lamellar ichthyosis (R. A. Kennis)

Robert Kennis Lamellar ichthyosis is more and more reported in the dog, especially in the following breeds: golden retrievers, American bulldogs, Jack Russell terriers and Yorkshire terriers. In golden retrievers, the disease is very subtle and is characterized by abundant squame formation; generally, there is no footpad involvement. Histological examination demonstrates no inflammation and a lamellar hyperkeratosis. Treatment options are mild antiseborrheic shampoos and moisturizing rinses. In American bulldogs the disease is quite mild: clinically, scales are more compact. In Jack Russell terriers, the disease is more severe. Treatment options are moisturizing rinses or baby oil to loosen the scales and then the use of more aggressive shampoos. Retinoids and vitamin A seem also to give promising results.

Robert Dunstan I advise the use of Goop®. It is an automobile industry product used to remove grease.

Further reading

Olivry, T., Poujade-Delverdier, A., Dunston, S. M., Fine, J.-D. & Ortonne, J.-P. (1997). Absent expression of collagen XVII (BPAG2, BPI80) in canine familial localized junctional epidermolysis bullosa. *Veterinary Dermatology*, **8**, 203–212.

Spirito, F., Capt, A., Ortonne, J. P., Guaguère, E. & Meneguzzi, G. (1999). Genetic basis of canine junctional epidermolysis bullosa. *Journal of Investigative Dermatology*, **133**, 9.

5.17

Histopathology of newly recognized skin diseases

Thelma Lee Gross[1] (Chairperson) and Ann M. Hargis[2] (Secretary)

[1] California Dermatopathology Service and Idexx Veterinary Services, West Sacramento, California, USA
[2] DermatoDiagnostics, Edmonds, Washington, Phoenix Central Laboratory, Everett, Washington, and the Department of Comparative Medicine, University of Washington, Seattle, Washington, USA

Feline herpesvirus-1-associated facial dermatitis (A. M. Hargis and P. Ginn)

Ann Hargis *USA* Feline herpesvirus-1 has been associated with a variety of disease syndromes in cats, most notably rhinotracheitis and conjunctivitis. Reports documenting cutaneous ulcers associated with feline herpesvirus-1 in domestic cats are rare. The reported lesions have been described as ulcerative, necrotizing, neutrophilic to mixed and multifocally distributed. In contrast, the cases in our study were different from those previously reported in domestic cats in that cutaneous lesions were localized to the face, some were dramatically eosinophilic and some were persistent. The prevalence of the cases in our study is also higher than expected from the rarity of reports in the literature.

Clinically, the lesions in our cats were ulcerative and crusted and were located on the haired skin of the face or the nasal planum. One cat had unilateral periocular lesions and one cat had a lesion on the soft palate. Some lesions were persistent and progressive. Microscopically, lesions consisted of necrosis, ulceration and crusting. Occasionally, microvesicular areas were seen in the epidermis. Mixed inflammatory cells, including eosinophils, were present in the dermis. In some cases the eosinophilic inflammation was prominent. Occasionally, collagen degeneration associated with peripheral macrophages and multinucleated giant cells was seen. Collagen degeneration was not a dominant feature and was considered secondary to the tissue eosinophilia. Some cats had eosinophilic folliculitis and furunculosis with follicular destruction and extrusion of hair shafts into the dermis. Intranuclear inclusion bodies were present in the epidermis, sebaceous gland and follicular epithelium in variable number. The inclusion bodies were amphophilic, filled the nucleus, and were associated with marginated chromatin and cytoplasmic swelling.

The infiltrate of eosinophils in these cases is not typically expected for viral infections. However, eosinophilic inflammation has been documented in influenza, rhinovirus and respiratory syncytial viral infections. Possible mechanisms contributing to eosinophil recruitment in viral infections include viral infected epithelial cell production of cytokines chemoattractant for eosinophils and viral production of proteins chemotactic for eosinophils. It is also reported that injection of herpesvirus into the skin of previously vaccinated cats may cause a hypersensitivity response associated with recruitment of eosinophils. Alternatively, the eosinophil inflammation may be due to a unique feature of the feline immune system, or the eosinophilic infiltrates may be present as a response to keratin in the tissue and may not be due to any influence of the virus.

The presence of herpesvirus-1 in our study was documented in three ways. The first was by histopathological examination; all cats in the study had intranuclear inclusion bodies consistent with herpesvirus inclusion bodies within epithelial cells in lesional skin. Secondly, electron-microscopic evaluation was performed on two cats. Ultrastructurally, lesional tissue had small numbers of keratinocytes with lysis of the nuclear matrix, peripheralization of chromatin and cytoplasmic swelling. Within these keratinocytes were individual or clusters of viral nucleocapsids of approximately 100–125 nm. The virons were round and comprised an electron-dense core bordered first by an electron-lucent zone and then by an electron-dense zone. The virons were consistent with herpesvirus. Thirdly, the polymerase chain reaction (PCR) confirmed the presence of feline herpesvirus-1 in seven of the eight cats tested. DNA sequencing was performed on selected cases.

The facts that most cats were adults, that lesions often developed in association with glucocorticoid therapy or crowded conditions, and that some cats had mild recurrent or chronic upper respiratory tract infection suggest reactivation of latent viral infection. Due to the prominent eosinophilic inflammation and low numbers of inclusion bodies, these cutaneous or oral lesions may be misinterpreted as allergic dermatitis or lesions in the eosinophilic granuloma group of disorders.

Trevor Whitbread *UK* mentioned that in the UK and some parts of mainland Europe, poxvirus infections in cats have eosinophil-rich histological lesions with necrosis. The virus inclusion bodies are different in that they are brightly eosinophilic but sometimes can be difficult to find. When inclusion bodies are difficult to find, the lesions are histologically similar to the herpesvirus lesions shown.

Edmund Rosser Jr *USA* asked whether the history indicated that, as kittens, the cats in the study had the more classic respiratory disease component of rhinotracheitis, conjunctivitis or glossitis. He had found such a history in a certain percentage of his cases.

Ann Hargis responded that a number of the cats in the study had a history of recurrent upper respiratory tract infection and that a few of these cats had been given glucocorticoid therapy. The recurrent respiratory tract infection, glucocorticoid therapy and possibly the stress of living in crowded, multiple-cat households in a few cases were considered possible predisposing factors in the development of herpesvirus facial dermatitis. Also, the history of recurrent respiratory tract infection and history of glucocorticoid therapy or a stressful living environment suggested the possibility of reactivation of latent viral infection as a cause of the facial dermatitis in some of the cats. In contrast, the dermatitis that developed in a 4-month-old kitten in the study may have been associated with a primary herpesvirus infection, not reactivation of latent viral infection. The kitten had an upper respiratory tract infection when found as a stray. Chemosis and conjunctivitis persisted in this kitten and the skin lesions subsequently developed after glucocorticoid therapy. Also, it was mentioned that the adult cats in the study had been vaccinated as kittens and adults with different types of vaccines, including intranasal vaccines in a few cats. No association with type of vaccine or recent administration of vaccine and the herpesvirus facial dermatitis was found.

Kai-Ning Tang *USA* asked about the location of the viral particles.

Ann Hargis indicated that in the electron micrographs, the viral particles were in the nucleus and were associated with lysis of the nuclear matrix.

Kai-Ning Tang asked whether viral particles were also seen in the cytoplasm and whether the envelope was identified.

Ann Hargis responded that Dr Pamela Ginn performed the electron-microscopic evaluations reported in the study and that viral particles were seen in the cytoplasm, but could not comment specifically on the envelope question.

Emily Walder *USA* indicated that immunohistochemistry can be used to identify inclusions or identify that inclusions are herpesvirus inclusions. She has been requesting a local human immunohistochemistry laboratory to apply a cocktail of human herpesvirus simplex-1 and herpesvirus simplex-2 and has been able to obtain a small number of positive results using that technique.

Ann Hargis commented that it can be difficult to establish the diagnosis of herpesvirus dermatitis in cats if inclusion bodies are not present histologically. When she was attempting to document the presence of herpesvirus in the cats in the study, she had difficulty finding a veterinary diagnostic laboratory that offered immunohistochemistry for feline herpesvirus. Since the completion of the study, she has learned of several veterinary diagnostic laboratories that have recently started to offer immunohistochemistry for feline herpesvirus. Also, originally she found only one laboratory providing PCR testing for feline herpesvirus but, more recently, additional veterinary diagnostic laboratories have started to offer PCR for feline herpesvirus. It therefore appears that increasing numbers of veterinary diagnostic laboratories are offering immunohistochemistry or PCR to aid in the diagnosis of feline herpesvirus infections.

Marianne Heimann *Belgium* inquired whether a sample collected via a swab would be enough to diagnose herpesvirus infection by PCR.

Ann Hargis recommended directing specific procedural questions to the laboratory to which the sample was going to be sent. One of the laboratories performing PCR primarily for herpesvirus keratitis accepted swabs, scrapings and biopsy samples. However, the laboratory reported that the larger the sample, the more likely they were to establish the diagnosis of herpesvirus infection. Therefore, a light swab over the surface of a lesion is more likely to produce a false-negative result than a tissue biopsy sample. To date, the veterinary laboratories performing PCR require submission of fresh, unfixed specimens. While it is possible to perform PCR using formalin-fixed, paraffin-embedded tissue samples, apparently it is harder to extract the DNA from formalin-fixed samples and these are more likely to result in a false-negative reaction.

Marianne Heimann asked about the use of culture media for submission of samples for PCR evaluation and what markers are used.

Ann Hargis responded that different laboratories might be using different types of PCR testing procedures. The laboratory that performed PCR on biopsy samples from some of the cats in her study was using a PCR specific for feline herpesvirus-1, which targeted the thymidine kinase gene of feline herpesvirus-1. Dr Richard L. Garber, a collaborator in the study, used both the PCR specific for feline herpesvirus-1 and a consensus primer PCR that is a nested PCR procedure. By DNA sequencing of the DNA regions amplified by the consensus primer PCR, feline herpesvirus-1 was identified.

Verena Affolter *USA* commented that for submission of samples for PCR, usually culture media should not be used. It is best to air-dry the sample and send it in a clean tube.

Judith Wilkie *Australia* asked, what would be the main criteria that would raise the index of suspicion that feline herpesvirus was the cause of the lesions in the absence of seeing viral inclusions.

Ann Hargis responded that recent necrosis of epidermis or adnexal epithelium and ulceration are features that may help to suggest feline herpesvirus infection.

Thelma Lee Gross *USA* inquired about differential diagnoses.

Ann Hargis replied that when there is eosinophilic dermatitis with eosinophilic folliculitis on the face, a principal differential diagnosis is mosquito-bite hypersensitivity. In her study, she also considered the possibility of facial dermatitis due to mosquito-bite hypersensitivity predisposing to the reactivation of a latent herpesvirus infection, similar to sunburn injury contributing to the reactivation of a latent herpes simplex-1 infection in humans. Clinically, in an attempt to assess the likelihood of mosquito bites contributing to the lesions in the cats in her study, factors such as the time of year when biopsy samples were collected (most of the samples in the study were collected during winter months), indoor versus outdoor housing (four cats were indoors exclusively or over 90% of the time) and the fact that one cat had one lesion limited to the oral mucosa were considered. Based on the combination of these factors, there was no substantial support to suggest coexisting mosquito-bite hypersensitivity in the cats in the study. So, in addition to the histological presence of necrosis and inclusion bodies, factors in the history may help with differential diagnosis in cases of facial dermatitis with eosinophils.

Emily Walder commented that to exclude indoor or predominantly indoor cats from the category of potential mosquito-bite hypersensitivity is inappropriate. In mosquito-heavy areas, mosquitoes can gain entrance into houses. There is no reason to presume that just because a cat is indoors it will not have a mosquito bite.

Trevor Whitbread commented that with the poxvirus infections, one striking feature is the necrosis in the follicles. It does seem to wipe out the follicles. He asked whether this was similar with the herpesvirus infections.

Ann Hargis responded that the inclusion bodies are found in the epidermis, follicular epithelium, and sebaceous gland epithelium, and the virus is associated with necrosis of the affected epithelial cells. The necrosis or destruction of the epithelial tissue is a feature that suggests herpesvirus may be the source of the inflammation and prompts her to search for the inclusion bodies if they are not readily visible.

Candace Sousa *USA* commented that from the clinical standpoint, it is interesting, if feline herpesvirus is a virus that may be latent in the trigeminal ganglia, that the lesions tend not to spare the median but are present on both sides. Usually the herpesvirus cold sores will be on one side or the other and respect the median plane of the face. Also, just one branch of the trigeminal nerve may be involved, as lesions may be restricted to the nasal planum and not affect the rest of the face.

Edmund Rosser inquired whether any of the cases presented clinically as unilateral upper lip indolent ulcer.

Ann Hargis replied that none of the cats in her study had ulcers of the lip.

Sherry Myers *Canada* mentioned that her laboratory in Saskatoon does have antibodies for feline herpesvirus and has had positive immunohistochemistry on a small number of feline cases that had inclusion bodies in epidermis and follicular and sebaceous gland epithelium. In one cat, the inflammation was not eosinophilic at all; it was totally neutrophilic. The cat had been treated with corticosteroids and she wondered whether the prior therapy had decreased the eosinophil migration into the tissue.

Ann Hargis replied that some of the cats in the study had been on glucocorticoid therapy which did not eliminate the presence of eosinophils in the tissue. It is not surprising that some cats with herpesvirus dermatitis do not have eosinophils as a component of the inflammation. The important point is to avoid the presumption that because eosinophils are present the inflammation must be due to an allergic or parasitic response or be part of an eosinophilic granuloma inflammatory reaction rather than a viral infection. Why the eosinophil number may vary from case to case is unclear.

Erythema ab igne (chronic radiant heat dermatitis) (E. J. Walder and A. M. Hargis)

Emily Walder Erythema ab igne (EAI) is a very old disease in the human literature but has only recently been described in veterinary medicine. Its many synonyms include ephelis ignealis (1835), ephelis ab igne (1902), erythema a calore (1963), reticular erythema of the lower back and 'toasted skin syndrome'. EAI is defined as an erythematous, reticulated, macular, often pigmented dermatosis occurring at sites of chronic exposure to moderate radiant heat of 32–41°C (approximately 90–105°F). If the temperature exceeds 44°C (112°F) at the point of contact, true thermal burn occurs. The most common sources in humans are open fires (coal, peat, fireplaces), stoves, hot-water bottles, heating pads and steam radiators. Sources in animals include heating pads, electric blankets, heat lamps, heat registers, stoves, radiators, refrigerators, cable television boxes and asphalt driveways.

Clinical lesions in humans classically involve shins, lower back or buttocks. Occupational exposure (e.g. in bakers and foundry workers) often affects the face and hands. Abdominal lesions of EAI are suggestive of serious internal disease, particularly pancreatic carcinoma. Clinical lesions in animals typically reflect exposure during lateral or sternal recumbency.

Radiant heat is infrared radiation (0.75–1000 μm wavelength) that emanates from one solid object, passes through air or a vacuum and is absorbed by an adjacent solid object. Infrared radiation penetrates skin and can cause damage to basal keratinocytes, melanocytes and blood vessels, as demonstrated in studies on infrared lasers. Single-stranded and double-stranded DNA breakage has been confirmed in bacteria exposed to infrared radiation at various wavelengths; this presumably occurs in all species. Interaction of infrared radiation and ultraviolet radiation is controversial; some reports indicate a protective effect by infrared radiation against ultraviolet radiation damage, while others describe exacerbation of epidermal and dermal damage with combined exposure. Cumulative DNA damage in EAI can result in carcinoma *in situ*; this is designated thermal keratosis (analogous to actinic keratosis). Thermal keratoses can progress to invasive squamous cell carcinoma in humans; this has not yet been described in animals.

The salient histological features in the epidermis are mild to moderate acanthosis, spotty karyomegaly, scattered atypical keratinocytes, mild to moderate basal cell apoptosis and vacuolar degeneration. There is attenuation of superficial dermal collagen with variable mucin deposition. Abnormal and often increased numbers of elastic fibers with deep eosinophilic staining ('red spaghetti') are pathognomonic for EAI. There is usually a mild interface to interstitial, mixed inflammatory cell infiltrate with melanophages and hemosiderophages.

EAI has several histological features in common with ischemic dermatopathies; this may reflect infrared radiation-induced vascular damage.

Typical examples of EAI (three dogs, one cat and one langur) will be presented. Most lesions will resolve after removal of the heat source or prevention of access to it.

Thelma Lee Gross commented that she may be missing the red spaghetti. The cases that she had seen, the cable-box cats, had more prominent fibrosis. The skin of these cats had more of a hyperkeratotic appearance. She asked whether the thermal keratosis is a later stage or is the result of a lower level of heat over a longer time, and whether anything was known about the difference between thermal keratosis and EAI.

Emily Walder replied that she really had no idea, that the investigation into the range of lesions that this disease produces had just begun. She also mentioned that if animals are lying in direct contact with the heat source (e.g. heating pads), another factor to consider is heat by conduction. The molecules in a warm object are vibrating at a higher rate than in a cool object. As soon as the molecules that are vibrating at a higher rate bump into the molecules of an adjacent cooler object, which is the dog or cat, the molecules in the epidermis and dermis also start vibrating at a higher rate. She could not find any specific reference describing the effects of conductive heat on damage to basal keratinocytes, dermal fibroblasts, blood vessels or elastic fibers. She believes there is a lot going on that is not currently fully understood.

Trevor Whitbread commented that the follicle atrophy was quite marked in most of the cases illustrated. He asked whether that was the usual finding, what the cause of it might be and whether vasculitis was a feature.

Emily Walder responded that those were very important questions, and she had not even thought about the adnexal changes until Ann Hargis suggested that these dogs had vascular lesions. The more Dr Walder looked at the sections, the more she realized that they almost all had some degree of what looked like ischemic dermatopathy. Because infrared radiation can cause damage to vascular endothelium, it is highly probable that these dogs do have concurrent heat-induced vasculopathy and these lesions are partially ischemic.

Verena Affolter inquired whether staining the sections for elastic fibers was performed.

Emily Walder replied that she had not done any elastin stains. It is very well documented in the human literature that these are definitely elastic fibers.

Ann Hargis commented that stains for elastic tissue on some of the cases were in progress, but the histology laboratory had technical problems with the quality of the elastic tissue stain and were re-evaluating their procedure before repeating the staining of the sections.

Emily Walder reassured the group that the fibers are quite striking, and that once one had been trained to look for the fibers, the changes were obvious.

Thelma Lee Gross commented that a worrying thing was how much one of the illustrated cases looked liked ischemic dermatopathy. Thus, some cases of EAI in dogs may have been missed. She was more confident of the diagnosis of EAI in cats, mainly because she does not have to worry about the 'red spaghetti'.

Emily Walder responded that the clinical presentation is so different from the other ischemic dermatopathies that they should never be confused.

Thelma Lee Gross replied that sometimes histories are not provided, or there is just a vague description of the distribution. She had certainly seen truncal ischemics, so it makes her a little bit insecure.

Kai-Ning Tang asked whether the damage to the basal cell keratinocytes is due to radiant heat or secondary to hypoxia.

Emily Walder responded that at least some degree of basal cell damage is a direct result of infrared radiation. It has been confirmed by other sources working with infrared lasers. It is known that infrared radiation, just like ultraviolet radiation, causes keratinocyte damage and can cause DNA damage to the keratinocytes. So there is no question about infrared radiation. However, what is not known is the extent to which secondary vascular damage will compound the keratinocyte lesions. There may be a two-pronged attack on the basal cell keratinocytes.

An idiopathic facial dermatitis of thirteen Persian cats (R. Bond, C. F. Curtis, I. S. Mason, E. A. Ferguson and J. Rest)

Ross Bond *UK* This study took the form of a retrospective review of case records of 13 cats. The work-up of these cases varied according to the individual clinicians and their practices, and also the owners' wishes, expectations and funds. However, a history was taken and a clinical examination was carried out in each case. The work-up included skin scrapings and cytology, fungal and bacterial cultures, hematology and biochemistry, feline leukemia (FeLV) and feline immunodeficiency virus (FIV) assays and skin biopsies.

We identified 13 cats (eight male and five female) that presented with progressive facial skin disease. The duration of skin disease prior to referral ranged from 3 months to 4 years. The median was 12 months. The age at onset of skin lesions ranged from 4 months to 5 years. The median was 12 months. In each case, the first abnormality noted by the owner was a black exudate or material in the periocular, perioral and chin regions. Initially these cats were non-pruritic. However, in each case, pruritus subsequently became a feature of their presentation, initially was mild but became moderate or severe. Some of these cats were euthanized because of the inability to control the pruritus. The affected skin became progressively inflamed and more widespread lesions developed over the face and head.

Clinically, the skin disease was confined to the head and neck region. Black exudate, which encrusted the lower portions of the hair, was present on the face and chin. Some of these cats also had lesions around the lip area and chin with quite tightly adherent black material. Some of these cats developed erythematous plaques in the preauricular area. Marked erythema, alopecia and evidence of self-trauma were also observed. Ceruminous otitis externa was present in seven cases. In summary, the clinical presentation is that of a black to brown exudate of the face, chin and ears, with varying alopecia, excoriation and erythema, depending on the stage of the disease. Submandibular lymphadenopathy was reported in five of these cats.

Microscopic parasites were not found (13 cats). Microbes isolated included *Malassezia pachydermatis* (six of nine), *Staphylococcus intermedius* (five of 10) and Gram-negative bacteria (four of 10). Peripheral eosinophilia was present in five of eight. Other tests yielding negative or normal results included dermatophyte cultures (nine of nine), FeLV/FIV assays (nine of nine), elimination diets (eight of eight) and intradermal tests (four of four). The diet trials were for at least 4 weeks and in some cases somewhat longer, but I cannot say that all of these cats were confined to the house during the testing period. None of these cats improved. There were no significant biochemical abnormalities.

Skin biopsies (nine cases) showed a hyperplastic, superficial or interface dermatitis. There were variable numbers of neutrophils, eosinophils, mast cells and histiocytes in the dermis. Sebaceous gland hyperplasia was seen and appeared more prevalent in areas where acanthosis was more prominent. The epidermal hyperplasia was marked and irregular and there was also a spongiotic and hydropic change in the basal layer of the epidermis and occasionally in follicular epithelium. A few apoptotic basal cells were also noted.

No satisfactory treatment regimen could be identified. Antimicrobial and glucocorticoid therapy, either alone or in combination, given systemically or topically, induced only partial responses. Black exudation accumulated again 1–2 days after washing. Because of the severity, four cats had to be euthanized.

In conclusion, the etiopathogenesis of this disease is unknown and requires further investigation. The black exudation may represent an abnormality of sebaceous gland function and a genetic basis seems possible.

Incidentally, a Persian cat with pemphigus foliaceus that, as an incidental observation, had black material on the face, was recently examined. The cat was given prednisolone and chlorambucil, and the black material disappeared. One cat was treated by a colleague with cyclosporine, with excellent results. Perhaps the geographical distribution of cases should be discussed.

Trevor Whitbread commented that he has also seen a lot of these cases and did not think he could distinguish these from any other case of facial dermatitis in a cat apart, perhaps, from the size of the sebaceous glands. He also mentioned that sebaceous gland size should be compared with age-matched controls and he did not think it was a real change. He then indicated that he hardly ever sees the interface change and does not think this is a real interface change. The lesions look like a hypersensitivity reaction to him.

Edmund Rosser stated that he has not seen this condition. What impressed him about the sections illustrated was that, although the cats were pruritic, the sections were relatively non-inflammatory. He inquired whether the non-inflammatory histological sections corresponded to the cats with less pruritus and the more inflamed histological sections corresponded to the cats with more pruritus.

Ross Bond replied that he could not specifically recall the stage of disease with the illustrations presented. However, he suggested that the assumption that the less inflammatory cases were an earlier and less pruritic stage, and the more inflammatory cases were a later and more pruritic stage, was probably correct. For the sebaceous gland size issue, it would clearly be nice to do some type of morphometric study to compare what a Persian cat's facial sebaceous gland looks like.

Thelma Lee Gross commented that the only thing she remembered seeing was really greasy Persian cats with diffuse sebaceous hyperplasia in all areas of the skin. That does not mean that these Persian cats don't start with a facially confined sebaceous hyperplasia that leads to the exudate and then secondary inflammation. She had seen two related cats, between 1 and 2 years of age, with a similar condition to that described, and thought that interface dermatitis was there.

Ross Bond stated that he could not prove the cats did not have allergic dermatitis. Ruling out a dietary sensitivity in a pet cat is not easy.

Ed Rosser indicated that a dietary trial of 4 weeks is not enough in some cases. Intradermally testing cats is difficult to the point that many people do not even bother because detecting weals can be difficult. Lack of response to corticosteroids, particularly if it is just oral prednisolone, is not totally useful. Many allergic cats are seen in which response to one form of corticosteroid is very poor but something else works quite well. However, in support of the exclusion of allergy, the early age of onset at 4 months is young for allergy, and he has never seen any other allergic animal where this black exudate develops.

Thelma Lee Gross inquired whether there is actually material on the surface that is visible histologically.

Ross Bond replied that there was histologically visible material on the surface.

Candace Sousa mentioned a pruritic cat that came to her on therapy for herpes keratitis. The skin lesions were not self-induced, as the cat was wearing an Elizabethan collar and the lesions continued to grow. The cat had demonstrable dermatophytosis which required shaving the cat and treatment for the dermatophytosis. She wondered about the possibility of an 'id' reaction, and if Persian cats are predisposed to dermatophytes, inquired what the 'id' reaction would look like.

Thelma Lee Gross replied that the 'id' reaction is a delayed hypersensitivity, spongiotic lymphocytic reaction, so perhaps fungal culture of the Persian cat haircoats in areas other than the face would be a useful additional diagnostic test.

Sonya Bettenay *USA* commented that when she was in general practice with an ophthalmologist, she saw a lot of Persian cats with periocular inflammation and one of the things she always remembered was black, thickened exudate. She wondered whether Persian cats produce black exudate when they get inflamed skin. Nailbeds will also produce similar material.

Ross Bond indicated he did not recall seeing any of this black material on the feet of the cats. One or two had some black material around the anus, but nothing in the toe webs.

Sonya Bettenay inquired whether an ophthalmologist had examined the cats.

Ross Bond replied that as he recalled a few cats may have had an ocular component but he was not involved with that.

Julie Yager *Canada* commented that the cases she has seen were spongiotic but not interface. The cases were very inflamed, much more inflamed than the pictures illustrated, and the inflammation was so mixed that it did not point in any one direction.

Equine spongiotic vesicular dermatitis (A. M. Hargis, D. Duclos, S. LeClerc and E. G. Clark)

Ann Hargis Over a 6 year period, seven adult horses of different breeds and sexes developed multifocal, exudative, often ulcerative dermatitis characterized by epidermal spongiotic vesicles and perivascular eosinophilic, neutrophilic and mixed mononuclear dermatitis. The breeds included two quarter horses, one thoroughbred, one miniature horse, one Appaloosa, one Arabian and one Morgan cross-bred. The horses ranged in age from 3 to 15 years. Five horses were geldings and two were mares. The clinical lesions were multifocal, sometimes involving the face, ears, neck, trunk and legs. Clinically, all lesions were described as exudative, oozing serum or weeping. The hair was matted with crust. Some horses had alopecia or ulceration. Pruritus was absent in four horses and present in three horses. Systemic disease was not noted. All horses were in contact with at least one other horse that did not have clinical lesions. Cutaneous lesions developed 1 week after vaccination in one horse. Two horses had a history of recurrent urticaria and one horse had nodules or welts at the time when lesions developed. Biopsy samples were collected in February, March, October and November. Two horses developed the lesions during two consecutive winters and were normal during summer months. Two horses had dermatitis, one for 6 months and one for 2 years.

Histologically, lesions consisted of intraepidermal spongiotic vesicles. Occasionally, a few neutrophils, eosinophils or mononuclear cells were in the spongiotic vesicular lesions. Some areas of vesicle formation contained a few acantholytic cells. Erosion and ulceration were seen. Proteinaceous fluid admixed with hair shafts covered the surface of some sections. The dermis had perivascular to interstitial neutrophils, eosinophils and mast cells. Dermal edema was variable between cases, but was more severe in the papillary dermis. In five cases, the papillary dermal edema was marked.

Avidin biotin complex–peroxidase staining for immunoglobulin G (IgG) was similar in all cases. There was no definitive evidence of specific deposition of IgG. There was immunoglobulin in the dermis, with secondary diffusion of immunoglobulin into intercellular areas of the epidermis.

A specific cause for the lesions in all horses was not identified, but all horses had dermal edema, especially in the papillary dermis, and inflammation suggestive of hypersensitivity. There was no known exposure to contact materials. With the exception of one horse in which lesions developed following vaccination, there was no known drug exposure immediately before lesional development, so spongiotic drug eruption could not be documented. The vaccination in one horse could have precipitated the lesions in that individual. Although acantholysis was occasionally seen, it appeared to be the result of spongiosis rather than loss of desmosomal or hemidesmisomal attachments. The lack of true acantholysis, plus the negative avidin biotin complex–peroxidase staining, essentially ruled out pemphigus and other disorders associated with significant acantholysis. Therefore, the lesions were not considered to be consistent with pemphigus foliaceus or vulgaris.

In summary, a unique exudative dermatitis characterized histologically by spongiotic vesicular dermatitis developed in seven horses. The lesions developed under circumstances suggesting that papillary dermal edema led to interepithelial edema, which progressed to the spongiotic vesicular epidermal lesions. Food allergy, atopic dermatitis and vaccination may have contributed to lesion development in three horses.

Finally, in the recently published special issue of *Veterinary Dermatology*, 'Stannard's Illustrated Equine Dermatology Notes' (2000), there is a discussion of exudative oozing urticaria that is very similar to the lesions just described.

Verena Affolter commented that she has seen two horses that were almost identical to the first slide. One of them belonged to a friend of hers, so she was able to follow the horse over 2 years. This horse had a food allergy and the lesions recurred on two occasions when the horse got into oat hay. As long as the horse is kept away from anything containing oats it is fine. Also, the lesions never began as urticaria. They started as small, markedly oozing crusty lesions, which did not bother the horse. The lesions were more cosmetic as the horse could not be shown. The histology was identical to what was shown.

Julie Yager commented that she photographed one of Tony Stannard's slides for the special issue of *Veterinary Dermatology*, 'Stannard's Illustrated Equine Dermatology Notes' (2000), and it had huge intraepidermal vesicles with few acantholytic cells, so the comparison of these cases and the 'exudative oozing urticaria' is very credible.

Sonya Bettenay mentioned that she had one section from a single nodule in a horse where there were a few acantholytic cells, but did not know whether there was any relationship between this case and those presented. She asked Danny Scott what he thought of this reaction pattern in one nodule.

Danny Scott *USA* said it was a common reaction pattern of the horse where spongiosis develops to the point of forming acantholytic cells, and he thought of a contact reaction.

Thelma Lee Gross remarked on the fact that the disease appears to be an inside-out disease, and the epidermal lesions are generated from dermal edema.

Possibly in some cases, the urticaria remains dermal but if there are other cytokines involved with some hypersensitivity reactions, the edema is more likely to escape, so there is a biphasic reaction.

Kai-Ning Tang inquired whether any of the horses developed signs of hematuria, and whether the hay was checked for blister beetles.

Ann Hargis responded that the hay was not checked for blister beetles and the horses were reported to be systemically healthy. In one of the horses that developed the spongiotic vesicular lesions over two successive winters, there was a concern that the horse might be eating different food in the winter, suggesting that a component of the food could be causing the lesions. For instance, horses might be given hay in the winter since they could not graze on fresh pasture. This horse was an expensive rodeo horse and was on the same special diet all the year round. Even so, because of the concern of a possible dietary factor causing the lesions, several different diets were tried in that horse and did not make a difference in the cutaneous lesions.

Thelma Lee Gross thanked the speakers and audience for their participation in the workshop.

Further reading

Stannard, A. A. (2000). Stannard's illustrated equine dermatology notes (Eds C. von Tscharner, J. Yager & G. Kunkle). *Veterinary Dermatology*, **11**, 159–223.

5.18

Topical antipruritic therapy

Rosanna Marsella (Chairperson) and Connie F. Nicklin (Secretary)

University of Florida College of Veterinary Medicine, Gainesville, Florida, USA

Rosanna Marsella *USA* Today we are going to talk about topical antipruritic therapy. Several people will share their clinical experiences. There are some studies but very few placebo-controlled studies, so we will primarily hear about clinical experiences. We have people here today from different parts of the world. They use different products and have different experiences, so hopefully they will contribute as well. I would like to thank EVSCO Pharmaceuticals for sponsoring this workshop. I will start by asking Sandy Merchant to talk about pramoxine.

Sandy Merchant *USA* I tried to get a little more scientific background, but I'll tell you what I like about it clinically. I like to use pramoxine in cases where I do not want to use topical hydrocortisone. That would be my product of choice, but if for some reason I do not want to use hydrocortisone, pramoxine is my second choice. It is not a '-caine' product like lidocaine or benzocaine. Therefore, you don't get the contact sensitization you get with those products. So, even if the animal is allergic to '-caine' products, it shouldn't react adversely to pramoxine.

I did some research and it is used a lot in people. They have been using it since 1953, and about 40 years later, we're finally getting around to trying it in animals. I am not sure why, although I would imagine it has something to do with marketing and research. Possibly, it's because in human medicine, they combine products like pramoxine and hydrocortisone and pramoxine and calamine. I think it would be perfect to do combinations in animals.

Pramoxine is not the end-all of antipruritic products but it's my topical choice if I can't use hydrocortisone. I really like the leave-on conditioner. It has a wonderful smell and the color of the product matches the color of the bottle. They did a very good job of marketing the leave-on product and it's what I tend to use. A lot of times, our dogs have secondary infections and are already using an anti-infective shampoo, so I follow it with the antipruritic leave-on conditioner. It does not work in all cases. There is no product available that when used alone will cure the worst pruritus. Pramoxine is a good adjunct.

I typically pick topical agents based on the case and the client. If I have a client who I think is willing to try different products if one doesn't work, I will sell them the spray or the leave-on and eventually we can find a treatment regimen that helps to alleviate some of the pruritus.

As far as products, there is only one leave-on, but between the shampoos, Dermal Soothe® (EVSCO Pharmaceuticals) or Relief® (DVM Pharmaceuticals), I do not have a preference. I think pramoxine is effective and will definitely use it before antihistamines. I am not a topical antihistamine fan, nor do I think oatmeal products provide much relief.

Marcia Schwassmann *USA* Do you mind going over the products you mentioned for those present from outside the USA who may not be familiar with the names?

Sandy Merchant The Relief line of products by DVM are 1% pramoxine, omega-6 fatty acids and colloidal oatmeal. The Dermal Soothe products are 1% pramoxine but they do not have the omega-6 fatty acids. They do have the oatmeal and some skin/respiratory factor.

Pramoxine sprays are nice instead of the lotions, since our patients have hair all over. Therefore, I think sometimes the sprays are better.

Rosanna Marsella How long do you think the effects last?

Sandy Merchant About 24–48 h. Sometimes I think it is also the action of applying the product and not just the product. I do not think there are any true adverse reactions to pramoxine. I think it is primarily the manipulation of the itchy skin in combination with warm water that makes the animal more pruritic. Therefore, I do not think I have ever really seen an adverse reaction to pramoxine.

Marcia Schwassmann Now I have a different view. I have had a significant number of dogs that not only were more pruritic but also actually turned red all over. In fact, I had one dog that had an exfoliative problem as well. I have clients use the leave-on conditioner as a lotion and I don't know if that has something to do with the reactions I've seen or not. Possibly it's because this product is not designed to be used like that.

Rosanna Marsella Have you tried using the pramoxine shampoo in those dogs to see if they reacted the same to the shampoo?

Marcia Schwassmann Yes, and they had no reaction to the shampoo.

Rosanna Marsella So it may not be the ingredient but the fact that it's being left on as a lotion.

Marcia Schwassmann I do not use pramoxine shampoo.

Tiffany Bogart *USA* When you use the conditioner as a lotion, do you have the client reapply the lotion every day? I have some experience where I have the client wet the dog daily to sort of reactivate the conditioner instead of applying it each day.

Cecilia Friberg *USA* I have some dogs where we have the clients apply it every day, and they haven't had any problems.

Ernie Smith *USA* There is a human over-the-counter product that I like for focal regions, called Itch-X®. It is a 1% pramoxine human product.

Sandy Merchant There is also a pramoxine foam preparation for human medicine, which I think would be good for some animals. The foam product is called Proctofoam®, which tells you where they are targeting. Tronolane® is another pramoxine product that contains no hydrocortisone, for humans. Another is Tronothane®, which does contain hydrocortisone. Fleet® Pain Relief is another human product and, as its name suggests, to those of us in the USA anyway, they are primarily targeting the anal region in human medicine. They also have a calamine combination for weepy lesions with anti-itch therapy.

I think it is strange that in people, they recommend avoiding contact with the nose or eyes, but applying it to the rectal area is satisfactory. They also suggest avoiding prolonged contact with pramoxine but do not elaborate on their reasons.

Rosanna Marsella Possibly they are worried about the development of contact allergies.

Emily Rothstein *USA* It is just a recommendation.

Rosanna Marsella Emily, would you mind telling us about your study with pramoxine?

Emily Rothstein About 5 years ago, I did a non-placebo-controlled, non-blinded study comparing the only two crème applications of 1% pramoxine available at the time, Relief and Dermal Soothe. Each has its own packaging and unique additives, as we discussed earlier, but otherwise they are the same.

We used 17 non-seasonally pruritic dogs that ranged from 1 to 6 years of age. All completed a food trial and were seen for their skin test. While we prepared their immunotherapy, the owners agreed that the dogs could participate in our study. They were free of infection and were not receiving, and had not recently received, any other medications. The dogs were all moderately to severely pruritic, which may have biased our study, since we are not sure how much topical therapy can help moderate to severely pruritic dogs, but all were glucocorticoid responsive. Each dog was randomly assigned to receive one product or the other first. This was not blinded, so the owners used the commercially available packaging and knew which product they were using. Both products contain 1% pramoxine and colloidal oatmeal. Relief has the omega-6 fatty acids, while Dermal Soothe has the skin/respiratory factor, whatever that is. The dogs were bathed twice weekly with baby shampoo. The conditioner was applied, rubbed in and then allowed 10 min contact time. The dogs were rinsed and drip-dried, or dried with a hair-dryer on cool setting if the owner did not want to let the animal drip-dry. The dogs were not towel dried. Owners graded improvement in pruritus as poor (0–25% improvement), fair (26–50% improvement), good (51–75% improvement) or excellent (>75% improvement).

In our study, the 17 dogs were of various breeds and had various responses on their skin tests. We did not compare the skin-test results at all. The dogs were of various ages and had been pruritic for 1–6 years. We did not control for any of those factors.

The results were as follows: no excellent results, four dogs responded better to Relief (graded as good responses by the owners), two dogs responded only to Dermal Soothe, one dog responded to both products and 10 dogs failed to respond to either product. Of the good responses, some were to the first product used, while others were to the second, so it's not suggestive that owners were merely happy with the first product they used. There was one complaint that the conditioners left the dog's coat greasy, but possibly these owners applied too much product, because there were no other cosmetic complaints. Most owners thought the coats looked silky and beautiful, even if the dog was still itchy.

There were five dogs in which the level of itch increased during the study. Four of the dogs were using Dermal Soothe, while one was using Relief. I do not think it was the pramoxine but probably the action of applying a topical product. It is possible that any topical product would have made the animals worse. The owners were instructed to use cool water, but owner compliance varies.

The key seems to be to find a topical product that owners are willing to use to help reduce the need for glucocorticoids and other medications. I will also use the leave-on pramoxine if I cannot use topical hydrocortisone. Just before I left for the meeting, Virbac provided some of their leave-on product (ResiProx®, Virbac Animal Health) for me to compare on a few dogs. Of course, they were different dogs and different scenarios, but I was able to use it in 10 known non-seasonal, non-food-allergic, non-infected atopic dogs in the midst of building up immunotherapy. All promised to call before I left, but I was able to get hold of only five and none of them was very impressed.

Robin Baldwin *USA* Is that just pramoxine?

Emily Rothstein In the ResiProx, it's pramoxine and oatmeal but I don't know if they have any other factors in their product.

Rosanna Marsella Have you ever used ResiSoothe® (Virbac Animal Health)?

Emily Rothstein I use it a lot. I like it.

Sandy Merchant I use ResiCort® (Virbac Animal Health).

Emily Rothstein I use ResiCort, but when I can't, I send the dogs home with ResiSoothe.

Rosanna Marsella How does ResiSoothe compare with ResiProx?

Emily Rothstein The owners of the five dogs I was able to contact before I left had already used ResiSoothe and it didn't work on them. However, those dogs had also received ResiCort previously and it only worked minimally. I haven't used ResiProx as often as I use ResiSoothe, so I really can't answer the question.

Rosanna Marsella How about Aveeno? Does anyone use Aveeno any more?

Marcia Schwassmann Yes.

Rosanna Marsella How do you ask them to prepare it?

Marcia Schwassmann Pretty empirically, especially since I've never done it. Basically, I tell them to put half a packet into a bucket of water and use it like a dip. Some clients make it up in a tub and put the dogs in the tub directly. I like the oilated version for dry, itchy dogs. I use it myself in the winter.

Rosanna Marsella Have you noticed excessive scaling when using this product?

Marcia Schwassmann If they use too much, yes.

Cecilia Friberg I sometimes recommend that clients put the Aveeno into a nylon stocking to minimize scaling.

Emily Rothstein OK, now that everyone has seen the bottles and had a chance to smell the products, which product do you like best? Relief? [About half of the group raised their hands.] Dermal Soothe? [The other half raised their hands.] How about packaging?

Sandy Merchant Since EVSCO revamped their look, I really like their packaging.

Rosanna Marsella Randy is going to talk about hydrocortisone.

Randy Thomas *USA* I'm going to talk about my resident research project at the University of Florida (UF) using a 1% hydrocortisone leave-on conditioner, which is ResiCort®. For some background, we decided to do this project because we knew that localized use of fluorinated glucocorticoids could cause adrenal suppression. Previously, a study using a fluorinated shampoo showed that product did not have problems. However, our concern was that even though 1% hydrocortisone is of low potency, if we spread it all over the dog, there might be some problems. The two goals of this study were to determine if this product was safe to use and what effect its use had on intradermal skin test (IDST) reactivity.

The study design was placebo controlled with three groups of dogs. There were two groups of normal dogs. One group of normal dogs was treated, while the other served as a control group. The third group was a group of treated pruritic dogs. I did not feel comfortable using a placebo on pruritic dogs in Florida. We felt it was important to look at safety in pruritic dogs because absorption through the skin may be different in pruritic or inflamed skin.

Basically, all dogs were bathed twice weekly with a hypoallergenic shampoo. The 1% hydrocortisone leave-on conditioner was applied to the treated normal dogs and the pruritic dogs after each bath. We aimed for approximately 300 mg hydrocortisone per meter squared of body surface. This was variable based on the size and shape of the dog, as well as hair coat length. The control group of normal dogs received the vehicle-only conditioner after their baths. On days 0, 14, 28 and 42, we ran complete blood counts (CBC), chemistry panels and an adrenocorticotropic hormone (ACTH) stimulation test looking primarily at parameters that might be related to iatrogenic Cushing's syndrome, including cell counts, and plasma concentrations of alkaline phosphatase, alanine aminotransferase (ALT), glucose, cholesterol, and pre- and post-ACTH cortisol. In addition, on those days, we performed a skin test using serial dilutions of histamine starting with 1:100 000, which is what we use clinically, and doubling the dilutions until we were down to 1:1 600 000. The thought was that while we may not get histamine suppression at the higher concentrations, we might at the lower concentrations.

The results of the study were, most importantly, that all of the mean blood work values, cell counts, etc., were within normal limits throughout the entire study. We did have some changes within the groups, but in the end, they are probably not clinically relevant, since all of the values were within normal limits. The mean pre- and post-ACTH cortisol levels also all stayed within normal limits. Nevertheless, the post-ACTH cortisol levels in the pruritic group were significantly lower throughout the study than the hydrocortisone-treated normal dogs. We saw some changes in the baseline cortisol levels in the treated group of normal dogs from the beginning to the middle of the study. In the pruritic dogs, the alkaline phosphatase values were significantly elevated after day 0, but again, these were all within normal limits. We saw no suppression of histamine, objectively or subjectively.

So, our conclusion was that using the ResiCort twice weekly is safe. There was the suggestion that absorption does occur in inflamed skin, and though we didn't measure this directly, our impression was that this product could be overused. As an example, we had one small dog with long hair that was very pruritic. Therefore, a lot of product was used in relation to body surface area. This dog had a flat ACTH stimulation test at the end of the 6 weeks. It returned to normal in 2 weeks. This shows that the product can be overused, but overall seems to be safe.

Since there was no suppression of the histamine, we decided that, based on that test, ResiCort should not have a huge effect on an IDST. However, I don't think that histamine suppression is a good measure of skin-test suppression. Therefore, we decided that skin-test suppression is something that needs to be looked at further using different antigens. In fact, there was a study presented that showed that using ResiCort did suppress type I hypersensitivity reactions using a different model, so it is something to keep in mind. I typically use a 1 week withdrawal of ResiCort before I perform an IDST.

All of my clinical experience with ResiCort is anecdotal. We did not look at efficacy during that study, but I will say that virtually every pruritic dog owner asked for more product at the end of the study and my own pruritic dog gets ResiCort quite a bit. Clinically, I think ResiCort is useful for uncomplicated, mild to moderate pruritic dogs, but just like all of the other products, there is some variation in response to treatment. In general, scabies dogs don't do quite as well as atopic dogs clear of secondary infections. I use it primarily as an adjunct therapy with immunotherapy, fatty acids or antihistamines. I think it's less useful for severe to marked pruritus or if there are secondary infections present. In fact, when clients tell me it's stopped working, I recheck the dogs and they usually have a secondary infection. I think the efficacy of ResiCort is more variable on pedal pruritus than pruritus in other areas. Adverse effects seem to be rare. I've never had a dog that gets more pruritic after using ResiCort. I have seen some that licked the product off and vomited, but mostly it is well tolerated. The study was funded by UF, the American Academy of Veterinary Dermatology (AAVD) and Allerderm/Virbac.

Rosanna Marsella Do you think that chronic use will predispose animals to secondary infections?

Randy Thomas I haven't seen that yet. We actually collected skin biopsies from the study dogs to look for subtle changes in the biopsies, but we did not get a chance to look at them. I have them with me in North Carolina. I haven't appreciated that it predisposes animals to secondary infections and, for the majority of the time, I don't use it more than once weekly.

Carol George *USA* I was wondering how often we should be using it.

Robin Baldwin I use it once or twice a week.

Cecilia Friberg I've used it daily.

Carol George All over?

Cecilia Friberg It depends on the area. Usually if it's required all over, then we use another treatment. If its used too much, some dogs get overhydrated skin that starts peeling.

Carol George Do you have them bathe the animal daily or just apply it as a lotion?

Cecilia Friberg Just as a lotion. Sometimes we have them wet the animal with a spray bottle and it tends to work better that way.

Dennis Crow *USA* I have used it on many animals as a spot treatment. It seems to me that small dogs actually respond better than large dogs. I've used it up to twice weekly on small dogs and daily on large dogs, and still the smaller dogs seem to respond better.

Marcia Schwassmann Of those of you who use it daily, have you seen any changes in the skin suggestive of iatrogenic Cushing's syndrome?

Rosanna Marsella I have seen it in other stronger steroids, especially in smaller dogs with cutaneous and systemic signs. I think it's size related.

Randy Thomas Has anyone used FS shampoo?

Rosanna Marsella I've used it quite a bit and I'm happy with it. FS Shampoo is a human shampoo product that is available only by prescription. It is quite expensive.

Randy Thomas Yes, it's about $25 to $28 per bottle.

Dennis Crow And that's for a 236–295 ml (8–10 ounce) bottle.

Randy Thomas I've only used it in some dogs that had intractable pruritus and we couldn't use systemic steroids because they were cushingoid when they came to us. In these cases, ResiCort did not work and it's my feeling that if the ResiCort doesn't work, then the FS shampoo will not have much effect either.

Marcia Schwassmann Is there anyone who uses any topical cortisone in very pruritic *Demodex* dogs?

Randy Thomas I have used ResiCort in *Demodex* cases.

Emily Rothstein Does it help?

Randy Thomas I think in some cases it makes the dogs feel better. All of these dogs are being treated with ivermectin and I don't think that the ResiCort slows the healing process.

Marcia Schwassmann I have used oral prednisone and ivermectin to treat some *Demodex* dogs.

Randy Thomas And we have had some chemotherapy dogs with *Demodex* and controlled it with ivermectin. Granted, that is a much more severe problem, but in the rare instances when I can't find anything else, ResiCort doesn't make them worse.

Rosanna Marsella I guess I try to stick with LymDyp® (DVM Pharmaceuticals). It works well if the owners are willing to do it.

Robin Baldwin Can you use LymDyp with amitraz or oral treatment only?

Rosanna Marsella Oral treatment usually, because most of the cases we see are on ivermectin or milbemycin so we don't use much Mitaban® (Pharmacia & Upjohn). Marcia, please tell us about your experience with lime sulfur.

Marcia Schwassmann Rosanna asked me to talk about LymDyp since she doesn't know many people who still use it. I live in Florida, it's warm year-round and I still use LymDyp. My clients are not excited about it. I usually have to twist their arms. I think it is interesting because it does five different things. LymDyp is antibacterial, antifungal, antipruritic, antiparasitic and keratolytic. I think it's a wonderful product, but its major problem is that it's not nice to use, so compliance becomes an issue.

I use it primarily for scabies in dogs. I usually give clients the option of LymDyp, explaining why I like it, or ivermectin: 90% of them usually pick ivermectin, especially after they smell the LymDyp. The clients I make use it are owners of dogs that have seizures. I think milbemycin is safer in these dogs. I know some people use fipronil and now there's selamectin (Revolution®, Pfizer Animal Health), so there are some more options, but I use LymDyp in old dogs that have seizures. I don't know if it's a southern thing or not, but we have some clients who firmly believe the old wives' tale that burnt motor oil kills mites. LymDyp appeals to these clients, though there are not many of them.

I use it for *Otodectes* in cats, though being a referral clinic we don't see much of it. If it's primarily facial, there is some concern about LymDyp in the eyes. What I use this most for is *Demodex* in cats: those with the short fat mite. Does this mite have a name?

Sandy Merchant It's *Demodex gatoi*. It was named at Louisiana State University.

Marcia Schwassmann So I really like LymDyp for cats because it's so safe. I've had only one case of generalized *Demodex* and that was the long skinny mite. Primarily I see *D. gatoi* in cats.

I forgot to mention, for scabies in dogs I usually dip the dogs once weekly for 6–8 weeks. If I found mites before, I'll scrape them again, though I do not usually find mites. I dip my cats once weekly for 4–6 weeks. I prefer 6 weekly, though I don't think I always get it. I scrape them after 4 weeks and haven't had a cat yet who still had mites after 4 weeks, but I still ask clients to dip for 2 more weeks. I try to get them back in after the sixth week for one last scrape.

Dennis Crow What dilution do you use?

Marcia Schwassmann I use 118 ml (4 ounces) per 3.79 l (1 gallon) of water. A lot of my *Demodex* cats seem to still be pruritic after the sixth dip, but I don't know if it's habit or the dip is drying, but the pruritus seems to fade after a few weeks.

Robin Baldwin Do you bathe them before dipping?

Marcia Schwassmann Yes, I do, if I can. I have them use a mild, non-medicated shampoo. I do not care what they use. And for cats that don't like to be bathed, I have clients use the dunk technique. Fill a plastic bucket with the dip, scruff the cat, dunk in the dip and let it dry in their carrier.

Sandy Merchant I know Karen, and for any pruritic cat that comes in and there's not an obvious reason why, she lime sulfurs every one.

Marcia Schwassmann So do I. Dr Karen Beale practices dermatology in Texas, USA, and her practice reported three cats in one household with *D. gattoi*, so it is potentially contagious. I had one the other day where they brought in a kitten. We couldn't find mites on the kitten, but the other cat did have mites, so we dipped them all. My record is a family with seven cats. One cat came in with *Demodex* but two more at home were mowing their bellies, so she actually dipped all seven cats four times.

I also use LymDyp in dermatophytosis. It's our old standby. We use it once weekly for 4–8 weeks or until we get a negative culture. The owners of long-haired cats do not appreciate this, so now we've been using Resizole® (2% miconazole leave-on conditioner, Virbac Animal Health) for those cats. Has anyone else done this? We've found that given the choice, even though Resizole is expensive, the owners choose it over lime sulfur. We use the Resizole weekly until the culture is negative. With cats with dermatophytosis, I use bathing a lot.

Sandy Merchant So do I, but it's really about decreasing environmental contamination. If I have a cat with a bad temper, I don't use any topical therapy. Everyone gets itraconazole and the environment is cleaned.

Marcia Schwassmann There is a poster downstairs that looked at household contamination after treatment, and even after cleaning, the households were still contaminated. And, if I remember correctly, houses with cats were worse than those with dogs.

The last thing I was going to mention was the use of lime sulfur in my nasty, smelly allergic dogs that are always loaded with yeast and bacteria. They are greasy and smelly, and I don't know how the owners can stand having them in their house. LymDyp gives good control on these dogs. It actually cuts down on the smell. The dogs are less pruritic and less scaly. I've used it in hyperpigmented and no hyperpigmentation cases, and it really works, although not in all cases. I use it once or twice a week, as needed. This is not a problem in Florida because of the humidity, but it might be in drier climates. It might be difficult to use this often. Lime sulfur, which is listed in the dermatology textbooks, also treats *Cheyletiella*, chiggers, lice and fur mites. I think we used it once during my residency for lice. I don't see much *Cheyletiella*, so I don't have any experience with that.

Cecilia Friberg I've used it in older dogs, where I was afraid to use ivermectin. It usually works, but you have to treat the environment. In some of our cats, we can't find mites on the cat, but when we do a tape preparation of the carrier, we've found mites in there. Now we always do a tape preparation of the carrier.

Marcia Schwassmann So, the advantages of LymDyp are safety and its antipruritic properties. If nothing else works, clients are desperate enough to finally try it, and it usually helps. The primary disadvantages are it smells, it's messy and it stains. I've had only rare instances of skin irritation. I've had more cats than dogs come back more pruritic after LymDyp. I've also had more trouble with the dip drying cats out more than dogs. If that's the case, I have the owner add non-scented bath oil (a couple of capfuls per gallon). I had one client who added oilated Aveeno and that seemed to help also.

Rosanna Marsella I use baby oil.

Marcia Schwassmann Is the smell acceptable?

Rosanna Marsella Yes.

Marcia Schwassmann The one cat that became ill was one of the seven mentioned earlier. It was vomiting and anorexic. I asked if it was grooming and vomiting the hair, but the owner said it wasn't grooming. So I suggested we wait and see, and the owner said she'd done it several times and the cat always had the same reaction. I think it is real.

Sandy Merchant I agree. I've had some practitioners call me with sick cats after lime sulfur dips. I think it's primarily ingestion. I tell all of my clients that the cat must wear an Elizabethan collar (e-collar) for 4–6 hours after the dip or until the hair is completely dry.

Marcia Schwassmann I have my clients watch their cats. If they groom a lot after baths or dips, I give them e-collars also. My thought is that if they lick it off, besides the fact that they may become ill, the lime sulfur is not on the skin doing its job.

Cecilia Friberg I have had some contact reactions. I use it at 177–236 ml (6–8 ounces) per 3.79 l (1 gallon) and have had some cats come back with very erythematous skin, so I tell clients to watch the animals carefully after using it.

Rosanna Marsella I increase the concentration also for those very pruritic animals. I have them use 177–236 ml (6–8 ounces) per 3.79 l (1 gallon) of water and dip the animal every 5 days.

Marcia Schwassmann Some other things to mention: this product stains. You must wear gloves. It will stain your fingernails yellow, not to mention the odor. I do not notice the odor on the animals once they are dry. Also, you have to remove jewelry. It will stain concrete and it reacts with porcelain. It also stains white coats yellow, although I don't think it's that obvious. It's more dingy than yellow.

I've had some questions about how careful you need to be using it around the eyes. I have clients use a sponge to dab it on the animal's face. I know Dr Gail Kunkle (UF, USA) had a colony of research cats with dermatophytosis and they just dipped them, including the head, with no problems.

Carol George Did they use lubrication to protect the eyes?

Rosanna Marsella Yes.

Marcia Schwassmann There is still some controversy as to whether that repels or traps agents.

Some miscellaneous things: when you have the diluted lime sulfur solution made up, it is stable for 2 weeks, according to the DVM people. Also, the spray has been taken off the market, apparently because they had some toxic reactions to the citrus scent. Apparently some cats were being bathed with a citrus shampoo, followed by the lime sulfur spray and they had problems. It is not likely to be brought back. I really like the spray for spot treatments. I think this is an excellent anti-*Malassezia* treatment and the spray worked really well for that.

Tiffany Bogart I worked for a shelter, and I would have the technicians make up a spray for spot treatment of those chronic neck problems in cocker spaniels. They sprayed them every other or every third day, and it worked really well to control them without oral medications.

Marcia Schwassmann The last thing I wanted to say was that we have a handout for our clients using LymDyp. It says the first dip should be made up using 59 ml (2 ounces) per 3.79 l (1 gallon) of water, and I think this is in case there is a reaction. All following dips should be made up using 118 ml (4 ounces) per 3.79 l (1 gallon) of water unless otherwise instructed. Please sponge onto and over your pet for 15–20 min. This does not apply to cats. Allow the pet to air dry. If the animal becomes red or itchy, please rinse several times and call our office. There is also a note to wear gloves and remove jewelry before using this product. It is recommended that this product be used outside only, and I believe that is primarily because of the smell. Dipping animals outside in Florida is not a problem, but it may be in other areas. In parentheses it says, 'will eat through porcelain and has a strong odor'. Repeat dip every 5–7 days unless otherwise directed.

Dennis Crow We had a client at UF who was instructed to use LymDyp for management of their atopic dog. The owner was allergic to oral sulfur drugs. We consulted a dermatology physician and they said though the risk was very small, there was the potential for a reaction. It was suggested that someone else dip the dog, while the owner avoided contact with it until the dog was dry. We managed that dog with weekly dips for a long time and they never had a problem.

Sandy Merchant We had a dog with oral erythema multiforme (EM) that somehow received topical sulfur and he developed EM again.

Verena Schaerer *Switzerland* There are other medications, like iodine or betadine, where people are allergic to the product, so you can't use it on their pets.

Dennis Crow Since then, I always ask people. I have had a handful of people that have said they do have problems and I don't send it home with them. I'll use something else.

Marcia Schwassmann In my practice, I was sending a client home with SulfOxidex® (DVM Pharmaceuticals) and he mentioned that his wife was allergic to sulfur drugs, and would this be satisfactory? I told him to consult his physician.

Randy Thomas How many people use LymDyp regularly? [Nine or 10 people indicated that they did.]

Verena Schaerer I would use it, but we do not have it any more. It used to exist in my father's time. I see it in a few of his books but you cannot buy it any more.

Marcia Schwassmann I had some people visit from Europe and they took a whole case back with them.

Dennis Crow I have had a few cases where clients were worried about all of the medications they were using on their pet and I explained to them that LymDyp is a natural product and they really liked that.

Anne Norton *USA* I have had a few clients who were like that with ivermectin. They just knew their dog was going to have a problem with it, so I gave them LymDyp. It's natural, safe and has few side-effects.

Rosanna Marsella Dennis, would you mind telling us about your nightmare case?

Dennis Crow I would love to. I have a photograph. This is Thumper Kissle. He is a male castrated bichon frisé. He presented to the UF when he was 6 years old. At about 1 year of age, he started with focal perianal and tailhead pruritus that was non-seasonal. I'll focus primarily on the topical therapies we used in this case, but first I'd like to briefly touch on some of the diagnostics. We biopsied this region initially and saw severe folliculitis and furunculosis with chronic changes including fibrosis and fibroplasias. We cultured a *Proteus* sp. He was treated with systemic and topical antibiotics for some time with no changes in his clinical presentation. Our primary rule-out in this case was food allergy. He went through elimination diets, including two Innovative Veterinary Diets (IVD), a home-cooked rabbit and potato and home-cooked peas and bean diet. All of these were good food trials, while he was clear of infection. Each lasted at least 8 weeks and there was still no improvement. He came to us having been on a skin vaccine for 2 years. The vaccine was based on an enzyme-linked immunosorbent assay (ELISA) that didn't really have any positives. We skin tested him and also had no positives, except a 2+ positive for flea antigen. Throughout the entire treatment, he was treated with Knockout® (Virbac Animal Health) spray once weekly, so there was good flea control. He lived in an e-collar for a long time.

The topical therapies we have tried include antibiotics, as I mentioned earlier, with no improvement. We tried Synotic® (Fort Dodge Animal Health) topically once daily for a month with no improvement. We tried a 1% hydrocortisone leave-on conditioner (Resicort®) on the back half of his body with no improvement. We treated him with Capsaizin P (0.025% capsaicin) ointment on the focal area twice and sometimes three times daily. Initially, his pruritus increased over the first week and then decreased slightly, but according to the owner, there wasn't much improvement. We tried lime sulfur dips and ivermectin at 100 μg/kg for 7–8 days, with no change. We performed cytology on many occasions, especially in the anal sac area. We even placed Panalog® (Fort Dodge Animal Health) into the anal sacs in the hope that it would reduce any inflammation that might be present instigating the pruritus, but it did not help. He was treated with 3 week courses of ketoconazole and itraconazole, with the thought that he might be hypersensitive to yeasts, but neither helped. We tried the entire gamut of tricyclics, although we have not tried the more specific serotonin reuptake inhibitors. We tried eight different antihistamines for 3 weeks each, with absolutely no improvement. He is a 33 kg dog and has been on 10 mg of prednisone daily for 8 months now. This allows him to go without the e-collar. We tried adding cyclosporine (Neoral®, Novartis Pharmaceuticals) in an attempt to reduce the prednisone dose, but after 3 weeks of 5 mg/kg cyclosporine they were still not able to reduce the prednisone dose from 10 to 5 mg. So, the only thing that controls this dog is prednisone. At this time, the owners are considering euthanasia as their only option.

Sandy Merchant I doubt this is a true neurogenic case like those sciatic nerve cases where they chew their toes off, but it might be something to consider. There is a γ-aminobutyric acid (GABA) product (Neuronitin®, Parke Davis) used in people with diabetic neuropathies. This isn't the region we would normally think about, but you might be at the point to consider using something that is for a true neurogenic pruritus.

Dennis Crow What do people think about the serotonin uptake inhibitors?

Sandy Merchant I would try those, but I would try the other drug mentioned above. Now, I know it's expensive, but these owners can't be too concerned about cost, based on their history.

Marcia Schwassmann Have you tried acupuncture?

Dennis Crow No, but the owner has brought it up. The dog has been to a chiropractor. This dog has had a full work-up including abdominal radiographs, ultrasound, etc., but we turned up nothing. The referring veterinarian had radiographs and suggested that the dog had some narrow spaces in the thoracolumbar spine, so the client took the dog to the chiropractor, with no benefit.

Marcia Schwassmann I do not know if acupuncture is considered topical therapy, but I had a case referred to me for a supposed lick granuloma. This was a German shepherd dog with hip problems and stifle surgery. He licked over one hip, not both, and I couldn't find anything skin related that might be causing the problems. Acupuncture is working well for that dog. I have also had a couple of other true lick granuloma cases where I felt it was more mental than physiological, and acupuncture is working well for them too.

Robin Baldwin Did the *Proteus* culture come back negative?

Dennis Crow Yes.

Rosanna Marsella Has anyone used capsaicin for lick granulomas? Are you happy with it?

Randy Thomas I think it works at least as well as everything else does. It works in about half of the cases.

Marcia Schwassmann Is everyone familiar with capsaicin?

Sandy Merchant It's a substance P inhibitor.

Rosanna Marsella Yes. It triggers the release of substance P in the skin so that eventually the substance P is depleted and the sensation of pruritus and pain should be diminished.

Marcia Schwassmann It is a hot pepper derivative.

Robin Baldwin Do you use it with bitter apple?

Randy Thomas No. I have them use the over-the-counter product.

Dennis Crow It was interesting because Thumper's owner was instructed to wear gloves when applying the capsaicin, but apparently she did not, because she called me a week later and her fingers were numb. She used gloves after that.

Rosanna Marsella What percentage do you use when you use it?

Randy Thomas I have them get the regular strength.

Sandy Merchant Regular strength is 0.025%. I don't think the 0.075% is good for dogs. It would probably be painful, since the 0.025% causes some burning.

Rosanna Marsella I've only used the lower concentration. I have used it for lick granulomas but now we are doing a study using capsaicin for atopic dermatitis. It is a double-blind, placebo-controlled, cross-over study, so that all dogs will get both treatments. So far, eight dogs have completed the study. The treatment period is 6 weeks, because it takes some time to deplete the skin of substance P. Then there is a 4 week washout period, after which the treatments are crossed over. We're primarily interested in pruritus, which is scored by both the investigator and the owner. At this point, the investigator's score of pruritus is lower in the capsaicin group, but this is not statistically significant. The owner's scores significantly increase after the first week and then there is a significant improvement by the end of the treatment. We'll see how the other dogs finish and if over time the numbers improve. I don't know if possibly we treated them for a longer period of time whether they would improve more.

When you use capsaicin for lick granulomas, how fast do you see improvement?

Randy Thomas All of my patients get an e-collar or a bandage for the first week. After the first week, the collar or bandage can be removed. Initially, I start with three to four times daily applications. Then, as they improve, I taper down to twice daily. After a couple of weeks, if they are still doing well, I'll reduce them to once daily. I've had a couple I've reduced to once to twice weekly. However, we've only treated about six cases. I've had some cases in which it didn't work at all, just like everything else.

Rosanna Marsella Have you seen any worsening, like a contact reaction? I know in people, especially with the higher concentration, they may develop a contact allergy to it.

Sandy Merchant There are initial sensations such as burning and itching that go away with time.

Randy Thomas I think they all get worse in the first week but I have not had any that got worse later on, though I have had some that never improved. I have not had what I would appreciate as a contact reaction.

Rosanna Marsella Have you seen any papular eruptions, as have been reported in people?

Randy Thomas No. The packaging even warns that it causes skin irritation, so if you don't discuss that with the owners, they won't use it. I've found that capsaicin requires more counseling than some of the other products, like Synotic® and Banamine® (Schering-Plough).

Verena Schaerer It also depends on the skin lesion. If it is a deep erosion, I use something else initially, until the wound heals to some degree. Otherwise, the owners are concerned when it becomes worse after applying the capsaicin therapy.

Randy Thomas My first choice is Bactoderm® (Pfizer Animal Health) for these problems. I use a few weeks or a month of antibiotic therapy before starting capsaicin therapy.

Marcia Schwassmann So you do not use capsaicin on the raw open area?

Randy Thomas No. I don't use it until after the wound has healed to a degree after antibiotic therapy.

Rosanna Marsella Or you can use it on the periphery of the wound. Applying it on the raw open area would be inhumane to me.

I have asked Cecilia to talk about topical therapy in horses. I don't know if you people see a lot of horses, but they always seem to be the forgotten species. We always talk about dogs and cats. So, Cecilia, please share with us some of your experience with horses.

Cecilia Friberg I think that the topical market is underutilizing the horse. Horse owners love to put things on their horses. They often have grooms that can do it even when they are not around and, therefore, compliance in horse owners is usually very good. The primary problem is first getting them to stop using all of the other material they are using. I think sometimes the horse's problem is a contact reaction overlaid on the original problem. I try to simplify the therapy and get them down to using just one or two products, so you have control over, and know, what they are using.

I've had a couple of horses where I think a secondary pyoderma was causing a lot of the pruritus, so I use a lot of the benzoyl peroxide shampoos. They seem to help a lot, probably not so much because of their antipruritic effects but because they help with the initial pyoderma. We all know the pruritic effects of pyoderma and I don't know many veterinarians who put their horses on 3–4 weeks of antibiotics, so the antibacterial shampoos help with some of those. Insect allergies are a very big part of pruritus in horses, so all topical products I use in horses are always topped off with a 2% pyrethrin spray to help with any reactions insects may cause.

The biggest group of antipruritic drugs in horses is the hydrocortisones. I don't like to go any higher than

1%. There are a lot of local practitioners who use betamethasone topically and I really worry about that. Many horses have manes that don't grow back and I really worry about wounds developing on the thin skin of the distal limbs.

There are not actually a lot of products out there specifically for horses.

Marcia Schwassmann I do not see many horses. What products are approved for use in horses?

Rosanna Marsella There is a 5% benzoyl peroxide shampoo called CytOxyl® (VetGenex). It's labeled only for use in horses and not dogs and cats.

Cecilia Friberg EVSCO has a 1% chlorhexidine shampoo for horses.

Dennis Crow VetGenex also has an oatmeal pramoxine and there's also a 1% hydrocortisone for horses. I don't know if it's a shampoo or a conditioner.

Rosanna Marsella Not many products labeled for horses can be used on dogs and cats. They usually come in gallon sizes, as well.

Cecilia Friberg So, like I said, I think the horse market is underutilized for topical therapies because horse owners like to put topical agents on their horses. I do not have any experience using lime sulfur on horses, but I imagine you could. That would be a lot of lime sulfur.

Randy Thomas I have. Actually, I had a student do it.

Rosanna Marsella I use things like SulfOxidex® and antiseborrheic, sulfur-based products, like Seba-Hex® (EVSCO Pharmaceuticals) or Seba-Moist® (EVSCO Pharmaceuticals).

Verena, what products do you have in Switzerland? We seem to talk mostly about products available here in the USA.

Verena Schaerer We have tar shampoos from Allerderm. We do not have lime sulfur, as I mentioned earlier.

Rosanna Marsella Do you use a lot of tar?

Verena Schaerer Quite a lot for scaly, greasy dogs. Occasionally, I have old dogs with seborrhea, and I use tar on them too. However, washing and treating dogs with tar is very drying. This is fine when the skin is greasy, but if not, you have to moisturize it. I have used skin oil used in human medicine and made a dilution, depending on the needs of the dog, and the skin was not greasy afterwards.

Rosanna Marsella Do you have any moisturizing products like HyLyt® (DVM Pharmaceuticals) in Switzerland?

Verena Schaerer We have Humilac® (Virbac Animal Health) spray that is very useful.

Marcia Schwassmann Do you have dog groomers where people can take their dogs to have them bathed?

Verena Schaerer They do exist.

Marcia Schwassmann Does it cost a lot of money for someone to take their big dog to the groomer?

Verena Schaerer Yes, that is a possibility.

Marcia Schwassmann I have a surprising number of clients that take their dogs to the groomer.

Verena Schaerer It is very expensive. I think sometimes that dogs are like horses. When you get the owners to stop using all the products they are currently using, the pruritus comes back under control. I have a question: do you think that the oatmeal shampoos are beneficial? I have treated several pruritic dogs with them and the owners were not impressed.

Sandy Merchant I think they are the lowest products on my list. I would use the topical steroids first, then pramoxine and finally oatmeal. I am not a topical antihistamine fan, so I don't know where that would fit in my list.

Marcia Schwassmann Are you talking about shampoos or do you use those things as rinses?

Sandy Merchant Both.

Verena Schaerer I'm scared of steroid shampoos because we really have to counsel the owners. I have seen dogs and cats that were not cushingoid but had lost their hair. Many owners use human products and feel more is better, and this causes problems.

Marcia Schwassmann Here, human products are much more potent than those we would use on animals. Is that the same in Switzerland?

Verena Schaerer That is true.

Marcia Schwassmann I have patients who come in and say that they've been using their psoriasis cream and it is obvious because the animal has comedones and no hair.

Verena Schaerer All of my clients work in a hospital setting and have access to all sorts of human products, and they self-medicate and make the problems worse.

Rosanna Marsella What kind of steroid-based products do you have labeled specifically for use in dogs? Do you have ResiCort?

Verena Schaerer Yes, that is commonly available. There are new ones, but for years you have been able to purchase steroid-based products for dogs.

Marcia Schwassmann Since it was brought up earlier, it made me want to ask a question. We have a number of moisturizing products available for dogs, but how many people actually use those versus telling people to buy some human bath oil, dilute it and use that?

Tiffany Bogart HyLyt EFA® (essential fatty acids, DVM Pharmaceuticals) shampoo and crème rinse are very popular and are coming out in a spray soon.

Emily Rothstein It depends on the client. Do they want to buy something else from you or would they rather buy it over the counter somewhere else?

Randy Thomas I try to make them use veterinary products, and I don't care if they buy it from me or from their veterinarian but I rarely tell people to buy human products for their animals. I don't even use Selsun Blue® a lot. We've spent so much time telling them about pH balance and not using just any product, and then if I turn around and tell them to use a human product, it confuses them.

Sandy Merchant And now there are reports that the pH of poodle skin is different from other breeds. Soon there will be shampoos for each breed of dog.

Tiffany Bogart I sell a lot of whitening shampoos for white dogs because as soon as people discover that it is specifically for white dogs, they want it.

Marcia Schwassmann Do they feel it really works?

Tiffany Bogart I use it a lot as a grooming shampoo for my boarders and I can tell a difference. They look better than when they came in, but it's just like everything else, you have to leave it on for 10 min before rinsing. It's the PearLyt HyLyt® (DVM Pharmaceuticals) shampoo for white dogs.

Rosanna Marsella We are out of time. I appreciate everyone coming and participating. Thank you.

5.19

In vitro allergy testing

Gail A. Kunkle[1] (Chairperson) and Diane E. Bevier[2] (Secretary)

[1] University of Florida, Gainesville, Florida, USA
[2] Purdue University, West Lafayette, Indiana, USA

Gail Kunkle *USA* I would like to take this opportunity to thank the Workshop Sponsor, VARL, and to thank you for coming. The handouts briefly give you a schedule of our plans that are of a slightly different style than other workshops you have attended. Instead of each speaker being followed by questions and discussion, I have set a very hard task for each of the speakers. I would like to especially thank those five speakers who agreed to participate. I proposed to all that they address a list of very pointed questions. These were:

(1) Describe your assay – immunoglobulin E (IgE) detection reagent (polyclonal, monoclonal, combination, other). If your assay is applicable to species other than the canine, what are your detection reagents in that case? Please discuss your readout reagent, your serum dilution, length of serum incubation and the reasons for these, as well as controls.
(2) Under the conditions in which your commercial test is run, what is the relationship between the test results and intradermal skin testing (IDST)? If IDST is used as the 'gold standard', describe the conditions under which your test can give a false-positive or a false-negative reaction. Your answer should address: the level of detection of assay (ng IgE, units, etc.), how you generate the cut-off values, the source, quality and potency of allergens used, the cross-reactivity of detection reagent for IgG and, if time permits, the effects of high total IgE and the presence of anti-carbohydrate IgE.

We will try to stay on schedule with questions following all speakers in a panel-like format.

Sola Alaba *USA* (VARL Laboratories) Since you have set the task of presenting all this information within 8 min, which is virtually impossible, I've tried to summarize as much as is possible. It is pertinent to appreciate several of the important distinctions that, put together, make the determination of allergen-specific IgE antibodies in the serum of dogs and cats quite unique and extraordinary. Foremost among these are the following facts.

Allergens are very complex mixtures of proteins, glycoproteins, carbohydrates and even nucleic acids. The Western blot profiles that are indicated on the slide show the complexity of allergen extracts. An individual patient can be sensitive to some of those molecules and not to others. Different patients are, therefore, not necessarily sensitive to the same allergenic molecules in an extract. Dogs and cats have exceedingly high amounts of circulating IgE antibodies in their blood. However, specific IgE antibodies constitute only a minute fraction of this circulating IgE. Different allergens have different levels of background that potentiate more or less non-specific IgE binding.

These facts constitute some of the fundamentals on which the VARL Liquid Gold® test has been engineered. The VARL Liquid Gold allergen-specific IgE test technically is not an enzyme-linked immunosorbent assay (ELISA). It is a liquid-phase enzymoimmunometric assay designed for the semiquantitative determination of canine and feline serum allergen-specific IgE. The technology is engineered not only to eliminate false-positive results but also to overcome some of the problems associated with solid-phase ELISA and radioallergosorbent (RAST) methodologies. These are some of the attributes uniquely engineered into Liquid Gold:

- All relevant allergenic molecules would be present in the test at the same stoichiometry as in the liquid extract.

- With the aid of Western blot, it can be ascertained that all allergenic molecules are present in every test so that sensitivity and consistency are not compromised.
- Conformational distortions that accompany the adsorption of allergens to a solid phase are avoided.
- Non-specific IgE sticking to a solid phase and leading to false-positive results can be eliminated.
- The amount of allergen in a test can be controlled and optimized initially when the patient has been on corticosteroids and also when specific IgG concentrations are very high.
- Dilution of serum samples should not be necessary since this practice compromises sensitivity and can lead to false-negative results.

My presentation will be limited to the left side of the panel for VARL Liquid Gold. On this slide is a representation of an allergen molecule with multiple IgE-binding domains. Allergens are three-dimensional molecules and having all these IgE binding sites available is a necessary prerequisite in order that the sensitivity of the assay is not compromised. Unlike a solid-phase method, where some of these epitopes may be occluded from binding IgE due to their attachment to the solid phase, liquid-phase technology guarantees that all the IgE binding epitopes are accessible.

The first step in the Liquid Gold technology is the attachment of an identifiable reagent in the form of biotin to the allergen. The allergen remains liquid. Each allergen is analyzed with Western blot using a serum pool from several dogs or cats to verify that all the repertoire of allergenic molecules is present. In the actual test, aliquots of liquid allergens are added to six wells of a microplate. The first set of triplicate wells is intended to measure the total amount of IgE detected against an allergen. The second set of triplicate wells serves as control wells to determine the level of non-specific IgE binding that may occur with regard to the patient serum and each and every allergen tested. This control is crucial to eliminate the possibility of false-positive or false-negative results. The patient serum reacts with liquid allergen in a homogeneous liquid-phase reaction. The patient serum does not need to be diluted. If dilution of patient serum is carried out (if there is not enough serum for a complete analysis), it may be diluted two- to three-fold.

During the 2 h incubation, IgE antibodies in the patient serum bind to their respective IgE domains. Non-specific IgE is also detectable in the microplate wells, along with the specific IgE binding to the allergens. After the allergen–IgE complexes have formed, the reaction mixtures are transferred to a new microplate. The wells of the new microplate have been previously treated to carry biotin molecules. Streptavidin is quickly added to the mixture transferred from the first microplate set of wells. The second set of triplicate wells that are intended for homologous controls for each test allergen do not receive streptavidin. During the 30 min incubation, streptavidin bridges the biotin on the allergen complex as well as the biotin on the well. The microplate is then washed to remove all unbound materials.

To quantify the amount of IgE anchored to the second biotin-carrying microplate wells, a cocktail of three monoclonal anti-IgE antibodies conjugated to horseradish peroxidase (HRP) is added and the reaction is allowed to proceed overnight. Following a washing step, enzyme substrate is added and the amount of color generated is measured in a plate reader. The intensity of color generated is directly proportional to the amount of IgE that reacted in the patient's serum. The mean absorbance obtained from the triplicate wells that served as homologous controls (wells that did not receive streptavidin) is subtracted from the mean absorbance of triplicate wells that did receive streptavidin. The net absorbance value is the true measure of the specific IgE present in serum to the test allergen. This net absorbance value is read against a standard curve that is constructed by reacting a calibrated control serum of different dilution with our control allergen, the house dust mite (HDM) *Dermatophagoides farinae*. The absorbance value obtained with each of the six calibrators is assigned to classes 1 to 6. Class 6 represents the highest IgE value and class 1 the lowest value. An absorbance value equal to two standard deviations above that obtained with our zero calibrator serum is assigned class 0. The zero calibrator is a pool of canine or feline serum that is negative to *D. farinae* both in Liquid Gold assay and by Western blot.

In the next couple of slides I will summarize the two studies that were carried out blinded. VARL Liquid Gold test for dogs was compared with intradermal skin testing using Western blot as the definitive standard. In both studies, Liquid Gold is 81% and 75% in concordance with Western blot, and the intradermal skin test was 74% and 29%, respectively. These data are approximately 8 years old. The Liquid Gold has undergone some re-engineering since that time. For example, we have switched from polyclonal to a cocktail of three monoclonal anti-IgE antibodies, and we now run homologous controls, i.e. each allergen is used as its own control, with the same patient serum and transfer of allergen–IgE complex reaction mixtures to a second microplate.

These steps have allowed us to virtually eliminate possibilities of false-positive results.

Catherine McCall *USA* (Heska Corporation) As the previous speaker noted, it is rather hard to address all these issues in such a short period of time, but the thing that is unique about the Heska Allercept test is that it uses IgE's own receptor as a readout reagent for IgE. The test is based on the use of a truncated extracellular portion of the α-chain of the human high-affinity IgE receptor. We adopted this agent because when we first started looking into developing a test for canine IgE we weren't very satisfied with the specificity of the commercially available polyclonal and monoclonal antibodies against canine IgE. The hallmark of our efforts to make this a very good test has been an emphasis on specificity, and the recombinant truncated α-chain of the IgE receptor binds a heat-labile antibody IgE in the serum of dogs, cats and horses. This is interesting, as although this is the human α-chain, it does in fact seem to bind IgE from other species. This isn't necessarily a reciprocal arrangement. For instance, the IgE receptor of the dog doesn't necessarily bind to human IgE. However, we found that this was a very useful reagent and that it will recognize IgE not only from humans but also from dogs, cats and horses.

Those of you who saw Wendy Lorch's presentation in the residents' forum have seen the work done using the assay. The recombinant truncated α-chain does not bind to highly purified canine, feline or equine IgG, which was what we were most concerned with. When we started to develop this assay, we felt that we had a reagent that was exquisitely specific for IgE and we weren't going to get false positives from cross-reactivity of the detection agent with IgG. We used this in a couple of standardized formats. It is a solid-phase assay and obviously the format we run in the commercial assay is looking for allergen-specific IgE where we have allergen on the plate. We come back with serum containing IgE and then the receptor and the labeled receptor, and our readout to pick up receptor bound to allergen-specific IgE in the assay is now streptavidin–alkaline phosphatase. We previously used a streptavidin HRP but, as I will come to later, we had some problems with that as an enzyme in these systems.

We can also measure total IgE, although this is less relevant in canine and feline populations than it is in humans. One can use the unlabeled α-chain to pull out IgE with very high specificity from serum and then come back with another anti-IgE agent. We now have a panel of monoclonals we've made that we are very satisfied with and we have made highly purified canine IgE standards so we can measure total IgE quantitatively when it is appropriate.

The assay itself is a standard ELISA apart from the unique IgE detection reagent. The allergen extracts we use are from Center Labs, which is a USDA/FDA licensed facility that has been producing extracts for human and veterinary use for many years now, with highly controlled production and quality control (QC) of allergens. The flea salivary allergens, which are also unique to Heska, are produced at our facility in Fort Collins, where between half a million and a million fleas a month work very hard to produce this allergen. The panel we run has 48 allergens. We currently have five fungi, five environmental allergens and regional panels with the appropriate weeds, grasses and trees for each region.

What is important is how we normalize the values every time we do a run. The optical density readout is normalized using a four-point calibration curve which is generated on each run, and we have a standard serum pool which allows us to do that so that any variations in the assay from day to day are normalized. The normalized value times 1000 is the EA unit value, which those of you who use the Allercept test will recognize is on the report form that you get. The cut-off for the assay was set by measuring values in the assay for 20 specific pathogen-free dog sera and 50 negative patient sera, and also heat-activated to make sure that we destroyed the binding site of IgE FcεR1α receptor. Technically, the cut-off for the assay is 100 EA but we erred a little bit on the safe side and used a cut-off of 150 EA. Subsequent experiments we've done using highly purified allergen-specific canine IgE show that this value represents between 150 and 300 pg/ml of specific IgE. So it's a very sensitive assay.

Everybody running *in vitro* tests, when they come to a specialist meeting like this, always gets asked how their test compares to IDST. The answer is that it probably depends on what population you look at, what allergens you're looking at and what time of the year it is. In many ways it's an almost impossible task to do, but let's quickly run through the pros and cons of these two widely used methods of looking at canine IgE. They both have pluses and minuses. An intradermal skin test obviously uses the appropriate target organ, can measure delayed reactions in addition to immediate, and should be more sensitive given that at a low serum IgE level you can probably still have fully loaded mast cells. However, it is subjective, is not easily usable and is a physical intervention. Data we've generated recently show quite clearly that when you skin-test an animal you boost its IgE response, so it's not a neutral test. It is relatively inconvenient, particularly for dogs. The *in vitro* test measures only serum IgE and only potential immediate reactions. However, it is objective, is reproducible when measured by all the laboratories represented here, requires only a blood sample, and is easy and convenient. So what everybody is interested in: if you are continuing to use the skin test as the 'gold standard' (we prefer to term it a reference comparison), when you see a discrepancy, why do you see a discrepancy? Why do you see what are termed false positives? Why do you see false negatives? False-positive *in vitro* tests occurred, particularly using the old polyclonal-based assays. There was a lot of cross-reactivity with IgG. The issue of high total IgE in serum has been brought up and we have some data to address that. The phenomenon we're interested in that may be giving potential false positives, or at least clinical false positives in assays, is the presence of IgEs that are reactive to carbohydrate cross-reactive determinants that are very widely distributed over plant and insect proteins. These are reported to be a source of false positives in *in vitro* tests in the human field and we have evidence that they may be so in the veterinary field also. False negatives may occur if you have very low serum IgE concentrations that drop below the limit of detectability.

Recently we've been looking at data derived from sera that were sent in from a number of clinics around the country. Analysis of these, comparing skin tests results and ALLERCEPT® results, is being looked at now, but here are some preliminary data. We've looked at 488 sera, 278 collected from November to March and 210 from April to October. These samples have come from all over the country from different clinics and from dermatologists using different kinds of intradermal skin test panels and methods. We tested all of them on their appropriate allergen panel for the geographical area. Obviously, the intradermal skin tests were carried out using each clinic's own panel of allergens and we've done comparisons where we have the same allergen. Therefore, approximately the same allergen was used for both the *in vitro* test and the skin test, for this is an issue when you use different allergen sources (most of the clinics use Greer allergens for skin tests, while we have Center allergens). Most of the clinics seem to be using mixed mite extracts, with only some of them using separate mite extracts. Most of the results that we got were with mixed mite extracts and we're comparing these to *D. farinae*. With fleas, there was a big discrepancy between the agents used: the skin tests used the whole body extract and we used flea saliva. Grasses, weeds and trees are approximately similar. We found that we could match allergens for 488 samples, which was a good number. We looked at whether the dog was positive to something over the year. One can see that a skin test will give about 80% positives, with a drop off in winter. The ALLERCEPT test shows approximately the same pattern. It is slightly lower than the skin test, but if you test in September, you're getting essentially the same number of positive animals. If you test in the depth of winter, the difference might be a bit bigger, which is what we've seen before. There does seem to be a seasonal variation, which you would expect given the varying allergen exposure. In fact, the skin test might be expected to pick up animals when the serum IgE is dropping. This is what happens when you look at the number of animals that are positive to HDM but the tests are reasonably parallel. Again, in winter there may be a bigger discrepancy between the two, but if you just look at prevalence the two assays are similar for HDM. So, despite the skin tests sometimes using mixed mites and our using *D. farinae*, they correlate quite well.

Now when you look at the comparison for fleas, the two tests seem to be fairly independent of each other. So, at some times of the year it looks like you'll pick up many more flea-positive animals with an ALLERCEPT and at other times of the year you'll be better off using a skin test. I think that this is a good example of trying to compare apples and oranges. You've got totally different extracts but, overall, averaging them across the year, they pick up approximately the same number of dogs. Now these are prevalences, the actual numbers of animals coming up positive. It doesn't necessarily mean these are the same animals that are coming up positive in both tests at any given time. To actually look at sensitivity and specificity, using the skin test as our reference standard, one can calculate sensitivity and specificity values across the whole year without reference to seasonal variations or allergens. We did this by looking at skin tests greater than 2+ and ALLERCEPT scores greater than 150, pushing the cut-off rate up a bit for both tests. The sensitivity ranged from 60% for HDM and Bermuda grass to 6% for cockroach. I don't know whether people are picking up spurious false positives to cockroaches or we're picking up spurious false negatives in the ELISA, but this allergen was the outlier. The specificity we've always pushed for in the ALLERCEPT test is very good. It ranges from 94 to 81%. If you want to pick up cockroach allergy, compared with skin tests it is an insensitive test, but the sensitivity with the other allergens and the specificity is really very good.

Why might discrepant results occur in skin tests and *in vitro* tests? Dogs and cats routinely have levels of IgE that would be pathological in a human. Could this affect the *in vitro* test? We've produced affinity-purified allergen-specific IgE from a large quantity of serum from our experimental flea allergy dermatitis (FAD)-affected beagles that is directed to the major flea allergen. We can then use this allergen-specific IgE to make a standard curve and, by running these standard curves, we determined our detection limit (in pg/ml). One can look at the 150 OD mark and calculate that the signal starts to be lost between 250 and 293 pg/ml. What's also interesting is that this allergen-specific purified IgE has been diluted out in serum that contains vastly different amounts of total IgE. The line shown here is diluted to serum that contains 0.1 μg/ml total IgE. This one here has over 320 μg/ml of total IgE. Thus, although there can be some differences depending on which serum you dilute them into, they are not related to the amount of IgE in the serum. In addition, although I haven't got the data here, if we plot out a series of 500 sera where we looked at the total IgE levels versus the number of positive allergens, there is absolutely no correlation.

One issue we think is very important potentially in canine serum IgE testing, and which is certainly of concern in the human IgE testing area, is the effect of anti-carbohydrate IgE. We are breeding high IgE beagles. If you immunize them within 10 days of birth they will make a high, persistent IgE response to whatever you immunize them with. These are laboratory animals, so they don't have any known exposure to other allergens. This puppy was immunized with *D. farinae*. In the ALLERCEPT FAD test, it is positive only to mites. This is its skin test with pollens. None is positive. It was previously positive to HDM when tested for that. This is not a littermate but an equivalent puppy immunized with one grass. It is positive in ALLERCEPT to all the temperate grasses that you would expect. It is also positive to taxonomically unrelated pollens, and we see about approximately 5–10% of animals submitted for ALLERCEPT testing with this pattern. This puppy has not been exposed to either weed or tree pollens but it's coming up positive to all of them. Why is this happening? When you skin-test this dog, it shows two positive grass reactions. If you skin-test it with the weeds or the trees, it is essentially negative, with possibly a very weak positive at the top dose. So this is genuine, heat-labile IgE, but it clearly hasn't been induced by exposure and it doesn't cause a skin-test reaction. This would be a classic case where you would get a major discrepancy between a skin test and a serum test. This has been reported recently in the human allergy testing arena. What is probably happening is that we are getting IgE directed to carbohydrate epitopes that are widely distributed on plant and insect proteins that are cross-reactive across taxonomic discontinuities. If an animal makes a substantial amount IgE to these, you will pick them up in any *in vitro* test, but they don't seem to be biologically active.

Per Matsson *Sweden* (Pharmacia Diagnostics) Thank you for inviting Pharmacia Diagnostics to the Fourth World Congress of Veterinary Dermatology. I am here to talk about the development of a new test for canine specific IgE. This development is actually an adaptation or line extension of the very well-known human S-IgE test, ImmunoCAP® from Pharmacia Diagnostics. The company has been providing S-IgE tests since 1972 and we produce and deliver tests to more than 4000 laboratories in more than 50 countries around the world.

The development of the canine assay is not done by Pharmacia Diagnostics alone. It is a collaboration between us, Pharmacia & Upjohn Animal Health and Antech Inc. In this presentation I have less than 10 min to explain how the assay works and why we believe we can transfer our experience from human assays into the animal area. I hope to get your feedback and a good discussion regarding the specific needs for the canine. I have selected a few slides from the handout you have received to exemplify the essence of this new test for canine specific IgE.

Testing for specific IgE is complex and difficult. Today's ImmunoCAP includes experience gained during about 30 years of research and development in allergy. Some basic facts of specific IgE testing include: IgE is one of five immunoglobulin classes, there is an extremely low serum concentration of specific IgE, the allergen source is complex and variable, there is a multitude of allergen sources and there is a diversity of patient IgE specificities.

All these facts need to be considered in order to develop sensitive, specific, truly reproducible, quantitative, convenient and reliable test systems for specific IgE. I will first focus on the allergen characteristics and the use of the ImmunoCAP. An allergen can be described with a few specific factors: there is no common structure, the molecular weight varies from 5 to 150 kDa, the isoelectric point is 4–7 and there are sequential and conformational allergen determinants.

Analyzing and understanding the allergen source is essential in order to correctly represent the allergen epitopes on the solid phase. Understanding the allergen also explains the need for a large solid phase such as the ImmunoCAP, which has a surface area and capacity much larger than any other commercially available

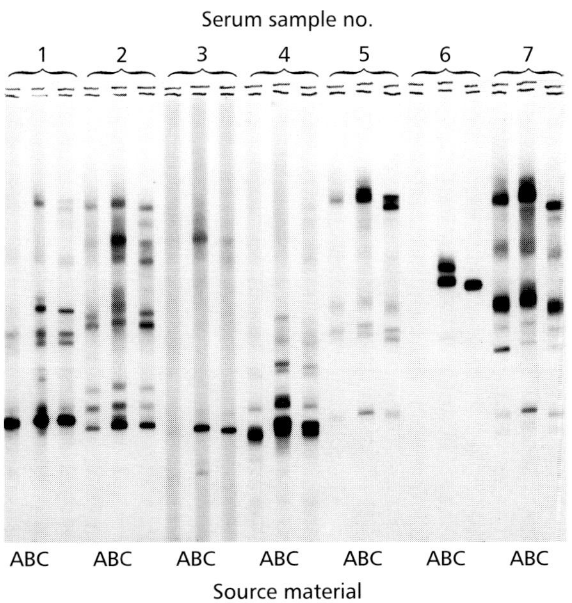

Figure 5.19.1. Comparison of three different sources of *Aspergillus Fumigatus* on exposure to seven different serum samples using ImmunoCAP® immunoblotting.

immunoassay. Figure 5.19.1 exemplifies the complexity of one allergen that has been blotted and exposed to different patient sera (1–7). Three different sources of *Aspergillus fumigatus* (A–C) have been extracted and blotted. As you can see, there is a high degree of variation both between patient samples and between the different allergen sources.

This very illustrative example shows the need for highly standardizing the allergen source and provides a solid phase with the ability to capture all different components in the allergen. At Pharmacia Diagnostics we routinely do this and we now have not only the scientific knowledge but also the long-term empirical knowledge of how different allergens should be treated to allow the reproducible manufacturing of stable ImmunoCAPs.

The ImmunoCAP assay design is very straightforward, with a few important steps:

- conditioning of the ImmunoCAP for running the assay
- addition of ~50 μl of patient serum
- incubation and washing
- addition of enzyme-conjugated anti-IgE antibodies
- incubation and washing
- addition of substrate, incubation and quantitative analysis.

After the careful selection of the allergen sources and solid phase comes an equally important step in the selection of the system to detect the amount of IgE bound to the allergens on the solid phase. Here, we have been required to develop and optimize a system different from the human S-IgE system. In the human system we have changed from using polyclonal antibodies to using monoclonal antibodies (mAb). By using mAb for the detection of IgE, we have accomplished an increased reproducibility in the system. For the development of the canine system we took a similar approach. We selected five well-characterized and available mAb against IgE. Out of those five we selected three for in-depth studies of how they interacted with the other components in the ImmunoCAP system. Out of these three candidates we have selected one to be used in the first generation of the canine ImmunoCAP system. This selection process includes:

- specificity for canine IgE
- cross-reactivity analysis of other immunoglobulins and potentially interfering substances
- sensitivity analysis

- background analysis
- quality and reproducibility of the enzyme-conjugated molecule
- reproducibility
- ease of manufacture.

After satisfactory development of the conjugated detection antibody the assay needs to be calibrated and a standard curve developed. We have chosen to develop an assay standard by using one allergen and well-characterized patient serum to ensure that the standard is valid and reproducible. We have also chosen to present the data as a percentage of the standard serum. This is a different way compared with the human system, in which we use a World Health Organization (WHO) standard material of IgE and we use the quantitative ability of the ImmunoCAP system. For the canine assay we have elected to use a relative standard based on material that we provide with the assay. The reason for this is that we have much less knowledge of canine specific IgE than human IgE. However, we encourage the future development of highly standardized materials QC in the canine situation. By working very closely with Antech and with the canine research community, we will be able to develop and improve the interpretation and assay standardization over the next few years. For example, we have for more than 10 years, together with our customers, been monitoring the human S-IgE assay performance. We are also very positive about this kind of development within the field of the veterinary diagnostic use of S-IgE. Figure 5.19.2 shows a graph of the reproducibility of the ImmunoCAP and the UniCAP systems.

Apart from being reproducible, we need to ensure that the assay behaves similarly with all different allergens, since we use only one allergen as our standard. On the human side, we have extensive experience that the ImmunoCAP shows parallelism between the variety of different allergens. Figure 5.19.3 shows an example of the parallelism obtained with the human test system. Our preliminary results indicate that we have a similar situation with the canine system.

A system for the determination of specific IgE also needs to perform well in the clinical setting. For example, we can again provide comparisons with

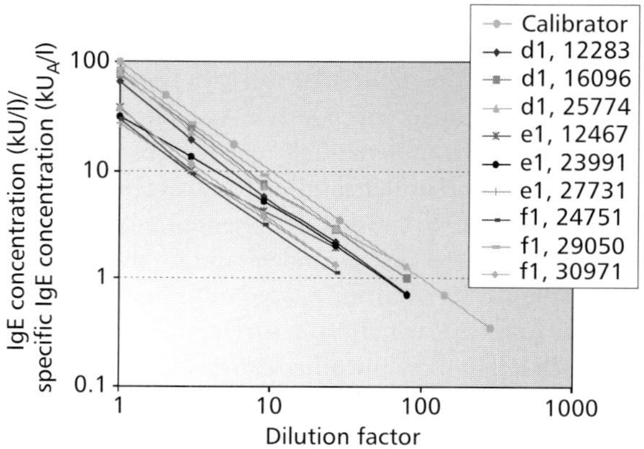

Figure 5.19.3. Quantitative parallelism obtained with the human test system.

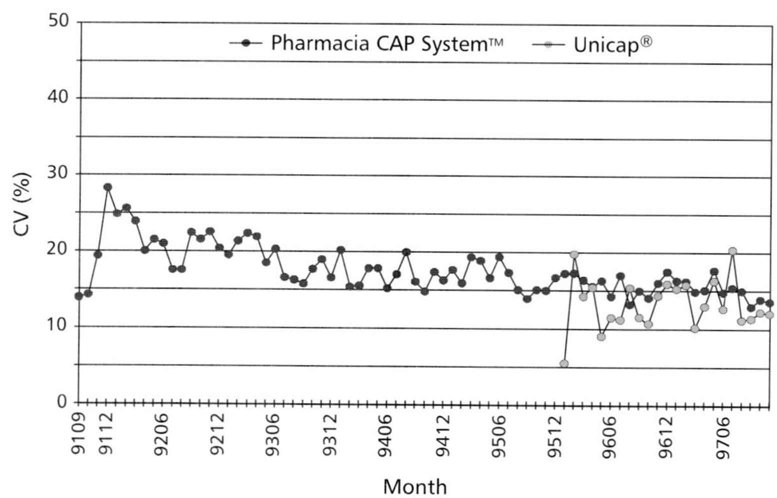

Figure 5.19.2. Reproducibility of the ImmunoCAP® and UniCAP® systems using pooled coefficients of variation (CV) of specific IgE from 9109–9711.

Table 5.19.1. Clinical performance of UniCAP allergen-specific diagnosis compared with clinical evaluation

	Positive	Negative	Total
Positive	1121	144	1265
Negative	360	3545	3905
Total	1481	3689	5170

examples of data from human test technology. In a very large clinical assessment of the ImmunoCAP system we have aggregated data from a number of allergen specificities compared with the clinical assessment of the patients. A total of 5170 individual ImmunoCAPs was analyzed, and the overall sensitivity was 89% and the overall specificity was 91%. The data are outlined in Table 5.19.1.

The canine S-IgE ImmunoCAP system has so far not been fully evaluated by comparing the assay results with clinical evaluation. However, the early assessments, analyzing 'negative' or at least well-defined healthy animals, indicate that the assay performs well.

We also compared 67 test results from clinical samples, allowing us to make a preliminary comparison between the canine ImmunoCAP system and another commercially available system. The data indicate that the systems compare reasonably well and the dynamic range of the PCS system indicates that it is greater than for the system under comparison (Figure 5.19.4).

In summary, I have presented an early but important development of the human ImmunoCAP system conversion to allow the analysis of canine specific IgE. This is an early development and I look to you as being part of the future development of this assay system. It is going to be important to obtain solid and relevant clinical samples to be able to thoroughly establish cut-offs and to decide which allergens are the most relevant to analyze in different dogs and at different geographical locations.

Bob Esch *USA* (Greer Laboratories) The previous speakers who extensively covered the technical aspects of immunoassays have simplified my job. So, I will only briefly describe our assay for allergen-specific canine anti-IgE antibodies. The anti-canine IgE antibody was produced in the rabbit and was affinity purified. The specificity of the anti-IgE antibodies is tested by reverse cutaneous anaphylaxis in normal dogs. Lack of reactivity towards canine IgG, IgM and

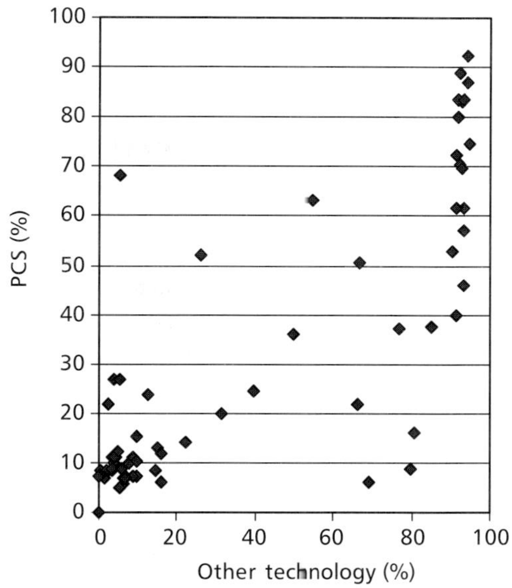

Figure 5.19.4. Evaluation of technologies: 67 canine test results.

IgA is verified by direct ELISA using solid-phase purified immunoglobulins. Our format is the direct-bind ELISA, developed in the 1980s and 1990s.

I want to spend some time on our scoring system and how we report IgE values. One of the differences between Greer's system and other scoring systems is that our system requires validation of each allergen with positive and negative sera. The first figure shows the IgE levels directed towards solid-phase short ragweed allergens by history-negative, skin-test-negative dogs, or the 'negative population', and by history-positive, skin-test-positive dogs, or the 'positive population'. An example of a similar study with HDM allergens is also shown. A score of 1 includes 99% of the positive population. A score of 2 would exclude greater than 95% of the truly negative population, but will also exclude about 10–15% of the positives. Finally, a score of 3 excludes 99% of the negative population. Clear cut-offs are not possible with any allergen as there is always overlap in IgE levels among clinically positive and negative dogs. So, basically ours is a statistical scoring system based on the probability of detecting or identifying a truly positive dog based on IgE levels.

In terms of reporting allergen-specific IgE values, we've looked at three different methods. The first is the % *R* value, which is based on the relative IgE level of the test serum with respect to the quantity of IgE in positive serum pool directed against the homologous allergen. This is the method we are currently using in our reports. The second figure shows the distribution of % *R* values towards four different allergens, *Alternaria*, *D. farinae*, ragweed and Kentucky blue grass. A second is based on a total IgE standard curve. The IgE values are reported in terms of mass units. When you compare these values obtained with the same serum samples with the % *R* values, what you see is that among the *D. farinae*-positive dogs there are two to three times greater apparent levels of IgE towards the mite allergens. Now, what is the clinical relevance of this apparent difference? We all know that the quantity of IgE antibodies directed towards an allergen doesn't necessarily correlate with the severity of symptoms. It is interesting that the IgE immune response to *D. farinae* is more robust than IgE responses to other allergens. A third method reports IgE levels with respect to the individual dog's total IgE level. The bottom panel of the figure shows the distribution of allergen-specific IgE levels reported as the percentage of total IgE measured in each positive sample. What stands out here is that there are some dogs that produce anti-*Alternaria* IgE antibodies accounting for more than 10% of their total IgE response. Again, very interesting, but the question is: what is the clinical significance of this?

Beat Bigler *Switzerland* (Imovet CAC) [Imovet CAC (Canine Allergy Control) Labor Laupeneck/imovet bg, Switzerland; www.laupeneck.ch] Small animal clinic (Kleintierpraxis) Laupeneck, Laboratory (Labor) Laupeneck and Imovet bg (selling test kits) are owned by Dr med.vet. Beat Bigler and Dr med.vet. Karl Güller. Kleintierpraxis Laupeneck and Labor have existed for 20 years and all three companies have been ISO 9001 certified since 1999.

Imovet CAC test system

- Allergens from Allergopharma (Germany), *Malassezia* (own), flea (Greer)
- monoclonal antibody (mAb): D9
- polyclonal antibody (pAb): anti-mouse IgG labeled with alkaline phosphatase (Jackson-Immuno-Research)
- semiquantitative system [no absolute values (lack of official accepted standards)]
- cut-off (IDST)
- same allergens (IDST, test system, hyposensitization).

Allergens

- Pollens [grass-mix (five grasses), rye, birch, hazel, mugwort, plantain, *Parietaria*]
- mites (*D. farinae*, *D. pteronyssinus*, *Acarus siro*, *Tyrophagus*)
- molds (*Alternaria*, *Aspergillus*, *Malassezia*)
- flea (whole body extracts).

Procedure

- Allergens as solid phase in microtiter plates (dry, possible storage of the plates for minimum 18 months)
- serum diluted 1:5, incubated in the wells (37°C, 30 min)
- wash
- mAb incubated in wells (37°C, 30 min)
- wash
- pAb incubated in wells (37°C, 30 min)
- wash
- DEA + p-NPP (25°C, 120 min)
- reading at optimum of our own control sera.

Quality

- No reaction with allergen-specific IgG (absorption of IgG with protein G does not influence test results)
- mAb rat anti-mouse (light chain) does not influence test results
- screening test (up to three different allergens in the same well) gives 98% agreement with single allergens in wells
- intra-assay and interassay differences in OD: 12%.

Comparing Imovet CAC with intradermal skin testing

In the northern part of Europe, 85% of dogs are only positive to HDM and storage mites. Thus, the most relevant allergens are mites:

- sensitivity: 75%
- specificity: 96%
- efficiency: 84%
- positive predictive value: 98%
- negative predictive value: 71%

Frustrations

- Human α-chain receptor labeled with human albumin and anti-human albumin labeled with alkaline phosphatase do not recognize canine IgE.

- The test system as described, but pAb labeled with peroxidase instead of alkaline phosphatase, gives positive reactions without any mAb against canine IgE.
- Forty-five dogs negative in the Imovet CAC test system become positive in 58% of mite results and 20% of pollen results, when changing the labeling of alkaline phosphatase to peroxidase: peroxidase gives nonspecific binding and unreliable results.
- pAb carried out in the goat, rabbit and sheep recognize dog serum with false-positive reactions in the test system.
- The test system with streptavidin/biotin gives a high background reading.
- Positive control serum of a competitive USA test system shows very weak or negative results.

Bruce Hammerburg *USA* I have to commend Heska for their heroic efforts in having a standard that really is a standard policy for these tests, and maybe that's one of the biggest barriers in doing your affinity isolation of IgE. I'm sure that being able to carry that through all your tests is difficult, though, with that affinity isolation. One question: did your affinity column antigen or allergen have the carbohydrate epitope that you're worried about or was it a recombinant?

Cathy McCall (Heska) The way we purified that is to use the *Escherichia coli* recombinant version of F1 that is the major flea allergen that isn't glycosylated anyway. So it's a nice clean system.

Bruce Hammerburg One of the systems that makes sense as far as you're talking about in the non-skin-reacting carbohydrate-specific IgE, though you do see it on your *in vitro* test, is the possibility that these are highly glycosylated smaller molecules and that you're getting more intramolecular cross-reacting, or binding ties up and doesn't allow intra-/inter-IgE binding on the surface of the mast cell. Thus, you're not getting cross-linking of your high-affinity receptor through the IgE. Your molecules are small and have the repeating epitope that binds that specificity on an individual molecule.

Cathy McCall (Heska) That's one possible reason. There is a lot of literature in the human area and the explanation that you can't physically cross-link just doesn't seem to be correct for whatever reason. Nobody really knows why these don't cross-link well. Ronald van Ree in Rob Alberse's group wrote an editorial on it last year: they are still looking for the reason why these anti-carbohydrate IgEs seem not to function biologically.

Bruce Hammerburg You may want to consider using a canine monoclonal-like IgE (heterohybridoma). The one that we made up is being produced now and basically we have the recombinant allergen for that as well. If someone is interested and wants to use that as a standard in their system it might solve a lot of other questions, and I think that might be important for the variation you see from serum to serum in these other questions that are going to be coming up. If you put that as an internal standard and then see how it reads out on your assay system, it might give you some valuable information about individual sera and how either autoantibodies or other things might be affecting the assay system that you have.

Don Wassom *USA* (Heska) Your comment is interesting, because one of the reasons we ended up going to the α-chain of the high-affinity IgE receptor for detection is that when we looked at a whole range of different monoclonal antibodies, some of them reacted with IgE and others didn't, and some of them reacted with IgE from certain patients and not from others. Realizing that perhaps not all IgE is alike, and certainly the specificities of the monoclonal antibodies are not alike, the receptor seemed like a good alternative to us. So my only caution is that using the heterohybridomas as a standard may work very well for some detection agents and not others.

Carol Foil *USA* I guess I'd like to see some of you who are using the solid-phase ELISA respond to the challenge of the ImmunoCAP about whether the appropriate epitopes are masked in your system or not. Do you have a specific response to that question?

Cathy McCall (Heska) I think it is very hard to check that you have all possible epitopes you need to pick up every possible animal in any system on any point. I think all *in vitro* systems are probably putting down the allergens with most of the epitopes intact, but each system may lose some epitopes. For instance, Western blot is a good idea but some allergens just don't show up on Western blot. The major flea allergen, for instance, does not show up on the Western blot, so we couldn't check flea saliva with it. Similarly, if you actually covalently couple allergens to any surface or you covalently label allergens, you potentially lose epitopes, so I think that every single system is probably showing a different array of epitopes: the system is losing some, maintaining others. Overall, what we're looking at are naturally sensitized animals that are producing IgE to a huge range of epitopes in each allergen system. There are probably enough epitopes left in everybody's system to pick up the majority of animals. Although there may be some very unusual animals that are highly focused on a couple of epitopes or a couple of proteins, or a couple of allergens that may be missed by any given system, I think most of us can probably be confident that the allergens coming down (whether they're on plates or CAP sponges or in liquid phase) probably present enough epitopes to pick up most of the sera of interest.

Per Matsson (Pharmacia) I can comment a little bit on that also. On the human side, we are having that type of discussion over and over. We have started to become a little more sophisticated in doing things like spiking and different allergens with, for instance, recombinant components. You can see in different systems when they do solution recovery that you don't have enough of certain allergens. That is, as you said, very tricky and you can normally, as a manufacturer, find patient sera that would support views either that someone else's system was poor and your system is the best or vice versa. The key thing is to be observant and check out the outliers, and then ask what it means clinically. It's difficult, but I think that what Catherine mentioned is true, that overall we're doing a reasonable job in identifying the right things.

Sola Alaba (VARL) I think it is a significant question because it's one of the factors that we considered in developing the liquid phase. We know definitely that not all proteins have the same propensity to bind sterically on a microplate. In fact, back in the 1970s it was pointed out very clearly that in technical building, when you use an antibody to determine how much albumin is bound on a solid phase and how much is available in liquid, you lose over 80% of the binding capacity when bound on a plate. Since allergens are very large there is a possibility that some of the molecules may not have any propensity at all to even stick sterically on a microplate. We believe that in the liquid phase we have all the binding sites of allergens in the original allergen extract.

Bob Esch (Greer) I agree with all three of them. These difficulties should be addressed during the assay validation process. When you test the truly positive serum samples and you only get 70% sensitivity it could be due to inadequate representation of the allergens. Among the 30 or so allergens that we've evaluated, maybe there were only two or three allergen systems where we saw that problem. Where we didn't have the adequate sensitivity, the problem was solved for the most part through fractionation or spiking.

Gene Nesbitt *USA* I have a question on molds. I know clinically there is fair amount of disagreement. As we look at the number of molds being tested on the various panels, you go from five to 15 or more. Some of us see a predominance of non-seasonally pruritic dogs and have a good response to hyposensitization to just mold preparations. I have some concerns that if we are not testing for molds are we really missing a lot? And if we are testing, how are we controlling for the false negatives?

Bob Esch (Greer) IgE towards molds is an interesting topic because it's very difficult to identify a truly mold-allergic dog. In many cases we can identify skin-test-positive dogs without a clinical history, or we can identify dogs where the clinical history points towards mold allergy, but we don't have skin-test positivity. When we did find skin-test-positive dogs, their specific IgE levels, history and apparent success with immunotherapy strongly suggested that they were truly mold-allergic dogs. Interestingly, many of them appeared to be reactive only to molds.

Sola Alaba (VARL) According to data that we have, mold hypersensitivity, specifically IgE to molds, does occur. It is quite common in some areas of the country and in some areas it can be predominant. We have found patients that tested positive strictly to molds only and have been hyposensitized successfully. The panel of allergens that we test for Cornell University contains quite a number of molds.

One observation that I wanted to bring up is that mold allergens especially are notorious for high backgrounds in solid-phase tests. We have observed that molds seem to non-specifically absorb IgE on a solid phase, which means that you really have to address this problem with very stringent controls. With Liquid Gold we have homologous controls to nullify such non-specific IgE binding. That is, each allergen is run as its own control against the patient serum through every step in Liquid Gold, but omitting streptavidin so that we can subtract that background from the final result.

Cathy McCall (Heska) I don't think we've seen that particular problem. When Heska first started to get into IgE testing, we brought in a technology that was based on polyclonal antibodies, and in that test, practically every dog we ran came out positive to *D. pteronyssinus* and a mold. This clearly wasn't reflecting reality as defined by skin testing. In the current assay, I think in the last couple of months about 18% of the serum samples submitted came up positive to one mold or another. But each individual mold of the five was only a few per cent. I second the problem of finding truly mold-positive dogs. It's like truly food-positive dogs which, as you know, is the other nightmare that we all share.

One anecdote I should repeat is that when we first started to develop the Heska test, we invited Harold Nelson from National Jewish, who's one of the experts in immunotherapy and allergen standardization in the human field. We asked him about testing for mold hypersensitivity and he said not to. He said there are approximately 40 000 species of described fungi and the allergy might be in the spores, while allergen extracts have to be derived from the mycelium and vice versa. He said the state-of-the-art of the field is 'rather poor', except in a few cases where recombinant allergens are defined. That is probably not a good reason for not addressing this issue, but it's going to require a lot of research in the dog to identify what are truly clinically important molds and allergens, so that we can make a relevant extract or a recombinant preparation. This is an area that needs addressing.

Sola Alaba (VARL) For a long time we've been using Greer allergens and have been pleased with the quality. On the aspect of molds, we have tested the allergens with Western blot and we know that there are some molds that may have allergenic molecules present, not just in the spores but also in the mycelium. Depending on the mold, you may need both the spores and the mycelium combined in the extract. I think that using the right extract is crucial.

Beat Bigler (Imovet CAC) I think there are a lot of different qualities in mold material and I think that the difficulty for the company is to produce allergen extracts. Perhaps we do not have the correct mold extracts in Europe because we see only a few dogs test positive for molds. It's very rare that we have problems with the background. My negative control serum is around 0.160 as optical density (OD). If we get higher than 0.18–0.2 then we have to discuss it with the technician. Our positive results start around 0.360–0.400. We have a clear cut-off between positive and negative sera. In our test system, the solid phase is not a problem. Our problem is that sometimes we have difficulties with sensitivity, and I'd like to ask if the other contributors see the same thing. Sometimes, we see dogs with good positive skin tests but completely negative results in our test system. I don't know if other people see this. What kinds of reactions are occurring in the intradermal skin test? Perhaps we see other kinds of immunoglobulins or a different IgE, which we cannot pick up with our test system. Normally, these dogs do well on hyposensitization.

Cathy McCall (Heska) Perhaps we shouldn't always compare *in vitro* and *in vivo* tests. I think the situation that you've just described is occurring at a time when the dog hasn't been exposed to the relevant allergen for a while and so the IgE is dropping. IgE levels in the serum have fallen below the detection limit of most assays, but there is still enough IgE on the cells of the skin if you do a skin test.

These data are from the flea saliva immunotherapy trial conducted by Ken Kwochka. These dogs, being evaluated at the Ohio State University, are extremely well-characterized flea allergy dermatitis (FAD) dogs. What we're doing here is looking at the beginning of the flea season when they haven't seen fleas since the previous autumn (May). If you do a skin test or run an ELISA, what percentage of FAD do you pick up? At the beginning of the season, 76% of these dogs are positive by skin testing but using our major flea allergen with an ELISA, only 15% of the dogs are positive. At the end of the season all of them are positive to the skin test and ELISA testing is identifying 70–80% of dogs that showed a positive IDST response. So I think a lot of this is simply a matter of the level of IgE. You can have the serum level dropping so far that you have to have an overly sensitive test to pick it up and get useful information. But, in the case of the skin test, because there is still IgE loaded onto the mast cells, one can still identify that animal.

Unidentified participant In all your allergens, you've mentioned pollens, dust mites, molds and a variety of other organisms, but you haven't mentioned humans or other animal cohabitants in the household.

Sola Alaba (VARL) We have a human dander test and if we look at the number of positive reactions, human dander and HDM are high reactors. It does make sense that the cross-species allergens in dogs, cats and humans are usually quite potent. In other words, humans are more potentially allergic to cats and dogs, cats to dogs, and dogs to cats. Humans are no exception to these other species.

Unidentified participant What is your level of reactivity to human dander in normal dogs?

Sola Alaba (VARL) Not very high. Actually, there are more reactions seen with dust mite than with human dander in non-clinical dogs. I have taken 275 serum positive dogs and I have bought human danders and have done ELISA, and none of the 275 had detectable IgE.

Bob Esch (Greer) The human dander extracts that we evaluated in our system could not be validated because we could not establish an appropriate positive control serum pool. This was either due to insufficient allergen content in our test extracts or because allergy to humans among dogs is rare. The reactivity of human dander extracts in skin tests has been reported to be as high as 50% or more among atopic dogs. We have found significant concentrations of histamine in some human dander extracts and this could have led to false-positive skin-test reactions. So, it would be important to rule out this possibility before anyone claims clinical significance of skin-test reactions to human dander extracts.

Beat Bigler (Inovet CAC) I have taken 275 serum samples of positive dogs and tested for human dander, and none had detectable IgE. You may think that my test system does not work, but I think that positive reactions in IDST are irritant and in ELISA peroxidase-positive reactions are not true IgE. We used cat saliva allergens from ALK, Denmark, in IDST and *in vitro*. At first I used a concentration of the allergen as in pollens and found a lot of positive cats. Later, we diluted the extract 1:10 and the positive IDST reactions disappeared. The higher concentration was only due to irritation. If there is an allergy against cat saliva, we should still find some positive dogs with the lower concentration. I do not believe that dogs can be allergic against cats.

Gail Kunkle I have one more question for Cathy about the pan-reactive carbohydrate. Have you had a chance to look at all this vast number of sera that are submitted to you? What kind of problems do you see to those kinds of reactions?

Cathy McCall (Heska) They occur in 10% of sera. This happens in every assay and I presume it's happening in the CAP. The paper addressing this last year was done with the CAP. I think what's important is whether it's clinically relevant or not.

Per Matsson (Pharmacia) On the human side, there's lots of controversy. In humans, we can see frequencies as high as 10% and we don't see the facts that are being claimed, so I think that it will take another year before we have a better solution on that issue.

5.20

Therapy options for canine pyoderma

Richard K. Anderson[1] (Chairperson) and Laurie J. Stewart[2] (Secretary)

[1] Angell Memorial Animal Hospital, Boston, Massachusetts, USA
[2] Veterinary Dermatology of New England, Acton, Massachusetts, USA

Richard Anderson *USA* Pyoderma is one of the most common and frustrating dermatoses seen by veterinarians in small animal practice. The disease is most often associated with a normal cutaneous commensal, *Staphylococcus intermedius*. The coagulase-positive staphylococcus population is probably transient on skin, resident on mucocutaneous areas, and seeded to the skin and hair by grooming. Overgrowth of commensals occurs as a result of disruption of balance of cutaneous ecosystems and/or failure of the host's defense response. Disease occurs when the virulence of the organism overwhelms the resistance of the host. The emphasis has been on the search for therapeutic agents to eliminate staphylococci from the skin in order to achieve a clinical cure. As this organism is a normal cutaneous microinhabitant and well adapted to its ecological niche, it is not surprising that in many instances it is not possible to achieve a permanent cure. Recurrence of clinical signs commonly occurs after treatment ceases.

Recurrent pyoderma should always be considered a secondary clinical manifestation of an underlying primary problem. Any plan for controlling the pyoderma without serious consideration of the predisposing diseases will fail. Some common predisposing causes include environmental factors (high heat and humidity), allergic dermatitis (including flea allergy, atopy and food allergy), endocrinopathies (hypothyroidism, hyperadrenocorticism), poor nutritional status, immunological incompetency, keratinization defects, ectoparasites (demodicosis, scabies) and inappropriate therapy such as excessive use of glucocorticoids. Bacterial hypersensitivity has been implicated in the pathogenesis of recurrent superficial pyoderma.

Treatment regimens must be aimed at attempting to correct the underlying cause and restoring cutaneous ecosystems to normality rather than the almost impossible task of permanently eliminating this organism. Therapy options we will consider include topical treatment, systemic antibacterial therapy, bacterial interference using avirulent variants of *S. intermedius* in order to prevent colonization by virulent pathogenic staphylococci and immune modulation.

Christine Rees *USA* Topical products are an important adjunctive therapy in treating canine pyoderma. Several different topical therapies exist. Therefore, for ease of discussion, the different topical therapies will be divided into two main groups, shampoo products and topical medications, and discussed individually.

Benzoyl peroxide is an excellent antibacterial agent that exerts its bactericidal properties by oxidizing substances. Benzoyl peroxide is also known for its follicular flushing, antipruritic, keratoplastic, residual (lasts up to 2 days) and degreasing properties. In one study, comparing a 3% benzoyl peroxide shampoo to three different antibacterial shampoos (0.5% chlorhexidine, 1% iodine as a polyalkylene glycol–iodine complex and 0.5% triclosan with 2% sulfur and 2% salicylic acid), benzoyl peroxide was the most effective in killing *S. intermedius* on canine skin. Skin irritation may occur in some dogs when benzoyl peroxide is used. Normally the skin irritation may be avoided by making sure that the shampoo product does not contain greater than 5% benzoyl peroxide. Another problem is that sometimes the benzoyl peroxide is too good a degreaser and causes excessive dryness.

Therese DeManuelle *USA* I like the 2.5% Sulfoxydex® by EVSCO.

Christine Rees Chlorhexidine has a broader spectrum of activity than benzoyl peroxide. Not only is chlorhexidine an antibacterial agent but it also has antifungal and antiviral properties when used at the appropriate concentrations. Chlorhexidine works by attacking the cell membrane of the bacteria, precipitating the intracellular contents and inhibiting adenosine triphosphate. This product has advantages in that it works well in organic debris and lasts for up to 2 days. Some debate exists over which concentration of chlorhexidine is the most desirable for treating canine pyoderma. Many of the newer chlorhexidine shampoos now contain 2% chlorhexidine, whereas in the past some products contained as little as 0.5% chlorhexidine. A product containing an even higher concentration of chlorhexidine is Maximum ChlorhexiDerm® 4% shampoo (DVM Pharmaceuticals). No efficacy studies have been published which compare the two different chlorhexidine concentrations (2% versus 4% chlorhexidine) in treating canine pyoderma.

Robert Schick *USA* I have not seen more benefit from the 4% compared to the 2% products of chlorhexidine.

Christine Rees Ethyl lactate is an antibacterial shampoo ingredient with mild follicular flushing action. This product is designed for treating surface and superficial pyodermas. Ethyl lactate hydrolyzes into lactic acid and ethanol. The lactic acid lowers the skin pH and results in inhibition of bacterial lipases. The ethanol renders fats soluble and decreases the amount of sebaceous secretions.

Patrick Breen *USA* Etiderm® makes a good long-term shampoo and it lathers better than benzoyl peroxide.

Christine Rees Bactoderm® (Pfizer Animal Health) contains the antibacterial ingredient mupirocin at a 2% concentration. Mupirocin has been shown to inhibit bacterial protein synthesis by reversibly and specifically binding to bacterial isoleucyl transfer-RNA synthetase. The spectrum of antibacterial activity of mupirocin includes both Gram-positive and Gram-negative bacteria. The main bacterium against which this product is marketed is staphylococcus species.

Patrick Breen I recommend using finger cots to dispense to owners, as the medical community worries about resistance in humans when using the veterinary product. I use it in the cat for chin acne and in dogs with recurrent pyoderma that is localized.

Richard Anderson I use isopropyl alcohol as a topical wipe to decrease bacterial carriage on lip folds and the anal area.

Terese DeManuelle We did a study at the University of California–Davis comparing enrofloxacin serum and tissue concentrations in control, superficial and deep pyoderma in dogs. In the study, both controls and those dogs with pyoderma were given enrofloxacin (Baytril®) at approximately 5 mg/kg daily. Morphometric analysis was performed on skin biopsy specimens to determine if there was a correlation between inflammatory cells and tissue enrofloxacin concentrations. There were no significant differences between serum enrofloxacin levels in the control dogs and dogs with pyoderma. Dogs with pyoderma had skin enrofloxacin levels that were significantly higher than control dogs. Significantly higher cutaneous levels of enrofloxacin were seen in deep pyoderma versus superficial pyoderma, supporting the hypothesis that the drug is concentrated within inflammatory cells and is unimpeded by granulomatous inflammation, fibrosis and purulent debris. A strong linear correlation was found between the number of inflammatory cells in skin and the concentration of enrofloxacin in skin.

I do not use fluoroquinolones in superficial pyoderma and would like to know what clinicians are using them for. I use them in dogs with deep pyoderma.

Otto Fischer *Austria* Enrofloxacin is commonly used in Austria and works well in superficial pyoderma.

Richard Anderson I use enrofloxacin in dogs with severe demodicosis, deep pyoderma and cellulitis.

Christine Rees I saw a dog on theophylline and enrofloxacin that had an abnormal electrocardiogram 1 week after starting the drug; enrofloxacin increases the concentration of theophylline. Central nervous system stimulation occurs in cats and they can act as if they are blind.

Terese DeManuelle The company has issued a warning that doses higher than 5 mg/kg in the cat can cause blindness.

Jim Jeffers *USA* Can you use fluoroquinolones with pentoxyphylline, since both are methylxanthines?

Terese DeManuelle I am not aware of a contraindication.

Otto Fischer A randomized prospective study was performed to compare the clinical efficacy of cephalexin, one of the most frequently used antibiotics for first-line treatment of bacterial folliculitis in dogs, with enrofloxacin, which has been introduced more recently in veterinary dermatology. Fifty-four dogs with clinical signs and cytology consistent with bacterial folliculitis were included; of these cases, 52% were recurrent (one to five relapses within the previous 12 months). Twenty-nine dogs received cephalexin (Rilexine®, Virbac) at 15 mg/kg twice daily, and 25 dogs received enrofloxacin (Baytril, Bayer) at 5 mg/kg once daily. Dogs were examined at days 0, 7 and 21, 35 and 49 if necessary. The pyoderma was treated until clinical recovery; antibiotic administration was then continued for 14 days thereafter, the maximum treatment period being limited to 9 weeks. Pyoderma lesions (papules, pustules, epidermal collarettes), erythema, pruritus and extent of lesions were scored on a 0 to 3 scale. Dogs that didn't improve until day 21 were classified as treatment failures and left the trial. Complete clinical recovery was defined as disappearance of pyoderma lesions (all reaching 0 score). When the score sum of pyoderma lesions was lowered to no more than 1, the case was classified as a clear improvement.

Fifty dogs completed the study. *Staphylococcus intermedius* was isolated from 79% of cases. The total recovery rate (complete clinical recovery plus clear improvement) was 92.6% in the cephalexin group and 91.3% in the enrofloxacin group. The results of our trial show that, despite many years of use, the efficacy of cephalexin remains at 90% and is as high as that of a third-generation quinolone, enrofloxacin. Therefore, cephalexin remains a drug of choice for first-line treatment of bacterial folliculitis in dogs, including cases of recurrent pyoderma.

Leena Saijonmaa-Koulumies *Finland* The difficulties in achieving successful management of recurrent pyoderma in dogs are well recognized. Continual, often lifelong, antimicrobial therapy is the cornerstone of the treatment. At the same time, the discussion of the risks involved in the heavy use of antibiotics is becoming more widespread, thus increasing the pressure on developing new strategies in the treatment of infectious diseases. In the future, bacterial interference may offer a means of control of canine pyoderma without antibiotics.

Bacterial interference can be defined as an interaction between two bacteria in which one bars the progress of colonization or infection by the other. The precise mechanisms involved in bacterial interference are still poorly understood. It is believed that masking the tissue receptors by competitive adherence and production of antagonistic substances, including antibiotics and bacteriocins, are of importance. Recent studies suggest that bacterial interference may also be mediated by the ability of one strain to inhibit the synthesis of virulence factors by the other.

Information gained by genetic fingerprinting of *S. intermedius* indicates that bitches are colonized by one or two dominant and persistent clones of *S. intermedius* and these are transferred to the puppies almost immediately after birth. This suggests that puppies could be colonized artificially at birth by the interfering strain. Alternatively, the colonization might be achieved by establishing the interfering strain in the bitches, from which these bacteria would be transferred to the puppies.

In dogs, evidence of the importance of mucosae as carriage sites for *S. intermedius* and its transfer to the skin has been obtained. Also, application of topical fusidic acid only at the mucosae has provided evidence that topical antibiotics are effective in elimination of *S. intermedius* from the mucosal carriage sites before establishing interfering strains of *S. intermedius* at these sites.

The problem of avirulent variants of *S. intermedius* needs to be solved before bacterial interference, using strains of *S. intermedius*, can be applied in the control of canine pyoderma. There is considerable evidence supporting the hypothesis that strains of *S. intermedius* may differ in virulence between one another and that the organisms that infect may be a subset of those that colonize; however, definitive studies are still lacking.

Christine Rees How did you treat the mucosa of animals in the studies?

Leena Saijonmaa-Koulumies One drop of fusidic acid eye-drops, which are licensed in Europe, was applied to each nostril, the anus and the vagina twice daily for 7 days.

Patrick Breen In chronic recurrent pyoderma where antibiotics work but the infection continues to recur and we cannot find a primary cause, immune stimulants are an option. I have used Staphage Lysate® (SPL, Delmont Laboratories) for over 20 years. The commercially available staphylococcal antigen product is prepared by lysis of whole *Staphylococcus aureus* bacteria, serotypes I and III, using a polyvalent staphylococcus bacteriophage. Both components are in the product, the lysated staphylococcal bacteria and the bacteriophage. SPL stimulates cytokines typical of the Th_1 pathway, to resist infections. Some of the mechanisms of action may include lysis of staphylococci by the bacteriophage, activation of macrophages, production of cytokines and stimulation of cellular immunity. The company is looking at including *S. intermedius* instead of the *S. aureus* currently in the product.

Initial treatment involves the use of antibiotic therapy along with the SPL at 0.5 ml twice weekly for 10 weeks. When a beneficial response is seen, the interval of injections is increased, along with increasing the dose to 1.0 ml every 3–4 weeks. The intervals between boosters with long-term therapy boosters are very dependent on the patient. Staphage Lysate may also be placed into antigen vials for immunotherapy for atopy with 10–20% added to the total volume. The concurrent use of Th_1 immunomodulators such as SPL with environmental allergens may lessen the symptoms of atopy and decrease staphylococcal infections. There is also interest in using the product topically on localized lesions such as medial canthus erosions and fold dermatitis.

David Ganfield *USA* Staphage Lysate has been used intranasally to reduce carriage sites of the staphylococcus.

Further reading

Ascher, F., Maynard, L., Laurent, J. & Goubet, B. (1990) Controlled trial of ethyl lactate and benzoyl peroxide shampoos in the management of canine surface and superficial pyoderma. In: *Advances in Veterinary Dermatology*, Vol. 1 (Eds C. von Tscharner & R. E. W. Halliwell), pp. 375–382. Baillière Tindall, London.

DeBoer, D. J., Moriello, K. A., Thomas, C. B & Schultz, K. T. (1990). Evaluation of a commercial staphylococcal bacterin for management of idiopathic recurrent superficial pyoderma in dogs. *American Journal of Veterinary Research*, **51**, 636–639.

DeManuelle, T. C., Ihrke, P. J., Brandt, C. M., Kass, P. H. & Vuillet, P. R. (1998) Determination of skin concentrations of enrofloxacin in dogs with pyoderma. *American Journal of Veterinary Research*, **59**, 1599–1604.

Kwochka, K. W. & Kowalski, J. J. (1991) Prophylactic efficacy of four antibacterial shampoos against *Staphylococcus intermedius* in dogs. *American Journal of Veterinary Research*, **52**, 115–118.

Rees, C. A. (1999) Noninsecticidal veterinary shampoo components. *Compendium of Continuing Education for the Practicing Veterinarian*, **21**, 55–63.

Saijonmaa-Koulumies, L. E. M. (2000) Bacterial interference in the control of canine pyoderma. PhD Thesis, University of London.

Saijonmaa-Koulumies, L. E. M. & Lloyd, D. H. (1995) Carriage of bacteria antagonistic towards *Staphylococcus intermedius* on canine skin and mucosal surfaces. *Veterinary Dermatology*, **6**, 187–194.

Saijonmaa-Koulumies, L. E. M., Parsons, E. & Lloyd, D. H. (1998) Elimination of *Staphylococcus intermedius* in healthy dogs by topical treatment with fusidic acid. *Journal of Small Animal Practice*, **39**, 341–347.

5.21

Dermatotechnology: computer, multimedia and Internet resources

David H. Lloyd[1] (Chairperson) and Christopher J. Chesney[2] (Secretary)

[1] Royal Veterinary College (University of London), North Mymms, Hatfield, UK
[2] The Mott Clinic for Veterinary Dermatology, Broadclyst, Exeter, UK

David Lloyd *UK* We live in an era of rapidly developing technology with the potential to greatly enhance our activities as dermatologists. I have selected four areas of technology for consideration today, which will be introduced by colleagues who are actively working with or developing new techniques. The topic areas are: non-invasive techniques for examination of components and changes within the skin, imaging the skin surface, image processing in histology and using the Internet.

Frank Niedorf *Germany* The principle underlying reflection spectroscopy is the analysis of the emission spectrum of reflected light. It enables non-invasive measurement of substances in the skin, which may include haemoglobin or drugs. Some of the light striking an object may be reflected or scattered, transmitted through the object or absorbed by it. Spectroscopy may use either transmitted or reflected light. Our study analysed the spectrum of reflected light. This spectrum, which contains information about the detected substances, is used for qualitative and quantitative measurements. However, there are many problems in studying biological material which, of course, has unknown absorbing substances, the path length is unknown and the tissue is composed of heterogeneous substances.

A first application of this new technique was the non-invasive determination of haemoglobin using the characteristic spectrum of oxygenated and non-oxygenated haemoglobin. The model used was the isolated, perfused, bovine udder. The problems described were overcome by the use of multivariate analysis. With special algorithms, some other applications were developed, for example, the determination of methadone, β-carotene or glucose.

Mary Dyson *UK* Ultrasound biomicroscopy or high-frequency ultrasonic imaging using ultrasound in excess of 15 MHz allows the visualisation of living skin at microscopic resolution. Healthy, damaged and repairing skin can be imaged, providing information previously only available from invasive biopsies. Ultrasound biomicroscopy is non-damaging and allows longitudinal studies of tissue changes to be made at the same or different skin sites; the progress of skin disease and the effects of therapy can be monitored in a safe, painless, rapid manner.

Recently developed portable pulse-echo equipment operating at a centre frequency of 20 MHz, with a resolution of the order of 60 μm, has been used to examine the components of intact, injured and repairing skin. The B-scans produced can be viewed in grey scale or in pseudocolour using a variety of palettes; they are digitised and can be transmitted via the Internet and used telemedically.

In intact skin, the stratum corneum can be distinguished from the living strata of the epidermis; the papillary and reticular regions of the dermis can also be identified, as can the panniculus adiposus and deep fascia. Blood vessels larger than approximately 60 μm can be visualised. Sweat ducts can be located. In damaged skin, eschar, clotted blood and oedematous sites can be imaged. As a wound heals, granulation tissue and scar tissue can be viewed and their linear dimensions measured. Fractal analysis is being examined as a potential method of quantifying changes in the pattern of the acoustic reflections obtained from these tissues as wounds heal. Ultrasound biomicroscopy has also been used to locate and measure foreign bodies and tumours in skin.

The potential role of ultrasound biomicroscopy in veterinary dermatology is great.

Genevieve Marignac *France* Can the ultrasound technique be used on hairy skin?

Mary Dyson One must clip the hair short, otherwise it creates an air space that causes reflections.

Manfred Keitzmann *Germany* We are looking at the effects on the skin of glucocorticoids. Among other things they increase the amount of water in the skin. Can this be measured?

Mary Dyson We can measure the thickness of the skin and this is equivalent to oedema. One can pick up changes in fluid, although one can't really see blood vessels themselves. So one cannot measure the water, but you can compare normal and abnormal.

Hans Koch *Germany* How does your technique differ from that of Hoffman and Aesuyer? Have you thought about using shorter wavelengths to analyse the epidermis with higher resolution? This might allow an *in vivo* diagnosis of some of the bullous diseases.

Mary Dyson Their group uses equipment with a frequency of 20 MHz, which looks at the epidermis only. We have a patented head, which produces something akin to a 'tuning fork' sound, rather than a 'bell'.

Pierre Cadot *France* This technique is like a sophisticated magnifying glass. Also, one can store and share images. One can appreciate the condition of the skin and hair, and may even see live parasites. The images can be shown to the owner, which greatly increases their co-operation!

I use a digital camera and a digital camera-recorder. This superseded the earlier use of a handy-cam with a miniaturised video camera. Because of movement by the observer and the animal, there is a limit to the magnification that can reasonably be used. However, the technique can be applied to various sized endoscopes. Some of these have a mirror to give a sideways view.

Images are captured with a video-capture board in a microcomputer. It needs a very large capacity hard disk and a CD writer unit. The total cost is between $7000 and $12 000. One must also record the site observed, using a simple dog-outline drawing. I take a general-view picture of the normal site, and then the magnified view. The method can be used, for example, to monitor healing over time, using serial pictures.

Lene Boysen *Denmark* During the past 10–15 years, image analysis of digital photographs has been used in human dermatology to assist the physician and the researcher in the description of skin. Recommendations have been made concerning the use of instruments such as the digital camera and image analysis. Only validated methods should be employed and certain factors, e.g. light conditions, should be controlled.

In order to introduce objective methods to veterinary dermatology, normal dog skin colour has been described using digital photography and image analysis. Two groups of dogs were used: eight German shepherd dogs and 10 dogs of mixed breed. The skin colour of six regions was measured by analysis of digital photographs and the results were compared to redness values obtained by colorimetry. The equipment used was a Kodak Nikon DCS 410 camera and Minolta CR 300 chromameter. The coefficient of variation of repeated measurements was below 10% for each technique. No statistically significant difference was found between right and left side measurements. Significant differences between regions were seen in both groups of dogs. The correlation of photographic redness values and values obtained by colourimetry was significant and positive in both groups of dogs.

The conclusion was that it seems possible to apply objective instruments, such as digital photography, to veterinary dermatology for skin colour quantification.

Hans Koch How do you provide standard distance from the lens of the camera to the skin as well as always the same angle, and what software do you use?

Lene Boysen I use a fixed shutter and lens aperture and I tape the focus ring to prevent movement. I now have a metal frame to hold the camera and to keep it at a set distance from the skin. The software is Adobe Photoshop or Image Pro-plus. The latter is more expensive but much more sophisticated.

David Lloyd In dermatology we commonly encounter large objects, such as ectoparasites, that we wish to examine in detail by microscopy and perhaps photograph. We also have problems with tissue sections containing features which, at high power, cannot be resolved in a single plane of focus or which are not flat, presenting the same problem. High power offers good resolution but also restricts the area of tissue that can be examined and recorded. Thus, it would be useful to have a method by which adjacent fields could be joined to create a single high-power image.

We have been using relatively inexpensive software (details from http://www.syncroscopy.com/syncroscopy/) to solve the problem of focus. A video camera attached to the microscope and a computer, with image capture board, are required. The specimen is then focused in the uppermost focal plane and the image captured. This process is repeated moving the focus down through the specimen and the collected images are assembled (*z* assembly) by an algorithm that retains only the focused components.

Assembling adjacent images (*xy* assembly) is more difficult. This can be done manually using image-processing software, but is quite difficult and very tedious. Solutions which employ expensive calibrated motorised stages can also be used. Powerful computers, which are capable of recognising tissue features and thus the anatomy of a specimen, can assemble adjacent images automatically without the use of calibrated stages [an image of a whole flea at medium power with combined *xy* and *z* assembly was shown to illustrate this]. However, as yet, these computers need to be specially built to enable rapid image capture and processing, and are quite expensive. In the future, it is likely that the costs of such computers will fall.

These techniques have great value in research and teaching and are a lot of fun for people who love beautiful images.

James Noxon *USA* The number of users of the World Wide Web (WWW) has increased so rapidly that estimates of the user numbers have been obsolete by the time they are published. It is sufficient to say that many veterinary professionals and pet owners have access to this information source. However, the use of the Web as an information source has positive effects and negative effects.

The uses of the WWW for information management can generally be divided into a number of areas based on the user, and include literature searches, acquisition or sharing of information about dermatology among professionals, and dissemination of information about dermatology from the veterinary professional to clients.

Literature searches can be performed on the Web using two types of search engine: the databases in literature and the general search engines (e.g. Yahoo). The database search engines include PubMed, a site where you may search for a keyword or words and then view the citation and occasionally the abstract. In PubMed (www.ncbi.nlm.nih.gov/PubMed/) you can order reprints for a fee. Other sites offer searches if the user subscribes to the site (e.g. Current Contents, www.isinet.com/). There are some free search engines such as Agricola (www.nal.usda.gov/ag98/) where you may view the abstract or simply the citation. After searching a subject at that source you would need to order reprints from a local library or other provider. One service, UnCover Web (http://uncweb.carl.org/), offers free searches without abstracts, but makes its money from its reprint delivery service.

There are many sites on the Web (home pages) that have been produced and maintained by professionals in dermatology. These most often originate from academic sources. Some sites contain case studies or photo libraries (e.g. The University of Iowa Department of Dermatology [tray.dermatology.uiowa.edu/home.html] and others are designed for residents or students of dermatology (e.g. *The Electronic Textbook of Dermatology*, www.telemedicine.org/stamford.htm).

There are also several dermatology journals with a presence on the Web. Most of these offer some type of search process through their archives, with the ability to put up citations and abstracts. Reprints are only available if you subscribe to the journal (e.g. *Journal of the American Academy of Dermatology*, aad.org). *The Archives of Dermatology* offers the entire article from their publication free of charge (archderm.ama-assn.org).

Information provided to clients falls into two main categories: client information materials and advertising. Often it is difficult to separate the two areas, since many companies provide information skewed to promote their products. Many practitioners have taken advantage of the WWW to offer client information about many dermatological topics. The danger in this area is the promotion of inaccurate material. Rarely are web-based client information materials peer reviewed. The authors may or may not even be identified and the credentials of the author are rarely mentioned. It is an area worthy of discussion.

David Lloyd Congress proceedings are now more and more commonly on the Web. The production for the first time of the World Congress of Veterinary Dermatology abstracts in a supplement to *Veterinary Dermatology* and its availability at the journal website simultaneously with the Congress is an example. *Veterinary Dermatology* is now fully on-line and the abstracts and the contents can be accessed at http://www.blackwell-science.com/vde/. This also gives access to the Blackwell Science literature portal and the *Synergy* literature searching system. Contents of *Veterinary Dermatology* issues can be searched and abstracts viewed. A powerful aspect of the search system is the ability to find other papers (in any journal) related to the topic of an abstract and to find other papers by the authors. Subscribers to the journal can also choose to have an electronic subscription to the journal and will then have access to the full texts of all the papers, including images. They can then also gain access to papers and publications by authors quoted in the references. In the future, this is likely to become the way in which many people access the literature. It is certainly very quick and efficient.

Mark Craig *UK* Does subscribing to *Veterinary Dermatology* at Blackwell@synergy entitle you to access only this journal or other Blackwell journals also?

David Lloyd It allows access only to *Veterinary Dermatology*, but you can view the contents of other journals and perhaps abstracts too.

5.22

Essential fatty acids: their many applications in dermatology

Petra J. Roosje[1] (Chairperson) and Michele R. Rosenbaum[2] (Secretary)

[1] University of Bern, Bern, Switzerland
[2] Veterinary Specialists of Rochester, Rochester, New York, USA

Petra Roosje *Switzerland* Essential fatty acid (EFA) use became popular in the mid-1980s. However, despite good results in published veterinary studies, clinical results are often disappointing. Most of the published veterinary studies on the use of fatty acids were not placebo controlled or double blinded.

EFA are polyunsaturated fatty acids (PUFA) that cannot be synthesized by the animal: linoleic acid (LA) for dogs and LA and arachidonic acid (AA) for cats. The mode of action of EFA is as follows: certain PUFA can bypass the δ-desaturase enzyme and these PUFA can compete with AA for incorporation into the cell membranes. This can induce a shift towards the non-harmful or less harmful released mediators. More specific PUFA exert effects on cyclic AMP (cAMP) formation and cell receptor expression and therefore can mediate activation and processing of cytokines via intracellular signal transduction. Eicosanoids are the prostaglandins, thromboxanes and leukotrienes that can be either pro- or anti-inflammatory. Omega-6 fatty acids consist of plant oils, while omega-3 fatty acids consist of marine fish oils and some plant oils. EFA are modulators of inflammation. Most of the veterinary studies have been performed in dogs and cats with allergic dermatitis. More recently, studies have shown that EFA may be useful in the treatment of dogs with nail disease, keratinization disorders, sebaceous adenitis and cancer. EFA have been shown to be immunomodulatory and increase $CD4^+$ T-cells in healthy beagles.

Our first speaker, Adrian Watson, will talk about supplementation of PUFA in small animal nutrition, followed by Kirstin Bergvall who will discuss EFA and their use in treating onychodystrophy. Annette Peterson will present her findings using EFA to treat mycosis fungoides in dogs, Margreet Vroom will discuss EFA in the treatment of atopic dermatitis and pruritic dermatitis in general and, finally, Jacques Fontaine will present controversies in the use of EFA over the past 10 years.

Adrian Watson *UK* (Waltham) I will present a background and historical summary of the reasons for supplementing PUFA in small animal nutrition. I will discuss the reasons for supplementation, the types of supplements available, the contents of supplements regarding their fatty acid profiles, the general efficacy of the different supplements available, potential problems associated with supplementation and future considerations in PUFA use.

Certain PUFA are essential to mammals because mammals cannot introduce double bonds at most sites in long-chain fatty acids, as they lack the position-specific desaturase enzymes needed. The minimum requirement for LA for dogs is 1.1 g/400 kcal and for cats is 0.5 g/400 kcal. No clear minimum has been established for α-linolenic acid (ALA) in dogs and cats. Cats have low activity of δ-6- and δ-12-desaturase and thus have a requirement for arachidonic acid, which is a downstream product of ALA metabolism, requiring δ-6-desaturase. The requirement for AA in cats is 0.02 g/400 kcal. Cats also are most likely to have a requirement for eicosapentaenoic acid (EPA) for similar reasons, but no minimum requirement has been established.

EFA deficiency can be caused by feeding poor-quality, low-fat dry foods (not a current problem in most cases), feeding low-fat and high-fiber reduced-calorie diets (fiber can prevent absorption of EFA) and oxidative damage to fats because of poor storage or insufficient antioxidants added to food (EFA are particularly susceptible to oxidative damage due to their high number of double bonds). EFA deficiency can also be caused by abnormalities in fatty acid metabolism due to hypothyroidism, atopic dermatitis (dogs with atopy may have a deficiency in the δ-desaturase enzyme which leads to a decrease in AA production, which is important in keratinocyte differentiation; supplementation with γ-linolenic acid [GLA] can bypass this enzyme deficiency), and seborrhea (dogs with seborrhea have increased incorporation of oleic acid instead of ALA into keratinocytes; supplementation with ALA can reverse this defect).

The clinical signs of long-standing EFA deficiency include a dull, dry haircoat, alopecia with poor hair regrowth, increased scaling and crusting with erythema and greasy skin, and secondary bacterial and yeast infections with resultant pruritus.

The skin requires EFA for many important functions, such as LA for the formation of ceramide-1, which is important in formation of lamellar bodies that are needed in forming the skin's permeability barrier, and AA, which is important in eicosanoid synthesis, and especially in the production of prostaglandin E-2 (PGE_2), which regulates keratinocyte differentiation. All PUFA that are incorporated into cell membranes influence membrane fluidity and thus the activity of membrane-bound proteins and receptors.

Polyunsaturated fatty acids are used to treat a number of inflammatory diseases due to their anti-inflammatory effects. Omega-3 fatty acids and GLA produce anti-inflammatory eicosanoids, while other omega-6 fatty acids produce proinflammatory eicosanoids. Both omega-3 and omega-6 fatty acids share the same metabolic enzymes without interconversion. Therefore, omega-3 fatty acids and GLA can be used to decrease inflammation in flea allergy dermatitis, atopy, food hypersensitivity and idiopathic pruritus. Supplementation options include high-quality, high-fat diets, food oils (safflower, sunflower oils) and proprietary supplements (DermCaps®, Efavet® capsules). Response to therapy is usually seen in 3–8 weeks.

Sources of AA include beef and pork tallow, while sources of LA include plant oils. Currently, many premium dog foods have increased the levels of LA. Based on levels of LA, sunflower and safflower oils are better sources than the proprietary products such as DermCaps®. Fish oil is a good source of ALA and its downstream products of EPA and docosapentaenoic acid (DPA). Flaxseed and soybean oil, as well as DermCaps and Efavet® capsules, also are good sources of ALA. Evening primrose oil (EPO) and borage seed oil are good sources of GLA. Premium dry and canned foods contain large amounts of LA but very little EPA or docosahexaenoic acid (DHA). Response to omega-6 fatty acid supplementation for EFA deficiency is overall very good. However, the optimal supplementation levels are not known for both omega-6 and omega-3 fatty acids. Some of our recent research has shown that supplementing above normal levels may be beneficial to the skin and coat, by making allowances for decreased EFA absorption during periods of ill health.

When using EFA for the treatment of inflammatory skin disease, there are many questions, including whether to use omega-3, omega-6 or a combination of fatty acids, the dosage, the ratio of omega-3 to omega-6 fatty acids and the treatment interval to effect. In the past, when scientific trials were carried out regarding the use of fatty acids to decrease pruritus, there was much variability in the study quality (most were not blinded or placebo controlled), length of study (1–9 weeks) and the results (poor to good response). More modern studies have been of much better quality. Logas and Kunkle reported, in a placebo-controlled, double-blinded cross-over study comparing the use of fish oil versus corn oil for the treatment of pruritic skin disease, that the fish-oil-treated dogs had improved pruritus and alopecia scores. Harvey (1999) in a study comparing treatment of atopic dogs with a combination of fish oil and borage seed oil versus olive oil, reported that the fish/borage oil-treated dogs had improved pruritus, erythema and self-trauma scores.

Although most are hypothetical and not proven, potential problems with EFA supplementation include increased caloric intake and resultant weight gain, increased need for dietary antioxidants, increased risk of pancreatitis due to increased fat in the diet, decreased platelet function with resultant increased bleeding time with omega-3 fatty acid supplementation, malodor from marine fish oil (MFO) supplements, increased tumorigenesis/metastasis in artificially induced tumors in rats and mice (not established in other species, or with naturally occurring tumors), worsening of pre-existing renal disease with omega-6 fatty acid supplementation, possible proinflammatory effects of omega-6 fatty acids, decreased omega-6 metabolism due to excessive omega-3 fatty acid supplementation, and resulting problems with the normal inflammatory response and in epidermal structure. Recent studies have shown that high levels of PUFA can increase the risk of atherosclerosis due to oxidation of low-density lipoproteins (LDL), with the formation of foam cells in the vascular endothelium.

Future considerations that I believe are important in fatty acid research include the influence of large doses of omega-6 on omega-3 fatty acids (Waltham is currently performing these studies), extending trials to 8+ weeks, performing trials using larger doses of fatty acids, such as 1.5 times to twice the recommended dose of MFO or EPO, and careful consideration of the background fatty acid profile of the study animals' diet, as omega-3 fatty acids can be stored in the body for long periods of time and may be carried over to the test base level. Other future considerations include further studies using the biochemical measurement of inflammatory markers, such as neutrophil-stimulated leukotriene levels and their response to fatty acid supplementation, as in the work of Campbell and Byrne, with the addition of correlation of these results with clinical pruritus scores, studies using an *in vitro* model of PUFA metabolism to measure the maximum level of omega-3 fatty acids that can be incorporated into the cell membrane, how this addition will affect performance of the membrane and how well these fatty acids can be removed from the membrane by phospholipases. We also need one unified efficacy assessment protocol in order to compare trial results. Finally, studies to examine breed differences in the absorption and response to EFA supplementation are needed.

Dottie LaFlamme *USA* (Ralston Purina Company) The current recommendations for PUFA supplementation are omega-3 or omega-6 fatty acids, specifically GLA. Why do you get the same beneficial effect from omega-3 fatty acids and GLA since they compete with each other, and since GLA is proinflammatory?

Adrian Watson My understanding of the pathway is that, although by supplementing with GLA you are providing a substrate for the proinflammatory eicosanoids, there is the possibility of the GLA being metabolized to PGE_1, which has a less proinflammatory role, leaving less GLA available to be metabolized to AA.

Chiara Noli *Italy* If you give both omega-3 and omega-6 fatty acids together, the omega-3 fatty acids use all the desaturase enzyme, so the GLA cannot be metabolized to AA using this enzyme, but instead is converted to the anti-inflammatory eicosanoids. So the combination of omega-3 fatty acids and GLA is good.

Giovanni Ghibaudo *Italy* Human atopic dermatitis patients lack the δ-6-desaturase enzyme, so GLA levels are low. By supplementing with GLA, we can bypass this enzyme deficiency. This enzyme deficiency is not documented in dogs, but the reasoning behind GLA supplementation is the same.

Kerstin Bergvall *Sweden* The question is, 'Why do I use fatty acids in the treatment of onychodystrophy?' First, I will start with a bit of history. In the early 1990s, Dr Danny Scott was speaking at a dermatology conference in Barcelona and he told us about onychodystrophy, a condition where dogs slough their claws and fail to regrow normal claws. Dr Scott claimed he had excellent results treating these cases with EFA (DermCaps). These results were later published with Dr Bill Miller in the *Journal of the American Animal Association* in 1995. In this paper, they treated nine dogs with DermCaps, two dogs with high-dose corticosteroids and one dog with vitamin E, and two dogs were not treated. All treated dogs responded well, while the untreated dogs continued to have signs of onychodystrophy. Follow-up was 2 years.

I recently had a similar case of onychodystrophy. It was a young, healthy, adult dog with sloughing, misshapen claws and failure to regrow them. In the past, this dog had been treated with many things and ended up being treated with corticosteroids, which he did not tolerate. We changed this dog from an alert, happy dog with painful feet into a sick, lethargic dog with comfortable feet. Eventually, the owners gave up and euthanized the dog. This bothered me since this was a very nice dog. So, after Barcelona, I decided to try EFA on my next case of onychodystrophy. The first five cases that I treated were described in *Veterinary Dermatology* in 1998. The dogs reported were two giant schnauzers (one male, one female), one German shepherd dog, one dachshund and one standard schnauzer. Two dogs, the male giant schnauzer and the German shepherd dog, were diagnosed histologically as having lupoid onychodystrophy.

The other three dogs were not biopsied. All dogs were otherwise healthy and had a similar clinical picture, with sudden onset of claw sloughing on all four feet with failure to regrow normal claws. The claws were dystrophic and appeared crumbly with splitting.

I treated these dogs with a commercial fatty acid supplement called Efavet (made by Efamol). All five dogs responded clinically in 11–15 weeks. When the Efavet was stopped in three dogs on four occasions, the dogs relapsed. This relapse was also seen in Scott and Miller's report in two dogs where EFA supplementation was discontinued. When these relapsing dogs were once again treated with EFA, they improved once more, both in Scott's report and in my cases. Two of the dogs initially were treated concurrently with prednisolone at 0.5 mg/kg every 48 h; there was no change in claw quality when this was discontinued. There was also no change in time to clinical remission in the prednisolone and EFA-treated dogs versus the EFA-only-treated dogs. For these five dogs, it seemed that the Efavet capsules improved the clinical condition. All dogs were initially started on Efavet-1® capsules, which contain EFA as well as vitamins and minerals. All dogs except for the standard schnauzer were later switched to the Efavet regular capsules (no vitamins and minerals added, except for a small amount of vitamin E as an antioxidant) without relapse or change in claw quality. So is it the low-dose vitamin E (0.1–0.24 mg/kg per day) or the EFA that are causing the improvement? It is probably the EFA, as the dose of vitamin E in the capsules is much lower than the usual therapeutic dose (400–800 IU/day) used to treat inflammatory dermatoses, but we don't know for sure.

So these are glorious results: I had five of five dogs, while Scott had nine of nine dogs respond to EFA supplementation. However, if you treat larger numbers of dogs, the figures are not that good. In my hands, not all dogs respond, but a good number of them do, so I always start with EFA treatment for onychodystrophy, as it is a safe and simple therapy. What about the dose and omega-6 to omega-3 ratio? This is always questionable. For my treated dogs, I used omega-3 fatty acids at 45–120 mg/kg per day. This is a much lower dose than what Dr Lewis reported using at a conference in England to treat onychodystrophy, which was EPA at 180 mg/4.55 kg with clinical response in 3–4 weeks. This is a much faster response than I observed. Double-blinded, controlled studies are needed to further investigate this treatment.

Annette Peterson *USA* How long do you try dogs with onychodystrophy on EFA before giving up and going to another treatment?

Kerstin Bergvall I use the EFA for 5 months. If there is no improvement at that time, I will try doxycycline or tetracycline with or without niacinamide, or pentoxifylline or corticosteroids.

Bob Brown *USA* Did you make any attempt to titrate down the dose of EFA to see what the minimum effective dose was?

Kerstin Bergvall No, we didn't.

Chiara Noli Did you treat any of your study dogs with antibiotics, because some of these dogs with onychodystrophy will respond to antibiotic therapy?

Kerstin Bergvall Yes, if bacteria were seen on cytology or culture, the dogs were started on antibiotics, but these five study dogs did not respond to antibiotics.

Margreet Vroom *The Netherlands* I also had a giant schnauzer with onychodystrophy, so maybe there is a breed predisposition. My case had a raging bacterial paronychia that was controlled with 8 weeks of antibiotics, but then the dog failed to respond to EFA therapy given for 3 months and tetracycline and niacinamide for 2 months. The owners did not want to treat the dog with corticosteroids, so the dog is living with abnormal nails. I am not sure that symmetrical lupoid onychodystrophy is one disease and this may explain why some dogs respond better to certain treatments than others.

Dottie LaFlamme Are there differences between responders and non-responders based on the fatty acid composition of their baseline diet?

Kerstin Bergvall What are needed are double-blinded controlled studies, where the dogs' baseline diet is strictly regulated.

Chiara Noli How many cases do you see a year of onychodystrophy?

Kerstin Bergvall I can't tell you for sure how many, but in Sweden there are many cases in certain breeds such as the giant schnauzer and the Gordon setter. The breeders admit there is a problem, because they hunt with Gordon setters and these dogs can no longer hunt.

Annette Peterson I came across the idea of using safflower oil (SFO) when I did a literature search on mycosis fungoides (MF) and I found two articles that described the use of SFO in treating cutaneous lymphoma cases in people. MF is an uncommon neoplastic skin disease and is an epitheliotropic lymphoma of T-cell origin that primarily affects older dogs. Treatment with chemotherapy or retinoids is often unsuccessful and survival time after diagnosis is 5–10 months. Fatty acid supplementation is used as an adjunctive treatment for a variety of neoplastic disorders in humans and no malignant cell line has been found which cannot be killed by at least one or several PUFA *in vitro*. The response to therapy depends on species, tumor type, number of double bonds, cell culture conditions and dose. Polyunsaturated fatty acids act by direct cytotoxicity by stimulating lipid peroxidation, as well as superoxide and hydroxyl radical formation. Rapidly dividing tumor cells are more susceptible to these effects. Polyunsaturated fatty acids can potentiate the effects of radiation and antineoplastic drugs. Antioxidants can inhibit these effects. Fatty acids can enhance macrophage function and can increase the production of lymphokines and interferon. PUFA can cause reduction in metastasis via increased PGE_1 production, which limits the aggregation of free-floating malignant cells to new sites.

SFO is derived from *Carthamus tictorius*, a relative of the thistle plant. SFO contains 76.4% LA. Commercial SFO contains 20–30% vitamin E. A genetically altered form of SFO is commercially available that contains 80% oleic acid and only 15% LA (Hain brand). Hollywood brand of SFO is the one you want to use: this contains the high percentage of LA. EPO contains 73.2% LA, while sunflower oil contains 66.4% LA. The first article that I came across was in the *South African Veterinary Journal*, by Williams (1988). The authors used Efamol G® capsules, which contained 40 mg GLA, 350 mg LA and 10 mg natural vitamin E in a gelatin/glycerin capsule. They gave a large empirical dose of 10–20 capsules daily to two dogs with lymphoblastic lymphosarcoma and saw a reduction in lymph-node size within 7 days. The dogs were euthanized for other reasons and necrosis of neoplastic cells was seen histologically. The authors felt this was a result of the Efamol supplementation. Even more interesting is an article by Iwamoto *et al.* (1992). Previous work by these same authors found that LA was probably the major component for anti-tumor activity in the small-intestinal mucosa, thus explaining the low incidence of small-intestinal tumors. They found that sodium linoleate was effective *in vitro* in killing human chronic lymphocytic leukemia lymphocytes, and that 200 μmol of LA can be lethal to a variety of tumors *in vitro*. Higher plasma levels of LA were obtained with oral administration of SFO than by injection. In their study, they used 3 ml/kg SFO orally twice weekly mixed in the food and they saw six of eight dogs with MF go into complete remission. All dogs had been previously treated unsuccessfully with other treatment modalities. The only side-effect seen was a transient increase in lymphocyte and leukocyte counts, and a transient mild decrease in alanine aminotransferase (ALT) and aspartate aminotransferase (AST) activities.

Their cases were as follows. Case 1: an 11-year-old shih tzu with lesions on the abdomen, prior treatment was isotretinoin and prednisone, treated for 2 years successfully with SFO, then euthanized for recurrence; case 2: a 15-year-old beagle with foot lesions only, a dramatic response to SFO but euthanized 2 months later for unrelated reasons; case 3: a 13-year-old golden retriever with lesions on the mouth, previously treated unsuccessfully with standard chemotherapy but which had a dramatic response to therapy with SFO, subsequently hit by a car, with no evidence of MF on necropsy; case 4: a 6-year-old boxer with lesions on the mouth, previously treated unsuccessfully with standard chemotherapy, in complete remission for 2 years at the time of the article; case 5: a 7-year-old golden retriever with generalized lesions, 90% regression of lesions but died 2 months later; case 6: a very young Rhodesian ridgeback with generalized lesions, previously treated with radiation and chemotherapy with no response and did not respond to SFO; case 7: a 13-year-old beagle with no prior therapy and good response to SFO; and case 8; a standard poodle with no prior treatment that also had a good response.

After I read these reports I decided to try this therapy on two dogs with MF confirmed by histopathology after obtaining skin biopsies. The first case was Dusty, a 9-year-old, female spayed Brittany spaniel with a 3 month history of circular, erythematous, scaly, alopecic lesions on the dorsum and parts of the rear legs. Previous treatment with griseofulvin, etretinate and prednisone did not result in improvement and lesions continued to progress. Dusty was then started on SFO, at 3 ml/kg orally twice weekly. Lesions improved by 25% after 8 weeks of therapy. Six months after starting SFO, a tumor developed near the base of the tongue, consistent with tumor-stage MF. After 7.5 months on SFO, more tumors and ulcerated lesions developed on the feet, causing lameness. Dusty was euthanized 9 months after starting SFO supplementation. However, I later found out that Dusty was on the genetically altered SFO with the high oleic acid content, rather than the desired natural product with high LA content. Dusty may have responded better if we had used the right SFO.

The second case was Beau, a 10-year-old, male neutered cocker spaniel with multiple alopecic plaques of various sizes on the head and dorsum. After 6 weeks on 3 ml/kg orally twice weekly, only three small lesions on the dorsum remained; the only side-effect seen was that a lipoma increased in size. Three months after starting SFO, there was no clinical evidence of MF and rebiopsy 5 months after starting SFO revealed no histological evidence of MF. Seven months after starting SFO, a new lesion, suggestive of lymphoid neoplasia on fine-needle aspirate, was noted on the front leg; this lesion resolved without additional treatment. After 19 months on SFO, no clinical evidence of MF was found. Beau's dramatic response to therapy was most likely due to SFO supplementation (in Beau we did use the right type of SFO, with high LA levels). SFO, containing high levels of LA, appears to be an effective, safe and inexpensive treatment alternative for the clinical management of MF in dogs. SFO deserves further investigation and comparison to other treatments for MF in a larger case series.

I have since consulted with other practitioners on several other cases of MF being treated with SFO and, so far, two dogs have not responded and one case is in remission after complete surgical excision, so it does not look like I can repeat the dramatic results that Iwamoto and his group had. But I believe that because SFO is cheap with no side-effects, it should be tried in these older dogs with MF, when owners don't want to pursue heroic, expensive treatments that may have side-effects.

Giovanni Ghibaudo It is important to make sure that the SFO is cold-pressed, otherwise it can lose all of its activity. PUFA have cytotoxic effects and in humans omega-3 fatty acids are used in the treatment of breast cancer or carcinoma and omega-6 fatty acids for the treatment of lymphoma. It seems that epithelial tumors are best treated with omega-3 fatty acids, and lymphoid tumors are best treated with omega-6 fatty acids.

Jacques Fontaine *Belgium* Omega-6 fatty acids, especially GLA, are very useful in association with classical therapy in the treatment of many cancers in humans, in order to improve response rates.

Giovanni Ghibaudo It is important to note that in humans they have found lower levels of fatty acids in tumor cells. Therefore it is important to give the right dose of fatty acids when treating cancer. I think we need to have studies done that measure fatty acid concentrations in tissues.

Marcy Murphy *USA* I just want to play devil's advocate here. It's very difficult to diagnose cutaneous lymphosarcoma (CL). In the cases that did not respond, were those tumor stage? These cases that you showed today looked to have very early-stage disease and may not have truly had CL.

Annette Peterson We did not do immunohistochemical staining, so the tumors could have been histiocytomas, but Bob Dunstan made the histological diagnosis and the dogs' age and clinical appearance fitted with CL.

Marcy Murphy Another interesting historical finding is that in many cases of CL, dogs have a chronic history of years of inflammatory skin disease. One of your cases was atopic and was treated with SFO, which is hopefully anti-inflammatory. There is some question of whether CL is neoplastic or inflammatory, so perhaps treating with anti-inflammatory substances may be helpful. These are just things to think about.

Margreet Vroom Unfortunately, I can't give you as good results as the previous speaker with the use of fatty acids for the treatment of atopy. I am in clinical referral practice, I see lots of atopic cases and I use fatty acids a lot. I have not done any placebo-controlled studies, and these are just some views from a practitioner. There are several short studies that report the efficacy of EFA to be 11–27% in allergic dogs and 50% in allergic cats. What do they mean by 'effective'? Is it no pruritus, less pruritus, less seborrhea or only improvement in coat quality? We can debate this. I think we would all agree that more EFA supplementation studies need to be done in atopic animals in which the fatty acid composition of the animal's baseline diet is included, as this is usually not done and is very important.

I want to present a case of a 2-year-old golden retriever with atopic signs (face, feet rubbing with superficial pyoderma and signs of otitis). As always, I began by excluding ectoparasites and I started the dog on a home-cooked hypoallergenic diet, which I prefer. There was no improvement at all. Then I tried this dog on a 12 week trial of Eukanuba Response Program® diet, which has high levels of EFA. After 6 weeks, the coat condition was better and there was less pruritus. After 12 weeks, we changed the diet back to the original diet (Eukanuba Regular®) to see if the high EFA-containing diet caused the decrease in pruritus and within 4 weeks there was more pruritus and the coat condition worsened. Also, at that time winter began, so we changed the diet back to the Eukanuba Response Program and, again, the pruritus lessened and the coat condition was better. So I concluded that the increased EFA in the diet did seem to make a difference in pruritus and coat quality in this case. However, I have tried EFA supplementation in many other atopic dogs that did not seem to respond at all. Owners are happy when the coat condition is better, but are frustrated when pruritus does not lessen.

So, if I have an atopic dog, I discuss a treatment plan with the owner: do we perform hyposensitization, or give EFA, antihistamines or corticosteroids? Because of the rather low success rate I have in my practice with EFA supplementation, many people do not choose to use EFA on their atopic pets, choosing other treatment options such as hyposensitization, antihistamines or corticosteroids. The problem with EFA is you need to give them for 12 weeks to determine efficacy, which is a long time to wait. Also, they are expensive. In my hands, although I do have some success in certain cases, the general low success rate does not make it one of my top choices for treating atopic dogs.

With regard to cats, I will tell you an interesting story. There was a cattery with eight Persian cats, male and female, all indoor. All cats developed pruritus and seborrhea. I examined all the cats carefully: there were no ectoparasites, and all cats were skin-scrape negative and fungal culture negative. Some, but not all, cats were put on a hypoallergenic diet for 4–6 weeks with no response. I was convinced this condition had something to do with an infectious disease, but I could not find anything. So we started the cats on EFA in a liquid form (Megaderm®, Virbac Animal Health) and all the cats improved: the coats became better with less pruritus. We discontinued this treatment and the pruritus and poor haircoat returned. The owner then resumed adding the EFA to the diet (she just added the oil to a communal big bowl of cat food, so since there was no individual feeding most cats were probably underdosed. After 2 years, the owner wrote to me recently that she changed the linoleum in the cattery, discontinued the EFA, and the cats remained normal. I am sure the EFA were helping these cats, but what the linoleum had to do with it, I don't know.

So my protocol for atopic cats is usually to start with antihistamines, since all owners hate corticosteroids. Some cats respond fantastically to antihistamines; some do not respond at all. Then, I try EFA if antihistamines fail, but palatability (fishy odor and taste), the huge capsule size and the long trial period of 12 weeks are problems when administering EFA to cats. In my experience, only 5–10% of atopic cats respond to EFA. Some newer products may have less of a fishy odor, so this might make them easier to administer to cats. So, I think that there is a place for EFA in veterinary medicine but the antipruritic effect is often disappointing. However, coat condition usually does improve, as does seborrhea sicca and oleosa. I also had a dog with skin problems and renal disease with a low glomerular filtration rate of unknown cause after a thorough work-up at the university in Utrecht, and after I started the dog on EFA for the skin condition, the creatinine became normal. This case may raise more questions than provide answers, but EFA may also be useful in the treatment of renal disease.

Jacques Fontaine Ten years after EFA were made commercially available, a lot of questions remain. The first question is: what is the best source of EFA? Is it special EFA-enriched diets or regular diets supplemented with EFA products? What is the best ratio of omega-6 to omega-3 fatty acids to reduce inflammation? What about supplementing with GLA, and what is the correct amount to use? The literature can provide some of these answers. Two papers reported good results in pruritus control by feeding diets containing an omega-6 to omega-3 fatty acid ratio of 5–10:1 (Scott *et al.* (1992) 44% response, including 11 dogs that did not respond to DermCap supplements; Schick *et al.* (1995) 45% pruritus reduction). However, some problems exist with these studies. These studies were not placebo controlled and pruritus is multifactorial, with yeast and bacterial infection, as well as food and flea hypersensitivities possibly playing a role, in addition to atopy. By changing the diet, food hypersensitivities may be controlled and this may play a role in the reduction in pruritus, in addition to any anti-inflammatory effects from the EFA in the diet.

In my opinion, EFA supplements are the best source of EFA for the treatment of canine and feline atopic dermatitis (excluding food intolerance) for the following reasons: good control of amount of EFA, better control of EFA source (omega-6 rich in GLA), better control of omega-6 to omega-3 ratio and better protection against oxidation than EFA-enriched diets. Should we use omega-6, omega-3 or a combination of EFA for optimal anti-inflammatory effects? When you have EFA deficiency in guinea-pigs, rats and dogs, it is more important to supplement with oral omega-6 than omega-3 to return the skin and hair structure to normal. Also, topical application of LA and AA results in local positive effects on the skin and haircoat. However, Logas and Kunkle (1994) showed that omega-3 supplementation can reduce pruritus in atopic dogs; yet Soyland *et al.* (1994) showed that neither omega-3 (fish oil) supplementation nor corn oil was helpful in human atopic dermatitis.

What is the best omega-6 to omega-3 ratio to use to maximally decrease inflammation? The optimum omega-6 to omega-3 ratio of between 5:1 and 10:1 was proposed by Vaughn *et al.* (1994), based on the measurement of leukotriene B-4 (LTB_4) in neutrophils and in the skin after artificial stimulation of the eicosanoid cascade. They found that diets with an omega-6 to omega-3 ratio of between 5:1 and 10:1 reduced LTB_4 production and increased LTB_5 production in neutrophils and in skin. But, are neutrophil levels of LTB_4 a good criterion for measuring inflammation? There are problems with this conclusion, based on human studies on atopic dermatitis patients. Neutrophils from atopic patients produce less LTB_4 than controls, and after 12 weeks of GLA supplementation in atopic patients LTB_4 levels in neutrophils increased by 56% despite clinical improvement. However, LTB_4 skin levels in atopic people are 100 times higher in affected skin than in normal skin. LTB_4 levels are also increased in the skin of atopic dogs. Recently, it was shown that in humans, the absolute amount of omega-3 fatty acid supplemented is more important than the omega-6 to omega-3 ratio in reducing inflammation and pruritus.

What about the dosage of EFA to use? In humans, the therapeutic effect of EFA supplements is observed with doses 70–160 times higher than those used in the dog. We must increase the recommended dose of EFA by at least two to five times the label dose for therapeutic benefit in dogs. This is not a physiological effect, but a pharmacological one that we are promoting by using these higher doses. High doses of omega-6 fatty acid supplementation do not promote the synthesis of proinflammatory substances, such as AA. Omega-6 supplementation, such as with GLA, results in only mild increases in AA. Arachidonic acid is needed for keratinization functions and is not a 'bad' fatty acid. In human studies, when atopics were supplemented with high levels of GLA, symptoms improved and there was only a slight increase in AA levels in the skin and in neutrophils. However, some problems can arise when large amounts of omega-3 supplements are given. The δ-desaturase enzyme has a greater affinity for the omega-3 fatty acids than for the omega-6 fatty acids. Thus, increased omega-3 intake can push the pathway to produce more omega-3 derivatives at the expense of omega-6 derivatives, resulting in a secondary omega-6 fatty acid deficiency. Supplementation with GLA in addition to omega-3 fatty acids bypasses the rate-limiting step of the δ-desaturase and prevents this omega-6 fatty acid deficiency. So, there is a synergistic effect with both omega-6 and omega-3 fatty acid supplementation. Weight gain and rarely pancreatitis are the only clinical side-effects in animals supplemented with EFA.

So, what is the best source of EFA? I don't know for sure. If a dietary source is used, a ratio of omega-6 to omega-3 of between 5:1 and 10:1 is recommended. A problem with EFA in food is oxidation of fats after the bag has been open for 1–3 months. Special packaging (not just a bottle that can be opened) is needed to prevent oxidation of fats, for both food and capsule/liquid sources of EFA. If supplements are chosen, they should contain top-quality EFA with both omega-6 (EPO, borage seed oil, blackcurrant oil, Argan oil as GLA sources) and omega-3 sources (marine fish oil, flax seed oil). If supplements are used, I suggest that you increase the recommended dosage. I never use EFA alone in my atopic dogs, because the success rate is too low. I suggest you use EFA in synergy with antihistamines or corticosteroids to reduce the dosage of steroids. EFA should be given for a minimum of 3 weeks, and probably more, before judging efficacy. I often use EFA to improve the cosmetic appearance of the skin and haircoat and to reduce hair shedding.

Further reading

Bergvall, K. (1998). Treatment of symmerical onychodystropy in five dogs with omega-3 and omega-6 fatty acids. *Veterinary Dermatology*, **9**, 263–268.

Harvey, R. G. (1999). A blinded, placebo-controlled study of the efficacy of borage seed oil and fish oil in the management of canine atopy. *Veterinary Record*, **144**, 405–407.

Iwamoto, K. S., Bennett, L. R., Norman, A., Villalobos, A. E. & Hutson, C. A. (1992). Linoleate produces remission in canine mycosis fungoides. *Cancer Letters*, **64**, 17–22.

Logas, D. & Kunkle, G. A. (1994). Double-binded cross-over study with marine fish oil supplementation containing high-dose eicosapentaenoic acid for the treatment of canine pruritic skin disease. *Veterinary Dermatology*, **5**, 99–104.

Schick, R. O., Schick, M. P. & Reinhart, G. A. (1995). Efficacy of an omega-3 fatty acid adjusted diet in pruritic dogs. *Proceedings of the 12th Annual Congress of the European Society of Veterinary Dermatology*. Barcelona, p. 245.

Scott, D. W., Miller, W. H., Decker, G. A. & Wellington, J. R. (1992) Comparison of the clinical efficacy of two commercial fatty acid supplements (Efavet® and DVM Derm Caps®), evening primrose oil, and cold water marine fish oil in the management of allergic pruritus in dogs: a double blinded study. *Cornell Veterinarian*, **82**, 319–329.

Scott, D. W., Rouselle, S. & Miller, W. H (1995). Symmetrical lupoid onychodystrophy in dogs: a retrospective analysis of 18 cases (1989–1993). *Journal of the American Animal Hospital Association*, **31**, 194–201.

Soyland, E., Funk, J., Rajka, G., Sandberg, M., Thune, P., Rustad, L., Helland, S., Middlefart, K., Odu, S., Falk, E. S., Solvolli, K., Bjorneboe, G. E. A. & Drevon, C. A. (1994). Dietary supplementation with very long-chain n-3 fatty acids in patients with atopic dermatitis – a multicenter study. *British Journal of Dermatology*, **130**, 757–764.

Vaughn, D. M., Reinhart, G. A., Swaim, S. F., Lauten, S. D., Garner, C. A., Boudreaux, M. K., Spano, J. S , Hoffman, C. E. & Conner, B. (1994). Evaluation of effects of dietary n-6 to n-3 fatty acid ratios on leukotriene B synthesis in dog skin and neutophils. *Veterinary Dermatology*, **5**, 163–173.

Williams, J. H. (1988). The use of gamma linolenic acid, linolenic acid and natural vitamin E for the treatment of multicentric lymphoma in 2 dogs. *Journal of the South African Veterinary Association*, **58**, 141–144.

Index